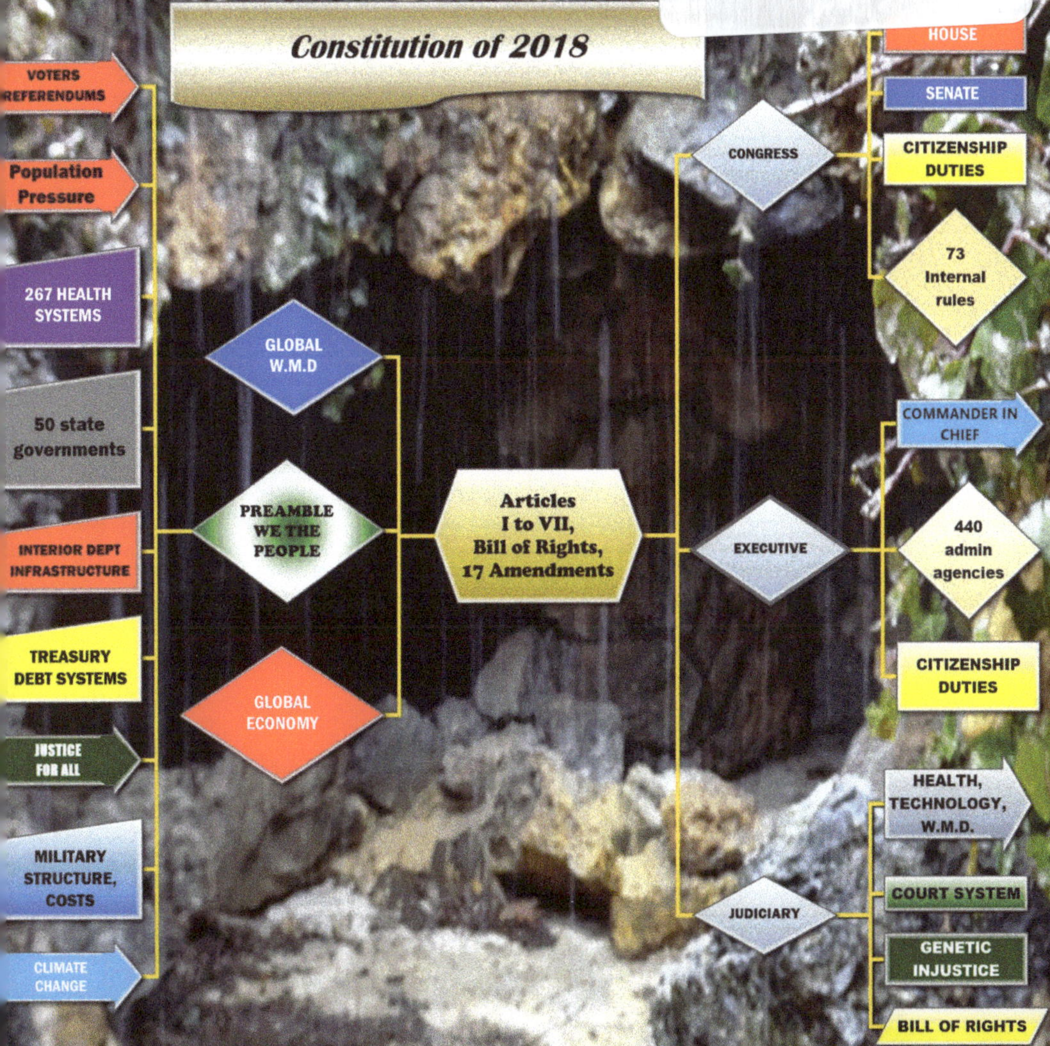

Constitution of 2018

HOUSE

SENATE

VOTERS REFERENDUMS

CITIZENSHIP DUTIES

CONGRESS

Population Pressure

73 Internal rules

267 HEALTH SYSTEMS

GLOBAL W.M.D

COMMANDER IN CHIEF

50 state governments

440 admin agencies

INTERIOR DEPT INFRASTRUCTURE

PREAMBLE WE THE PEOPLE

Articles I to VII, Bill of Rights, 17 Amendments

EXECUTIVE

CITIZENSHIP DUTIES

TREASURY DEBT SYSTEMS

GLOBAL ECONOMY

HEALTH, TECHNOLOGY, W.M.D.

JUSTICE FOR ALL

COURT SYSTEM

MILITARY STRUCTURE, COSTS

JUDICIARY

GENETIC INJUSTICE

CLIMATE CHANGE

BILL OF RIGHTS

Chronicles of the Kwedake Dikep

A TimeLIne of the Indian Spring on the Capitol Hill

TL of 2018

Robert J. Thayer

Chronicles
of the
Kwedake Dikep

A TimeLine of the Indian Spring on the Capitol Hill
TL of 2018

Robert J. Thayer
TL of millennium 6

For permission to use material from this book, including graphics, contact:

Kwedakedikep@earthlink.net

NOTICE TO THE READER   SPECULATIVE CONTENT DISCLAIMER

The Publisher has taken reasonable care in the preparation of this book, but makes no expressed or implied warranty of any kind and assumes no responsibility for any errors or omissions. No liability is assumed for incidental or consequential damages in connection with or arising out of information contained in this book. The Publisher shall not be liable for any special, consequential, or exemplary damages resulting, in whole or in part, from the readers' use of, or reliance upon, this material because Constitutional change has a clear precedence and history of a traumatic process.

Independent verification should be sought for any data, advice or recommendations contained in this document. In addition, because of its futurist speculative nature, no responsibility is assumed by the author or publisher for any injury and/or damage to persons or property arising from any methods, products, instructions, ideas or other speculations contained in this publication.

This publication is a collage of opinions expressed by the author while researching the system dynamics of the US Constitution. The opinions are contact quotations from many internet newspaper and documentary sources under conditions of 'fair use' extraction and under conditions of the MIT Intellectual Commons license educational process. As the author retains all 'work in progress' rights associated with speculative literature, some items are entered as 'common use' knowledge found on the internet and therefore do not necessarily follow the rigid permissions required for specific intellectual property. The content of the Chronicles of the Kwedake Dikep is sold with the clear understanding that the Publisher and Author are not engaged in rendering legal or any other professional services.

Library of Congress Cataloging-in-Publication Data:

Available on request, Robert J. Thayer

Chronicles of the Kwedake Dikep, A Timeline of the Indian Spring on the Hill,

Time Line 1965 to Time Line 2022 / Robert J. Thayer (author)

ISBN-13: 978-0-99-706541-1 (E-book)

ISBN-10: 978-0-99-706540-4 (paperback)

Abstract, sort of

The Chronicles examine the possibilities of an addition, not a singular amendment, to the American Constitution for establishing a freedom that could not have existed before the twenty first century. The medical and genetic technologies have advanced during the last generation to the point that a health or wellness right can be established for all citizens. The only real way of determining this feasibility is by examining the dynamical arrow of time of the U.S. Constitution and especially the remarkable 'set' of concurrent, paralleled wisdom 'entities' expressed in the 52 words of its Preamble. No other document's stated purpose had managed set expressions of Justice, Tranquility, Common Defense, General Welfare, Liberty and Our, note Our, Posterity that defined the basis of a successful society when there had been no real precedent in history before it.

The Chronicles were then created as expressions of *in situ* observation of the dynamical interaction of the 'entities' or 'phenome' that each of the six declared covenants represented. These were then introduced into the processes of Complex Adaptive Systems methodologies the author had become aware of over many years, based largely on experiences at Harvard, MIT and oceanographic research travels around the world. At some point in the early 21st century, it became apparent that the Constitution had not foreseen some of the vast medical, scientific, social, communication, and genetic processes that had appeared and equally important, Americans had become uncertain about the constitutional basis of society resulting in a gridlock or paralysis of both its Common Defense and General welfare directives. These combined into the need for a change in the Constitution, but could modern operations research define what that change might be? Could many of the 'entities' of governance be recombined into some form of Wellbeing 'right' that addressed the new technologies on an evolutionary timeline that was now 70,000 years along?

The specific Wellbeing right is intended to give genetic security to the unborn human throughout its initial physical development through modern technologies that will free the person from the molecular deformities that have accumulated since the end of the interstitial or Ice Age 10,000 years ago. The human race has within its means the ability to create a better image. That image becomes a matter of a conferred Right that is extended to all citizens conceived within the jurisdiction of We the People. The Article VIII then confers the governance authorities of We the People to their various governance processes both national, state and community with the intention of creating a continuous evolutionary process of Wellbeing. The role of the citizen is defined in terms of this new Right and, as has always been true, the citizen is the agent of change that makes any of the rights work. But how to make a dynamic this complex understandable to a people and society who had no previous history-based experience with it?

This timeline methodology chapters are the same in all Chronicles for continuity reasons. The TimeLine of 2018 further examines the methodology of bringing about a Constitutional Convention and the inherent dangers in that process, along with the 'our Posterity' need for an addition for a 'Wellbeing' Article VIII to the American process. Previous Chronicle incident observations indicate that a scientific reductionist analysis might not be the perceptional mode that operations research into a wellbeing right is optimal; that a 'sense' of the domain(s) can also optimize, which many people do anyway with some accuracy. So did the Founders.

Acknowledgements

The purpose of this research into constitutional dynamics was to determine if there was an 'order' to the complexity of the Constitution. Many thanks to the arrival of the World Internet System, from which the 'systems' of the world became accessible and Jay Forrester's original MIT research into 'World Dynamics' did not need to be limited to a discrete set of timelines from the 1970s. This was because of the introduction of the Massachusetts Institute of Technology OpenCourseWare online courses from the Sloan School of Management, Physics Department, Health Sciences and Technology, Biological Engineering, Brain and Cognitive Sciences and several other departments. Their course updates from 2007 on (thank you, Provost Brown) gave a timeline observation of various disciplines that was unusually useful to one who knew what to look for in the MIT environment. The Chronicles were not possible without access to many sciences and perceptions at the same time, especially for one who did not have the math IQ center developed in the brain.

Special thanks are given to the 2000 era online news media of Washington DC, as they provided insights into modern constitutional applications of healthcare, economics and politics. The Washington Post was especially helpful in that its commentators covered a wide range of constitution related subjects, although they were not exactly looking at their efforts from a constitutional relevance standpoint. Online news sites of The Hill and Roll Call supplied a close timeline of the Congress itself, which in turn showed the dynamics of the Kwedake Dikep itself.

Also, special thanks to the staff and facilities of the Library of Congress, The National Archives, the Congressional Research Service and the Congressional Budget Office where the on-going Constitutional research into the timeline sequences of the three branches of American governance was carried out. The endless forbearance of the U.S. Capitol Police and the Architect of the Capitol staffs is also appreciated during image 'shoots'.

The media of other urban centers such as New York City, London, Los Angeles, Tokyo, Jerusalem and Hong Kong also showed the Common Defense interactions of Americans with other regions.

The work and graphics were created by the software products of ABBYY, Adobe, Calibre, Cyberlink, Mathworks, Microsoft Office, NVidia, Octave, Smartdraw, SAS, Paint.net, and Pinnacle.

The search engines of Wikipedia, Thomas, Global Security, Janes, Stratfor, Milnet, NARA, LLC, Questia, Acadamia and Nexus are also very much appreciated as the large-scale CAS perception of the Constitution needed them just to start.

The forbearance, and occasional political tolerance, of all kin and relations is also acknowledged.

Contents

NOTE: for those interested in year to year tracking of the Constitutional dynamical systems, you can go directly to the chapter on Summary sets at the end of the yearly Chronicles. For searching, combinations of the Preamble Six [JU], [TR], [CD], [GW], [LI] or the date 2018.nn.nn field will find specific speculation data. Page numbers are given per chapter as a reader courtesy on estimating time for inspecting a content group.

Introduction

The Cambridge Electron Accelerator at the northern edge of the Harvard campus had many complex systems of people, electronics, microwaves and a ring of magnetic fields. These were all magically combined in a system that was designed to hold free electrons that were being accelerated so that they could break up atoms and measure the resulting energy levels of many different 'particles'. But this facility was so complex that it was difficult to know what the entire dynamical system was doing at any one time. Therefore, the systems were monitored by people in a control room in those days and there were no central computer banks that did this for the scientists and engineers. There were glowing tube lights with numbers and digits all about measuring the various values of the hundreds of components and people had to memorize whether they were 'within parameters' at any time.

But the other end of this complex Accelerator had a large experimental floor in which the very high-powered electrons were magnetically deflected into various nuclear and unstable matter in order to produce the very intense particle bombardments that showed on readouts and photo tracks. All of these experimental areas and the magnetic tubes coming into them produced intense radiation and therefore required a safety officer to ensure that no one slid by the lead-filled concrete blocks or walked through the wrong access tunnel.

This experimental area, which normally ran 24-7, had one other feature of significance. It allowed the safety officer to sit and study anything he desired from one night to the next and perhaps do a walk-in on a course of interest the next morning in the lecture halls on Oxford Street. This included the Science Center with math and physics and cosmology, the Museum of Natural History, the Peabody Museum and the Divinity School that dated back to 1630. The combination was a fairly intense concentration of human diversity for one who had already lived among Japanese, Comanche, Hawaiians, Koreans, Panamanian San Blas, Good ol Boys, and semi-Puritan New Englanders. Oxford Street also started at Kirkland Street, which was a short walk (or the proverbial stone's throw in the late 1960s) from a dormitory an ancestral cousin, Nathaniel, had built there in the Yard.

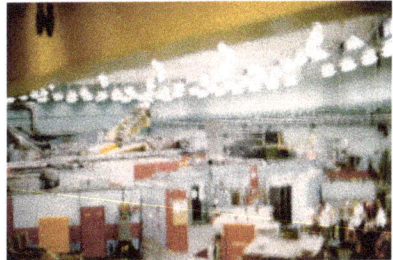

In 1970, the complexity and strife of the Yard's previous few years was beyond comprehension in terms of the other human societies that had been encountered. Going from an intense military environment of the Vietnam conflict to one of riots and the evolving Harrad Experiment with new chemicals can be a bit confusing. People were looking for new solutions all around and so was one sitting in a particle physics lab reading about the 'dynamics' of planet earth. That including some articles about 'system dynamics' that were being discussed at the Accelerator lab and down the street at the Massachusetts Institute of Technology. Some lectures were suggesting that the 500-year-old scientific method of deductive reasoning did not work as the complexity of a system increased and the particle physics researches were beginning to find holes even in MC squared. How would you define a phenomena that was appearing simultaneously in different systems when there was no measurable connections between them and 'C' was based on time? Or when one cannot account for the gravity of the universe by the 'particles' in it? Even if you couldn't do the math, they were interesting questions.

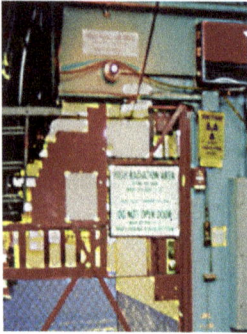

Worse, humans simply didn't fit into any system of coherence even when the researches of Darwin, Mendel and Watson said there was in the mysterious double helix of DNA and many people had begun to worry about that, especially one who had seen some very negative ripple effects among those he encountered in his travels. A group at MIT had begun to formerly research system dynamic phenomena in large systems of people and these quiet readings about it in a complex physics environment might have caused an 'enlightened moment' about things that appeared to be beyond comprehension.

A closer look involved the research of Jay Forrester at MIT and his studies of 'urban dynamics' with Mayor Collins of Boston. He had also developed a ferrite memory that let him 'store' data about systems, which was of considerable interest to people attempting to visualize 'nuclear' activity, including at a fog-shrouded Los Alamos. Even so, how could you sum the energies of a complex society like Boston with an 'agent of change' history going back several centuries?

I had just transited from possibly traumatic military service in Asia and Washington DC and knew where governmental hearings were being held on the Hill after many Common Defense security related visits myself while assigned to the Pentagon. It was an eye opener concerning the OTHER value of the Constitution, General Welfare, when an article about Jay Forrester appeared.

Jay Forrester, at a U.S. House of Representatives subcommittee hearing on urban growth, 1971:

> Our social systems are far more complex and harder to understand than our technological systems. Why, then, do we not use the same approach of making models of social systems and conducting laboratory experiments on those models before we try new laws and government programs in real life? The answer is often stated that our knowledge of social systems is insufficient for constructing useful models. But what justification can there be for the apparent assumption that we do not know enough to construct models but believe we do know enough to directly design new social systems by passing laws and starting new social programs?

But the government had caught up with me again about this time and the Accelerator was closing due to its funding being transferred to a much larger ring facility at Batavia, Illinois, which itself would eventually be replaced by a much larger proton accelerator ring at CERN, Switzerland. The operations research was continuing in Cambridge, but the anomalies concerning the basis for society had begun to develop some definitions and because of family matters on Cape Cod, I became interested in a research facility called WHOI some miles from history related places like Hyannis Port (which had interesting residences accessible from Lewis Bay and a private airline to Washington nearby) and Plymouth Rock (15 miles from our ancestral home in 1641AD). I did not quite realize I was signing on at the Woods Hole Oceanographic

Institution as a technical crew member in the traditional manner of ships acquiring 'crews'. But the vessels were named 'RV' for Research Vessel and not 'HMS' for His Majesties Ship of 1812 sailor impressing or kidnapping fame, so the opportunity to examine more of the world as a dynamical system, and perhaps aid your own society, was too ordained to pass up. These scientific ships too were complex systems and looked upon the entire world in an 'in situ' context if you survived the process of docking in strange places, or bad weather, or running into and over some anti-submarine warfare activity where megatons were involved. But all of the Earth science disciplines such as geology, microbiology, weather and oceanography came and went on the RVs and they also were an enlightenment concerning molecular complexity and 'systems'.

Meanwhile, Forrester and his group had begun to define operations research with the publication of several defining treatise including *Urban Dynamics* and *World Dynamics*. I had two copies of each book over a period of years and during some 600,000 miles of travel, all of them managed to disappear along with my 'dot connect' notes to the 9-inch floppy disks the HP computers I was responsible for. The HP computers were being used to store ocean related data, but had word processors as well. The *Dynamics* books basically said what complex systems were in 1971. 01.01:

1. System: A system is a set of entities, real or abstract, comprising a whole in which each component interacts with or is related to at least one other component.

a. Environment: The system must be understood in the context of an environment, which is not part of the system itself.

2. System of Systems: Some of the entities composing the system are themselves systems.

3. Complex: The system exhibits emergent behavior which arises from interrelationships between its elements; this behavior is of greater complexity than the sum of behaviors of its parts and not due to system complication.

4. Adaptive: The system is adaptive; the behavior of entities or sub-systems and their interaction change in time possibly resulting in a change in the way the entire system relates to its environment.

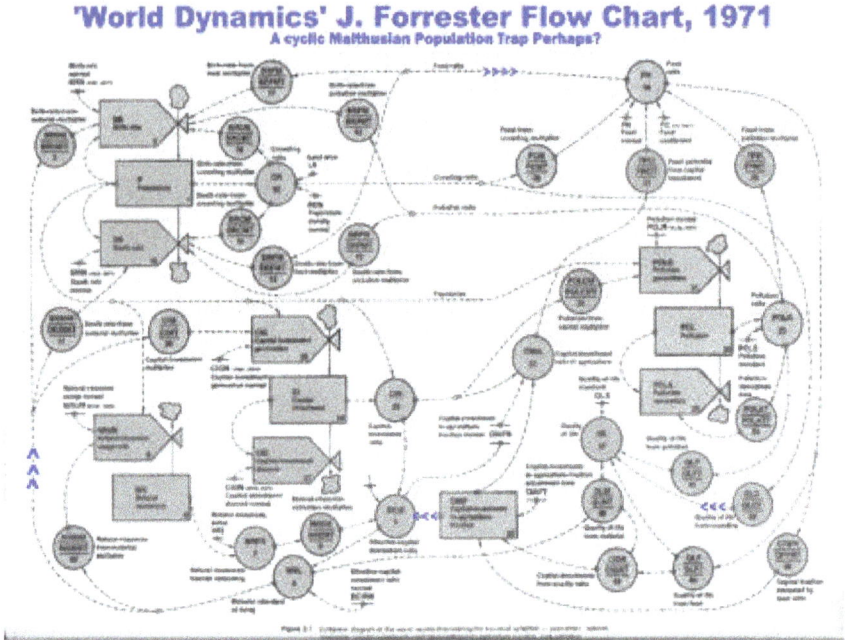

Figure 1.   Jay Forrester Original

The groups shown in blue would qualify as systems of systems within a 'world' environment.   The 'systems' being looked at are the rectangular blocks such as Population, Death rate, Pollution, and Capital Investment.   Into this is the interactive conditions of 'adaptive change' over time, where a loss of value in one of the circular representations has cascade or ripple effects in other parts of the system of systems. Obviously, the ripple effects of sudden loss of food supply would be drastic for population and capital and cycle back to the inability of societies to stay together. Testing this original Malthusian process in different societies was a very appealing idea, along with intelligence gathering on societies.   Oceanographic ships went to these societies all the time, but what eventually became plain was that human societies do not base their existence on food supply alone.

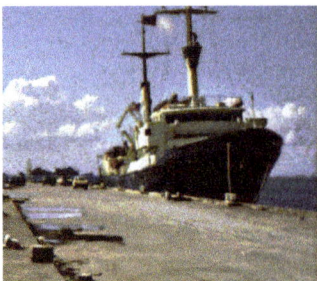

I am applying this concept of Complex Adaptive Systems (CAS) to not only the oceanographic research aboard ship but to the peoples visited ashore.   That attitude of viewing a person as a dynamic system of molecules would not make one popular with the ladies, including biologists, by the way. It did not take any math to see that many areas of the world except possibly America had fallen into deep Malthusian Population Traps (MPT) from which only eternal strife and violence emanated, much of which involved Zenophilia or ethnic MPT motivation. Zenophilia is a 2010AD term for genetically passed on 'race fear' that couldn't be accurately defined until a method called fMRI scans of the brain appeared in the 1990s. Even without an MRI, everyone on earth knew what ethnic aggression systems were and what they did to humans. A Forrester fifth order differential involving birth rates being equated to the combined food, energy, health and productivity 'entities' concerning MPT was barely calculable on the early HP 2100 computers but could stimulate some 'complexity' understanding. The early HPs could certainly contain lists of observations on societies along with other data.

Unfortunately, collecting data like this had certain Cold War espionage appearances, especially in places like Singapore, Hong Kong, and Tehran, Frankfurt a Mein, Cape Verde, Lima and Jerusalem. The copies of the *World Dynamics* with various references to the floppies got confiscated or lost in baggage. The floppies and tapes themselves were stored in safe areas of the computer decks until the ship returned to Woods Hole, sometimes along with bottles of Glenmorangie malt Scotch. At least most of the time. The floppies could then be printed out ashore, all they really indicated was that a 'system of systems' pictured in *World Dynamics* definitely could not be defined by component or regression analyses. Oh well, the biological researches at Woods Hole were beginning to re-define molecular complexity all over the oceans anyway with unknown dynamical systemic issues ahead. That research included virtually all of the Mother Earth systems of oceanography, molecular biology, geophysics and global warming trends.

One expedition by Robert Ballard on the RV Knorr in 1977, was especially meaningful. I had the duty of monitoring the satellite radio system at Woods Hole on this occasion (which I also did on the ship transmitter end during various expeditions) when a series of images of the 'alien' life forms 6000 feet down in the Galapagos Rift appeared from Ballard's expedition. There was a great deal of excitement and speculation about the images of 'black smokers', crabs, mussels and various life forms pictured around the heat vents of the Rift. Most of the biological community were examining the molecular breakdown of life that did not require sunlight or oxygen to exist as a form of reduction analysis. But when the images were spread on a table, I saw a new *coherent system of life* that operated independently of other systems of life. The effect of seeing that system within systems was profound for one who had been studying human dynamical systems on the side and one who knew of the *other Rift,* the Great Rift Valley of Kenya where someone or something may have said 'let there be light'.

At some point, the pressure (and changes in government research funding again) to look at system complexity entities outside the pleasant, if monastic, society of Woods Hole and Cape Cod became stronger and I applied for work as an analyst at MIT. This was at the top of the Greene Building where a new sea surface research system was being installed that had advanced graphics simulation ability. In 1981, it was nearly impossible to perceive that a home computer in 2011 or a hand held 'tablet' in 2016 would be able to do the same simulations as a computer room full of electronics. I also discovered an 'in situ' research environment on ships might leave one out of a math loop for complexity and programming of computers. This research simply confirmed the

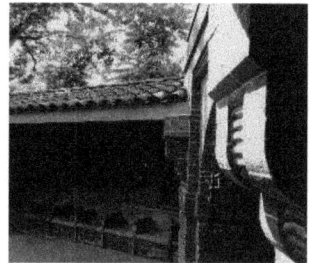

suspicions that the world was a far more chaotically organized dynamical system than most thought, weather patterns included. The MIT campus in 1982 was well along into various studies of Operations Research at Sloan, biomedical laboratories with advanced molecular technologies and as funding changed again, eventually for me led to a plasma fusion research computer administration where entire DEC computer systems were taking data from large complex systems called Tokomaks, which in theory would produce thermonuclear fusion energy someday. It also led to frequent visits to Washington and Hawaii on family matters.

The Washington visits re-established interest in a little-known dynamical system called the Constitution and curiosity as to why it had lasted so long regardless of the trials put to it, including the ongoing struggle between Liberty, Rights and Common Defense. A little organization across the street from the Capitol was called the Library of Congress and held many resources available to researchers, as did George Washington University, which had several entire centers on Law and the dynamics of politics using the law. One only needed to inspect the course material on Constitutional law and visit a nice little book store on F Street, two blocks from the Executive Office Building to get a 'feel' for current thinking. Most, however, didn't seem to equate a document carefully penned in September 1787 with the social processes of 'law' in the 1980s. Wondering in and out of the White House also produced a 'feel' of the power it held, although much different than security visits of 1965.

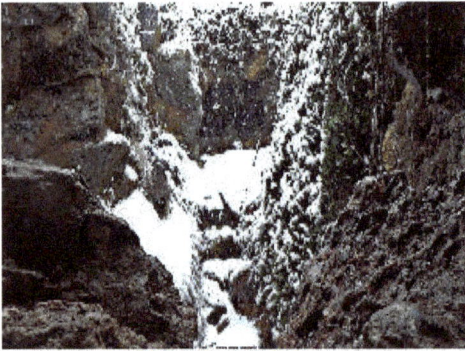

The Indian Spring on the Hill.
The ancient Kwedake Dikep of the wandering Iroquois Peoples

But a strange thing happened in the mid-1980s that would change the dynamics of Humanity for much of the future. One of the computers I was responsible for had direct 'wired' links to several other places doing fusion research. I sent or controlled messages to administrators in Palo Alto and Los Alamos (along with a cryptic electronic address in northern Virginia) asking for fusion data results the various groups at MIT were interested in and was pleasantly surprised to see data streams almost immediately. They called this the DARPAnet and for the first time I realized that I could not identify a 'person' anymore unless he was a proper electronic symbol.

The physicists were looking at very complex systems of thermonuclear interactions being 'downloaded' which, oddly enough, looked quite similar to the energy fluidity of four-dimensional ocean systems previously encountered. As I was a systems analyst, I was more interested in the *patterns* of systems and not necessarily the details of each. The math was entirely different (which I wasn't good at), even if lucidly described in a little Albany Street first floor library on thermonuclear dynamics. That was the first place I saw the term 'Bell's theorem' and its concept that complex entities could be co-existent or parallel, not just hierarchical and linear.

As a large digital tape library, including descriptions of molecular structures, soon developed in the lab computers I was admining and with a new Tokomak under construction, some further thought on social entities existing as coexistent rather than sequential was needed and why such entities needed 'time' in their definition. Many political, religious and economic theories looked quite different if the time factor was removed. This led to a further examination of one of the most successful dynamic social systems in history; the society created by the 1789 Constitution. Did its balanced and parallel processes give society its success? Was there really any coherence to systems the Cro-Magnon perceived or used?

The newspapers of Gutenberg's printing press form were beginning to show signs of stress as media forms became more electronic in the 1980s, but their archives concerning Capitol Hill were also beginning to open up electronically. MIT's library system went 'online' during this period and access to many disciplines became available on TV tubes that fortunately did not have the continuous interruption cycle of the 'Main Stream Media' as some had begun calling the air networks, which themselves qualified as complex systems within systems. Learning and perception itself began to speed up almost exponentially, almost of it were an ordained process itself. But that data availability also allowed access to data about one's own genealogy and the part that DNA pattern had played in the formation of a new Republic, such as in its few and short wars (if compared to European and Asian systems of mass murder, anyway). It also led to family discoveries, including an unusual 'wanderlust' pattern over several centuries. Considering the Cro-Magnon (and other) DNA migrations, the thought occurred that DNA itself created systems within systems and could be manipulated for good and evil just like anything else the Cro-Magnons touched.

The chaos of world politics of the period was perceived as more dangerous than most realized as interaction with people who were politically and militarily motivated increased. A little brick-walled oasis with an ancient Indian spring in the middle of this chaos was revisited and triggered some thoughts concerning war and the Cannon Office Building's Armed Services Committee conference rooms that had been seen and absorbed as memories in the 1960s. No one had called this pleasant, quiet place a Di'Kep for many centuries in the early 1990s. Other Constitutional matters like the idea of blocking proposed legislation from editing in a computer system days before a vote wasn't too popular, even if it had 'obvious' value.

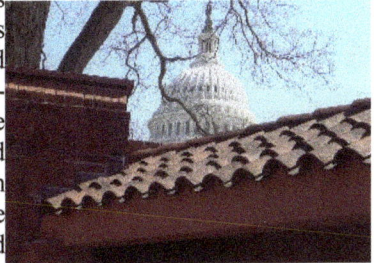

The visits to the Di'Kep only indicated a complexity level that was truly dynamic, even to the level where sub-systems resembled a cloud in a bottle. A blatantly primeval invasion by an FBI profiled serial murderer (a negative progression system itself?) named Saddam Hussein didn't help 'constitutional research' either; reacting to the real world had a serious habit of getting in the way of its fundamental values like Justice, Liberty, and especially Common Defense. How does one defend through Common Defense if the majority 'systems' of the world are determined to destroy the values of Justice, Liberty and Tranquility found in the American Constitution.?

The advancing sciences indicated that the venerable Constitution of We The People was clearly being threatened even as inefficient 'systems' of totalitarianism began to be seen for what they were; something from a primeval past. An impressive description of social dynamics by William Strauss and Neil Howe called *Generations, the History of America's future, 1584 to 2069* appeared in 1991. It had some Appendices, one that defined the 'dynamic' of generations, including a 'Cohort

Generation' which defined all the people of a given age group in a period of history as a generation. But there was also an attempt in Appendix B to define generations of the Executive branch and how the elected Presidents affected the Nation. This was a very interesting dynamical idea because it defined the government as a 'system' not necessarily based on politics of the moment which certainly fit with the Constitution as a 'set' of near independent processes. 'Generations' from 1584 easily translated into the 'our Posterity' dynamic of the Constitution's Preamble Unfortunately, the authors in 1991 could not have envisioned what the Internet technologies and Humane Genome mapping would do to the future they said would extend to 2069, nor what the effect of consuming all available energy on a planet would do.

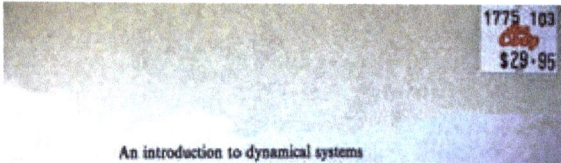

1775 103
$29·95

An introduction to dynamical systems

At this time, government funding for particle research caught up with me again and choices to pursue research on the Constitutional systems became mandated. It is difficult to leave an environment like MIT, but that really wasn't where the idea of Constitutional Dynamics could be researched, especially when Jay Forrester's researchers over in Sloan didn't even have such a discipline. The term 'free-lance' writer/researcher entered the picture, even if the economic value 'Gross Domestic Networth Index' or GDNI was less and in Washington DC of the 1990s, GDNI needed careful nurture.

It was becoming fashionable for some to use a GDNI reference to define the confusion of the Marxist, Keynesian, and Friedmanist economic macro systems in the USA in terms of the 'Networth' of an individual after all liabilities had been subtracted from his productivity, whatever that actually was in system dynamics. In any case, a move to the District of Columbia area, with the aid of far-roaming relations there, was initiated so that a certain Library of Congress, a Congressional Research Service and a new Archives of the US could be more closely examined for the history and dynamics of three branches of government with human rights imbedded. But how was such a dynamical system even visualized? Scientific systems integration that had once been a lab environment was rapidly coming to the home and individual computers. So were software mechanisms such as many Agencies in the District area had begun to use and these modelling technologies supplied a basis for virtually any visualization. A very sophisticated group known as the NRO did this very well. So a very serious examination of 'Constitutional Dynamics' developed.

Note Forrester's original idea: "1. System: A system is a set of entities, real or abstract, comprising a whole in which each component interacts with or is related to at least one other component. a. Environment: The system must be understood in the context of an environment, which is not part of the system itself." How does that apply to a 'system of systems' like the American Constitution when the environment is always part of the 'systems' of the North American continent?

Using the original concept of the Complex Adaptive Systems (CAS) philosophy in a somewhat speculative Constitutional environment such as the Kwedake (or better known as the Capitol Hill) is the result of research into the historical relationships between the American Society and the advances in human technologies, especially those concerning the evolution of the biological body, the molecular mind and the resulting advanced Being, sometimes known as Human Being, a total entity, rather than Homo sapiens, the 'wise man'. It is an attempt to closely follow the original intent of the American Constitution to recognize the evolving Human Rights that establish an advanced basis for human cooperation. That cooperative awareness is one of the principal reasons Human Beings have advanced so rapidly over the last seventy thousand years and may have culminated in the Constitutional covenants of Justice, Tranquility, Common Defense, General Welfare, Liberty, and Posterity that have served the Americans so well.

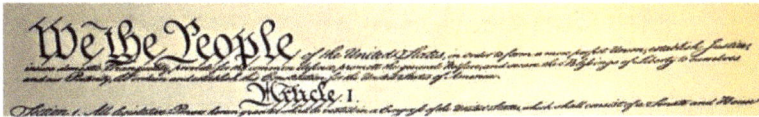

The Preamble to the Constitution is many times taken for granted and many assume that the Declaration of Independence was incorporated into its wording but that actually didn't happen. The Preamble wording was almost an afterthought by the Committee of Style in the Constitutional Convention of September 1788. They had been so busy writing and re-writing the Articles of the Constitution, with many debates on the wording, that they had overlooked the inclusion of the purpose or intent of the Constitution. What was striking for one investigating dynamical systems from an engineering or systems analyses approach was that the wording of the Preamble had compressed six major dynamical systems into a coordinated entity of intent with 52 words. It stated in order to establish a more perfect Union, a given as far as the Convention intent was concerned, that six conditions had to be met. They were (1) establish Justice, (2) insure domestic Tranquility, (3) provide for the common defence, (4) promote the general Welfare, (5) secure the Blessings of Liberty to ourselves, and (6) our Posterity.

Now, one could say that the six conditionals were arbitrarily perceived by someone in this century because the use of capital letters to emphasize an important subject in the 1700s meant that *only* those capitalized were significant. In that case Union, Justice, Tranquility, Welfare, Blessings of Liberty (for individuals especially, from the Declaration of Independence) and Posterity would be considered equally important in the minds of the Style Committee. There was no emphases whatever on common defence and Posterity wouldn't be separated from Liberty for individuals. But no matter how they are emphasized, the 6000 year history of the world had shown with virtually no exceptions that without a balanced implementation of both common defense and general welfare together, a society would fail within a few generations because neighboring societies that did balance them would simply absorb the entity that didn't have them. A person being exposed to both Common Defense in the Pentagon and General Welfare at the Cannon Office Building, could not help but note the conflicts of the two. Even with the Tranquility of the Dikep just a hundred yards away, it had always been difficult to balance the two.

In the 1700s, Common Defense and General Welfare were happening all over Europe, China, Africa and the native societies of the Western Hemisphere. Justice, Tranquility, or Posterity could not exist without Common Defense and General Welfare as *Prime Directives* of a society, but Liberty had not even become a concept in 1776 or 1788 because of worldwide slavery, serfdom or indentured servitude.

Liberty could not even exist unless the other conditionals already existed, and that included a society that held to 'our Posterity'. The Preamble had emphasized 'our Posterity' as an end product, so perhaps some other dynamic besides living from one minute to the next was also at work in the Philadelphia of 1788. But could each complex adaptive conditional be measured as subsets of a dynamical system called a nation and what other subsets besides them could also be integrated into a balanced Union or complex adaptive system?

Note again the definitions being used in this study context, slightly different from Jay's in 1971:

A system.

A group of molecular or quantum structures that operated as a single function that was dependent on its existence by co-existence with other systems with different functions. Each function is distinctive but requires co-existence. There is no limit on the size of the components or 'elements' of a system, either quantum or cosmic in scale.

System of systems.

The reduction analysis of something into its various parts. A human person is a system of systems that starts with a few conception molecules, begins multiplying through DNA programming into increasingly complex subsystems basically divided into body systems, mind systems, environment systems and spirit systems that integrate the other subsystems. When the Human Genome mapping was completed in 2010, some 700,000 subsystems had been catalogued for humans. A human family develops as a system of systems and perhaps qualifies as the nucleus of positive energy or wealth development. This might lead to 'systems' of governance like those leading up to the Constitution in the 1700s.

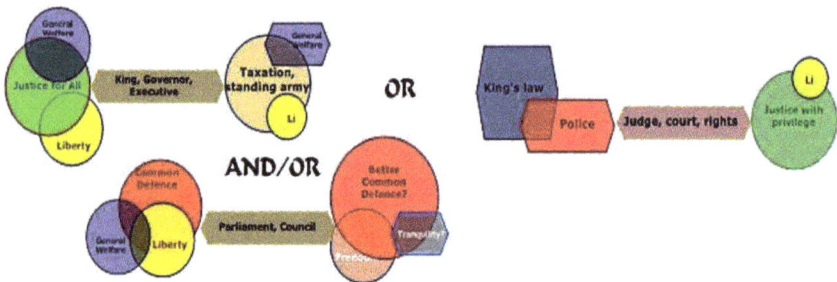

Governmental Organization to 1700

A Dynamical System.

A set, usually defined mathematically, of unified systems that create an interactive environment for other combinations of systems. A solar system is a dynamical system, as is a galaxy of solar systems, or a human tribe or city state is. A group of city states becomes a set when they join in a common function. The Constitution then creates a Dynamical System through its Union of states.

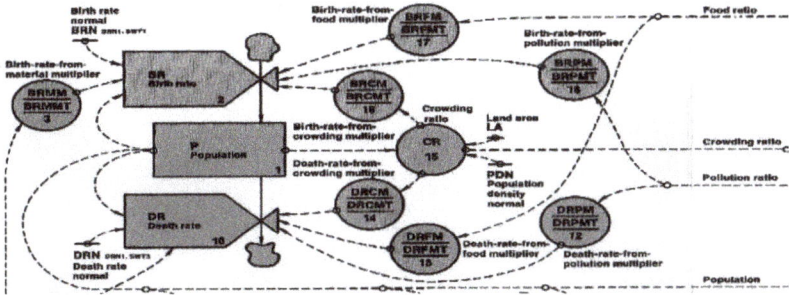

But a quick look at Jay Forrester's original mapping of a society shows three primary conditions (birth, population, and death) and a number of variable conditions that together qualify as a 'system of systems' just in the initiating of the timeline. The timeline with the other 'system of systems' constitutes a true Dynamical System. A dynamical system can exist in time as an entity of its own with 'self organizing' features and energy levels. It can also have enough energy to feed back on itself and grow more dynamical as an evolutionary system

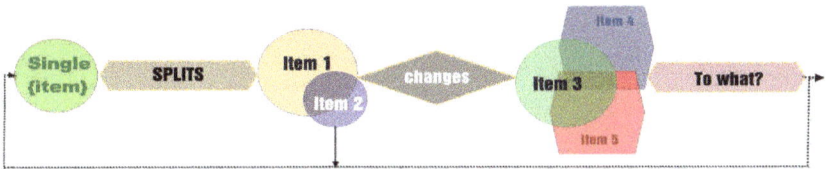

ITEM CHANGES TO SOMETHING ELSE,
BUT WITH AN OPTIMIZATION LOOP?

But suppose one visualized the Constitution in the same way with modern (2005) Venn charts? A Venn chart simply illustrates how groups of 'things' interact at any moment, while a flow chart such as in *World Dynamics* shows interaction of 'things' going –in a logical direction.

A person can visualize this for just about anything (see Methodology, next chapter, for explanation of symbols in the graphics); family, household (complex), transportation (very complex in city states), or government (complex sets of complexity).

In the Venn charts, how does Justice and Liberty evolve into a positive our Posterity that builds a better generation later? Obviously General Welfare or Common Defense as a single item couldn't produce our Posterity with a better value than before, especially if each only produced more of itself. How does a singular Phenom or thing evolve into a coherent group of things through time? How does a single cell a billion years ago continually evolve into more complex DNA 'systems' that eventually combine into a human dynamical system with hundreds of thousands of molecular parts? And don't say it doesn't matter; even if you only exist from one minute to the next in thinking, you wouldn't be here if a positive evolution of those 'systems' didn't exist.

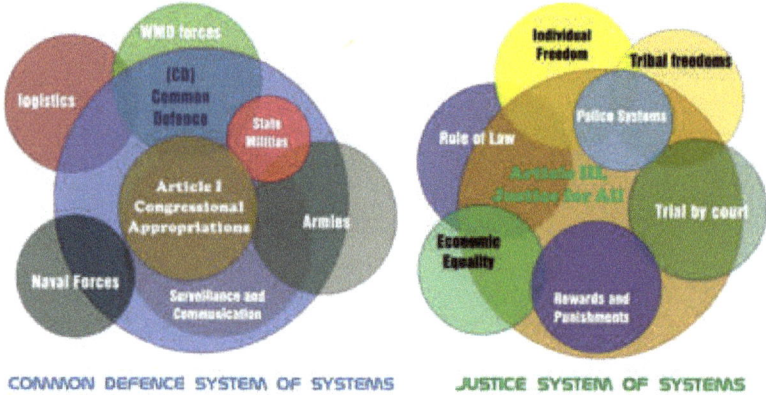

COMMON DEFENCE SYSTEM OF SYSTEMS   JUSTICE SYSTEM OF SYSTEMS

The problem with this analytical process becomes fairly obvious when one tries to break a CAS down into its components, the process almost all humans use to evaluate something. Note the 'common defense' and 'justice' Venn charts of the complex breakdowns of its component systems. Even the smallest component, such as 'militia' can be further broken down into complex items, especially if one adds the Second Amendment right to possess weapons as a Justice system.

Article I has the empowerment of congress to make appropriations and just the common defence components are extremely complex. But Article III, involves the Supreme Court and its authority concerning [JU] or justice for all. It gets even more complex because the components of the original Justice intent involve virtually all of the Bill of Rights, along with the Supreme Court's rulings over a century that initiated the 27 later Amendments. The 14th Amendment's due process concerning life, liberty and property (from the Declaration of Independence which was NOT law) has had dozens of complex plus and minus interpretations since 1868. But the checks and balances of the Constitution's directives demonstrates and proves the theory that it, as a complex adaptive structure, is a very positive societal mechanism.

Albert Einstein, First Impressions of America, 1921.00.00:

> Nothing is more destructive of respect for the government and the
> law of the land than passing laws which cannot be enforced.

And he also said: "Everything should be made as simple as possible, but not simpler." That is just a reflection of the complexity he had encountered (as told by his son, Eduard, in Woods Hole) in the cosmos of a beautiful simplicity called 'energy = mass times light squared' for Relativity. The EPR process he developed would remain too complex even for an extended neural brain like Einstein's, as his son's allowed research on that brain showed. And then there is the *System's Bible* by John Gall in 2002 which had the fairly famous comment: "A complex system that works is invariably found to have evolved from a simple system that works. A complex system designed from scratch never works and cannot be patched up to make it work. You have to start over with a working simple system." In the 20th century the argument could be made that dividing government into three separate balancing entities in 1789 was NOT starting over with a 'simpler' system. A king, caliph, emperor, duke or lord proprietor with life and death power over everything WAS simple and inalienable. A permanently owned veto power by some biped or other on everything actually does stabilize things, but to what point?

By the start of the 21st century, this curiosity about the Constitution would lead down a path that involved the intricacies of the process as well as the actual effects of any given combination of the values of the Prime Directives. The 'details' devil was in any other conditions that might aid or usurp its demonstrated positive processes. This inquisitiveness led to studying the government from the position of an 'outsider', which can also be interpreted to mean that you were spying on the government, not necessarily attempting to aid the process.   But as one who came from a long line of people who liked Liberty and Justice, what others might think had to be put aside or 'cherry picked' just in order to 'see' the process of governance and whether there was some fundamental good or evil in its future direction or 'our Posterity'..

But the need for a modern methodology for 'sight' was becoming clearer with each passing year, especially as some of the older assumed values of the Constitution begin breaking down under the speed of new technologies used as weapons became apparent. [CD] and [GW] could be permanently unbalanced.

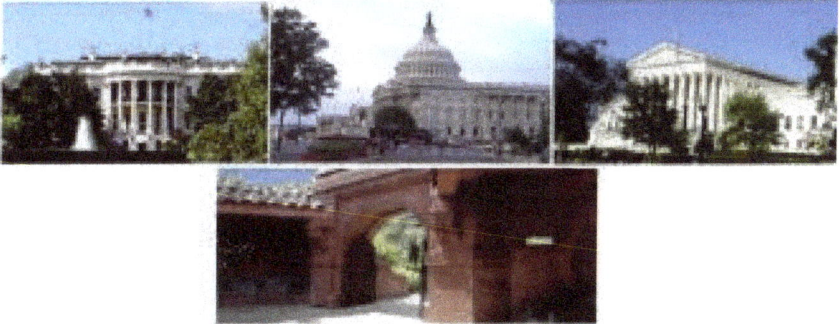

Constitutional Dynamics Pre-history

Researches into the creation of the Constitution will lead one into what can only be defined as a systemic quagmire. Over the years, there are hundreds of interpretations and literary cross references in the thousands that attest to the fascination with a document of governance like no other before it. Aristotle had produced a description of social systems, *Politics*, in the 5th century before the Common Era that described the various city states (earlier mindset of the *Urban Dynamics* by Forrester?) and what people agreed to as governance then and how they related to each other. It is interesting that one Hippocrates had compiled a description of the 'systems' in a human body by this time, even when he couldn't define them as a huge complex entity of dynamic molecular systems.

Neither did a parallel 16 volume medical effort by Zhang Zhongjing in China describe molecular systems, but the interest in the human, and possibly non-human, sub-systems was well established and more detailed than descriptions like Aristotle's of politics or Sun Tzu's *Art of War*. People along the Han and Yangtze Rivers were more interested in *War* than in health books or books by the *other* Tzu, the *Tao Te Ching*, which had a dynamic of its own. The rule by force of arms was absolute and universal until the 1500s when the freezing climate of Europe caused them to wonder about the planet in new ships and come upon a land that was itself becoming unpopulated because of the icy conditions where food could not be grown.

Magna Carta of England, June 1215, carried over to the Bill of Rights:

39. No freemen shall be taken or imprisoned or disseised [removed from his property] or exiled or in any way destroyed, nor will we [the king] go upon him nor send upon him, except by the lawful judgment of his peers or by the law of the land.

The concept of the 'divine right' of kings, emperors, czars, caliphs and oligarchic nobilities did not really come into question until the latter half of the second millennium, about the time of a drastic climate change in the 1500s. This climate change, a world temperature drop of just one degree average, cause virtually all of the European fiefdoms to be unable to produce the necessities of survival for their 'serfs' and the system began to break down amid intense strife and persecution. The idea of an 'agreement among peoples' began with a spiritual literary analysis by one Martin Luther that was tacked on a church door in 1517. It was the first systemic dynamic of the separation of the 'spirit', the 'state', and the 'individual' that had become obvious to so many. The concentration of everything into one political hierarchy had been shown to be dysfunctional and the cold of a mini-ice age only proved it to those who began to flee to places like the Caribbean, then to other warm parts of the earth such as India and Polynesia.

In the 1600s, the devastation of the climate shift began to subside, or humans began one of their remarkable adaptions to it. The New World fostered many new concepts concerning society as many new things about humanity were discovered. The English Revolution, which made many other revolutions pale by comparison to its violence, first brought about a very brief idea called the *'Instruments of Government'* that lasted from 1653 to 1657. It was quickly suppressed by both the Round Heads of Cromwell and the Cavaliers of Charles I because no one could deal with the idea of 'separation of powers'. Power is absolute. Everybody knows that. Especially if YOU want it.

But a strange thing happened to those who were fleeing this English Civil War, including a large clan of Thayers who were too good with leather crafting and matchlock muskets to be left alone by either Roundheads or Cavaliers, and these Thayers then came to places like Salem and Boston and Braintree in the Massachusetts Bay Colony. The Thayer 'freemen' were similar to those who came to New Amsterdam, Montreal, Philadelphia, and Williamsburg. But not Charleston and St Augustine? They brought with them that simple idea of the "agreements with separate powers' and began applying the idea of dynamical city states with voting 'freemen' that Aristotle had described. Might not have had a choice; many of the city states of North America were only connected by ship. Even in 1650, only the Powhatten of the Chesapeake, the Iroquois from the North and the Cherokee from the South wondered by and camped by the Kwedake Dikep between the Anacostia and Potomac Rivers. That nice little place on a hill would one day be called 'The Hill' or Capitol Hill. But in the "world dynamic' that was coming, the hunter gatherer with a stone club and flint arrow, whether Iroquois or Powhatten, would be no more.

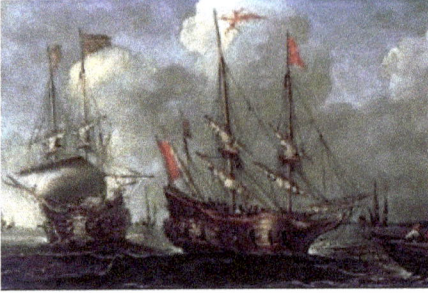

By 1600, the Europeans had begun their great expansion into the world and they had used the fundamental concept that if you could occupy some area and had the force of arms to hold it, you could extract 'wealth' from the people and molecules of the area. A concept fundamentally no different from the attacking Neolithic tribes that had survived the Ice Age 10,000 years before, except that that the process was now organized into dynamic systems.   The weapons and social organization of the Europeans had changed drastically, and this allowed for the misnamed 'colonialism' to expand. An English invention called the 'volley fire' of cannon and musket by many at once could not be overcome by individuals like Shaka of the Zulu or Chief Powhuten of the Iroquois or Takirau of the Maori no matter how physically and mentally able. But had that murderous ferocity of the European mini ice age caused another dynamic to appear concerning the consensus idea of a 'Republic' with Justice for all? Or was cold and hunger just Malthusian population pressures that created the ferocity as it appeared in the Mongols of the 1200s before and the Persians 1500 years before that? And would the rapidly expanding heat waves after 1800 cause another form of ferocity?

1653, Instrument of Government, veto power carried to the Constitution?

XXIV. That all Bills agreed unto by the Parliament, shall be presented to the Lord Protector for his consent; and in case he shall not give his consent thereto within twenty days after they shall be presented to him, or give satisfaction to the Parliament within the time limited, that then, upon declaration of the Parliament that the Lord Protector hath not consented nor given satisfaction, such Bills shall pass into and become laws, although he shall not give his consent thereunto; provided such Bills contain nothing in them contrary to the matters contained in these presents.

Instruments of power or rule first appeared described as a 'dynamical system' about this time, first by one Blackstone in 1769 and then by one Ben Franklin who had returned from his European 'studies' in the 1770s, and who possessed a copy of the 'Instrument of Government'. Others also had begun to call for a 'system' that reflected the original full citizenship participation of the Greeks 2000 years before with a Union of various democratic city-states. Those city-state freedom ideas had eventually been removed by such as Philippe and Alexander of Macedon in the ancient days, leading to feudal systems of organization that were 'universal' on Earth, including within such States created by the Emperors of Rome, Byzantine, Tang of China, Abbasid of Persia, and much later, by the Hapsburgs of Europe.

Even these empires had systems of 'justice', 'tranquility' and 'common defense', but rarely combined them with a system of 'Liberty'. Systems of indenture and slavery were norms on planet Earth and Liberty could not be allowed to exist. They also had engineering systems of 'health' such as sewage, roads, hospitals and postal letters. Emperors and royal families had one thing others didn't have; they had time to learn and many times put knowledge about systems to good use. But economic 'systems' were developing in parallel with the political and the two were no longer the same. The encrypted letters of the Knights Templars in the 1200s was one of the earliest systems to combine communication, gold and geography into a 'system' of international wealth transfer. This dynamic, very dynamic, system was so good that it was arbitrarily seized by the kings of France and Germany whose treasuries were depleted. The massacres of the Templars was just 'normal' conduct for European rulers into the 1400s. And so was the narcissistic mismanagement of regions though debts by many such rulers, an item that had become despised by immigrants to North America.

But only the Americans of the 1600s and 1700s began to think of a dynamical system of governance based on Liberty, Justice and Equality even as they engaged in the shipment of gold and tobacco to Europe and manufactured goods back to Africa and America, where they were in turn sold for other 'goods'.

Ben Franklin, 1774.09.00:

> This will be the best security for maintaining our liberties. A nation
> of well-informed men who have been taught to know and prize the
> rights which God has given them cannot be enslaved. It is in the
> religion of ignorance that tyranny begins.

The Americans and Europeans also became aware that they could control the elements, as Franklin did with lightening and spectacles for reading, Jenner and Pasteur did with vaccinations and some Pennsylvanians and Kentuckians began doing with 'long rifles' instead of muskets. In the 1600s, standing armies in battle went from a few thousand to 100,000 and by the time of Napoleon in 1812 had reached 400,000. Vaccination or molecular enhancement of the human immune 'system', a reaction to the intense plaques of that time, was the most important development, as it would eventually save the lives of some half billion people. The feudal world of individual power ownership acquired by force was being challenged, but power owners seemed to find new ways of controlling people; usury, indenture, health and standing police forces being some of them. Some people needed controlling as the genetic effects of one born with Anti-social Personality Disorders and other forms of inherited violence would one day show. The Industrial Revolution began in this century and new forms of wealth and land use made many aspects of Feudalism obsolete but also made the world's urban population traps more severe, as one Malthus described. During this period of extreme weather change and human change from 1400 to 1800, many conditions of feudal ownership of 'property' in a human society were challenged and many ideas of the Dark Ages came into question as Galileo, Descartes, Newton and many others reacted to the disintegration of life in the 1600s.

Even though people operated as mutually cooperative systems for thousands of years in common defense and general welfare, the dynastic processes were not really defined. Indeed, most human societies such as the Tang of China, the Romans of Europe and Africa built great cities but left few engineering drawings of 'systems' in the records of history. The descriptions of histories until the 1700s had remarkably few perceptions of organized systems, almost as if the perception of structures hadn't evolved. The 'Constitutional Dynamics' sequence indicates a randomness that might have been because people were reactive to day to day survival and nothing else even when their perception of organizations was developing. The idea of a Union among peoples that had a common intent had not really existed before.

Constitutional Dynamics Chronology to 1800s

The timeline for the development of the Constitution isn't too long as a process of evolution and history. Many cultures of the world had 2000-year chronicles of various cycles of rise and fall, with documentation of their 'systems'. By the 1600s, there was still no real rise and fall of a dynamical system of democracy with separation of powers and reasonable equality of rights among members of society. There are some thousands of books on the event progressions leading up to the establishment of the Constitution as a form of democratic self-rule but few that define the resultant Constitution timeline as a 'dynamic'. The timeline is included here as a brief glimpse of the process, while visualizing it as an accumulation of dynamical systems. In dynamical systems perception, it is important to remember the *process* and not the details of it.

1642. Henry Parker. *Observations*, about English separation of power,1642.00.00:

But now of Parliaments. Parliaments have the same efficient cause as monarchies, if not higher. For in truth, the whole kingdom is not so properly the author as the essence itself of parliaments, and by the former rule 'tis magi's tale because we see ipsum quid quod efficit tale [it is greater because itself produces it]. And it is, I think, beyond all controversy that God and law operate as the same causes both in kings and parliaments, for God favours both and the law establishes both and the act of men still concurs in the sustentation of both. And (not to stay longer upon this) parliaments have also the same final cause of a monarchies if not greater, for indeed public safety and liberty could not be so effectually provided for by monarchs till parliaments were constituted for the supplying of all defects in that government.

1661. Massachusetts General Court, 'concerning our liberties', 1661.00.00:

1. Wee conceive the pattent (under God) to be the first and maine foundation of our civil politye, by a Gouvemor & Company, according as in therein exprest.

2. The Gouvemor & Company are, by the pattent, a body politicke, in fact & name.

3. This body politicke is vested with power to make freemen......

6. The Gouvemor, Deputy Gouvemor, Assistants, & select representatives or deputies have full power and authoritie, both legislative & executive, for the gouvernment of all the people heere, whither inhabitants or straingers, both concerning eclesiasticks & in civils, without appeale, excepting lawe or lawes repugnant to the lawes of England....

8. Wee conceive any imposition prejudicial to the country contrary to any just law of ours, not repugnant to the lawes of England to be infringement of our right.

1663. Regis, King Charles II, Lord Proprietor of Carolina, 1663.09. 04:

4. We shall, as far as our charter permits us, empower the major part of the freeholders, or their deputies or assembly-men, to be by them chosen out of themselves, viz: two out of every tribe, division, or parish, in such manner as shall be agreed on, to make their own laws, by and with the advise and consent of the Governor and council, so as they be not repugnant to the laws of England, but, as near as may be, agreeing with them in all civil affairs, with submission to a superintendency of a general council, to be chosen out of every government of the province, in manner as shall be agreed on for the common defence of the whole; which laws shall, within one year after publication, be presented to us to receive our ratification, and to be in force until said

ratification be desired and by us certified; but if once ratified, to continue until repealed by the same power, or by time expired.

1669. John Locke, Constitution of Carolina, concerning 'Lord Proprietor' ownership of persons:

> Sixteen. In every signiory, barony, and manor, the respective lord shall have power, in his own name, to hold court-leet there, for trying of all causes, both civil and criminal; but where it shall concern any person being no inhabitant, vassal, or leet-man of the said signiory, barony, or manor, he, upon paying down of forty shillings to the lords proprietors' use, shall have an appeal from the signiory or barony court to the county court, and from the manor court to the precinct court.. Seventeen. Every manor shall consist of not less than three thousand acres, and not above twelve thousand acres, in one entire piece and colony, but any three thousand acres or more in one piece, and the possession of one man shall not be a manor, unles it be constituted a manor by the grant of the palatine's court.

1695. William Penn, a proposal for a Union in the colonies, 1695.00.00:

> A brief and plain scheme how the English colonies m the North parts of America—viz., Boston, Connecticut, Rhode Island, New York, New Jersey, Pennsylvania, Maryland, Virginia and Carolina— may be made more useful to the crown and one another's peace and safety with an universal concurrence.
>
> That their business shall be to hear and adjust all matters of complaint or difference between province and province. As,
>
> 1st, where persons quit their own province and go to another, that they may avoid their just debts, though they be able to pay them;
>
> 2nd, where offenders fly justice, or justice cannot well be had upon such offenders in the provinces that entertain them;
>
> 3rd, to prevent or cure injuries in point of commerce;
>
> 4th, to consider the ways and means to support the union and safety of these provinces against the public enemies.
>
> In which congress the quotas of men and charges will be much easier and more equally, set than it is possible for any establishment made here to do; for the provinces, knowing their own condition and one another's, can debate that matter with more freedom and satisfaction, and better adjust and balance their affairs in all respects for their common safety.
>
> That, in times of war, the king's high commissioner shall be general or chief commander of the several quotas upon service against the common enemy, as he shall be advised, for the good and benefit of all. ....

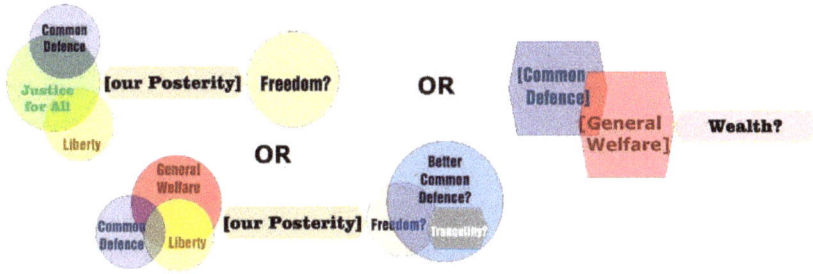

Constitution System of Systems Interaction

At this point in time, the North American colonies each had a governor and an assembly of representatives with the laws and leaders appointed by the king and parliament of England. The 'common enemy' as William Penn, Governor of Pennsylvania, put it was the French and Indians, along with Caribbean pirates and slavers. There was also the problem of lawlessness made easy for criminals, many of whom were indentured 'serfs' from Europe, being able to move from province to province in the 'wilderness' of the coastal regions. Commercial enterprises were also being heavily taxed with the income going to the home country, without visible benefit to the local city-states. A tradition arose that commerce should not be subject to *any* taxation, leading to a large amount of political debate in the colonies. No taxes, of course, must abolish the idea of both common defence and general welfare in order to be true.

But there was an increasing need for 'systems' that organized people's behaviors and relations with each other. This was more apparent to immigrants coming to the colonies of North American because the vast majority were fleeing an extreme environment of feudalism in Europe. As early as 1600, they had begun looking for some structure that was better and included such things as equal justice, economic freedom, and yet retaining some of the 'tribalism' found in European communities and cities.

The early communities had 'militia' made up of citizens who worked together to defeat intruders such as the Iroquois and Cherokee and built European walled towns and forts against such intruders. There is a need to keep in mind that the Native cultures in North America were hunter-gatherer tribes similar to those of Europe and Asia 7000 years before. There is only one way a clash of cultures like that can turn out. It might have taken an Iroquois Chief a whole hour to figure out that ten of his beaver pelts would get him a new Sheffield, England hand axe he appropriately called a tomahawk.

The Europeans had 'sheriffs' whose main occupation was returning serfs, slaves and indentures to their owners, along with bringing peace to communities. They had masons and carpenters who could build 8 bedroom homesteads for large families because many knew what inflectional accidents, influenza, smallpox, and cholera were going to do to those families. These communities created assemblies, schools and churches in the same building because there was no real separation of church and state in their eyes, even if the combination had been disastrous for a thousand years in Europe, China and the Arabic empires.

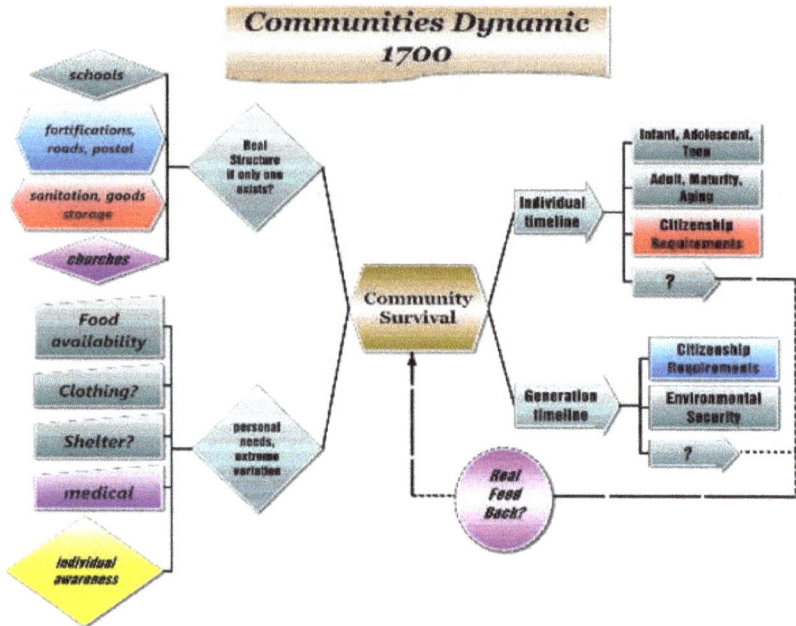

Communities Dynamic 1700

1766. William Pitt, House of Commons, concerning separation of powers, 1766.00.00:

There are many things a parliament cannot do. It cannot make itself executive, nor dispose of offices which belong to the crown. It cannot take any man's property, even that of the meanest cottager, as in the case of enclosures, without his being heard.

1776. from the Declaration of Independence, 1776.07.04:

In every stage of these Oppressions We have Petitioned for Redress in the most humble terms: Our repeated petitions have been answered only by repeated injury. A Prince whose character is thus marked by every act which may define a Tyrant, is unfit to be the ruler of a free people.

1776. from the town's Assembly of Concord Massachusetts, lack of government, 1776.10.21:

At a meeting of the Inhabitants of the Town of Concord being free & twenty one years of age and upward, met by adjournment on the twenty first Day of October 1776 to take into Consideration a Resolve of the Honourable House of Representatives of this State on the 17th of September Last the Town Resolved as followes—

Resolve 1st: That this State being at Present destitute of a Properly established form of Government, it is absolutely necessary that one should' be emmediatly formed and established.

Resolved 3d. That it appears to this Town highly necessary & Expedient that a Convention, or Congress be immediately Chosen, to form & establish a Constitution, by the inhabitants of the Respective Towns in this State, being free of twenty-one years of age and upward, in Proportion as the Representatives of this State formerly were Chosen: the Convention or Congress not to Consist of a greater number than the house of assembly of this State heretofore might Consist of, Except that each Town *8c* District shall have the Liberty to Send one Representative, or otherwise as Shall appear meet to the Inhabitants of this State in General.

1777. Articles of Confederation, 'Perpetual Union between the States', note friendship, 1777.11.15:

Article III. The said states hereby severally enter into a firm **league of friendship** with each other for their **common defense**, the security of their liberties and the mutual and **general welfare**, binding to assist each other against all force, or attacks made upon them, or any of them, on account of religion, sovereignty, trade, or any other pretense whatever.

1786. James Madison, letter to Thomas Jefferson, concerning the Constitutional Convention, 1786.10.27:

Hence was embraced the alternative of a Government which instead of operating, on the States, should operate without their intervention on the individuals composing them: and hence the change in the principle and proportion of representation.

This ground-work being laid, the great objects which presented themselves were

1. to unite a proper energy in the Executive and a proper stability in the Legislative departments, with the essential characters of Republican Government.

2. to draw a line of demarkation which would give to the General Government every power requisite for general purposes, and leave to the States every power which might be most beneficially administered by them.

3. to provide for the different interests of different parts of the Union.

4. to adjust the clashing pretensions of the large and small States. Each of these objects was pregnant with difficulties.

The whole of them together formed a task more difficult than can be well conceived by those who were not concerned in the execution of it. Adding to these considerations the natural diversity of human opinions on all new and complicated subjects, it is impossible to consider the degree of concord which ultimately prevailed as less than a miracle.

This Constitutional Convention came together in Philadelphia with a reluctant George Washington as one of its delegates. Washington had a pronounced interest in his Mount Vernon estate activities, along with rheumatism, and the calls for the convention had begun in April, 1787 at the start of planting season. But this time also allowed Washington to gather together the 'intelligence' of the dynamic failure of the Confederation of States and its Congress in New York, which many times could not even get delegates from nine states in attendance long enough to have a quorum or voting power. Much of this 'intelligence' was from newspaper deliveries at Mount Vernon but also lengthy letters from delegates, especially Jon Jay, Henry Knox, and Washington's neighbors Madison and Mason. Mason opposed such a Convention, fearing too much government and Madison favored it, having seen what Europeans were doing to a Nation that couldn't defend itself or even bring 'tranquility' between its member states. Washington went to the Convention with accurate summaries of what a 'government' free of feudal totalitarianism and economic anarchy would look like. He might have been known for being the Commander in Chief of the Revolutionary War in the years before, but the ideas he brought to the Convention really were those of the 'father of his country'.

1787. We the People, September 12, Final Draft, 52 words.

Gouverneur Morris, Deputy of Pennsylvania, at the City Tavern, Philadelphia, with the Committee of Style for the wording of the new Constitution's Preamble, which the Committee of Detail writing the Articles had left to them on September 9. Signed and sent to the States for ratification, September 17, 1787.

> **We the People** of the United States, in Order to form a more perfect Union, establish **Justice**, insure domestic **Tranquility**, provide for the **common defence**, promote the **general Welfare**, and secure the Blessings of **Liberty** to ourselves and **our Posterity**, do ordain and establish this Constitution for the United States of America.

From an operations research viewpoint, and almost all other readings of it since 1787, this wording of the Preamble said more than many books in the previous thousand years. It described a **people**, not an individual king, or ownership oligarchy, as the basis for a system of systems. It described the systems of **Welfare** and **Defence** as necessary components of a people, which were obvious to all in that year, but added subsystems like **Justice, Tranquility,** and **Liberty** as conditions of a functioning human society. No society had such a subsystem definition before, even as it might have included one or the other in its values. Societies of the Nile, Euphrates, Ganges, Yangtze, Han and Danube Rivers all had philosophies reflecting this or that form of Justice or Welfare or peace or dynasty progression. But none had ever linked all five to our, and note our, **Posterity.** A common path of evolution for a system of **We the People?**

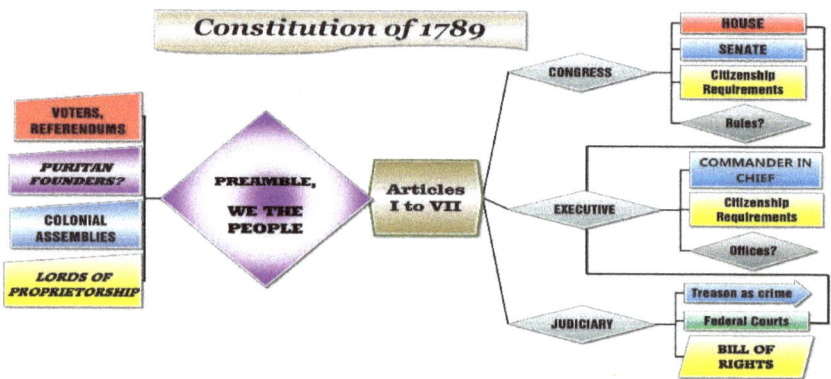

Figure 3.   1789 Constitution Model

There had been some discussion about what qualified as a nation and the first Preamble draft had included all of the States as the primary 'systems' as the purpose of the

Constitution, but this was later changed with a flourish to We the People. For operations research types or system analyst types, this Preamble Six would not have been very obvious as a system of systems. But in the case of one who had the Internet open to him and was experienced in its search technologies as well as those of Thomas in the Library of Congress, it became apparent that the Preamble Six was more than the sum of its parts, as complex adaptive system theory advocates. Searches of words, philosophies and constitutional facts indicated a striking anomaly in the Six intents of the Preamble. Dating back to the Hindi Vedas, the Egyptian Book of the Dead, the Chinese Taos and the various Bibles and Qurans, it became clear that the Preamble Six had managed to compress something like two-thirds of the written knowledge of Humanity into 52 inter-related words, with six intents each a dynamical system itself.

1789. Hamilton, Federalist no. 37, concerning the Constitutional Convention, 1789.01.11:

Would it be wonderful if under the pressure of all these difficulties, the Convention should have been forced into some deviations from that artificial structure and regular symmetry, which an abstract view of the subject might lead an ingenious theorist to bestow on a Constitution planned in his closet or in his imagination? The real wonder is, that so many difficulties should have been surmounted; and surmounted with a unanimity almost as unprecedented as it must have been unexpected. It is impossible for any man of candor to reflect on this circumstance, without partaking of the astonishment. It is impossible for the man of pious reflection not to perceive in it, a finger of that Almighty hand which has been so frequently and signally extended to our relief in the critical stages of the revolution.

There were many inputs into the Convention of September 1787 in Philadelphia, with some delegates very unhappy about the 'Confederation' that has no authorities to do anything above what the traditional 'Lords of Proprietor' in each community of property ownership desired. That was still the way it was done by the Feudal societies of the world and that would still be the case in many for hundreds of years to come. By 1789, the idea of a mercantile 'Lord' had begun to appear, and the wildernesses of North America made that almost a necessity if one was to begin a growth process in a new society. But such is not mentioned anywhere in the Constitution; indeed, a 'Lord' was actually prohibited from existing by Article I, Section 9. Washington, Adams and Jefferson could easily have been defined as feudal Lords of Proprietor even as they crafted a Constitution that denied this. Madison, who formed the Bill of Rights while inheriting a slave plantation, noted that this constitutional process was unusually unique even if he had serious reservations about it.

Echoing many at the Convention, Hamilton summed it nicely: "The real wonder is, that so many difficulties should have been surmounted; and surmounted with a unanimity almost as unprecedented as it must have been unexpected." Was some other 'dynamical system' present during the Constitution's formation?

1787. Brutus, Antifederalist no. 33, power of taxation, 1787.12.27:

…. Besides, in the very clause which gives the power of levying duties and taxes, the purposes to which the money shall be appropriated are specified, viz., to pay the debts and provide for the common defense and general welfare.'" I would ask those, who reason thus, to define what ideas are included under the terms, to provide for the common defense and general welfare? Are these terms definite, and will they be understood in the same manner, and to apply to the same cases by everyone? No one will pretend they will. It will then be matter of opinion, what tends to the general welfare; and the Congress will be the only judges in the matter. To provide for the general welfare, is an abstract proposition, which mankind differ in the explanation of, as much as they do on any political or moral proposition that can be proposed; the most opposite measures may be pursued by different parties, and both may profess, that they have in view the general welfare and both sides may be honest in their professions, or both may have sinister views. Those who advocate this new constitution declare, they are influenced by a regard to the general welfare; those who oppose it, declare they are moved by the same principle; and I have no doubt but a number on both sides are honest in their professions; and yet nothing is more certain than this, that to adopt this constitution, and not to adopt it, cannot both of them be promotive of the general welfare.

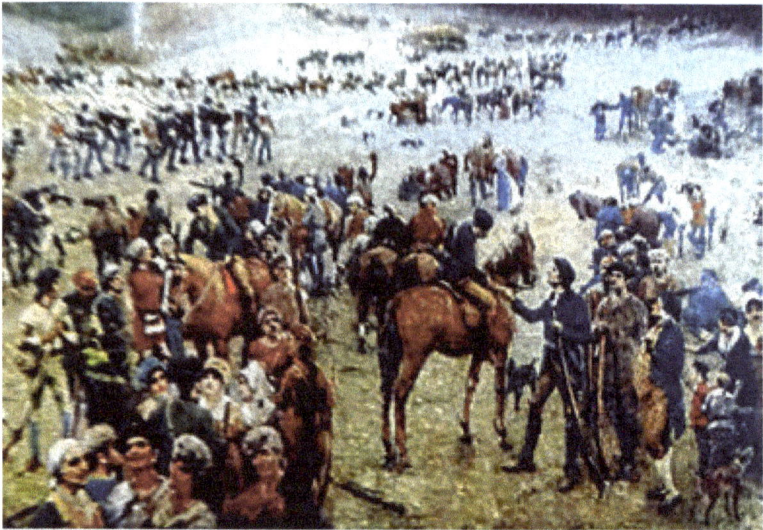

1780s. What Next?

1788. Alexander Hamilton, Federalist no. 85, final remarks on the formation of the Constitution, 1788.08.13:

> It may be in me a defect of political fortitude, but I acknowledge that I cannot entertain an equal tranquility with those who affect to treat the dangers of a longer continuance in our present situation as imaginary. A nation, without a national government, is, in my view, an awful spectacle. The establishment of a Constitution, in time of profound peace, by the voluntary consent of a whole people, is a prodigy, to the completion of which I look forward with trembling anxiety. I can reconcile it to no rules of prudence to let go the hold we now have, in so arduous an enterprise, upon seven out of the thirteen States, and after having passed over so considerable a part of the ground, to recommence the course. I dread the more the consequences of new attempts, because I know that powerful

individuals, in this and in other States, are enemies to a general national government in every possible shape.

The final Convention process took place in Philadelphia in September of 1787 and concluded on the 17th, with the signing by thirty-nine delegates, with some thirteen leaving without signing. There was not a unanimous agreement on the Constitution, especially since George Mason, who did not sign, had already made major objection to the fact that giving so much central power to a government meant that the ordinary citizen would not be protected in his person, place or property. European parliaments had routinely removed the rights and property of political opponents for capricious reasons and the French King Louis 16th could issue something called a 'letter de cache' that was a blank letter with his seal and signature. The owner could fill in the 'conditions' above the signature as he pleased, which could include the acquisition of a neighbor's property and wife.

In 1787, the lack of protections for citizens and in some cases, the state oligarchies of the 'Lords of Proprietorship' that John Locke had described as a 'system of governance' for imperial colonies, had become the main reason for not ratifying a federal government with new (and feared) powers. This in turn, led to a very intense ratification debate throughout the Nation, including the very lucid 'system progression' debates of the Federalist and anti-Federalist Papers created after the Convention of 1787.

1788. James Madison, Federalist no. 38, concerning a Bill of Rights, 1788.01.15:

> Such a patient and in such a situation is America at this moment. She has been sensible of her malady. She has obtained a regular and unanimous advice from men of her own deliberate choice. And she is warned by others against following this advice under pain of the most fatal consequences. Do the monitors deny the reality of her danger? No. Do they deny the necessity of some speedy and powerful Remedy? No. Are they agreed, are any two of them agreed, in their objections to the remedy proposed, or in the proper one to be substituted? Let them speak for themselves. This one tells us that the proposed Constitution ought to be rejected, because it is not a confederation of the States, but a government over individuals. Another admits that it ought to be a government over individuals to a certain extent, but by no means to the extent proposed. A third does not object to the government over individuals, or to the extent proposed, but to the want of a Bill of Rights. A fourth concurs in the absolute necessity of a bill of rights, but contends that it ought to be declaratory, not of the personal rights of individuals, but of the rights reserved to the States in their political capacity. A fifth is of opinion that a bill of rights of any sort would be superfluous and misplaced, and that the plan would be unexceptionable but for the fatal power of regulating the times and places of election.

Even though the Constitution had been written and signed by September 19, 1787, the debates over it would last another two years and result in the Federalist and anti-Federalist Papers being published all over the new Union. Ben Franklin's *Almanac* would show the need for national roads in order to speedily communicate, roads which were brought about officially by one President Eisenhower in the 1950s. The Papers indicated just how much depth of knowledge had gone into the creation of the

Constitution. Items referred to the Greek 'democracies', where slavery was normal and human rights were governed by the proficiency of the swordsman. Items referred to the absolute need for separation of powers into three branches, something that would be nearly universal on planet earth in the year 2000, except among the totalitarianists. Items like 'General Welfare' and 'Common Defence' were debated extensively in the Papers but more about *HOW* they should exist, not *IF*. But people in each of the States, no longer colonies, recognized almost immediately that the new government did not protect them as individuals against the excesses of government or the Lords of Proprietorship that interstate commerce was creating. Something more was needed and a Bill of Rights, which sort of existed in some state constitutions, was considered by people to be necessary in order to agree to the full national Constitution.

In 1788, the issue of human Rights involved both Liberty [LI] and Justice [JU], but was also very much a concern of Common Defense [CD] in the question of standing armies or professional military. The issue of being 'impressed' into military service would be a matter of contention worldwide for all centuries to follow and the term 'draft' would cause as much strife as the term 'slavery'. By 1864, during the Civil War, The Draft would be causing riots in dozens of American cities on both sides because no one in his right mind would seriously consider that a blue row after a grey row of slaughter was a legitimate form of Common Defense. The idea of Rights was also a matter of debate as to whether a king or emperor or even a parliament could bestow natural rights at all. The facts that no spiritual scripture anywhere in history, Vedas, Taos, Torah, Bibles, or Qurans, had ever said that a human right was 'divinely' natural were oddly overlooked. Was it overlooked because a citizen of the new Republic that looked around and saw the other people coming and going around him didn't have a real definition of 'human' and therefore you couldn't actually define 'human rights'?

During the Constitution debates, a set of 'Rights' were introduced by James Madison but were not considered by the Convention. Technically, the ninth state to ratify the Constitution made it lawful and that was New Hampshire on 1788.06.21. It was lawful for the Deputies to become Representatives and the first order of business was considering a bill of rights. This was used by Mason and other anti-federalists in arguments against Ratification with considerable success. So Madison, in the new Congress of June 1789, submitted 12 Articles for inclusion in the as yet unratified constitution.

He submitted them as Articles, but this was changed to Amendments to the existing Constitution, not as Article level authorities of the Constitution like I, II, and III. That would make individual rights subordinate to the Article authorities of Common Defense [CD], General Welfare [GW] and Justice for all [JU]. Human Rights were NOT created equal to the Constitution as many through the centuries assumed afterwards. By December 15, 1791, only ten of the Amendments were added, largely from the Virginia work of George Mason, with one of the rejects added in 1992 as the 27th Amendment and another involved use of population as the measure of the number of Representatives was rejected, which became totally and physically impossible at the Kwedake Dikep by 1929 when the number of House members was limited to 435. This meant that a Representative would be accountable to an ever-increasing number of people, with gerrymandering or adjusting congressional districts by states becoming a national pre-occupation by 2010.

Madison also had originally wanted some form of the Declaration of Independence included in the Constitution as a 'rights' amendment, but this didn't show up until after the Civil War extreme re-evaluation of Rights. In 1868, the 14th Amendment's first clause described the 'due process' conditions of a citizen's rights and privileges concerning life, liberty or property, along with equal protection for all, a clear [JU] condition. But it also defined 'citizenship' as a birthright within the jurisdiction of the United States, so how is one born a citizen if neither parent is within the citizenship jurisdiction of the United States? And if one is seeking Justice for all, why doesn't a human right protection apply equally to relations between citizens the way it does between a 'government' and a citizen? Especially true if the rights violator is a citizen who had taken an oath to defend and protect the entire Constitution. With all of its complexity, the Bill of Rights brought ratification of the Constitution to New Hampshire, the 9th state required and to Virginia, the 10th state to vote it in to make it the foundation of We the People and [OP], our Posterity as a dynamic system.

1789. George Washington, first inaugural address as President, 1789.04.30:

> "By the article establishing the Executive Department, it is made the duty of the President "to recommend to your consideration, such measures as he shall judge necessary and expedient." The circumstances under which I now meet you, will acquit me from entering into that subject, farther than to refer to the Great Constitutional Charter under which you are assembled; and which, in defining your powers, designates the objects to which your attention is to be given. It will be more consistent with those circumstances and far more congenial with the feelings which actuate me, to substitute, in place of a recommendation of particular measures, the tribute that is due to the talents, the rectitude, and the patriotism which adorn the characters selected to devise and adopt them.

Washington clearly understood that in establishing the three branches of government in a Great Charter that he was not a King in any way, nor did he or any others own the power they were creating by the formal referendum and consensus of 1791. But already, the ambitions of many individuals were appearing in the new electoral process in which many did believe that political power was an extension of property, the same as it had always been. But was power considered a form of property because the enhancement of property such as described by John Locke and Adam Smith required an organizational perception ability that was 'superior' to other perceptions? Such survival modes of the hunter-gatherer tribe's instinctive reaction to surroundings or the serf's building of families that could produce food beyond a coming year for many were not the same as perception of systems that the new government's three branches required. Going from chief to sheriff to nobleman to king did not require the same organizational skills that operating as a senator, representative, or president possessed. In the following years, contrast in organizational ability would continually affect the dynamics of governance for the Nation.

The ups and downs of the new 'Republic' were directly related to the perception of three branch governance of huge territories that oddly enough contained the representatives of nearly all human societies by 1830. In 1808, shortly after a term in Article V of the new Constitution allowed, the trafficking of slaves on the high seas was prohibited by law and naval ships were sent to the African coasts to prevent it,

along with that of the Barbary pirates. Several months later, the English parliament
did the same. A judiciary system was created by the new congress almost immediately
and it was supported enough to have courts and 'marshals' in all states and territories.
In 1813, a government in happy isolation had little understanding of what a European
standing army could do to them and watched helplessly as a British force casually
marched across from Chesapeake Bay and burned its new capitol. Common Defense
[CD] was difficult to establish when a congressional session lasted only two months
and a President James Madison, the Constitutional Article II military Commander in
Chief, did not actually know what an 8-pounder caisson was even when he signed
appropriations for them.

1835. Alexis de Tocqueville, *Of Democracy in America*, 1835.07.00:

> From Canada to the Gulf of Mexico one still finds some half-
> destroyed savage tribes that six thousand soldiers push before them.
> To the south, the Union touches at one point on the empire of
> Mexico; it is from there probably that great wars will come one day.
> But for a long time still, the barely advanced state of civilization, the
> corruption of mores, and misery will prevent Mexico from taking an
> elevated rank among nations. As for the powers of Europe, their
> distance renders them not very formidable.

> The great happiness of the United States is therefore not to have
> found a federal constitution that permits it to sustain great wars, but
> to be so situated that there are none for it to fear.

> No one can appreciate more than I the advantages of a federal
> system. I see in it one of the most powerful combinations in favor of
> human prosperity and freedom. I envy the lot of the nations who
> have been permitted to adopt it. But I nonetheless refuse to believe
> that confederated peoples could struggle for long, with equal force,
> against a nation in which governmental power were centralized.

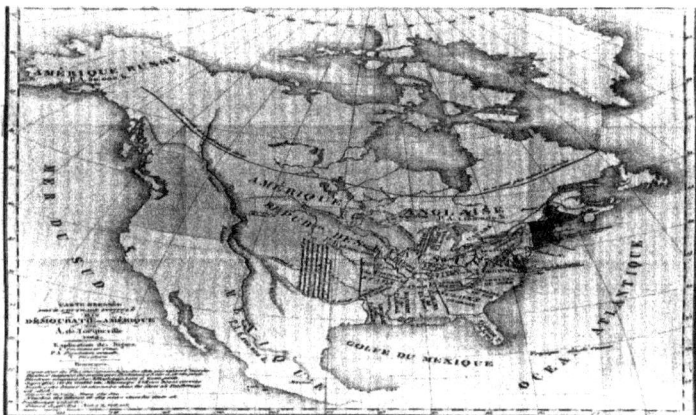

Image courtesy of Special Collections, Joseph Regenstein Library, University of Chicago

The people that, face to face with the great military monarchies of Europe, would fragment its sovereignty, would seem to me to abdicate by that fact alone its power and perhaps its existence and its name.

Admirable position of the New World that enables man to have no enemies but himself! To be happy and free, it is enough for him to wish it.

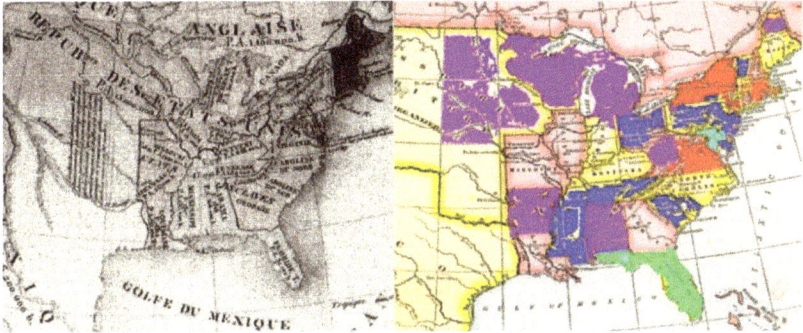

By the time of Alexis de Tocqueville, the main ideas of the US Constitution (Justice, Tranquility, Common Defense, General Welfare, Liberty and Posterity) had been pretty well established in not only the original 13 Colonies, but in the rapidly expanding Columbia, Missouri, St. Lawrence and Mississippi river societies. But de Tocqueville's prophetic intelligence analysis of the American People and its Constitution for the French government also had another side written by his companion, **Gustave de Beaumont, on the dismal prospect of slavery destroying the Republic and this was the one submitted to that government.** That might have led to the activities of one Emperor Maximillian in Mexico in re-imposing 'traditional' imperialist power in North America. A modern operations analyst might ask, in the 1835 context, how does one balance Common Defense's inability to 'sustain great wars' with General Welfare's 'in favor of human prosperity and freedom'?

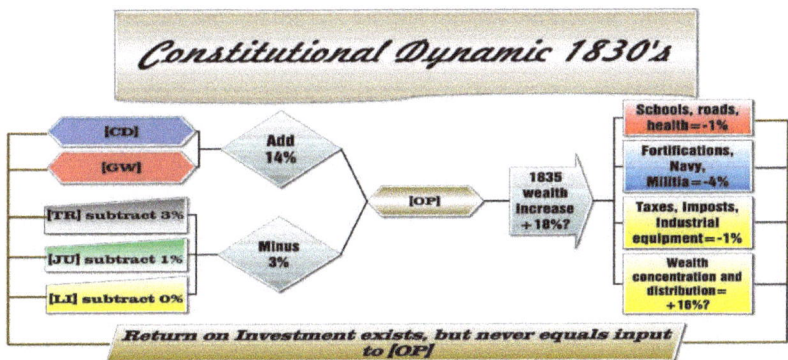

Figure 4. 1830 Dynamics Model

Just looking at these conditions as 'sets' of a dynamical system requires one to remove himself from the process in order to visualize it properly. And the 'speculation rule' applies, where one does not make any dogma decisions about what is seen. Many of the documents even in the mid-1800s written into the Congressional Record were of the dogma *details* of the rule of law and did not reflect a fact that the dynamic of the Constitution was actually the basis for rule of law, not the other way around. That problem of rule of law verses constitutional intent involving slavery occupied a large percentage the entire activity of the 3 branches in this period even as the Nation grew enormously with the Industrial Revolution and Midwest river regions added as States. But wealth supporting the government?

By 1840, John Jacob Astor owned two fifths of Manhattan Island including what became Central Park, along with most of the rail and ship transport to the Island region of New York. His net worth in 2000 AD dollars would have been equivalent to $130 billion and this allowed him to make loans to various governments for 'interest'. Whether this activity came under some authority within Article I remained a matter of concern. The cotton producers along the Mississippi at Natchez and New Orleans owned about half that, with other areas in industrial growth conditions acquiring wealth guaranteed by the 'peace' of Common Defense and freedom to own anything created by General Welfare and Liberty. But where was Justice and Tranquility in this equation, especially when everyone believed our Posterity would take care of itself and the need for [CD] was nearly non-existent except for British Canada and Spanish Mexico?

Lady Freedom 1845

Both Astor as owner of industries and the Mississippi slave labor 'Lords of Proprietorship ' from medieval times had very different views of what life was like, and both could see systems of wealth under [CD] and [LI] but perhaps no 'sense' of constitutional Justice for all [JU] or even nationhood beyond state Tranquility [TR]. Much too early for a concept of universal wellbeing. [{WB}].

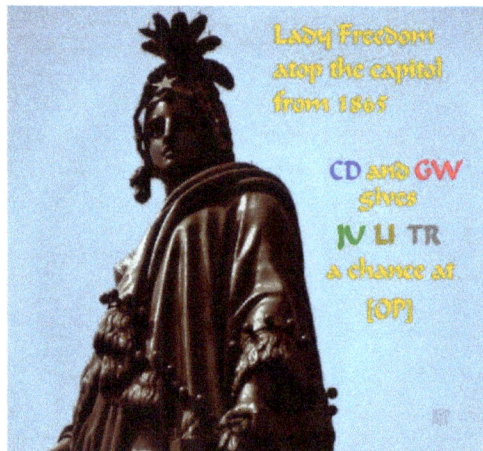

Lady Freedom atop the capital from 1865

CD and GW gives JV LI TR a chance at [OP]

'Sensing' Methodology in Constitutional Chronicles

Methodology generally means the way that something is analyzed or perceived but also how an objective is obtained. In a family of four, methodology for doing things usually centers on improving the conditions for living as the births occur but this can be a fairly chaotic set of processes. Nearly all of the 'methodology' is focused toward acquiring the means to live from one month or a year to the next, but rarely for a lifetime. But the more people involved, the more complex this analysis becomes, especially in forming human organizations. Armies solved this chaos methodology by organizing people into groups with very specific functions of force. It is simply easier to direct this force if each group has a specific function and visualizing the methodology becomes more certain at any time. But an agreement to form a social organization that, in 1787, was spread across an area twice the size of Europe requires a methodology of compromise forming into imperfect but not chaotic systems. The methodology for such a 'system' required defining each part and merging them from essentially nothing, but many in operations research analysts will happily tell you that the simpler the system you start with the more successful it can be.

The methodology of visualizing the constitution became as important as the 'data' of events under which the constitution was formed. But once formed, the Constitution needed to be analyzed in modern 21st century terms and the methodology used was that of a complex system being broken into its active components, but not 'reverse' engineering. The Constitution was far too involved to be called a 'simple' complex system. The Chronicles needed to visualize a 'dynamic' in space-time, which was something most scientists at MIT, GWU, Stanford, around the world and even Social Darwinists were doing routinely by the 20th century. An example was the fact that such visualizing and measuring of Cro-Magnon DNA in the 21st century would doom the previous 1800s concept of Social Darwinism had not yet appeared, nor was 'survival of the fittest' considered a system in the Complex Adaptive System (CAS) molecular definition sense. For systems analysts or the new operations research engineers, the 'dynamic' non interaction rule was become a major issue as Forrester saw it would when he said in *World Dynamics*:

"Our social systems are far more complex and harder to understand than our technology systems. Why, then, do we not use the same approach of making models of social systems and conducting laboratory experiments on those models before we try new laws and government programs in real life?"

But note Murphy's Law on complexity:

> A complex system that works is invariably found to have evolved from a simple system that works. If there is a possibility of several entities going wrong, the one that will cause the most damage to the system will be the one to go wrong.

Worse, the scientific rule was that in order to visualize a phenom or 'dynamic entity' or Gell-Mann's 'schema', the measurer couldn't become part of the 'dynamic' for the same reason that one cannot see the forest because of the trees. So if one looked at the processes of the constitution not from a 'tree' position of what could it do for me, the traditional voter, lobbyists or representative approach, but from what a process (the grove of trees) contributed to a sum making up the forest. How does one pick the 'one to go wrong' in complex systems? That is what 'e Pluribus Unum', from many: one, meant. In the 20th century, 'from many, one' was applied to virtually all nuclear and molecular structures in space-time as a complex system. It was reduced to its components, something any kid learns in school but rarely applies to himself. Since Homosapiens became increasingly sophisticated bundles of molecular structure over 70,000 years, perhaps the 'system' methodology should be derived from the math and structure of a quantum or sub-nuclear level as the ultimate reduction to parts.

So what was the method for visualizing a dynamical system generally being used? The purest mathematicians of the 1970s didn't seem to quite have a visualization mechanism for complex processes but many, including the military organizations of a mathematician named Omar Bradley, were using 'symbols' on a map to describe conditions of warfare. One Eisenhower, along with Bradley and Patten, had even added symbols from weather patterns to the symbols of fleets, air wings and divisions and battalions to a map known as D-Day, 1944.06.06. The combination of weather 'symbols' and force 'symbols' told them the 6th of June was their 'optimized' time period and in that instance, proved true. So perhaps the use of symbolic visualization could be successful, judging from the results on that D-Day on Normandy and might apply to something like the Constitution.

Jay Forrester's staff had adapted symbols to visualize his flow diagrams in *World Dynamics* and these consisted of a circle as a 'connector' between different processes, a rectangle for any process, an 'arrow block' that indicates a changing process and arrowed lines to show the flow of the system. These were well known symbols and such flow symbols have not changed much, only added to over the years. An 'ellipse is used to show a resulting process or an end process. A diamond becomes a symbol for 'decision' or 'change of state'. A hexagon shows a process 'mechanism' that is always in operation, such as 'our Posterity', where an ellipse isn't used because the process doesn't end. The 'arrow block' can be a resulting process as well but is also on-going. There is also a 'document' symbol which is a process or a 'baseline' for the larger dynamic being visualized. The Constitution is, of course, an ultimate document symbol because it is the baseline for a very large number of processes over a long time. In the graphic shown for a simple generic process, a dynamic system is shown being processed by a 'system activity' to create two dynamical systems that are affects of a 'decision'. This decision then leads to an altered original dynamical system with new processes in it. The new combination then leads to a possible new process that is fed back to the original, creating a dynamic loop for either a positive or negative dynamical super system of various parts.

A family might look something like a super system in a graphic. A man and a woman become a dynamical system, create a lifestyle together, and through decisions, create a larger dynamical system with children and wealth. Try to visualize two adults with thousands of molecular structures each getting together to form a dynamic system that might be even more complex. Then some idea of the complexity involved appears, noting that people have dealt with this 'system' for thousands of years. The resulting new process feeds back into the original with varying degrees of value or energy and without respect for time. The 'family' dynamical system can occur in one year, five years, or twenty years with only minor variations in the 'decision process' super system. But that balance can quickly disappear in a hostile environment beyond the families' control or because the cooperation level among its members ceases. Each family works that out as a survival process and purpose as they defined it, much as a constitution defines things for a much larger group.

But in 2000 AD, if an analyst applied those symbols to the Constitution's Preamble 'Six' as a 'super dynamical system', what would it look like? The diamond becomes the 'decision' for the interaction of [CD] and [GW] as the prime necessity for the system, but also the 'decision' for various inputs or compliments such as [LI], [JU], [WB] and [TR]. Wellbeing [WB] is a theoretical addition to the Constitution as an Article VIII but has existing components in the American 'system' in a nearly unbelievable jumble such as Social Security Disability, Medicare, Veterans Administration, and a Department of Health and Human Services. Each CAS is shown as a manual input process with a slanting block but not as continuous update survival mechanisms like the hexagons of [GW], [CD] and [OP].

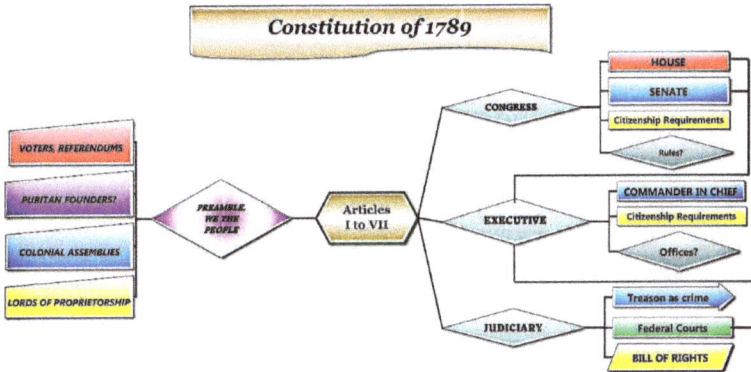

We the People of the United States, in Order to form a more perfect Union,

(1) establish Justice, [JU]

(2) insure domestic Tranquility, [TR]

(3) provide for the common defence, [CD]

(4) promote the general Welfare, [GW]

(5) secure the Blessings of Liberty to ourselves [[LI] and

(6) our Posterity, [OP]

do ordain and establish this Constitution for the United States of America.

In this 'Constitutional Dynamic',   the sets Common Defense (blue) and General Welfare (red) are shown as 'prime directives' that need to be balanced within any given generation or perhaps two. Both are termed 'prime directives' simply because all successful societies in history had BOTH as balanced components of civilization. Virtually no society in history had lasted longer than three generations without bringing about or correcting to an equilibrium of the two. That included centuries-long 'dynasty's' in which an appearance of equilibrium formed but closer examination shows the 'dynasty' suddenly changing without balancing the two primes. In very many cases in history, the societal degradation was due to the 'emperor's' inability to 'sense' that [CD] and [GW], along with the Justice domain [JU] were changing. Those dynasties in many cases operated only with the CD and GW and little else as they were attacked by other societies operating with variations of the two. It never failed to help the balance if you could take resources of other societies, the 10,000 year old solution to tribal poverty.

But the Constitution had added other intentions of purpose, Justice (green), Tranquility (grey), and Liberty (yellow).   In a rare perceptional instance in 1787, the intent of these items was attributed to 'our Posterity' (gold) as the purposes of a representative form of governance for a society.   I know 'gold' has connotations when applied to Posterity, but the rest of the spectrum wasn't available at this writing. The idea was to attempt to see an 'entity' in society as a vectored dynamic that could be changing in real time . This 'seeing' or 'sensing' of a condition with both past and future quantities is essentially what happened at the First Convention in 1787. The Preamble context led to a 'sensing' of the need for three branches of government and specific [CD] and [GW] authorities for each, along with the innate 'sensing' for Justice and Tranquility.

About the only quantity anyone could apply to the various directives at this speculative stage was adding or subtracting *something* from the total effect of the directive. [CD] can be sensed as a composite of many {subsets} of conditions needed to protect society.   Since a completely open mind was required just to look at the interaction of the dynamic 'sets', speculating on an add/subtract value appeared appropriate. In fact, such individualized, subjective perception might even be required if the processes are to eventually reach a calculated consensus such as what American voters do.   There is also the little matter of populations using an innate genetic ability to do what is called Motivated Reasoning where the consensus is arrived at for the pure instinctive benefits of a group.   Many of the Founders, if not all, were concerned about this idea of 'mob rule' as much as they were about totalitarian reasoning in the interests of a 'nobility'.

There were very many perceptions of the system dynamics through history, that implied an *innate* sensitivity to one's abstract surroundings that was operating on a different level than any 'food radar' that operated with a range that was inversely proportional to the square or cube of the distance Some samples are:

Justice Steven Breyer, *Active Liberty,*

Interpreting Our Democratic Constitution, 2005, Epilogue Page 133:

> Judges can explain in terms the public can understand just what the Constitution is about. They can make clear, above all, that the Constitution is not a document designed to solve the problems of a community [TR] at any level—local, state, or national. Rather it is a document that trusts people to solve those problems themselves.[CD] and [GW] And it creates a framework for a government that will help them do so. That framework [{branches}] foresees democratically determined solutions, protective of the individual's basic liberties [LI]. It assures each individual that the law will treat him or her with equal respect [JU]. It seeks a form of democratic government that will prove workable over time.[OP]

Would this literary form of a perception or sensing of Liberty in the Constitution have an expression such as:

[GW] balance [CD] cause→ summing of Σ[LI] [TR] [JU]approximates ≈ [OP]less than or no change or greater than >0<n some vector?

Larry J. Sabato, A More Perfect Constitution,

chapter concerning a 21st century Convention, Page 220:

This [a single senate Amendment in a Constitutional Convention process] shows the complexity involved in constitutional revision. The courts, ultimately the Supreme Court, would have to decide this question (probably after Wyoming or another small state mounted a challenge to the proposed Senate amendment) and other dilemmas would have to be similarly resolved judicially. As the founders could have told us, Constitution making is thorny and perilous. **Yet all of the most vital and rewarding elements of nation building are thorny and perilous.** Let's remember that the founders of the Republic undertook the job under far more difficult conditions and without the benefits of an **educated electorate** and modern marvels of communication and composition. Surely, then, with all our blessings of **wealth, training, and technology** we can endeavor to make some modern improvements on their work."

Would this perception be expressed as a General Welfare domain [GW] with various relevant{subsets} such as:

[GW]cause→[JU{wealth}]><n→causes[TR{education}]<n+[TR{infrastructure}]ap proximates ≈ [OP] a long-term improvement

It does not take much to 'sense' the components of a dynamical system. Homosapiens have been doing it since they discovered that rice and wheat grew in weather cycles where THEY could control the outcomes, more or less. The key of the qualia opservationis was not to get into the 'swamp' but to see the *relations* involved

It is very important to understand that the following methods used to analyze the Constitutional dynamic include some highly speculative observations in the Chronicles called the 'Opservationis' or qualia instances in order to differentiate them from a pure commentary on an existing governance or social process. Many of the 'entities' within modern legislation could be found in the speculative visualizations of the Congressional Budget Office and Congressional Research Service of the Library of Congress but were detail reduction visualizations rather than 'system' visualizations. Again, the idea in the Chronicles is to use a system visualization rather than a component visualization. Most people do that well but also use a self/others filter when perceiving their surroundings, a not too accurate visualization, as history will attest. Speculation of timelines may even be a form of IQ that is under development in this post Ice-age period of 2000.

There have been many recent books about revising the Constitution since it was becoming obvious that things were beginning to change for better AND worse at the same timeline as the Internet, streaming media with no captive audiences, suitcase weapons of mass destruction, hyper speed computers that could control the sale of stocks and bonds, genetic manipulation of the human and animal DNA structures that might become evil weapons began to rapidly take hold by the early 21st century.

Those massive social, economic and technological changes were going to alter many things, including how the three branches of the Constitution interacted with a very close world society that had never existed before. The Chronicle Opservationis are seeing a real time condition of the media. That allowed an analyst to measure various governmental processes against some combination of the six intents of the Constitution, and also against common thought.

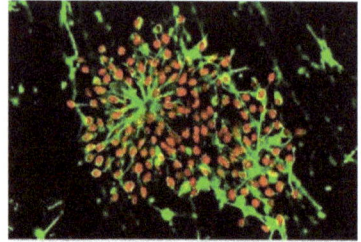

2010.02.15: Dynamical system of a human brain cell. Trillions required to make a brain 'system', thousands of cell systems to make a person.

With this much evolving complexity in a singular being, what then is a 'person'?

Image courtesy of Zhang and Hu, Univ. of Wisconsin, Madison

One of the problems of the 21st century was that many people, and their representatives, could not grasp the intricacies of governance in order to make common sense decisions. After about 1995, there were consistent complaints not only by the media and elected Representatives but across political and cultural spectrums concerning 'mismanagement'. But was it a system failure of the Constitution or just that the various CAS conflicts had become more precisely defined? In order to establish the 'dynamic' visualization process, an absolute necessity for change in this century, a timeline is also necessary since it involves an 'in place' or *in situ* perception of an ongoing Constitutional dynamic that is inherent in the instances described in the Kwedake Dikep Chronicles.

Murray Gell-Mann, Complexity and Complex Adaptive Systems,

'definitions' of, Santé Fe Institute, 1992:

> I favor a **comprehensive point of view** according to which the operation of CAS encompasses such diverse processes as the prebiotic chemical reactions that produced life on Earth, biological evolution itself, the functioning of individual organisms and ecological communities, the operation of biological subsystems such as mammalian immune systems or human brains, aspects of human cultural evolution, and adaptive functioning of computer hardware and software. Such a point of view leads to attempts to understand the general principles that underlie all such systems as well as the crucial differences among them. The principles would be expected to apply to the CAS that must exist on other planets scattered through the universe. Most of those systems will of course remain inaccessible to us, but we may receive signals some day from a few of them.

Gell-Mann's ' comprehensive point of view' has been essential to human evolution because it is the neural definition of human 'pattern recognition' that allows one to read an entire web page at a few glances, or recognize a hostile intent in a predator's face, or perceive a group of legislative {subsets} in an appropriations bill. Such views are carefully reflected in a book by Ray Kurzweil in 2012.

https://en.wikipedia.org/wiki/How_to_Create_a_Mind :

> Kurzweil describes a series of thought experiments which suggest to him that the brain contains a hierarchy of pattern recognizers. Based

on this he introduces his Pattern Recognition Theory of Mind (PRTM). He says the neocortex contains 300 million very general pattern recognition circuits and argues that they are responsible for most aspects of human thought. He also suggests that the brain is a "recursive probabilistic fractal" whose line of code is represented within the 30-100 million bytes of compressed code in the genome.

Kurzweil then explains that a computer version of this design could be used to create an artificial intelligence more capable than the human brain. It would employ techniques such as hidden Markov models and genetic algorithms, strategies Kurzweil used successfully in his years as a commercial developer of speech recognition software. Artificial brains will require massive computational power, so Kurzweil reviews his law of accelerating returns which explains how the compounding effects of exponential growth will deliver the necessary hardware in only a few decades.

The Wikipedia description of one book showed links to 14 separate complex qualia and would easily qualify as a linked complex system in one paragraph. But sensing the entities in that paragraph show that complex pattern recognition *can* be an analytical tool. In the case of the Chronicles, the pattern recognition process focused on the dynamics of the Constitution, along with speculation on the patterns of Wellbeing evolution such as 2018.08.14:07:24 and 2018.09.04:08:06 below. And adding a 'spirit' [ξ] element of mind, body and 'soul' might be considered frivolous or irrelevant except that there is too much literature about it to be ignored.

2018.08.14:07:24 [ξ] >3 [WB]>2⋈ [GW]>3⋈ [TR]<1 [LI]>3[JU]<2 ≈ |OP|>1

Balingit, WaPost, 'Do children have a right to literacy? Attorneys are testing that question.':

"The case illustrated a conundrum that has vexed education advocates for decades: Neither the word "school" nor "education" appears in the Constitution, and federal courts have largely shied from establishing a special right for children to receive an adequate education. [ξ] >3 [WB]>2 That has posed formidable hurdles for those who turn to the courts for help[JU]{n}<2 when their school buildings are falling down [TR]<1, or their children are enduring long stretches in classrooms without real teachers, or even when they see evidence of discrimination."

There is this persistent belief among some that anything they want to do is automatically a 'right' to do it, [LI]>6and there are dozens of 9-0 Supreme Court decisions that say that just ain't so. If the 'right' wasn't specified by a majority referendum of two-thirds of We the People as in the original Bill of Rights, then it doesn't exist [JU]{n}>3. That includes the 14th Amendment's citizenship and due process clauses, which are widely regarded in the judiciary system as human rights even though they were created by less than 10 percent of the citizens at that time. Doesn't mean it was a bad idea, just that the 14th doesn't meet the standard of a right that is given to the people by the people. [GW]⋈ [TR] [LI][JU]

Several of the author's case samples indicate that the problem might have been a neural cognitivity issue of the brain and not a read/write memory problem. What might be useful in this century, and you couldn't have done it before this one, would be to make 'cognitivity' a right because the brain had been cured of anomalies at conception or birth. That would involve a whole body 'wellbeing right' as an amendment to the Constitution with a two-thirds acceptance, but at least it would be a clearly defined right $\sum[\xi]>3$ [WB]>3. The term 'wellbeing' is used to imply that the entire molecular growth of the fetus is enhanced from conception, not just some 'component' treatment the way its done now.

And

2018.09.04:08:06 $\sum$ [WB]>1⋈ [GW]>3⋈ [TR]<1 [LI]>3⋈[JU]<1 ≈ [OP]>2+[ξ]>?

Ed Rendell in TheHill,'3 ideas that beat single-payer to reform health care':

"Third, Congress should study ways the federal government can help drive down the prices of pharmaceuticals[OP]>2+[ξ] for Medicare and Medicaid, to help reduce overall costs for both programs. This would dramatically reduce the cost of both government programs [GW]{n} and would not be a totally unique approach, since the Department of Veterans Affairs [CD]{n} already has that right."

The easiest way to do this pharma cost is to apply the Constitutional authorities in Article I for enhancing the national infrastructure by applying an 'eminent domain need' condition to molecular enhancements like drugs. [TR]{n} [GW]{n} A pharma company could spend $500 million on just the new laboratories to develop a single drug because the research must be carried out in a total health-isolation[TR]{n} environment. Just the testing with human participants might cost half a million more per test patient and the minimum statistical requirement might be a thousand patients. [LI]<3?

An eminent domain release of the drug patent after production begins would lower the costs to everyone in need, but it wouldn't be Justice to simply steal the pharma product. If Justice is served, [JU]{n}<1 eminent domain for the General Welfare would mean that the federal government would compensate the pharma company research costs on any drug development and compensate for the loss of profit due to the exclusive patent rights removal. This compensation could be two billion dollars in cost to the government but would introduce an immediate savings to the health casualty because of the open manufacture. That savings might be $50,000 per person per year [LI]times 500,000 citizens[GW]{n} or $25 billion. 70 million Americans [OP]take medication based on exclusive patents every year. As long as the original pharma research costs are covered by justifiable rewards, who would lose by an eminent domain process in the Congress [LI][n}<3, which MUST make the specific appropriation in each case?

If one looks at the subset 'elements' closely, there will be a strong desire to attach reductionist detail level to the series as [XX]{n1}+{n2}+{n3}≈ to get a possible qualia value of the whole. I have attempted to carefully avoid this in the estimates of the qualia progress (→, ↔) because they might interfere with the pattern recognition of the system, very much in the manner of the genetics-based facial pattern recognition of humans to focus on the eyes for emotional interpretations. This involved an arbitrary numeric constant set from 0 to 6 that was sensed rather than calculated through reductionism. This was sensed in such a manner because both a element progression and a direction were involved in space, very much like a tensor. If one goes back over some of the Solvay Conferences, especially after 1918, he will find that 'sensing' of nuclear and cosmological entities was very much in evidence because of the 'uncertainty principles' involved.

Since a consensus mode is being used to describe constitutional domains in the modern era, it was necessary to apply 'common sensing' of items just as the original Founders did in the Federalist and anti-Federalist Papers that led to referendums on the constitution and the Bill of Rights. The Papers did go into some detail concerning aspects of the Constitution but in the Chronicles, there has been a reasonable attempt to perceive elements or qualia in terms of modern consensus such as noted here in Justice Breyer's and Larry Sabato's discussion. In many cases, references have been made to online databases that have citations that represent a sensed consensus of a given {subset} group. The internet or literary reference consensus citations are not reproduced here for the sake of simplicity because the Constitutional model itself was so complex.

The idea is to use a pattern recognition with general dot-connecting mechanisms and attempts to adhere closely to this method were followed. This would almost certainly have had to be the case where the additional Article VIII with its multiple 'consensus' requirements for a whole mind, body, consciousness structure $\sum [\{WB\}]>l\bowtie[\{\xi\}]$ multiplied by 300 million or more $[GW]\{n\}$ is involved. But one can also 'sense' the need for the next 'methodology'.

CAS Principles:

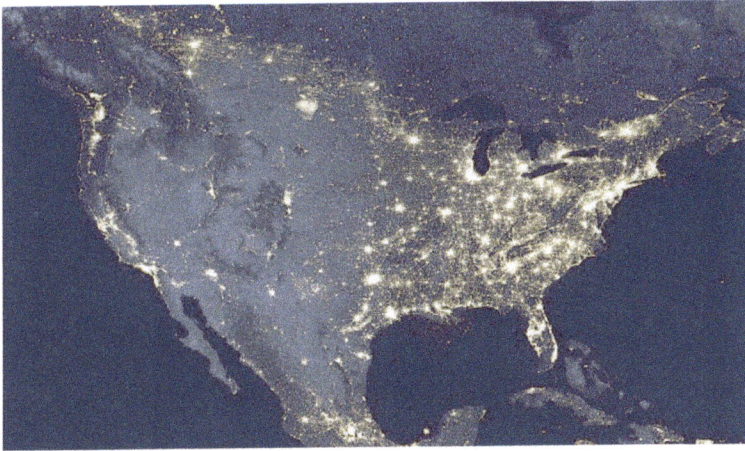

Figure 5. CAS from sea to shining sea

Complexity is difficult to sense by humans, but they do it reasonably well in just about all of their endeavors. Just defining something like Justice [JU] takes considerable effort, in many cases the perception requires a 'jury' of twelve people to decide the events that created an injustice to one of its kin. The perception can be wrong in many cases, but the First Constitution established an entire system based on the idea of fairness and no harm between individuals and in very many cases it was far superior to the decisions of a totalitarian 'lord', just more complex. Plus, the element of changing as circumstances changed (adapting to...) made the justice process even more complex because in order to determine a better future, one would have to rely on 'precedent' or the past. The number of elements needed to bring an equilibrium into peoples' affairs became multiple systems each with many interacting qualia of their own. Note the consensus on what a complex system is from the internet database.

https://en.wikipedia.org/wiki/Complex_adaptive_system :

> The study of CAS focuses on complex, emergent and macroscopic properties of the system.[7][10][11] John H. Holland said that CAS "are systems that have a large numbers of components, often called agents, that interact and adapt or learn".[12]

> Typical examples of complex adaptive systems include: climate; cities; firms; markets; **governments**; industries; ecosystems; social networks; power grids; animal swarms; traffic flows; social insect (e.g. ant) colonies;[13] **the brain and the immune system; and the cell and the developing embryo**. Human social group-based endeavors, such as political parties, communities, geopolitical organizations, war, and terrorist networks are also considered

CAS.[13][14][15] The internet and cyberspace—composed, collaborated, and managed by a complex mix of human–computer interactions, is also regarded as a complex adaptive system.[16][17][18] CAS can be hierarchical, but more often exhibit aspects of "self-organization".[19]

(1) Its experience can be thought of as a set of data, usually input / output data, with the inputs often including system behavior and the outputs often including effects on the system. The problem is that subsystem elements are so numerous that ordinary math doesn't work well, even if people can 'see' such systems in other people.

(2) The system identifies perceived regularities of certain kinds in the experience, pattern recognition, even though sometimes regularities of those kinds are overlooked or random features misidentified *as* regularities. The remaining information is treated as random, and much of it often is.

(3) Experience is not merely recorded in a lookup table; instead, the perceived regularities are compressed into a schema [subset of a systemic something]. Mutation processes of various sorts give rise to rival schemata. Each schema provides, in its own way, some combination of description, prediction, and (where behavior is concerned) prescriptions for action such as [JU] and [TR]. Those may be provided even in cases that have not been encountered before, and then not only by interpolation and extrapolation, but often by much more sophisticated extensions of experience.

(4) The results obtained by a schema, element, or phenom in the real world are then fed back as 'energy' ($[\{\xi\}]$?) to affect its outcome again. Some refer to this as a 'positive feedback loop'. The balance of [CD] and [GW] into our Posterity is such a loop, but could you enhance it?

(5) The interactions have regular components but also have 'non-linear' components that can be either positive or negative to the other components. A CAS is dynamic, not static, and is therefore not at all linear. This can lead to serious misconceptions on the *balance* of [CD] and [GW], as history has shown.

The Opservationis, taken at random from media accounts of activities and compared to overviews of histories of the three branches of governance or human history, should (probably?) give an estimate of any social process the Americans were involved with and how they might relate to the Preamble's Six conditionals. At that sensing point, the individual is analyzing a CAS with varying degrees of interaction and understanding.

But one must understand that there is also a secret history of decision making in all governments that has affected the relation of [CD] and [GW] and [JU]. That is indicated in the Chronicle researches such as *For the President's Eyes Only* by Christopher Andrew and *The Wizards of Langley* by Jeffrey Richelson and in *Voices of Terror* by Alter Laqueur. A major question of the 'dynamics' operational research involves whether a given decision was actually made in some context of the Preamble Six or whether some other dynamic was at work, such as economic, spiritual, evolutionary, or technological or even individual ego aggression.

Any of these could be 'sets' or 'schema' within some CAS and most people would have a tough time interpreting them because they are not in the realm of their 'common sense' sensing. The secret decision making has to be taken into account, because sometimes the timeline pre-emption of chaos ($[TR]\rightarrow<0?$) can be accomplished without interfering with the balance of [CD] and [GW]. Unfortunately, the number and type of what was being called Complex Adaptive Systems involving the Preamble Six kept increasing into the 21st Century, so that balancing was put in the position of having to continually re-act to forces outside its Constitutional system. Not the best Our Posterity path, especially when a far more complex CAS involving the molecular combinations down to a quantum level was appearing as well during the early 2000s. That involved summing $\sum [\{WB\}] > 1 \bowtie [\{\xi\}]$ with all of the subset elements in a human body: . https://en.wikipedia.org/wiki/List_of_systems_of_the_human_body into a CAS [{systems}] with all other people in a context of three branches of government.

Gaustello, *Chaos and Complexity in Psychology*, 2009, Chapter 1, p4:

> Our notions about the nature of a system have shifted as well. In Newton s view of a mechanical system, the function of the whole can be understood by understanding the function of each of the parts. A correction of a flaw in a system can be accomplished by removing and replacing one of its parts. **In a *complex adaptive system* (CAS), however, the whole is greater than the sum of its parts. This description should surely ring familiar to psychologists because of the Gestalt laws of perception.** The parts of the system, perceptual or otherwise, interact with each other, shape each other, and pass information around, and they are not replaceable or removable without fundamentally altering the dynamics the system as a whole. Furthermore, attempts to correct "flaws," or to change otherwise a part in a CAS, often do not succeed because the parts adapt in such a way as to protect the system from the intrusions of the outside tinkerer.

Kaplan, Schroeder, *Keeping Faith with the Constitution*, 2010, p153:

> A century later, Americans continue to face the task of applying the Constitution to new contexts. William Faulkner famously wrote: "the past **is** never dead. It's not even past." And so we still face some **of** the questions raised by *Weems*. How does the Constitution apply to United States-controlled territory overseas—for example, the naval station at Guantanamo Bay in Cuba or the Bagram Air force Base in Afghanistan? Does the Eighth Amendment forbid repeat offender laws that impose draconian punishments for minor offenses? Are there punishments that may not be imposed under any circumstances, beyond the punishments already forbidden under existing case law?
>
> **More broadly, the Constitution's text and principles must be adapted to changes in the world. Constitutional law has only begun to consider the array of issues arising from the omnipresence of computers.** How should First Amendment principles of free speech apply in cyberspace? To what extent do constitutional principles restrict government surveillance of electronic communications? Should the various doctrines governing campaign finance law apply to candidates' use of the Internet? Or should campaign finance law be reconsidered in light of changes in modern communications and media?

> Moreover, how should changes in scientific understanding inform constitutional law? The Constitution has long recognized principles of liberty and autonomy with respect to intimate matters of family life. How do those principles apply to abortion and end-of-life issues in light of medical advances and our evolving understanding of human development and cognition? **Scientists have managed to sequence the entire human genome and are now poised to elucidate the genetic bases of disease, behavior, and even cognition. What constraints does the Constitution impose on the government's collection and use of Human DNA?** What powers does the Congress have to under the enforcement clause of the Fourteenth Amendment to regulate state use of genetic testing?

The question arises as to what qualifies as a complexity model of evolution involving the now quantified, not counting 'junk' DNA sequences in the Genome, that ensured molecular level quality to that very same human DNA. In 2010, Stefan Thurner of the Santa Fe Institute wrote a chapter on this CAS perception. In his contribution to the compilation *Principals of Evolution*, 2010, he described '4.2 A General Model for Evolutionary Dynamics' and said :

> New things such as species, goods, and services, ideas, or new chemical compounds often **come into being as (re)combinations or substitutions of existing things.** …. New species, goods, compounds, etc. "act on the world" in three ways: **(i)** they can be used to produce yet other new things (think of [sense?] modular components), **(ii)** they can have a negative effect on existing things by suppressing (or outperforming) their (re)production, or **(iii)** they have no effect at all [sense this?]. In the following we refer to species, goods, compounds etc. genetically as "elements"

Such "elements" easily describe the six covenant [{sets}] in the constitution as CAS modular components operating in real time.

(i) is a domain [NN] transiting toward a new condition of the same domain toward a new [NN], (ii) is a [NN] domain with 'elements' that are less than 0 as a condition, which means that there are element changes of state going to a lesser state or even non-existence, and (iii) is a NO change of state in [NN] regardless of the domain combination or even the {subset} movements. The Standard Model equations Thurner used in '4.6 Toward a Unified Mathematical Framework'. are very similar to those used in this speculation. The intent is to visualize a dynamic model without direct quantifying of its conditions.

The idea is to 'sense' the balance between any given combination of the Preamble domains without losing their relation in space and time. This is where any domain [NN] progresses toward, or into, or out of, another condition in a context of 'space' (We the People) and 'time' (year.month.day:hours:minutes). The term ' ⋈ ' is used in the Chronicles to designate a balanced union within the Preamble Six, although it is nearly equivalent to the set theory symbol(s) for union '∪'. Example:

[GW] ⋈ [CD] = {A (t) ∪ B(t) ⋈ C(t)}.

The ' ⋈ ' is used as a *specific* Preamble balance, not just a union of parameters.

The conditions of the domains mean that some form of 'balance' is required for the two prime directives [GW] and [CD] and then a progression ↔ for any {subfunctions} of each domain. Those could be positive, no change, or negative going as >0<.

As before imagine that at each time each element i experiences one of three scenarios, (i) creation $\sigma_i(t) = 0 \to \sigma_i(t+1) = 1$, (ii) annihilation $\sigma_i(t) = 1 \to \sigma_i(t+1) = 0$, or (iii) nothing $\sigma_i(t) = \sigma_i(t+1)$. Suppose the existence of a function $f_i(\sigma(t)) : \{0, 1\}^N \to \mathbb{R}$, which indicates which of the transitions (i–iii) takes place. Let $f_i(\sigma(t))$ indicate the following:

$$\text{(i)} \quad f_i(\sigma(t)) > 0 \Rightarrow \sigma_i(t+1) = 1,$$
$$\text{(ii)} \quad f_i(\sigma(t)) < 0 \Rightarrow \sigma_i(t+1) = 0,$$
$$\text{(iii)} \quad f_i(\sigma(t)) = 0 \Rightarrow \sigma_i(t+1) = \sigma_i(t). \tag{4.9}$$

For (i) or (ii) a transition occurs if $\sigma_i(t) = 0$ or 1, respectively. That is, if $f_i(\sigma(t)) \geq 0$ the system evolves according to

$$\sigma_i(t+1) = \sigma_i(t) + \Delta\sigma_i(t) \quad \text{with} \quad \Delta\sigma_i(t) = \text{sgn}\left[(1 - \sigma_i(t))f_i(\sigma(t))\right]. \tag{4.10}$$

Figure 6. Standard Dynamics Model

Note the same modelling in the Preamble Six, where a {>[X](n)↔0↔<[X](n)} type of perception is used. Assume the resultant [OP] is in the (t) or related (n) time factor. This might work out as a series of progressions in which the >0< is almost a vector showing the movement without quantifying. In the Constitution, (t) works out as a two-year and four-year electoral cycle, not useful for modern Our Posterity planning. Again, a need to 'sense' the [domain] process for operations research 'satisficing' or optimization reasons. You want to see Common Defense in such a manner at (t) that it doesn't remove Justice or Tranquility with the same (t) but acts in concert with them. Because you are looking at relations of the domains in each other's context, would the model {>[ ](n)↔0↔<[ ](n)} applied to the Preamble Six look like:

(i) [GW{n}]> ⋈ [CD{n}]> → Σ[TR]>n [LI]<n+[JU]>n ≈ [OP]>n

(ii) [GW{n}]<0 ⋈ [CD{n}]>0 → Σ[TR]<n [LI]<n+[JU]>n ≈ [OP]=0

(iii) [GW{n}]<3 ⋈ [CD]<1 → Σ[TR]<n [LI]<n+[JU]>n ≈ [OP]<n

In visualizing combinations of all three transitional states (i to iii) of the Preamble Six, the model will show that if the subsets of both Common Defense and General Welfare approach zero in effectiveness, then the other conditions like Justice will also have little effect. If [GW] and [CD] subsets are reasonably balanced, (i), then transitions among the three other domains will have a strong effect on the [OP] outcomes. The same ups and downs occur as [GW] and [CD] become increasingly unbalanced, (iii), leads to a lessening of options in Our Posterity. Each is a CAS in its own progress and most people can recognize the CAS progression intuitively as being the right or wrong direction for the Nation as a whole [OP]>0<. Note the sensing described in https://en.wikipedia.org/wiki/Pattern_recognition_(psychology) as far is seeing what might happen in any of the combinations.

A Gallop poll in 2018.10, https://news.gallup.com/poll/244367/top-issues-voters-healthcare-economy-immigration.aspx , just before the mid term elections indicated that various aspects of healthcare were a very strong 80% concern for voters, with the economy and immigration {subsets} closely behind. That would qualify those items as a three fourths consensus even with statistical errors. But {health} is a CAS in itself according to the poll consensus and it might affect each of the Six domains, noting that immigration and {items} of 'the economy' are in [GW{n}]. Suppose that a [WB{n}(t)]>0< domain set were added to the visualization where healthcare as perceived affecting the entire [OP] process? The resulting CAS might be seen as :

https://www.complexityexplorer.org/explore/glossary/391-complex-system :

> A system composed of a large number of interacting components, without central control, whose emergent "global" behavior—described in terms of dynamics, information processing, and/or adaptation —is **more complex than can be explained or predicted from understanding the sum of the behavior of the individual components.** Complex systems are generally capable of adapting to changing inputs/environment and in such cases sometimes referred to as complex adaptive systems.

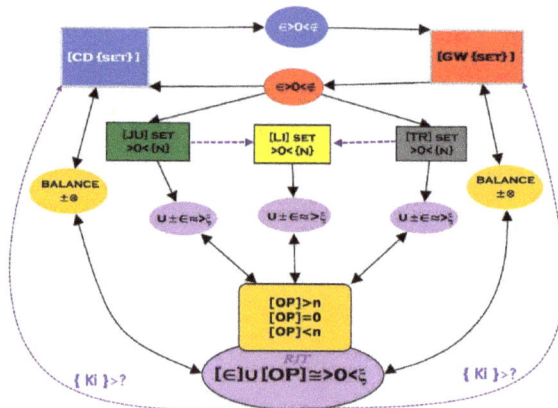

Figure 7.   CAS healthcare model

Wellbeing in a context of the Preamble Six covenants' interactive [domains] certainly meets the modeling principles of a Complex Adaptive System. It might be the future domains are too complex even for the innate sensing abilities of ANY homosapien. How, then, does one solve CAS problems?

Methodology Progression of the Chronicles and Readings

In applying complex adaptive systems ideas to **We the People,** it was necessary to develop methods for doing this that did not really appear before. There were many statistical studies and incremental histories and political biographies that described America but few that showed the relationship to the Constitution. You could find very extensive details of the Revolutionary Period and subsequent generational periods after. The Library of Congress with its Congressional Budget Office and Congressional Research Service and the Administration's yearly summaries of various activities showed just how complex the dynamics of governance had become. Americans, by 2005, had begun to react to this complexity by increasingly conservative interpretations of where the Nation should be going, and this included some very wishful thinking about returning to the good old days of yesteryear when simple dogmas of the 1890s and early 1900s could still actually solve or ignore problems.

A timeline progression is included here to show simply that the processes were gaining in complexity and that some new constitutional mechanisms might be necessary in the coming century.

Timeline 1965.

As an electronic countermeasures 'probie' assigned to the Pentagon, this required access to the meetings and offices of the DOD Secretaries, NMCC, Congress and the White House in order to give electronic security to various principles of the government. It allowed a 'feel' for the power of decision making simply by watching the process without being directly involved. But these meetings also indicated to a 25-year-old the bewildering complexity involved. The question arose: how do people make complex decisions? Recognizing the decision-making of the Executive branch as a life and death process, the dynamic cannot be forgotten or even laid aside temporarily. But observing complex decisions will also simply trigger the innate curiosity about humanity. Reading the *Art of War* by Sun Tzu and *A Soldier's Story* by Omar Bradley concerning logistical organization and intelligence use in war (along with learning Russian and Korean for other 'duties')

Timeline 1975.

The 'lost' years. Malthusian Population Traps and tribalism everywhere in the 600,000 mile journey on research ships as shipboard 'geek'. Chronicles of the Population Traps and various world conflicts could be compared with systems engineering and theory. But were they lost years at the Kwedake Dikep too, with intense inflation, population stresses and 'old boy' conflicts? Handy little pocket definitions book that could go anywhere called *The Constitution of the United States, an Introduction*, by Floyd Cullop. It contained the first instance where the Preamble had been broken down into its six intents or directives. But don't carry such a book near totalitarianists.

Many of the systems of the 1970s had been altered by the cultural shifts of the 1960s and the Cold War's Mutually Assured Destruction, along with the advent of genuine mass communication that caused a severe Constitutional misconception of power by a president and intensification of elective propaganda wars. A disappointment after reading Article II and its CD and GW relationships.

Timeline 1983.

Inspection of government processes and a voluntary commitment to an original oath to protect and defend the US Constitution. Research at the Boston Pops suddenly involved a lawful (that is, constitutional) order to proceed with an analysis of the Common Defense and General Welfare prime directives and protect them as needed. Readings: *Generations in History, an Introduction to the Concept* by Esler and *Reality vs. Myth* by Cline concerning organizational structure. Also, *Hawaiian Mythology*, Beckwith, concerning fisherman-gatherers, which was appropriately done on Waimea or Kona beaches.

Weather dynamics research at MIT's Greene Building and introduction to the operations research group down the street. Weather was becoming predictable at this point and some of the 'system' of dynamic force had become mathematically definable and visible on computer screens. But did weather have parallel systems that were ALWAYS in conflict like people had?

Timeline 1990.

Use of MIT operations research group's activities to visualize the six ideas of the Constitution. Inspection and use of the 'process' modelling graphics of Shlaer and Mellor at Lawrence Berkeley Laboratory. Graduate student library at the MIT Albany Street Plasma Fusion Center, various research modes. A 'letters' book, *The Origins of the American Constitution*, by Michael Kammen showed many of the reasoning processes of the Constitution, including [CD and [GW] balance, but modern [CD] was nearing a sea change as the Soviets became bankrupt enough to contemplate MAD as a reality. Could world dynamics 'accidently' wipe out the six covenants of the Constitution or worse, distort them into a totalitarian hypocrisy?

Timeline 2000.

Studies of Common Defense as a prime directive. Use of Santa Fe Institute (near Los Alamos nukes, nice place) methods of system dynamics, such as discussed by Murray Gell-Mann and John H. Miller's *Complex Adaptive Systems*. Serious evaluation of 2001 and subsequent Common Defense activities in relation to the Constitution. But subordinate General Welfare entirely to the point there was no balance? Definition of Constitution's Preamble and the resulting six major purposes of the Convention of 1787.

[CD] requires re-evaluation of Bill of Rights [LI] and [JU] conditionals, but how much? Election census gerrymanders changing balance of [GW] and [CD] toward over weighted [GW]?

Timeline 2005.

Investigation of US Constitution as a form of 'system dynamics' and the relation of economics which played an enormous part of the General Welfare prime directive but didn't actually appear in the intent of the Constitution. A limited definition of 'wealth' systems is taken from Eric Beinhocker, *The Origin of Wealth*. It gave researcher regressive analysis to Marx, Keynes and Freidman 'system models' but only indicated that 'wealth' meant political power, not the other way around. Why wasn't 'power' a separate entity from 'wealth? ' Evaluation of many proposed changes to the Constitution, some reflected the Preamble's six intents, some not. Change the intent of the Constitution from six ideas that represented over half of human wisdom?

Timeline 2007.

What is the constitutional relevance of Friedmanist economics to laws that removed the authorities of Article I, powers of the Congress? If Milton Freidman's *Capitalism and Freedom* is actually being implemented in law, how is it constitutional when it's advocates say that economics are not subject to 'interstate commerce' regulation by a legislature? Does the Patriot Act and various military operations in the ancient Levant of Abraham, Iraq, actually have an Article I basis and were [CD] imperatives of the attack enough to set aside the 4th and 14th Amendments?

Timeline 2008.

Definition of 'General Welfare' prime directive during a recession. Attempts to align Andrew Napolitano's *Constitutional Chaos* discussion of rights and the Bill of Rights in terms of post 09.11.2001 attempts to carry out the prime directive of Common Defense. Careful evaluation of Justice Stephen Breyer's notes in *Active Liberty, Interpreting our Democratic Constitution.* Very heavy election turnout might enhance [GW] and [JU] but not {CD] or [OP]?

Symbolic use of the Preamble Six such as [GW] and [JU] began in notations at this time. None of the six had quantitative values, just relevance to specific Chronicles and their impact on Our Posterity.

Timeline 2011.

Research on additions to the constitution, including *Article VIII* addition for healthcare as a 7th intent of the Constitution. Affordable Care Act formation and debate in Congress, with [GW] and [JU] as main [OP] components. No Tranquility at all in this debate. The world can't really be falling apart on its own. Would a new constitutional addition, Article VIII (not an Amendment) that accounts for the new technologies in medicine, genetics, diagnostics, imaging, internet and lethal droids change the timeline path of the Americans and perhaps the Cro-Magnons away from its randomized HAR1 mutations? Inspection of Nick Lane's *Life Ascending, The Ten Great Inventions of Evolution* and especially the chapter on 'consciousness' and how 200,000-year DNA progressions might be the same as [OP], our Posterity, in the Constitution.

Timeline 2012.

Darmend Ripple Effect on genetic health and the molecular basis of Creation. Darwin's concept of survival of the fittest not working well in the molecular biology world, inferior mutations rampant and might be a serious [GW] and [TR] issue.

TLO Speculation: Primitive Mesoliths become aware that they can dominate humanity through totalitarian technologies, form alliances of terroristic state power for the purpose of ending the advance of humanity. They as individuals cannot co-exist with an advancing human race and their survival is dependent on keeping Humanity enslaved to its primitive past. A [CD] overview of this process world-wide might indicate an intelligence failure because the priorities of such communities are ignoring the possible effects of growing totalitarian use of technologies.

Review of Chester Antieau's A U.S. Constitution for the Year 2000, essays in Balkin and Siegel's 2009 The Constitution in 2020, and essays of many in Chaos and Complexity in Psychology, The Theory of Nonlinear Dynamical Systems by Gaustello, Koopmans and Pincus as part of the [TR] and [GW] components.

Extreme electoral unhappiness as We the People attempt to re-establish balance between [GW] and [CD] with [JU] and Friedmanist economics, whose 'free wealth' conditionals actually are not part of the General Welfare directive of the Constitutional system, even if equated with [LI] and [JU].

Timeline 2013.

Inherited medical problems causing increasing expenditure in birthing, youth.

[CD]	model	related
[GW]	model	related
[JU]	model	related
[LI],	[TR]	related

[WB] related. Model for current health care costs and projects. Terrorist use of genetic and germ warfare. See Hammond, *Guns, Germs, and Steel, The Fates of Human Societies,* Chapter How to make an Almond, 1999, [CD] and [JU] also CAS interactive.

See Germs, Biological Weapons and America's Secret War, 2001, Miller, Engelberg, Broad. Review of Nessa Carey's *The Epigenetics Revolution, How modern Biology is Rewriting Our Understanding of Genetics, Disease, and Inheritance,* 2012. Genetic Manipulation, epigenetics, rapidly becoming a [CD] issue instead of a [WB] or [OP] issue?

[OP], [WB] and DRE interaction. Wording of Article VIII compared to older Constitutional sections, deliberate vagueness and care for Posterity evaluation.

Timeline 2014.

Darmend Ripple Effect on genetic health and the molecular basis of Creation. Darwin's concept of survival of the fittest not working well in the molecular biology world, inferior mutations rampant and might be a serious [CD] issue. Speculation: Primitive Mesoliths become aware that they can dominate humanity through totalitarian technologies, form alliances of terroristic state power for the purpose of ending the advance of humanity. They as individuals cannot co-exist with an advancing human race and their survival is dependent on keeping Humanity enslaved to its primitive past. [DRE] activities of Mesoliths compounding in many areas, along with MPTs. See *Age of Sacred Terror* and Robert Baer's *See no Evil,* 2002

[CD]	model	related
[GW]	model	related
[JU]	model	related
[LI],	[TR]	related

More Constitutional change study. Chester Antieau's *A U.S. Constitution for the Year 2000,* essays in Balkin and Siegel's 2009 *The Constitution in 2020,*

Andrew Napalitono, *Constitutional Chao*s, Chapter 13 and essays of many in *Chaos and Complexity in Psychology, The Theory of Nonlinear Dynamical Systems* by Gaustello, Koopmans and Pincus as part of the [TR] and [GW] components. John Holland, *Signals and Boundaries*, Chapter 13, Ontogenetic Sequence.

Wellbeing comparison between *Landmark, The inside story of America's New Health-care Law,* Washington Post Staff, 2010, timeline for implementation and actual EHR processing of 6 million. Special analysis of [GW] and [WB] effects on children in CHIP program, but exchange systems already too expensive for Posterity 'plus' effects.

Common Defense comparison of Bradley's Normandy combined arms operations (air, land, sea, special ops) with Petraeus' Iraqi 'surge' tactics with close support of combined arms technologies (satellite, air, land, drone, asymmetric, sigint) when 'war' was not defined by Article I, Section 8

USA Demographics based on DNA history show surprises, much tribalism.

Low voter turn-outs may be serious [OP] problem. Extreme electoral unhappiness for [TR] and [LI] as We the People attempt to re-establish balance between [GW] and [CD] with [JU] and the Friedmanist economics, which actually are not part of [GW]. See *That Used to Be Us, Chapter 'Whatever It Is, I'm Against It'*, Thomas Freidman and Michael Mandelbaum, 2011, very negative [TR] and [OP] effects. Is balancing of [GW] and [CD] instinctive with Americans during voting?

Constitutional evaluation, [CD], [GW], and [JU] components, of world Friedmanist effects on Article I and [WB]. TLO used: *The Heritage Guide to the Constitution, 'The Meaning of the Constitution'*, Edwin Meese III, 2005, [GW] and [CD] require limited government during current timeline?

Citizen relationship between [WB] and [GW] when narcissism is involved. TLO reference: Selfish Gene and *Genethics*, Suzuki and Knudtson, 1990

Analysis of Article VIII wording, should 'wellbeing' be intentionally vague so that [OP] can evaluate better?

Timeline 2015.

Review of 'covert' decision making and relation to prime directives [CD] and [GW]. *Spycraft* Wallace & Melton 2008. [WB] as weapon by toties. *See No Evil* Robert Baer p 151. *Spies The Rise and Fall of the KGB in America* Haynes Klehr and Vassiliev Chapter 6. AnQuanBu (Chinese) influences in American elections after 2008?

Review observations prior to Recession *The World is Flat* Thomas Friedman 2007 p 533.

Technology review of sociological models that affect [WB] and politics. Models may be inducing lack of common purpose in North America.

Bioethics concerns at a molecular level. *Intervention in the Brain Politics Policy and Ethics* Robert Blank (AUS) MIT Press 2013.

Modern definition of 'rights' analysis in terms of [TR] [LI] and [JU] *An introduction to Rights* William A. Edmundson et al especially chapters 07 and 11 2012.

Timeline 2016.

Review of *Epigenetics Evolution,* Carey, Chap 12, esp Nature Neuroscience.

Optimization theory, *Mathematics for Operations Research.* Marlow, OR summation to 1980.

Quantum Biology: Life on the edge of a storm, Chap. 10, McFadden et al in notes for consensus to 2014.

Quantum Enigma, Rosenblum & Kuttnet, 2006, Chap 14 and 15. Chap 'Suggested Reading' as consciousness 2006 consensus.

DMAIC flow chart symbols (not OR consensus), Identifying Causes Chap 8, *Lean Six Sigma Packet Toolbook* George Group, 2005. ToolBook is a reduced consensus of DMAIC.

Thinking in Systems, Meadows, 2008, Notes and Appendix are Systems consensus following J. Forrester's original ideas.

The Energy of Life, Guy Brown, Appendix is consensus thru 1999. Not detailed in molecular biology but general public history of molecular perception.

TOL: Constitutional process far more complex than anticipated.

Timeline 2017.

Masha Gessen, *The Future Is History, How Totalitarianism Reclaimed Russia,*

Elisabeth Rosenthal, *An American Sickness: How Healthcare Became Big Business and How You Can Take It Back,* 2017,

Yuval Noah Harari , *Homo Deus: A Brief History of Tomorrow*, 2017, Harari presents three possible futures: In one, humans are expendable. In a second, the elite upgrade themselves, becoming a species that sees everyone else as expendable. In a third, we all join the hive mind.

Hillary Rodham Clinton, *What Happened*, 2017, The defeated presidential candidate offers a guide to the contemporary political arena and directly addresses how she was treated because she is a woman.

Yaneer, Bar-Yam, Dynmics of Complex Systems, 1992, Chp 6 'Life I, evolution and chp 7 biology'. Style is pre-quantum.

Wikipedia, *Dynamical System*, pdf, 2017. Very technical, no popular perception. Hamiltonian manifold description might apply to [CD], [WB], [JU] interactions in 'human' systems.

On Human Rights, Griffin, 2008, Rights Discrepancies chap 11. Democracy and Rights, chap 14. Notes from chap 11 on qualify as consensus.

Some Final Twists, chap 14, *Ratification,* Maier, 2010. Notes on chap 14 and epilogue qualify as consensus on first convention.

Chap 4 Road to Amending, *The Second Constitutional Convention*, Labunski, 2000. General consensus on 2nd Convention. Notes on all chapters qualify as consensus on Second Convention thru 2000.

Review of *An Introduction to Rights*, several insights thu 2004, notes are limited consensus on human rights, not molecular in nature. Whole body entity discussion. Still valid?

Editor Marks, HU school of Public Health, *Health and Human Rights, Basic International Documents,* 2012, 'II. Basic Texts in Bioethics', text listings of documents, overall is consensus of 'rights' through 2012.

Timeline 2018.

An Introduction to Bioethics, Shannon and Kockler, 2009. Summary of Issues and parameters, too early for consensus.

Meltdown: Why Our Systems Fail and What We Can Do About It, Clearfield and Tilcsik, 2018, Notes as Consensus?

Responding to Imperfection - The Theory and Practice of Constitutional Amendment Levinson (edit), 1995. Chap 11 towards a theory of Constitutional Amendments.

Scale: The Universal Laws of Growth, Innovation, Sustainability, and the Pace of Life in Organisms, Cities, Economies, and Companies, Geoffrey B. West, 2017

Who We Are and How We Got Here: Ancient DNA and the New Science of the Human Past, David Reich, 2018. Consensus on DNA history in social groups. Wide DNA variations noted. Genome is game changer for rights.

Leiyu Shi, *Essentials Of The U.S. Health Care System, 2018,* references as consensus.

Congressional Research Service, 2018 health legislation and national security reports.

The standard Model is a description of the universe and shouldn't be ignored in the molecular evaluation of homosapien 'systems' and their inherent but randomized health. See:

https://en.wikipedia.org/wiki/Mathematical_formulation_of_the_Standard_Model

Research Timeline to be continued.

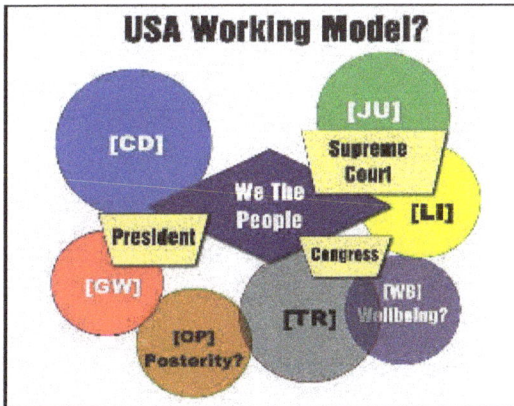

OVERVIEW 2018.01 to .04

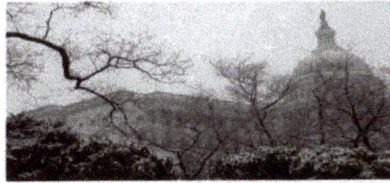

TIME LINE 2018.01.NN

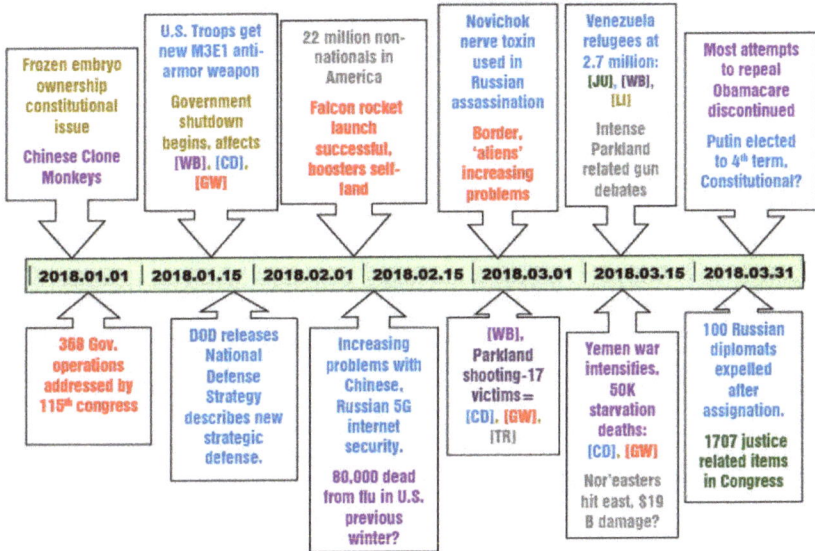

| Frozen embryo ownership constitutional issue

Chinese Clone Monkeys | U.S. Troops get new M3E1 anti-armor weapon

Government shutdown begins, affects [WB], [CD], [GW] | 22 million non-nationals in America

Falcon rocket launch successful, boosters self-land | Novichok nerve toxin used in Russian assassination

Border, 'aliens' increasing problems | Venezuela refugees at 2.7 million: [JU], [WB], [LI]

Intense Parkland related gun debates | Most attempts to repeal Obamacare discontinued

Putin elected to 4th term, Constitutional? |

| 2018.01.01 | 2018.01.15 | 2018.02.01 | 2018.02.15 | 2018.03.01 | 2018.03.15 | 2018.03.31 |

| 368 Gov. operations addressed by 115th congress | DOD releases National Defense Strategy describes new strategic defense. | Increasing problems with Chinese, Russian 5G internet security.

80,000 dead from flu in U.S. previous winter? | [WB], Parkland shooting-17 victims = [CD], [GW], [TR] | Yemen war intensifies. 50K starvation deaths: [CD], [GW]

Nor'easters hit east, $19 B damage? | 100 Russian diplomats expelled after assignation.

1707 justice related items in Congress |

[GW]>3⋈ [CD]<1 = ∑ [TR]<1 [LI]<3⋈[JU]>1 [WB]>?→ [OP]<2

[CD]<3 ≈∑ [OP]<2 [WB]<1⋈ [JU]>2 ⋈ [GW]>2→[TR]<2

[TR]<2≈[WB]<2+[CD]<3 ⋈[GW]- [JU]<2→[OP]<?

[JU]<2→ [OP]>1 ≈ [WB]<2⋈ [GW]>1⋈ [CD]<1 [TR]>2 [LI]<3[ξ] <1

[LI]<3≈[TR]<2[WB]<2+[CD]<3 ⋈[GW]-[JU]<2≈[ξ] >1≈ [OP]<?

[WB]>1⋈ [GW]>3⋈ [TR]<1 [LI]>3⋈[JU]<1 ≈ [ξ] >1 [OP]<2

[OP]<2 ≈∑ [TR]<3 [LI]>3⋈[JU]>1....[GW]<2+[CD]>2

| [Common Defense, CD]
▽△ ▽
△
[General Welfare, GW] | { Justice, JU }
▽△
≃ { Tranquility, TR } ≅ [our Posterity, OP]
▽△
[Liberty, LI] |

Figure 8.   Overview 2018.01

TL Opservationis 2018.01

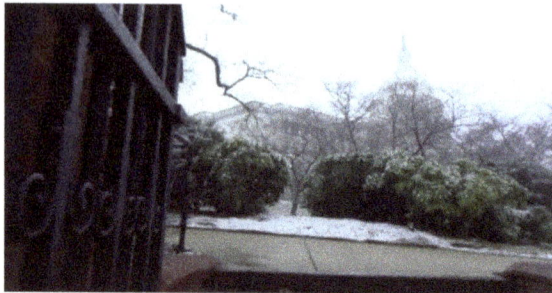

2018.01.01:10:15 |GW|<1 |CD|<2] [JU|>n |OP|:<3

Ginsberg and Ereli in TheHill, 'It's past time to investigate Iran's 'summer of blood':

"History has taught us that the only way to stop brutal leaders from using murder as a tool of repression is to investigate and hold them accountable for their crimes."

Constitution of Iran, as Amended, 1989.08.17:

Article 37: Innocence is to be presumed, and no one is to be held guilty of a charge unless his or her guilt has been established by a competent court.

Article 38: Prohibition of torture All forms of torture for the purpose of extracting confession or acquiring information are forbidden. Compulsion of individuals to testify, confess, or take an oath is not permissible; and any testimony, confession, or oath obtained under duress is devoid of value and credence. Violation of this article is liable to punishment in accordance with the law.

Article 39: All affronts to the dignity and repute of persons arrested, detained, imprisoned, or banished in accordance with the law, whatever form they may take, are forbidden and liable to punishment.

Article 40: No one is entitled to exercise his rights in a way injurious to others or detrimental to public interests.

The interpretation of the 'rights' Articles is done directly on the orders of the Guardian Council who are appointed by the Majlis and not by a people's referendum. Since all of these rights' are found in Quranic revelation, but not necessarily in the Sunnah of the first Caliphs including Ali ibn Abi Talib, systemic abuse of these rights by ANY persons or groups within the Iranian government would mean that these Pasdaran people who carried out the violations of the Constitution have renounced that Constitution and the Quran.. How is it that, without a Constitution validated and upheld by popular referendum and Quranic belief, a condition of national 'sovereignty' exists in the regions occupied by Majlis members of the Pasdaran violators who implemented the executions? Can other nations recognize 'sovereignty' when there is no valid constitution in existence?

2018.01.03:05:00   [WB|<3 |GW|<3 |CD|<1 |TR|<3 |LI|<3 |JU|>n |OP|<2

President Trump, National Security Strategy, 2017.12.30:

"Th e United States faces an extraordinarily dangerous world, filled with a wide range of threats that have intensified in recent years. When I came into office, rogue regimes were developing nuclear weapons and missiles to threaten the entire planet. Radical Islamist terror groups were flourishing. Terrorists had taken control of vast swaths of the Middle East. Rival powers were aggressively undermining American interests around the globe. At home, porous borders and unenforced immigration laws had created a host of vulnerabilities. Criminal cartels were bringing drugs and danger into our communities. Unfair trade practices had weakened our economy and exported our jobs overseas. Unfair burden-sharing with our allies and inadequate investment in our own defense had invited danger from those who wish us harm. Too many Americans had lost trust in our government, faith in our future, and confidence in our values."

Reasonably accurate in a context of foreign items affecting the six parameters of the Constitution.

2018.01.10:06:45 |WB|<3 +|GW|<n⋈ |CD|<n+ |TR|<3 |LI|<3⋈|JU|>n =|OP|<2?

M. Bloomberg, BloombergOpinion, 'A Seven-Step Plan for Ending the Opioid Crisis More treatment, stronger oversight. And above all, bolder leadership.':

We must stop doctors from over-prescribing opioids.

Insurers and pharmacy benefit managers must better oversee opioid prescriptions.

We must hold pharmaceutical companies accountable for the supply of prescription opioids.

We must start treating those with addiction disorders when they come in contact with emergency rooms, hospitals and clinics.

We must stop stigmatizing the medications that have been proven to help people recover.

We must develop better data.

We must do more to block the importation of heroin .

All of the above, but within the authority of the current Constitution and Bill of Rights?

2018.02.07:00:00 [WB]n+[CD]<1.....[LI][TR]-[JU]<3+ [GW]>1=[OP]<2

JHU, Bloomberg School of Public Health, *The Characteristics of Pandemic Pathogens*, Executive Summery, Recommendations to Prepare for GCBR-level Microbial Threats:

> Preparing for GCBR-level microbial threats as a class is a complex endeavor, with many facets, challenges, and priorities. The following are recommendations that emerged from this study:

> Preparedness against GCBR-level threats should first be focused on those pathogens with the characteristics that are most likely to result

in GCBRs. But the work should be flexible enough to encompass new knowledge of pathogens and resist focusing entirely on lists of specific proscribed potential microbial agents. The most probable naturally occurring GCBR-level threat that humans face is from a respiratory borne RNA virus, and so this class of microbes should be a preparedness priority. However, because other classes of microbes (viral and other) still possess some ability to incite a GCBR-level event, they will continue to merit significant study and appropriate preparedness efforts.

Historical pathogen list–based approaches should not stand as permanent fixed ideas that stultify thinking on pandemic pathogens. An active-minded approach that seeks to root the pandemic potential of pathogens in their actual traits is one that will foster more breadth in preparedness and proactivity. Incorporating this approach would require a major change in thinking and resource allocation.

Given the greater concern for respiratory-borne RNA viruses, improving surveillance of human infections with this class of viruses should become a higher priority. Currently, such a system exists for influenza, but other viruses, such as parainfluenza, coronavirus, and RSV, are not given the dedicated resources necessary to track their epidemiology, clinical characteristics, and microbiological traits. Future efforts could build on the success of influenza surveillance and incorporate additional high-priority viruses.

An increased emphasis on developing a specific pipeline of antiviral agents for RNA respiratory viruses would add resilience against these potential GCBR agents. Today, no such antiviral agents exist outside of influenza that possess high efficacy. Broad-spectrum therapeutics should be pursued given their potential value, even if the likelihood of identifying such medicines remains low. Narrow-spectrum agents should be pursued because of the increased likelihood of identifying candidates.

Vaccines against RNA respiratory viruses should be pursued with increased priority, as no highly efficacious vaccines, including against influenza, are commercially available today. Vaccines could be used to quench nascent outbreaks or to pre-vaccinate target populations. Ongoing efforts to create a universal flu vaccine should continue and be supplemented, given the risk of a novel influenza A virus to cause a GCBR.

A clinical research agenda for optimizing the treatment of respiratory-spread RNA viruses should be funded by pharmaceutical companies and medical research agencies and pursued by clinical centers. Important research questions regarding supportive and adjunctive therapy, intensive care unit interventions, and antiviral therapy should be addressed and answered. As many of these viruses circulate and cause disease, there is an opportunity to systematize their study in order to prepare for a GCBR from this class. From these efforts, treatment protocols could be developed for various syndromes caused by this class of microbes that could be relied on for routine clinical care as well as during an emergency outbreak situation.

Research that could increase the pandemic potential or risk of respiratory-borne RNA viruses or the orthopox viruses should undergo special review, given the potential consequences. Such work should be performed under the appropriate biosafety level protocols.

Pursuing microbiologically specific diagnoses of infectious disease syndromes in strategic or sentinel locations around the world should become more routine, especially now that diagnostics are becoming more powerful and available. Since it is unclear where the next pandemic pathogen will appear and because there are countless undiagnosed severe infectious disease syndromes (including sepsis, pneumonia, meningitis, and **encephalitis**) in every hospital and clinic in the world, we need to do more to understand these causes of undiagnosed infectious syndromes, some of which may be the result of a novel GCBR-level agent in its first forays into humans or a changing spectrum of illness in a known agent.

TLO: Some people are concerned about the right things in the pandemic(s) timeline. Are encephalic effects automatic with GCBRs? If so, when do the human haters start to manipulate that?

2018.01.11:10:12 [WB] ⋈ [GW] +[CD] |TR| [LI]<2 |JU|<2 ≈ |OP|<1

Javanbakht in WaPost, 'Why psychiatrists should not be involved in presidential politics, psychiatric diagnoses should generate empathy, not scorn':

"In the considerable fallout that followed Fact's provocative cover story, the APA formally stated that it is unethical for psychiatrists to give a professional opinion about public figures they have not examined in person and from whom they have not obtained consent to discuss their mental health in public."

Without proper neurological scan with a functional MRI and brain/blood biopsy, the chances of a psychiatrist accurately evaluating someone from a distance are quite low. He is almost certainly going to introduce his own environmental screens into the perception without the molecular-level evidence to make the evaluation. The same should be true of a court or even an impeachment. Political behavior under conditions of continual stress cannot be ascribed to a molecular degeneration harmful to others and no ethical person, including politicians, should even try.

TL Opservationis 2018.02

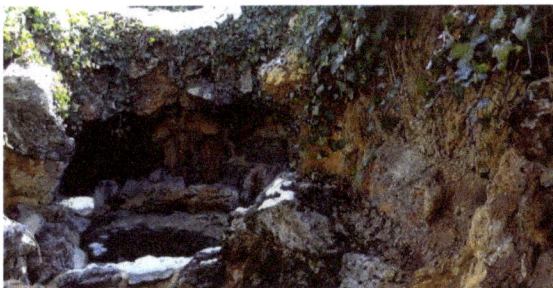

2018.02.01:08:30 |WB|>2 ⋈ [GW] +|CD| |TR|>2 ≈ |OP|>2

Bershidsky, BloombergView, 'How Amazon & Co. Could Fix Health Care':

"Lower pay than in the rest of the U.S. health care economy would be justified by having to do zero insurance paperwork -- something that forces U.S. doctors to hire extra staff and waste precious time. The companies would merely set pay levels based on tasks performed -- something that, in much of Europe, falls to health care providers' unions to negotiate with the government or with payer pools. That's the system the joint venture would ultimately end up with. Amazon's tech could help track the tasks in real time."

This combination of corporate entities also has the ability to automate the HC system to the point that not only puts doctors in a 'pay- per-cure' (as opposed to pay-per-service) process, it can automate many diagnostic processes to the point that employees and families can engage in very positive pre-emptive self-health. It helps to have employees who are young and healthy to start with, as nearly all of the million employees involved would be, but allowing them to have full mind-body scan diagnostic rooms in the work place (instead of going to offshore hospitals?) would create a national infrastructure model that employees were responsible for their own health as much as the HC system. Preemptive, droid administered health systems might cut overall costs by half and the model might be cloned into a national self-care system that actually was profitable.

2018.02.03:08:23 [LI][JU][TR]>3≈ WB]n

Luke O'Neil, Boston, in WaPost: 'I love the New England Patriots. That's why I need them to lose the Super Bowl.':

"But now it's gotten to the point where writers are contacting ethicists to ask if it's okay to cheer for the Patriots, and otherwise decent New England natives are pledging to donate to charity every time the team scores as a form of penance for their fandom. There's a common expression in Boston media about this sort of thing: "They hate us 'cause they ain't us." I would probably edit that down by four words."

People in operations research can easily use the term 'Patriots' to define a successful team of problem solvers intent on a common goal. A Patriot is an unselfish member of a team that has united to solve a problem by giving more to his 'nation' than to himself, just as the Continental Army at Valley Forge did in1778. It is the same term involving an unselfish contribution making the whole greater than the parts (e pluribus unim) that can be used for a corporate think tank group or a modern special operations team or a hospital surgery staff. Or a football team that has united with a common Patriotic purpose without groupy narcissistic personalities, the well-known Achilles heel of failed, decadent organizations in American society. Obviously, the self-indulgent narcissists of America cannot stand the idea of Patriotic self-sacrifice within a team spirit and therefore must hate the very idea of disciplined, altruistic AND very successful Patriotism. Conclusion: only decadent self-loving groupy 'members' serving their own purposes could hate Patriots.

2018.02.06:07:10 |LI|<1|TR|<2|WB|>1+|CD|<3 ⋈|GW|>1-|JU|<2≈|OP|>2

Editorial Board, WaPost, 'The immigration bills in Congress aren't perfect. That's okay.':

"But the deal he [the president] has proposed and is insisting on goes much further than that. Yes, he has offered a path to citizenship for 1.8 million dreamers, but Democrats are highly unlikely to support his quid pro quos, which would not only crack down on illegal immigrants but also slash legal immigration to levels unseen in decades — a policy goal that was never part of Mr. Trump's rhetoric as a candidate."

With an estimated 43 million bipeds in this country who don't have a 'legal' status (previous WaPost article), isn't 'a path to citizenship' the actual problem that needs solving? The condition of Dreamers and half a dozen other categories of American space occupiers wouldn't exist if the issues of citizenship had been resolved 30 or 40 years ago. While there is some strong Justice and Liberty components in the current bills, they do not actually solve the larger citizenship problem that faces the nation.

Even a very strict DNA and loyalty oath definition of naturalized citizenship based on the mind-body 'character' of the immigrant might cause most of the 43 million bipeds to obtain citizenship and have voting rights, but that is not covered by the current bills. Their wording, in fact, might extend the non-citizen status to millions more rather than welcome them as conscious, literate Americans who are defined citizens. Defining citizenship was a clearly worded naturalization authority in the Constitution, not the endless reaction to border jumpers the actual citizens have spent their lives and incomes dealing with.

2018.02.11:07:10 |WB|<2⋈ |GW|<3⋈ |CD|<1= |TR|<1 |LI|>3⋈|JU|>1

Wang and Berman, WaPost, 'Las Vegas shooter was sober, autopsy finds, leaving his motives a mystery':

"The doctor described Paddock as "odd," noting that he believed that Paddock may have had bipolar disorder but refused to discuss the topic, the Las Vegas police report said. The doctor said Paddock refused antidepressant medication but accepted prescriptions for treating anxiety. Paddock appeared to be afraid of medications, the doctor told investigators, and would often refuse to take them."

The fact that the 'odd' conditions lasted several years, including his social interaction with others, might indicate a mild form of bipolar disorder called Cyclothymia that doesn't have the noticeable mania/depression swings of full bipolar. Cyclothymia would be consistent with the ups and downs of a frequent gambler also. It just puts a person in a perpetual state of being 'sick' or 'hurt' and this in turn can lead to a 'defense' reaction that is violent, although extremely rare. Cyclothymia is mild enough that it won't appear in a biopic analysis of brain tissue or diagnosis, but the 'defense' reaction might show up as a desire to 'get' the people causing the feeling of 'hurt'.

Unfortunately, people with Cyclothymia are also subject to autosuggestion from others and there is a possibility that someone else, even in the cyber-media, might have suggested the path he took to him. Note the careful planning over months, which implies a repeated or reinforced autosuggestion.

2018.02.11:23:10 [GW]|<3⋈ |CD|<2 ≈ ∑ |TR|<3 |LI|<3⋈|JU|>1 |OP|<4

Samuelson, WaPost, The one-word reason Congress's debt deal should worry us (Prudence):

"Deficit financing has become the mother's milk of politics. Compromise occurs by mutual forbearance. "Each party is giving the other its wish list with all the bells and whistles included and asking future generations to pick up the tab," notes the CRFB's Maya MacGuineas."

Bible's Habakkuk 2:6:

Will all these victims of his greed not take up a taunting song against him,

And in mocking derision against him Say, 'Woe, for judgment comes, to him who increases that which is not his—

How long will he possess it? And woe to him who makes himself wealthy with usury.

2018.02.12:00:00 |JU|<1[LI|>2|TR|<3⋈[WB|>1≈[GW]>3⋈ |CD|<1....|OP|n

Samuelson, WaPost, 'This is what an immigration policy for the 21st century should actually look like':

"As a group, there are now more than 43 million immigrants in the United States, legal and illegal, representing about 13 percent of the population, reports the Migration Policy Institute, which generally supports looser policies. The U.S.-born children of immigrants constitute a group almost the same size. This means that about a quarter of the total U.S. population are either immigrants or their offspring."

If you have an American economic system that is producing several hundred robots a day to do routine maintenance and fabrication of its human AND material infrastructures because humans SHOULDN'T be doing that type of labor, the addition of ANY immigrants who can't be citizens is pointless and dangerous for the society and the individual. Of the quarter of the population that is immigration related, how many could actually qualify by testing as citizens? Worse, how many are currently legally on voting registration lists under 'sanctuary' even when they have no concept of citizenship either in America or their origin? 60 million people, 1st and 2nd generation, who have no cultural belief in any constitutional governance but can 'vote' as some Great Leader tells them to?

The commonly held myth of skin tone 'culture' being a criteria for voting is not supported anywhere in the Constitution even with gerrymandering, only legitimately defined citizens are authorized to vote in this representative republic. But a non-citizen certainly can participate in the economy and culture under the Article I, Section 8, clause 4 'uniform Rule of Naturalization' authority as a 'US National'. A US National could easily be defined by law as one who is transitioning back and forth, provided he has taken a polygraphed oath of allegiance to protect BOTH societies as he is able and has established citizenship 'roots' in the American society.

Speculation:

But one of the definitions that might be needed in the future would be whether the individual biped coming across a border has all 49 genomic conditions known as Human Accelerated Regions (HARs) of DNA that actually defines such a biped as a real human being. HARs involve DNA that allow a special ankle and upright back for mobility, intestine sophistication that allows digestion of almost anything, and consciousness with literacy itself. There is nothing in the Constitution that suggests the 49 HARs defining humanity can't be conditions of citizenship.

2018.02.14:10:12 |CD|<3 ⋈ |GW|>1-[JU]>2|TR|<2≈|OP|>3

Thiessen, WaPost, 'There's another memo on the Russia investigation. This one demands answers.':

"The FBI "relied heavily" on the Steele dossier to obtain warrants for surveillance of Carter Page, a marginal former Trump campaign adviser, the senators write. Moreover, they say, the FBI did not have "meaningful corroboration" of Steele's claims when it submitted its application to the Foreign Intelligence Surveillance Act court."

Carter Page already had a FISA warrant for surveillance issued against him in 2013 and 2014, which when combined with ANY later 2016 international activities of a political nature, would easily have been justification for issuance of a new warrant. The existence of the Steele dossier, not its contents, would have justified the warrant in an election year and would not have required 'corroboration'. In the upcoming election period starting next month, the Americansky security services might need a blanket warrant on international contacts in order to protect the public's voting rights.

2018.02.15:07:15 |LI|>1|TR|<2|WB|<2+|CD|<3 ⋈ |GW|>1-[JU]<2≈|OP|>3

Carney, TheHill, 'Immigration fight down to the wire':

"McConnell teed up procedural votes on four proposals Wednesday evening: the Grassley bill, a separate plan from Sens. Christopher Coons (D-Del.) and John McCain (R-Ariz.), a proposal from Sen. Pat Toomey (R-Pa.) that would crack down on sanctuary cities, and a placeholder for the Collins proposal."

No matter which version of the 'alien occupier' problem (all 43 million?) is cleared by the Senate, it will not solve the non-citizen voter registration problem unless they ALL have some form of DNA-based identification card saying they are a lawful 'national' in the USA. Without the clear ID card indicating status, non-voter interference in citizen's rights make Russian and Chinese political interference look tame. Congressional authority is clearly defined by Article I, Section 8, clause 4: 'establish an uniform [NOTE uniform] Rule of Naturalization'.

2018.02.16:10:28 LI|>4|TR|<3+|CD|<3 ⋈|GW|<1?-|JU|<2≈|OP|<3

McArdle, BloombergView, 'We Need Everyone at the Immigration Table':

"To disagree with Douthat and Linker, then, you need to argue, not just that the restrictionists are propounding bad policy, but that the restrictionists must be shut out, delegitimized, anathema. Practically, this is a silly argument as long as they are able to capture the White House and dozens of Congressional seats. But in a way I didn't appreciate ten years ago, it is also corrosive to our civic institutions."

NOTE 18 U.S. Code § 611 - Voting by aliens, 1996:

(a) It shall be unlawful for any alien to vote in any election held solely or in part for the purpose of electing a candidate for the office of President, Vice President, Presidential elector, Member of the Senate, Member of the House of Representatives, Delegate from the District of Columbia, or Resident Commissioner, unless—

(1) the election is held partly for some other purpose;

(2) aliens are authorized to vote for such other purpose under a State constitution or statute or a local ordinance; and

(3) voting for such other purpose is conducted independently of voting for a candidate for such Federal offices, in such a manner that an alien has the opportunity to vote for such other purpose, but not an opportunity to vote for a candidate for any one or more of such Federal offices.

The article misses the point entirely with a circular argument that a person occupying space in America automatically has voting rights BECAUSE he has stepped off a plane or boat or crossed a border and is therefore entitled to the rights of citizenship so that he, or any of the other 43 million aliens has a voice on further stepping across the border.

A person needs to be a citizen in order to vote or change the policies of the country, as the laws of the country say. It has nothing to do with skin tone. The commonly held myth of skin tone 'culture' being a criteria for voting is not supported anywhere in the Constitution even with gerrymandering, only legitimately defined citizens are authorized to vote in this representative republic, noting that there has never been a functioning democracy above the size of a city-state.

But a non-citizen certainly can participate in the economy and culture under the Article I, Section 8, clause 4 'uniform Rule of Naturalization' authority as a 'US National'. A US National could easily be defined by law as one who is transitioning back and forth, provided he has taken a polygraphed oath of allegiance to protect BOTH societies as he is able and has established citizenship 'roots' in the American society.

One of the citizenship definitions that might be needed in the future would be whether the individual biped coming across a border has all 49 genomic conditions known as Human Accelerated Regions (HARs) of DNA that actually defines such a biped as a real human being. HARs involve DNA that allow a special ankle and upright back for mobility, intestine sophistication that allows digestion of almost anything, and consciousness with literacy itself. Making Immigration from one Malthusian Population Trap to create another as an end onto itself is not bio-ethically rational in a democracy. There is nothing in the Constitution that suggests the possession of all 49 HARs defining humanity can't be conditions of citizenship PRIOR to the alien movement into this country.

2018.02.16:21:01 |OP| ≈∑ |TR|>3 |LI|>3⋈|JU|>1….|GW|>2

Pegden and Procaccia in WaPost, 'There's another way to solve gerrymandering':

"This property holds when both parties employ their best possible strategies, which might make use of sophisticated algorithms and detailed information about voters."

According to the federal Constitution, each 700,000 people is entitled to one Representative, with each state, note state, entitled to a minimum of one, regardless of population size. The idea then would be to insure, mathematically ruthlessly, that a Representative actually represented a majority of the citizens (constitutionally valid voters) and not some faction within the District, which the two-party formula won't do. Obviously, that representative ideal would screen out any population distribution that did not have a 'bell curve' spectrum of voters that could represent 51 percent. Perhaps a 'Rule of Fives' distribution is required in which the two major parties, independents, unaffiliateds AND 'No Confidence' (NC) are given a chance at true representation. If a candidate got more 'No Confidence' votes than party or independent vote combinations, he would automatically be eliminated for two subsequent elections, but the NC distribution would have to be in the calculation.

The Rule of Fives would also require a mathematical calculation (Huntington-Hill method?) that took into account five possible votes by the 700,000 based on the previous census and a State authorization based on the previous two federal elections. If a state commission calculated 700K people according to a truly representative Rule of Fives, they couldn't calculate a District without a demographic center, so odd district configurations couldn't be created in the states with 5 or more Districts. End of the gerrymander?

TLO: The Rule of Fives are an attempt to have continuous representation of a census defined population. Each of the two primary political entities, independents, other political entities AND No Confidence are a numerical distribution of an entire population. Not based on any economic, ethnic or physical combination, although these might be in the 'spectrum'.

2018.02.18:09:53 |CD|>3 ≈|OP| Ξ|WB|<2+|LI| ⋈|GW|≈ |JU|

Ignatius, WaPost, 'The lessons the United States should learn from Raqqa':

"Another moral is that it's a mistake to let a determined adversary like the Islamic State ever gain control of an urban center like Raqqa, or Mosul in Iraq, which was also cratered in its liberation. Once committed fighters take over a city, they can be rooted out only at great human cost."

It is hard to grasp the idea that there are 'humans' who get pleasure from creating the pain and suffering and death of people to the extent that they hide behind humans as shields and leave behind the traps for mass murder. Yet every totalitarian force that has ever come down the road has managed to have large numbers of such 'humans' in their convoys. Not the same as a disciplined army on the march that abides by rules of engagement.

Speculation:

In the not too distant future, military organizations who wish to keep civilians AND themselves alive in a world of making small WMD in every basement or garage, they will very quickly discover that a robot that can selectively, very selectively through AI brains, root out some pathological killer who hates life itself is much more efficient than risking lives. If that robot has the killing efficiency of the sci-fi 'terminator', it just might save lots of lives (as would an AI-enhanced droid in a hospital) but would it then become the victim of human hackers like those now so busy at their own forms of destruction?

2018.02.18:22:05 |CD|>1+|WB|<2 ≈|OP| Ξ |LI| ⋈|GW|<2≈ |JU|<4

Diehl, WaPost, 'The nuclear agreement is 'the worst deal ever' — for Iran':

"What this tells us is that one of the best ways to counter Iran's interventions in Iraq, Yemen and Syria is to ally with the large bloc of Iranians who oppose them. In part that means helping Iranians find out what their government is up to; the news that it was planning to cut food subsidies while increasing spending on the Revolutionary Guard was one of the triggers of the protests."

The reason for so much opposition to the Pasdaran (Iran's Revolutionary Guard economic elite) excursions into other countries is obvious even to Iranian citizens without media discussion. Well-dressed Pasdaran soldiers are being supported with minimum pay vouchers of $1500 a month and any over-the-border Pasdaran 'proxy' soldier is getting about half that from the Iranian treasury. Even a foreign fighter for the Guard or a member of the Basij militia get about twice what the average Tehran worker gets, and he knows it.

If you start doing the numbers, you will find that a Pasdaran operating outside Iran's borders costs about $400 a day to logistically feed and equip, with Guard troops inside Iran only slightly less. There are 300,000 Iranians in these categories and that works out to $120 million a DAY or about 20 percent of Iran's real GDP. American overseas funding in the same military categories is three hundredths of one percent of GDP, and even though both countries borrow the money to finance these, the effect on Iran is a constant drain on the banks, making nearly any private sector operation difficult or borderline bankrupt because of the lack of capital. And any Iranian can see that.

2018.02.21:16:20 |OP| n?≈Σ |TR|>3 |LI|>3⋈|JU|>1....|GW|>2

Andrew Van Dam in WaPost, 'Using the best data possible, we set out to find the middle of nowhere':

"We focused our analysis on that previously impossible search for the most remote places in the contiguous United States, using a variant of the methodology the researchers used. Like them, we attempted to measure a place's distance from any densely populated spot within a metro large enough to provide key goods and services."

Very nicely done, but the 'algorithms' in use suggest a more important calculation could be made. Suppose you used a population spectrum algorithm similar to these that could calculate the 'nowhere point' at the exact center of each 700,000-person federal Representative District? If you then calculated a five-section bell curve political spectrum consisting of Republicans, Democrats, Independents, Unaffiliated, and those with 'No Confidence' votes, you would be able to calculate the truly representative boundaries of each District without gerrymandering. Perhaps the authors of this article could go back to the touch screen and run a really important calculation on the 'middle of'.

2018.02.22:21:13 |OP|<2 ≈∑ |TR|<3 |LI|>3⋈|JU|>1....|GW|<2+|CD|>2

Evan Bayh in TheHill, 'New poll reveals why Founders would be worried':

"The bipartisan House Problem Solvers Caucus and several bipartisan groups of senators have each proposed plans that would marry these two ideas together, comprehensively saving the Dreamers and protecting the border. But Washington remains mired in disagreement, unable to move forward on any specific plan. That's not because a grand compromise on border security and immigration would mark bad policy. It's not because the compromise offends any particular constituency. It's just because, well, that's Washington."

The Founders would have been very worried because their checks and balances to reach a rational solution of 'federal' level problems had simply disappeared in this century. But they did debate the idea of putting 'citizenship' definitions in the Constitution but decided not to (thanks, Ben) because it was obvious the definitions would change over time. They nicely opted for an authority of the Congress 'to establish a uniform Rule of Naturalization' rather than birth citizenship. And this proved correct as wave after wave of immigrants stepped off a one-month boat trip. They would never have anticipated a immigration need for an Afghan translator serving our military or a need for asylum from Latin Conquistadors overrunning some county somewhere or a naturalization need for a skilled worker because our own society was too media-decadent to produce them. It really is time to create a 'uniform Rule of Naturalization'.

Speculation:

Suppose modern biomedical technologies on DNA Identification were used to create a 'green' card (555 nm, the exact middle of the color spectrum) that expressed a Condition of Naturalization? There are some 50 categories of alien residents created by the various waves and a single uniform ID card showing what the status is, including those with a presidential or gubernatorial pardon status, might be made a requirement for residency and work regardless of the time involved. That smart card would make the person or visitor an 'American National' which would cover all of the 43 million 'aliens' coming and going from the country. It happens that the military common access card (CAC) is already in wide use and is 'smart' with a 64 mbyte chip. There is no reason at all that a USNational card could not be created with DNA data concerning the Human Accelerated Regions (HARs) that truly identify a person as a homosapien, even if such data and health related to the HARs require 2000 mbytes.

Addressing two current 'wave' problems with three-year extensions is laudable, but a much more 'uniform' solution based on 21st century no-doubts DNA technology would go much further in solving the true Naturalization problem.

2018.02.23:07:10 |CD|<3 ⋈|GW|>1-|JU|<1|TR|<2 ≈ |OP|<1

Blackwell and Gordon in TheHill, 'Russian attacks on America require bipartisan response from Congress':

"With Mueller's confirmation that Russia manipulated this system, new legislation is needed to identify political ads paid for by foreign countries, root out fake accounts and disinformation, and review algorithms to prevent Russia-funded propaganda arms like RT and Sputnik from figuring prominently in news feeds. The Honest Ads Act, cosponsored by Sens. John McCain (R-Ariz.), Mark Warner (D-Va.) and Klobuchar, would close the loophole in current law by requiring social media platforms to identify the sponsors of political advertising, as is already required on radio and television. Its passage would be another step in the right direction."

This Honest Ads Act, S.1989, has specific language concerning the people who must place their names on the political ad regardless of the format used, because previous versions of FEC regs were only concerned with 'paper' ads, not electronic. The language should hold up under Judicial review, although that might be why only the payer of the ad is required on the ad. Most scientific, newspaper and other 'info' related articles also have the author listed in the item and there is no Constitutional reason that both the author and the payer could not be prominently displayed in the political ad. This might ensure clear references for the voter, since the author might need to be identified as an American Citizen or resident National.

As for a bipartisan response to the Slavic (Attila?) attacks on democracy, the additional $4.8 billion allocated to East NATO operations might have included an AUMF for the physical deployment of fully equipped U.S. Cyber Command 'technical' units in those areas around St. Petersburg and Odessa. But the wording of a cyber related AUMF and/or an AUPF (Authorization for the Use of international Police Force) might require some Congressional authoring skills the Founders couldn't even dream of.

2018.02.25:08:15 |LI|<3|TR|<2|WB|>1+|CD|>3 ⋈|GW|>2-|JU|<1≈|OP|>3

Schoen in TheHill, 'gun safety':

"The evidence suggests America has reached a tipping point. According to an October 2017 Gallup Poll, over six in 10 registered voters cited >>gun control<< as one of the most important factors they considered when selecting who to vote for and 24 percent say a candidate must share their views on >>gun control<<.

Consequently, >>gun safety<< is shaping up to be a major electoral issue in the 2018 midterm elections that could potentially win Democrats back the House."

The author is equating 'gun safety' with 'gun control' and anyone who has ever fired a ballistic device such as a handgun, shotgun, or even a bow and arrow knows the two are not the same at all. 'Gun control' is a totalitarian mechanism for population intimidation and is used to ban all weapon possession except by state-controlled militia. The ruling king's (emperor, commissar, oligarchy, elite, whatever) 'ban' mechanism is exactly what the 2nd Amendment was designed to prevent and the idea of using gun control laws to effectively ban weapons has been routinely tossed by the Supreme Court.

But what would happen if you had a national referendum on a 'gun safety' mechanism that mandated the safe keeping of all weapons, ammunition AND household toxins like opiates, insecticides, antihistamines or bleach/ammonia? There might be a surprise or two by such polling because most gun owners have lockups for weapons and would vote to make them mandatory, possibly insisting cipher lock cabinets be mandated for 'safety'. It might also be a surprise that the voters in general would NOT vote for the mandatory lockup of household toxins.

It is also noticeable that, statistically, many of the weapon mass-abuses of this century have occurred in areas of the Nation under the political control of liberal or 'enlightened' segments who do not wish to equate mental illnesses with an habeas corpus or involuntary restraint problem. From the standpoint of the national Common Defense covenant in the Constitution, it would be difficult to decide whether unrestrained mental illness or unrestrained profiteering in a fully saturated arms market is the real problem that needed 'control', but it still might be a referendum issue.

2018.02.25:22:19 [WB]|<3+ |LI|<3|TR|< ⋈|GW|>2-|JU|<1 ≈ |OP|>3

Editorial Board, LATimes, 'Editorial: Los Angeles' homelessness crisis is a national disgrace':

"Skid row is — and long has been — a national disgrace, a grim reminder of man's ability to turn his back on his fellow man. But these days it is only the ugly epicenter of a staggering homelessness problem that radiates outward for more than 100 miles throughout Los Angeles County and beyond. There are now more than 57,000 people who lack a "fixed, regular or adequate place to sleep" on any given night in the county, and fewer than 1 in 10 of them are in skid row."

National problem based on illegal immigration, or is it a 'symptom' of the rapidly increasing economic inequality that makes housing costs inflate locally at 8% per year? Loss in human capital or not because of health issues?

2018.02.28:07:30 [WB]n+|CD|<1…..|LI|>3|TR|-[JU]<1+ [GW]>1=|OP|>2

Ignatius, WaPost, 'The crown prince of Saudi Arabia is giving his country shock therapy':

"MBS said that a "shock" was also needed to check Islamist extremism in the kingdom. He said his reforms, giving greater rights to women and fewer to the religious police, were simply an effort to reestablish the practices that applied in the time of the prophet Muhammad."

MBS and company could do worse. Most of the extremist sentiments of both Sunni and Shia versions of the Prophet's Revelations developed in the 1700s and 1800s, not during the Medina period when the Revelations created the Constitution of Medina. Those later extreme sentiments were designed to give absolute control of every person's wealth to a national government rather than create conditions where the Ruh or Holy Spirit could develop in a person and a community. In many 'States' after the 1800s, the obsession with state wealth caused the totalitarian 'Caliphate' mentality rather than a spiritual infrastructure of peaceful Quranic Revelation as in the al jihad al akbar.

It was this fundamental diversion from the spiritual Quran that created unnaturally cruel fascist entities like ISIS, Taliban, Baathists and Pasdaran. Any return to the peaceful community building by Mohammed bin Salman that allows the Holy Spirit to enter into the children is welcome. When the Prophet said 'be like me in your life', he didn't mean acquire wealth by force, the al jihad al asghar, or grow beards or carry swords or enslave women. He meant let the Ruh force enter in to your life as it did him.

TL Opservationis 2018.03

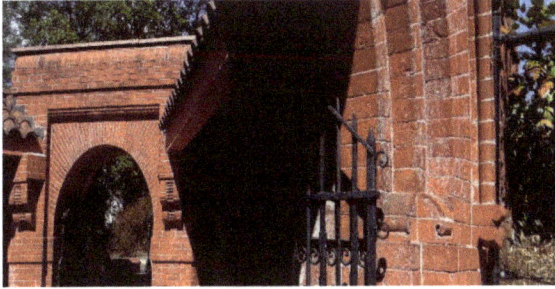

2018.03.01:07:20 |CD|<1 ✉|GW|>1-|JU|<2|TR|<2≈|OP|>1

Lane, WaPost, 'We got China wrong. Now what?':

"Instead, the Cold War's dramatic end spawned a new and loftier rationale for the policy, which had acquired a life of its own. Americans believed that history might be flowing inevitably in favor of free markets and free elections. All we had to do was stay patient, maintain our influence and let China evolve. There would be no long-term conflict between U.S. self-interest and U.S. values.

The fact that this also happened to be the position most congenial to American business, hungry for access to China's cheap labor, seemed like a feature, not a bug.

Now it's evident China has been gaining leverage over the political and economic leaders of the United States and has learned how to make them defer to its norms."

President Xi Jinping 'thoughts to be included in the Chinese Constitutions', both Party and National, 2018.02.28:

> Item 13. Promoting the building of a community with a shared future for mankind.
>
> The dream of the Chinese people [socialism with Chinese characteristics] is closely connected with the dreams of the peoples of other countries; the Chinese Dream can be realized only in a peaceful international environment and under a stable international order. We must keep in mind both our internal and international imperatives, stay on the path of peaceful development, and continue to pursue a mutually beneficial strategy of opening up. We will uphold justice while pursuing shared interests, and will foster new thinking on common, comprehensive, cooperative, and sustainable security. We will pursue open, innovative, and inclusive development that benefits everyone; boost cross-cultural exchanges characterized by harmony within diversity, inclusiveness, and mutual learning; and cultivate ecosystems based on respect for nature and green development. China will continue its efforts to safeguard world peace, contribute to global development, and uphold international order."

Now what? NOTE:' We will uphold justice while pursuing shared interests, and will foster new thinking on common, comprehensive, cooperative, and sustainable security.'

Why is Socialism with Chinese Characteristics a shared interest or a common, sustainable security? Would it be better than the constant indecision on security by your own government?

2018.03.04:10:02 ∑ |LI|>3|TR|<2|WB|<2+|CD|<3 ⋈ |GW|-|JU|<2≈|OP|<?

Ana Marie Cox, WaPost, 'Trump actually thinks executing drug dealers would help. That's the problem.':

"There's no real need to explain why the execution of drug dealers is a bad idea, though it is a very, very bad idea. The country has already tried an aggressive enforcement approach to drug crimes — the four-decade-plus war on drugs — and among experts and law enforcement officers , it is almost universally acknowledged as a massive failure in economic and practical terms."

The 'war on drugs' never applied the necessary crime against humanity criteria the 1998 Rome Statute Section (k) against a WMD chemical distributor, whether it was permanently disabling drugs, radiation or poisons being created. Possibly wasn't systematized enough. Although many of the addicted distributors need treatment (regardless of skin tone) rather than imprisonment, the manufacturer and distributor of the WMD substances is not in that category. That form of genocidal predator, and his capital or media supporters, has engaged in a systematized attack on humanity no different from using VX neurotoxin bombs against Syrian towns. The neurological effects, whether slow or fast, are identical as far as a human brain is concerned and constitute a crime against humanity. It is not a matter of punishing or deterring a cartel-level WMD maker as it is permanently removing him and his co-conspirators from contact with the human race.

Speculation: since advocacy of leniency for a distributor of 'pleasure' is because the advocate needs that 'pleasure' (that is, he has adapted to the drug-food), could any person who wants easy availability of WMD devices be taken seriously as an advocate of Justice for all 'humans'?

2018.03.05:08:10 |LI|<1|TR|<2|WB|>1+|CD|>3 ⋈ |GW|>1-|JU|>2≈|OP|>3

Carney, Theill, 'Gun debate: Here are the proposals that Congress is considering':

"Background checks:

Senate Democrats are demanding more extensive background checks on gun purchases.

Schumer, outlining his caucus's three-part plan, said Trump should "at a minimum" support closing "loopholes" by requiring background checks for all firearms sold at gun shows or over the internet.

"I think the president knows he could show real leadership by bucking the NRA, providing cover for his Republicans and getting something actually done," he told reporters.

Schumer didn't say if Democrats would offer Manchin-Toomey as their background check legislation or file a separate piece of legislation.

A Quinnipiac University Poll released late last month found that 97 percent of Americans — including 97 percent of gun owners and 97 percent of Republicans — support requiring a background check on every gun sale.

White House Press Secretary Sarah Huckabee Sanders said on Friday that the president is "not necessarily" pushing for "universal" background checks.

"Certainly, improving the background check system. He wants to see what that legislation, the final piece of it looks like," she told reporters.

It is noticeable that there are no provisions in these legislative domain sets to protect citizens under the 4th and 5th Amendments, only to 'regulate' under the 'well regulated militia' concept of the 2nd Amendment. The background check conditionals all involve increasing the capabilities of the FBI's National Instant Background Check System, which any Sequoia-class supercomputer and 5G internet structure would help, but it would still remain in the FBI's criminal investigation jurisdiction. That in turn, because of lax data security and FOIA abuse, could turn the NICS into an automatic criminalization apparatus by the future 'deep state' and such Federalist abuse is the main objection of even the 97 percent of gun owners who approve of background checks.

Blue-state extremists already violate the 4th Amendment 'effects' protection of gun owners by publishing originally 'secure' data through FOIA abuse and there is no reason to believe they wouldn't do that on a national NICS scale if given the chance.

Speculation:

In order to protect the individual's Bill of Rights, it would be necessary to insure that the information in the NICS is secure, especially if a person IS denied a purchase permit on the local end of an internet query to it. If the person does have some noticeable or recorded mental disorder that the seller of the gun has reasonable cause to deny purchase, it might be that he is eligible for a 'witness protection' status while the attempted purchaser immediately acquires a 'fugitive' status because of the attempt to become dangerous. Under FBI and ATF rules, the individual MUST commit a crime in order for them to intercede, but would that be true of a Federal Marshal engaged in 'fugitive' interdiction? Even missing persons qualify as fugitives.

Suppose that the NICS data was sent through a cyber-protected channel to the Marshal Service General Council office and it was authorized to issue a 'fugitive' warrant through a local deputized entity, along with witness protection compensation for the source? This would take the matter of the Background Check out of the criminal justice domain set until a Marshal deputy had determined probable cause and effect but would still allow for temporary restraint of a disturbed person while protecting the rights of all others involved. Would that solve the 'red flags' and 'straw purchases' issues as well? School (or hospital or subway) safety is aided by the 'witness protection' status of the seller, but only insured by the genetic therapy elimination of the neurologically disturbed themselves, which might be a century away.

Banning pre-trial 'gossip' on such cases with sealed warrants would be a further protection of the Bill of Rights, but you would never get for profit First Amendment media to agree.

2018.03.07:00:00 |WB|<3⋈ |GW|<1⋈ |CD|<1≈ |TR|<1 |LI|>4 ⋈ |JU|<1

Armstrong, CRS-LSB10049, Responding to the Opioid Epidemic: Legal Developments and FDA's Role:

According to the Centers for Disease Control and Prevention, "115 Americans die every day from an opioid overdose," and deaths from prescription opioids have more than **quadrupled since 1999**. The epidemic's origins are complex, with fingers pointed at pharmaceutical manufacturers and distributors, addicts and dealers, health care professionals, and insurance companies. Like the causes of the opioid epidemic, any solutions to the problem will likely involve many actors, including the federal government. The Food and Drug Administration (FDA)—the executive agency charged with protecting the public health by ensuring the nation's drug supply is safe and effective—has developed an "opioids action plan," discussed in more detail below. Nonetheless, questions remain as to what actions the agency should take and whether the agency's existing authorities are adequate for addressing the crisis. This Sidebar provides an overview of FDA's existing authorities, the historical context for the opioid epidemic, and the agency's current plan for combatting the opioid epidemic, concluding with an examination of the broader legal questions concerning the crisis.

The agency's plan includes:

1. consulting with an advisory committee prior to approving an NDA for an opioid without abuse-deterrent properties;

2. developing additional warnings and safety information for certain opioid labeling;

3. strengthening post-market requirements to require, for example,

the study of the long-term effects of using extended-release/long-acting opioids;

4. updating the REMs program, such as by requiring sponsors to fund continuing medical education for prescribers;

5. expanding access to abuse-deterrent formulations (ADF) of opioid medications by issuing draft guidance on the agency's recommendations for approving such drugs;

6. supporting better treatment for opioid abuse, such as expanding access (e.g., over-the counter availability) to overdose treatments and opioid alternatives; and

7. reassessing the risk-benefit approval framework for opioid use to account for the current understanding of the risks associated with opioid use and misuse.

'quadrupled since 1999'?   No chance under [wellbeing] conditions, artificially contrived? Sellers engaged in a crime against humanity, even if they are non-governmental actors? 'Systemic' crime criteria is there.

2018.03.09:08:17 |CD|<3 ⋈|GW|>1-|JU|>2|TR|<2≈|OP|>1

Gibney, BloombergView, 'A Summit Failure Would Hurt Trump More Than Kim':

"In both cases, he would not be able to move ahead effectively without the support of South Korea, Japan and other U.S. allies. China and Russia, each with huge stakes in the future of the Korean Peninsula and vetoes in the United Nations Security Council, also need to be on board."

The 'huge stakes' of China and Russia involve having entire government directorates doing nothing except attempting to humiliate the 'temporary' leadership of the Americans. Large amounts of the propaganda by these ministries is specifically designed to demean and make ineffective the activities of an American leader, no matter what party. Note the continuous, well orchestrated slights directed toward the previous two presidents when traveling overseas.

If the objective of the 'huge stakes' oligarchies is to prove that an elected leader is always dysfunctional, then those countries would advise their proxy leader in their northern Korea provinces to engage in a humiliating dialog that scams the American and does nothing constructive. That would demonstrate to all Asians that the junfas, khans, emperors and czars that have always ruled Asia can demean democracies at will and the 'old ways' are inherently stronger than some peasant willing to give up power.

2018.03.15:22:10 |CD|> ≈|OP| Ξ|WB|+|CD| ⋈|GW|≈|OP|

Ignatius, WaPost, 'Putin has finally gone too far':

"A joint statement denounced the attack as "the first offensive use of a nerve agent in Europe since the Second World War" and called it "a breach of international law" that comes "against the background of a pattern of earlier irresponsible Russian behavior." That strong language warrants action by NATO and the United Nations."

A neurotoxin WMD attack against one is an attack against all. Even with deniability, the attack justifies retaliation in kind, the same as such mass murder did in World War I. The Syrian Baathists could not be using chemical agents without support of a UN Security Council veto backing them up, but the use is still crimes against humanity. There is clear evidence that the totalitarianists are experimenting with neurotoxin WMD as a terror weapon against populations that might oppose the ruling 'tribe'. The same ruling tribe mass murder mentality also exists in Korea and China and they all seem more than happy to say 'so what'. Not a nice world under production and the only fix might be retaliation in kind.

Maybe someone should show anti-government populations how to REALLY defend themselves against toxic toties with the same chemicals. But it won't be me opening that century-long can of vipers.

2018.03.17:06:15 |OP|<2 ≈∑ |TR|>3 |LI|>3⋈|JU|<1....|GW|<2

Kabaservice in WaPost, 'The old tea party may be over, but the new one is at peak power':

"Despite the tea party's provenance as a conservative movement, there was little about past political patterns and practices that it wanted to conserve. Activists hoped not only to "throw the bums out" but also to get rid of anything that passed for the status quo."

The 'status quo' should be in the six covenants of the Constitution Preamble; Justice, Tranquility, Common Defense, General Welfare, Liberty and Our Posterity. You can be a conservative right up to the point that you take an oath to protect those covenants and then carry out a political act or agenda that demolishes any one of them. 'Liberty' somehow comes out as placing personal wealth gain as the objective of political office such as in Russia or China? 'Tranquility' somehow comes out as making each state a sovereign nation ruled by a one-party oligarchy? 'Common Defense' somehow occurs when irreversible debt finances international contractors? A 'conservative movement' that dismantles national infrastructures somehow believes in 'our Posterity', which means leave something better for future generations?

One thing is certain: you can't be an office-holding constitutional conservative and a made-in-Asia anarchist at the same time.

2018.03.18:07:19 |OP|>3⋈|GW|>1-|JU|<2

Troianovski, WaPost, 'Russia scrambles to get voters to polls to legitimize election ahead of expected Putin landslide':

"But at 10 a.m. Moscow time, Central Elections Commission Chairwoman Ella Pamfilova said, nationwide turnout was 16.55 percent — more than double the 6.53 percent at that time in the previous presidential election, in 2012."

At that rate of participation in the vote, it is likely that 64 million Russians will actually vote, out of a total of 114 million eligible voters. If the 'landslide' holds at 61% for Putin, he will get a minimum of 39 million votes, which would be about one third of the eligible voters but nearly two thirds of the actual voters. So that would indicate sufficient popularity that a 'no confidence' vote didn't materialize. In elections where there is only a one-party state in effect, a 'no-confidence' vote would require at least half of the no-shows AND at least half of the actually voters to disavow the leading candidate. 51 percent of the no-shows is 26 million and 51 percent of the voters is 33 million, so there is not enough for a no-confidence vote by the Russian We the People.

It is interesting that the entire election process cost some 32 billion rubles or 3,523,575,000 Chinese Yuan (USD 556 million). That is about the price of two advanced surgery hospitals, one half a mobile MSKT missile launcher, or one third the cost of safety shielding for the Novichok toxin production facility at Krasnoarmeysk in the Moskva District.

But what could Americans do with the $3 billion they spend on elections if they didn't have to?

2018.03.18:22:03 |TR|<2 |LI|>2 |JU|<2 ≈ |OP|<1

Marcus, WaPost, 'Trump had senior staff sign nondisclosure agreements. They're supposed to last beyond his presidency.':

"This is extraordinary. .... And while White House staffers have various confidentiality obligations — maintaining the secrecy of classified information or attorney-client privilege, for instance — the notion of imposing a side agreement, supposedly enforceable even after the president leaves office, is not only oppressive but constitutionally repugnant."

There are also a number of laws that prohibit an government individual from profiting by transfer of information or job-gained expertise to a 'competitor' that are easily within employment contractual conditions. The EOP 'competitor' can be any foreign head of state or his 'gang'. Transferring sensitive, personal or classified information for profit from the EOP to the public media is a form of espionage and should be treated accordingly. The EOP, regardless of the occupants, is not a cackling hen house for neurotic gossips.

As for the constitutionality of 'leaks' under the 1st Amendment, keep in mind that a malicious gossip in the EOP who profits from his stories almost certainly violates the 4th Amendment 'papers and effects' protections of the employees working in the White House complex, with the exception of elected office-holders who gave up that protection when they became a public candidate. Technically, any non-elected who is mentioned in a gossip book or media segment can sue for violation of his 4th Amendment based privacy. But should that 'leaking' for profit be prohibited only if the non-disclosure contracts have a sunset clause that causes the contract to terminate one election cycle after the events? It stops being malicious gossip four years later and becomes historical (or hysterical?) research at that point.

But free speech for instant profit and gratification like it has been since the internet came into existence is protected by ALL of the Bill of Rights?

2018.03.20:12:05 |CD|<3 ⋈|GW|>1-|JU|<2≈|OP|<2

Ka Zeng in WaPost on U.S. tariff processes:

"According to the Foreign Trade Highlights published by the Census Bureau, the two countries now have five commodities that show up on each country's list of top imports/exports. This is up from just two overlapping products in 1996. While that number indicates an increasingly competitive trade relationship, it still falls below that for other U.S. trading partners such as Japan (eight overlapping products) and Britain (nine)."

If one uses the original Ricardo model for international trade, the idea was that a trade balance, note balance, of goods was achieved when each country had goods from different sectors that the other country did not produce. The effect of the Ricardo model was that the trade of mutually exclusive goods was greatly beneficial to both societies and did not produce an impossible trade balance. That model proved correct up to the point that a national government subsidized its goods in order to maintain a monopoly on the product. England did that in America for nearly a century (1750-1850) and Japan attempted it for decades (1970-1990).

At this time, the Beijing government has been subsidizing some eight product categories through interest-free loans in order to prevent other countries from developing overlapping product facilities of their own. Cell-phone technology is an example: one major cell phone manufacturer produces its electronic parts for one tenth the offshore price of the device, virtually guaranteeing no possible competition.

At that point, state subsidy of product manufacture, the Ricardo model breaks down and it becomes essential for other societies to either tax-subsidize the new facilities for products or equalize, through tariffs, the incoming 'dumper' products. A return to a Ricardo balanced economic wealth transfer is essential for the relationship of both societies.

2018.03.21:07:10 |JU|<2|LI|<2|TR|<3⋈[WB]<2 ≈ [GW]?

Dershowitz, TheHill, 'Trump is right: The special counsel should never have been appointed':

"But these [cultural?] views are not supposed to influence their decisions. In our age of hyper partisanship, the public has understandably lost confidence in the ability and willingness of our leaders to separate their political views from their law enforcement decisions. This is not all attributable to the appointment of the special counsel, but the criminalization of political differences on both sides of the aisle has certainly contributed to the atmosphere of distrust in our justice system."

In a 'system' where partisan control of propaganda is the objective, it might be very difficult to get a 'commission' to adhere to an oath to defend and protect the constitution above all else, especially when such a commission allows day to day access to 'lobby' influences, including foreign, inside the Beltway. Note the Warren Commission of 1964.

A properly convened and isolated grand jury with subpoena powers and severe 'obstruction' criminal penalties attached (the obstruction of justice might include contempt of constitution charges as well as normal usurpation of Justice charges) might have a much better chance at protecting the integrity of the Republic form of governance guaranteed by Article IV. It shouldn't matter what criminal activity is exposed, whether relevant to Constitutional integrity or not; a grand jury of citizens, not 'commission experts', might have a better chance at the truth.

2018.03.23:07:35 |OP|<n?

Gerson, WaPost, 'The 'DO NOT CONGRATULATE' leak shows the White House is panicking':

"Into this vacuum of plausible explanation have flooded other theories. "I think he is afraid of the president of Russia," former CIA director John Brennan recently speculated. "The Russians may have something on him personally that they could always roll out and make his life more difficult.""

Considering the Russian secret police's tradition of compromising 'enemies of the state' with defamation and lies, not to mention toxins that cause brain damage, it wouldn't be surprising at all that they went after an American who was naive enough to wonder about Russia without protecting himself. A certain Clinton managed that by using an unsecured Blackberry cell phone at various east European and Asia airports under FSB technical surveillance. It would have taken Russian 'mercenaries' under the GRU almost nothing to set up video capture minicams of the activities of one Kata Sarka in Moscow's hotels in 2013. Did the GRU pick up something interesting then?

In any case, once the Article II Oath of Office is taken to 'preserve and protect', anything previous to that doesn't count if one really is a president.

2018.03.23:07:10 |CD|<3 ⋈|GW|>1-|JU|<2|TR|<2 ≈ |OP|<1

Vanita Gupta in WaPost, 'The bitter lie behind the census's citizenship question':

"Not only is the constitutionally mandated census central to apportioning political power at every level of our representative form of government, but also the data collected influences the allocation of more than $675 billion in federal funds every year, along with countless policy and investment decisions by government agencies, nonprofit organizations and private enterprise."

Pew Research Center, from U.S Census data, chapter 5 'U.S. Foreign Born Population Trends':

"Even so, the five U.S. counties with the largest foreign-born populations in 2013 (Los Angeles County, Calif.; Miami-Dade County, Fla.; Cook County, Ill.; Queens County, N.Y.; and Harris County, Tex.) accounted for fully 20% of the U.S. immigrant population. The population has become more dispersed since 1990, when the top five counties accounted for 30% of the immigrant population."

If these five counties, note counties, account for 20% of the immigration population, 4.4 million, they might also be the 'sanctuary' for elements that are absorbing, not contributing, $135 billion out of the $675 billion in 'allocations'. That has little to do with reasons for not determining the citizenship status of people occupying American space, which the Pew Research and many others describe as 44 million including tourists, green card holders, and 'aliens'. The tax revenue appropriation per county is under the Article I, Section 8 authorities of the Congress, not the enumeration clause of Section 2.

The Constitutional point of the Census was to define the political authority of CITIZENS in the United States, not the civil rights of transients coming and going across the borders. Citizenship is a constitutionally valid determination of the Census, regardless of how money distribution is apportioned among counties.

2018.03.30:18:10 |CD|<3|LI|>2 ⋈|GW|<1-|JU|>2|TR|<2≈|OP|<3

Megan McArdle, WaPost, 'Should paying even a paltry ransom to hackers be a federal crime?':

"We don't need to ensure that no victim pays; we just need to make the payoff sufficiently uncertain that it will no longer be worthwhile for attackers to invest their efforts."

In cyberspace, because of its obvious advantages for sociopathic aggression including various forms of extortion, the normal system of human justice tends to break down because you can remain anonymous while operating there. In the case of cyber-crime, the idea of normal Justice, innocent until proven guilty (sorry, that is NOT in the Constitution) should be reversed. It is necessary that such a crime as cyber-ransom must assume that the 'victim' has arranged for the distribution of the ransom to be to HIMSELF or co-conspirators. This is actually occurring in many 'raided' financial institutions and corporations. The corporate officer almost always has an insider in the organization that has allowed the 'raid' through arranged security failures, and is therefore guilty unless he can prove otherwise. Assuming the guilt of the insider as a benefactor will almost certainly reduce cyber-crime to the pre-internet levels and is perfectly in keeping with the Constitution's current jurisdiction.

2018.03.31:07:20 |GW|>1-|JU|<2|TR|<2 ≈ |OP|<3

Editorial Board, WaPost, 'The Parkland shooter should not face the death penalty':

"The horror of that day is without dispute. So, too, is the need for serious legal consequences..... But will killing him serve justice? Even proponents of the death penalty (which we decidedly are not) are hard-pressed to justify its use on those who suffer from mental illness."

Never again be in a position to harm others? There are indications that the family he was born into may have genetically based mental disorders and that his condition(s) were amplified by that environment. And the only suggested remedy by 'society' was incarceration in some form even before he committed the mass-violence. What if he had been detected and treated during toddler stages? Would all of the 'ripple effects' of several thousand damaged neural structures in his mind never happen if he had treatment available to him? Suppose the parents had a predictive DNA testing that indicated their 'marriage' might have unfortunate genetic consequences? Are incarceration remedies of the 1800s still appropriate?

Opposition to the 'death penalty' is clearly indicated here since there is no point in seeking social vengeance against someone born without a conscious understanding of himself. But the constitution says no cruel and unusual punishment is allowed and this means that any form of incarceration IN HIS PRESENT STATE is a cruel and unusual punishment. You could easily make the case that if he is deemed by experts to be incurable or terminally ill through unconsciousness that 'assisted termination', not a punishment, IS appropriate. Many of the definitions and procedures for assisted suicide being developed in many states might also be appropriate in cases of incurable brain damage, the same as for cancer or dementia conditions. But it would take a 'jury' of wellness experts to determine that, not a jury of peers, and there is currently no such medical jury system defined by the Constitution.

OVERVIEW 2018.04 to .07

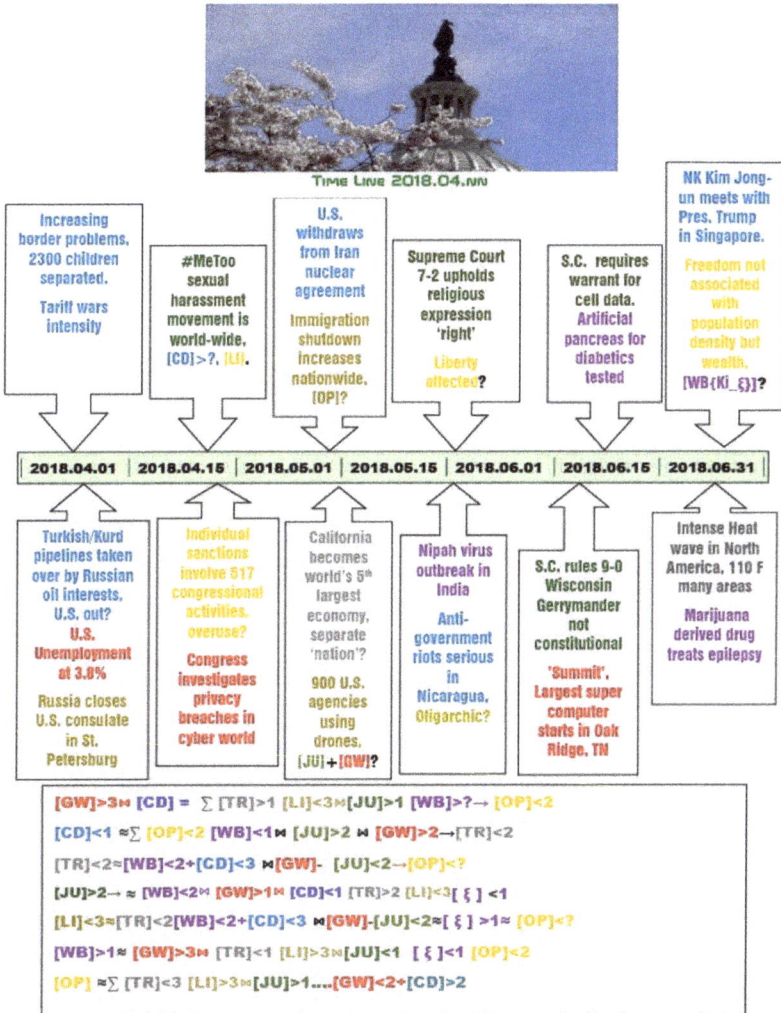

Time Line 2018.04.nn

| Increasing border problems, 2300 children separated. Tariff wars intensity | #MeToo sexual harassment movement is world-wide. [CD]>?, [LI]. | U.S. withdraws from Iran nuclear agreement Immigration shutdown increases nationwide, [OP]? | Supreme Court 7-2 upholds religious expression 'right' Liberty affected? | S.C. requires warrant for cell data. Artificial pancreas for diabetics tested | NK Kim Jong-un meets with Pres. Trump in Singapore. Freedom not associated with population density but wealth, [WB{Ki_{}]? |

| 2018.04.01 | 2018.04.15 | 2018.05.01 | 2018.05.15 | 2018.06.01 | 2018.06.15 | 2018.06.31 |

| Turkish/Kurd pipelines taken over by Russian oil interests, U.S. out? U.S. Unemployment at 3.0% Russia closes U.S. consulate in St. Petersburg | Individual sanctions involve 517 congressional activities, overuse? Congress investigates privacy breaches in cyber world | California becomes world's 5th largest economy, separate 'nation'? 900 U.S. agencies using drones, [JU]+[GW]? | Nipah virus outbreak in India Anti-government riots serious in Nicaragua, Oligarchic? | S.C. rules 9-0 Wisconsin Gerrymander not constitutional 'Summit', Largest super computer starts in Oak Ridge, TN | Intense Heat wave in North America, 110 F many areas Marijuana derived drug treats epilepsy |

$$[GW]>3\bowtie [CD] = \sum [TR]>1\ [LI]<3\bowtie[JU]>1\ [WB]>? \to [OP]<2$$

$$[CD]<1 \approx \sum [OP]<2\ [WB]<1\bowtie [JU]>2\ \bowtie [GW]>2\to[TR]<2$$

$$[TR]<2\approx[WB]<2+[CD]<3\ \bowtie[GW]-\ [JU]<2\to[OP]<?$$

$$[JU]>2\to \approx [WB]<2\bowtie [GW]>1\bowtie [CD]<1\ [TR]>2\ [LI]<3[\ \xi\ ]<1$$

$$[LI]<3\approx[TR]<2[WB]<2+[CD]<3\ \bowtie[GW]-[JU]<2\approx[\ \xi\ ]>1\approx [OP]<?$$

$$[WB]>1\approx [GW]>3\bowtie [TR]<1\ [LI]>3\bowtie[JU]<1\ [\ \xi\ ]<1\ [OP]<2$$

$$[OP] \approx\sum [TR]<3\ [LI]>3\bowtie[JU]>1....[GW]<2+[CD]>2$$

Figure 9.   Overview 2018.04

TL Opservationis 2018.04

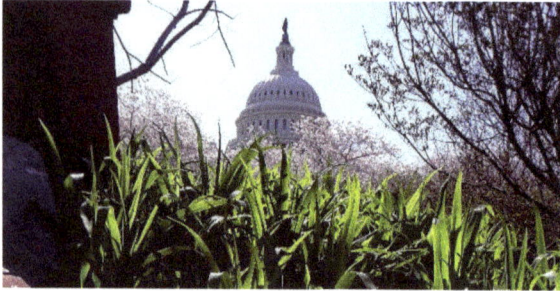

018.04.01:08:10 |LI|<1|TR|<2+|CD|>3 ⋈|GW|>1-[JU|<2≈|OP|>1

Thomsen, TheHill, Census advisers say decision to add citizenship question based on 'flawed logic':

"The panel, which includes top economists and demographers, also said the wording of the question should have been tested, and that the bureau should start doing so immediately."

The 2010 census short form asked the following ten questions ONLY:

How many people were living or staying in this house, apartment, or mobile home on April 1, 2010?

Were there any additional people staying here April 1, 2010 that you did not include in Question 1?

Is this house, apartment, or mobile home: owned with mortgage, owned without mortgage, rented, occupied without rent?

What is your telephone number?

Please provide information for each person living here. Start with a person here who owns or rents this house, apartment, or mobile home. If the owner or renter lives somewhere else, start with any adult living here. This will be Person 1. What is Person 1's name?

What is Person 1's sex?

What is Person 1's age and Date of Birth?

Is Person 1 of Hispanic, Latino, or Spanish origin?

What is Person 1's race? Does Person 1 sometimes live or stay somewhere else?

Speculation: Why is the short form asking for information about 'race' and 'national origin' but NOT citizenship when only citizens are allowed to vote? The enumeration clause in Article I, Section 2 clearly intended that everyone be counted even if he didn't have voting rights. The concept is that a 'representative' could represent the interests of a district population regardless of the number of actual voters (currently pretty poor in some states if eligible voters are compared to votes counted) and the actual voters were, through various amendments, defined as citizens. Why shouldn't the question of 'citizen' be on a short form if race and national origin, which cannot by law be 'represented', are on them?

2018.04.02:21:35 |TR|<1[LI|>3 →|WB|<2 [GW]|<1◄|TR|>1=|OP|<?

Parsons, WaTimes, 'Over 70 percent of Americans see media as 'fake news,' a Monmouth University poll shows':

"A majority of Americans — 77 percent — said traditional news outlets are "fake news," according to a Monmouth University poll published Monday.

Twenty-five percent say that **"fake news" is a story where the facts are incorrect,** while 65 percent say it is editorial decisions made by various outlets. Thirty-one percent of people believe this happens "regularly," and 46 percent say it's occasional.

A vast majority point to social media as a major problem. Sixty percent say the sites are "partly" responsible for spreading fake news, and 87 percent say outside groups are trying to push fake news stories on sites like Facebook and YouTube"

Reasonably accurate. But OK in the 1st Amendment? TBD.

2018.04.04:00:00 |WB|<2◄ [GW]|<2◄ |CD|<3 |TR|>1=?

ScienceDaily, 'New coronavirus emerges from bats in China, devastates young swine

Identified in same region, from same bats, as SARS coronavirus

Source: NIH/National Institute of Allergy and Infectious Diseases. Summary:

A newly identified coronavirus that killed nearly 25,000 piglets in 2016-17 in China emerged from horseshoe bats near the origin of the severe acute respiratory syndrome coronavirus (SARS-CoV), which emerged in 2002 in the same bat species. The new virus, called swine acute diarrhea syndrome coronavirus (SADS-CoV), doesn't appear to infect people, unlike SARS-CoV.

China bats carrying more than one virus? But only affects animals even if there is close human contact with bats, as in a lab? [OP]<n?

2018.04.06:14:20 |LI|>1|TR|<2|WB|<2+|CD|<3 ◄|GW|>1-|JU|<2≈|OP|>1

Tonette Walker in TheHill, 'We now know the importance of trauma-informed care, but there is more work to be done':

"Research shows when a person has one ACE [Averse Childhood Experience], they are more likely to have another two or more. The most recent national data indicate that almost 25 percent of children in the United States have experienced at least one ACE and almost 22 percent have two or more. In Wisconsin, these rates are lower than the national average, at 21.2 percent and 20.3 percent, respectively.

When trauma is experienced as a child, the unmitigated toxic stress created by these experiences can change brain chemistry, shape educational outcomes, and influence a person's future health and well-being. Research also shows a strong link between the number of ACEs and adult health. As the number of reported ACEs increase, so does the person's risk of cancer, diabetes, depression, alcoholism, drug use, smoking, suicide, homelessness, and more."

Those ripple effects, DNA based or other wise, are pretty severe even if only 10 percent of a state population is affected. And even if there is a desire to 'toughen-up' a kid as he grows up, you might still have to watch carefully for the ACE. Football concussions being just one example. An upbringing by parents with inherited sociopathia might be another. But one of the largest issues from a Capitol Hill view is 'research shows'. There really isn't any healthcare information protection available to prevent predators from making an ACE or PTSD episode sequence worse because he can access the health data of any individual within his 'range', such as a certain Olympics-related doctor had in nearby Michigan.

What might be useful is for state level governments to come to a 'constitutional census' on what qualifies as protected DNA, EHR, ACE and other information about human beings that, as our Russian and Chinese friends have demonstrated, can be used to attack them with. The fact that a multi-state system of 'research shows' implies that individual information was easily accessible without any cryptographic or identity screening of the unfortunate people.   In the modern age, shouldn't there be at least some 10th Amendment state extension of the 4th Amendment 'effects' protection that makes abuse of health information a violation of a person's Bill of Rights because such abuse adds an ACE?

2018.04.08:06:10 |CD|<3 ⋈ |GW|>1-|JU|>2|TR|<2≈|OP|<2

DeBonis, WaPost, 'Congress is back at work, without much legislating on the agenda':

"An absence of hard deadlines and the political realities of an election year mean that the $1.3 trillion spending bill that President Trump begrudgingly signed into law last month is probably the last significant legislation to pass Congress before voters go to polls in November."

New, valid AUMFs not even on the radar? No wonder the Commander in Chief has to withdraw from Syria, Afghanistan and the Ukraine. The is no longer a constitutionally valid authority for the use of military force in these areas, maybe not even a Congressional authorization to stop Russian/Syrian/Iranian chemical warfare attacks on civilians as crimes against humanity. One half of the Congresses Article I authority, general welfare and/or common defense, is not even being considered this year?

2018.04.13:08:24 Σ|CD|<3 ⋈ |GW|<1|WB<3-|JU|>2 |TR|<2≈|OP|<2

Editorial Board, WaPost, 'A few cruise missiles from Trump won't stop Syria's war crimes':

"Mr. Trump does have an advantage that Mr. Obama lacked: Thanks to the capture by U.S. and allied forces of a large part of eastern Syria, the United States has the capacity to stabilize at least part of the country and has leverage in demanding an acceptable outcome to the war."

Syria maintains 11 major chemical facilities , including one at the Russian naval base at Latakia. A much larger complex had been built in the western foothills of Aleppo, but it appears to have been degraded by various asymmetric operations and might be little more than a buried VX storage facility. The other ones around Homs are still very active but appear to be focused on World War I style chlorine production, which is very dangerous but not in the same class as VX, which is lethal at 6 mcg. Only the facility near the 'friendly' embassies in Damascus appears to be experimenting with VX. The use of chlorine sometimes means the intent is not to kill, but to permanently 'punish' a human who might oppose the ruling oligarchy or tribe such as the Alawite in Syria. You can't get chlorine out of the lungs once it is breathed in.

If we had enough troops or allies, the only way to stop chemical crimes against humanity is the physical occupation with force of each chemical facility and the space within a radius of 5 miles. Otherwise, you would be telling the criminal elite that they are ALLOWED to and have a 'right' to create WMD facilities. Surrounding nations might not even need a Security Council resolution to use occupying force; under Article 51, preemptive closure of the facilities is automatic since crimes against humanity removes all sovereignty from the perpetrator.

2018.04.11:10:35 |WB|<2⋈ |GW|>3⋈ |CD|<1 |TR|>1 |LI|<3⋈|JU|>1 ≈ |OP|<2

DePetris in TheHill, 'The US has nothing left to gain in Syria — but much to lose':

"To maintain a U.S. military presence in the country indefinitely would be the worst policy option to pursue. Countering transnational terrorism and protecting the homeland from planned attacks from radical Islamic extremists is certainly a U.S. national security interest."

You can't have it both ways. The 'transnational terrorism' is being carried out by an illegitimate clique occupying Damascus as its continuous experimentation with neurotoxin WMD on slave populations indicates. The fact that this Shiite clique is being aided and protected by two other nations also engaged in neurotoxin experimentation on opposition peoples indicates that it isn't just radical ISIS-type elements that are a 'national security interest'. It is the totalitarian belief in their own divine authority, such as the 'right' of life and death control over all humans, that is the enemy of our democracy and the rule of constitutional law.

That Caliphate mentality, whether you call it Czar, Emperor, Pharaoh, Fuhrer or Supreme Leader, that allows a 'sovereign' to kill his 'serfs' cannot be tolerated in a modern world with some 2700 molecular combinations of poison, radiation, gas, or germ WMD being built in national sanctuaries, sometimes in a Leader's own private medical facility. The existence of such a facility, including the 11 known facilities in Syria, is sufficient reason to declare an area de-sovereignized or without legitimate government, making the region's WMD locations occupiable by police force from lawful nations. If humans continue to allow ANY creation of WMD facilities under no lawful control, it is as if inviting the very primate 'divine power of kings' to attack them in the future. There are strong reasons, such as preventing crimes against humanity, for American military force to be present in Syria on a permanent basis, especially if they are protecting and aiding a local International Criminal Court process. Not a loss there.

2018.04.18:10:20 |WB| <3⋈ |GW| <2+|CD| |TR| |LI|<2 |JU|<2 ≈ |OP|<1

Wootson, WaPost, The disturbing reason behind the spike in organ donations':

"They were able to identify more than 7,313 donors who had died from drug overdoses, resulting in nearly 20,000 transplants, CNN reported. From 2000 to 2017, the number of overdose-death donors increased by 17 percent every year. In comparison, donations from people who had died in traumatic injuries increased by 1.6 percent."

Speculation: No obvious appearance of a dot-connected 'system' of for-profit induced overdoses to create available transplants, but the possible revenues from 20,000 organs actually might be $700,000,000. If even a tenth of the fentanyl/opioid overdoses were artificially induced in unsuspecting citizens for the purposes of acquiring organs, the profits in the dark-side of health care could be pretty high. Unfortunately, the agencies that might do the dot connecting on what amounts to a possible crime against humanity are being systematically defunded and reduced in personnel. Is that a coincidence unrelated to the increase in overdoses?

License with a certification on training with the weapon as specified by the majority of state laws. That is, in order to disqualify 'buffoons', not to mention serial mass murders, the concealed carry individual would have to have the training and discipline of a licensed gunsmith (type 1 License) in order to cross through federal border conditions, such as a state or territory or federal land boundary.

2018.04.19:09:53 [OP] n? ≈ ∑ |TR|>3 |LI|>3⋈|JU|>1....|GW|>2

Jackman, WaPost, 'Police chiefs implore Congress not to pass concealed-carry reciprocity gun law':

"Texas is a state that takes gun ownership seriously," said Houston Police Chief Art Acevedo. Texas requires an applicant to receive training and demonstrate proficiency with a weapon before receiving a permit. "Until we have that kind of standard nationwide," Acevedo said, "we should not be forced to accept reciprocity with places where any buffoon who has a pulse gets to carry a gun."

Pretty good advice supported by a three-fourths majority of states, which coincidentally is enough of a referendum vote to alter the meaning of the 2nd Amendment according to the requirements of Article V. But you wouldn't need a Second Constitutional Convention to satisfy both the Common Defense requirement of the Constitution and the 2nd Amendment 'right' to possess a concealed weapon WITHIN a state. To carry the weapon across a state line, you should need a Federal Firearms License equivalent to a 'type 1 dealer'

2018.04.25:13:06 [OP|n ≈ ∑ [WB] ⋈ |TR|>3 |LI|>3⋈|JU|>1....|GW|>2

Moss, BloombergView, 'Australia Shows Compulsory Voting Is No Cure-All':

"Turns out it's not so simple. Compulsory voting in Australia hasn't diminished polarization; it's merely masked it. That's one of the sobering conclusions reached by Lachlan Harris and Andrew Charlton, who analyzed electoral data and summarized their work in a Sydney Morning Herald article this month. Both have the benefit of an insider's perspective, having been aides to former Prime Minister Kevin Rudd."

From the Sydney Morning Herald, concerning the 2016 Australian Election Study:

> "In the 21st century, these binding forces have weakened and voters
> have become more disparate. Fewer people are members of

churches, unions, service and community groups. Rather than watching the evening news on TV, many Australians now get most of their news through personalised social media feeds, which can reinforce group-think among ever-more partisan communities.

The internet is the new political battleground. Political differences are being exploited by organisations that target individuals using data from Facebook, Twitter and massive email databases. Rather than prosecuting a single public manifesto, political warfare now involves personalised messages directed at the known fears and prejudices of individual voters with unprecedented precision."

Do the Aussie folks sound familiar? 'Personalised messages directed at the known fears and prejudices of individual voters' almost certainly will create dissension in a society as it did in the decade preceding the American Civil War. Much of those electronic 'messages' systems weren't even from within the American society in the last election.

But what has that to do with mandatory voting?   The higher the number of voters in an election, the higher the representative nature of the candidate who is elected. That is a major attribute of a constitutional democracy even with attempts to subvert it by foreign totalitarians.   If you were going to worry about something, worry about why that mandatory voter doesn't have a 'no confidence' choice that would eliminate candidates operating on fake news agendas. The 'no confidence' voter option should eliminate those who can't possibly represent anything except themselves.

TLO: This 21st century internet communication might require a much more sophisticated [WB] component by ALL citizens.

2018.04.25:20:18 |OP|n?

Dionne, WaPost, on Emmanuel Macron speech at Joint Session:

"Still, the French president said last week that in light of the many forces undermining democracy around the world, he did not "want to belong to a generation of sleepwalkers." On Wednesday, no one missed his sense of urgency."

Pretty good joint session of the Congress, even with a fair amount of agreement on the content. Not too many people around these days that can speak and think eloquently for the world's rational middle in two languages, let alone have the substance come out the same in both.

2018.04.26:07:16 [WB]>2⋈ [GW]>2⋈ [CD]<3

Aki Peritz in WaPost, concerning agency partisanship:

"When the institution itself speaks, that's a different story. It is inappropriate for the official social media mouthpiece of the CIA to speak out in favor or against anything expressly political. The agency's current director, Mike Pompeo, appears to understand that: The State Department's Twitter feed is not campaigning for Pompeo to be confirmed as its next secretary."

Picking or supporting a leadership candidate from within an executive branch agency might not even be constitutional. There is no devolved authority from Congressional lawmakers or the CinC authority of the Executive that can authorize such a internal 'vote' for a candidate. Picking its own leaders isn't even a matter of supplying non-policy intel to the Branches of governance, it is simply assuming an authority it doesn't have. Even if you excused out of the Constitutional box 'instances' of reacting to totalitarian attacks (who almost certainly are imminent dangers to the Nation), you would not acquire an authority to advocate publicly for an INTERNAL leader, but might advocate for a group of possible external candidates who had been 'vetted' internally. You might not even have to discuss how they were 'vetted', but could you do that for an internal candidate at all?

 If it is a domestic process, rather than operating in areas of unconstitutional anarchy, strict adherence to protecting the Constitution as employee oaths require is the only option.

2018.04.30:09:31 [WB]>2 ≈ |LI|<I⋈|JU|<3....|GW|<2

Samuelson, WaPost, 'There's a genuine solution to our health-care problem':

Many health-care experts believe that high prices — hospital and doctors' charges — as opposed to more utilization of medical services are the main reason that U.S. health spending outstrips costs in other advanced societies, says Miriam J. Laugesen of Columbia University's School of Public Health and author of "Fixing Medical Prices: How Physicians Are Paid."

There are other tomes that also agree with this approach;   Ezekiel Emanual's "Prescription for the Future" and Paul Starr's "Remedy and Reaction". One of the fundamental problems has been the 'facility' costs of the health care process that 'businessmen', doctors or otherwise, must pass on to the patient charge system in private insurance and Medicare. This is the 'ill-defined conditions' costs listed in the per illness costs to the Nation, which is $290 billion a year with circulatory diseases (heart) second at $270 billion. Ill-defined conditions include misuse of Emergency Rooms and hospital administrative cost to cover the un-insured.

One of the items being suggested is that rather than continually adjusting to the inflation of costs by providers (which has a simple greed factor as well), that the Feds pickup the costs of the healthcare infrastructure itself, which is easily with the Constitutional authorities of Article I, Section 8. The idea of mandating the Medicare fee system can be instituted as a condition of support for the facility costs, which for some doctor/providers can be 60% of his overall costs.   Facilities include standardization of record keeping, another major problem that causes mis-diagnostic deaths of some 30,000 a year. Just the healthcare facility electrical bills might be $70 billion a year. If the Feds or States combine to enhance or remove the overhead costs, it might become immediately apparent exactly who is profit motivated rather than cure motivated.

TL Opservationis 2018.05

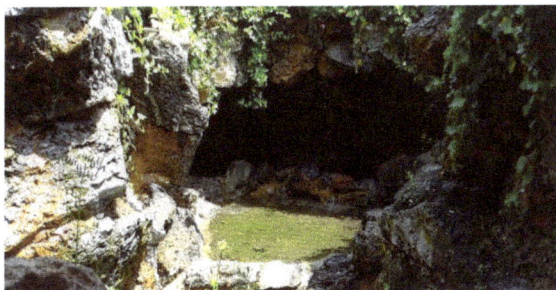

2018.05.01:06:33 |CD|<1 ⋈ |GW|>2-|JU|>2|TR|<2≈|OP|>3

Chalafant, TheHill, 'Federal 'turf war' complicates cybersecurity efforts':

"As it relates to intelligence-sharing and mission, DHS has long struggled with turf wars, first as the new kid on the block, then constant changes at the leadership levels, vacancies and lack of a clear chain of command at the middle management level," said Norton."

The problem with government cybersecurity is that you might WANT 'turf' compartmentalization so that methodology can't be compromised as it was with cyber tools and apps information released from the NSA by totalitarian sympathizers. There are several instances where humint activities in various agencies remotely picked up on cyber breaches in other agencies and were able to exploit them without disclosing their processes and there is little reason to change that to some concentrated super office that is going to be immediately targeted by the toties.

It might be better if the Congress created classified 'Authorizations for the Use of Cyber Force' that defined the compartmented 'turfs' of various agencies and their reporting chains of command. These AUCFs might also include specific definitions of cross-over authorities where an investigative cyberforce inspects another agency and rights are not abused within a constitutional context by rogue employees.

But the AUCFs will not change the real problem that has appeared in the last 20 years; the constant change-over of people and political agendas that create the chaos where cyber security, and other national securities, can not be carried out effectively. The only cure for that is an executive AI android in each SES office that has an un-erasable memory and a 40 year non-disclosure cyber encryption app that only a new CES can read. Only the President, Vice President and Speaker can possess the decrypt keys for the SES android. The only question then is how long the new SES can learn from the android to prevent the chaos the the toties love to inflict on their enemies.

2018.05.02:07:14 |LI|<1|TR|>3|WB|>2+|CD|>1 ⋈ |GW|>1-|JU|<2≈|OP|>1

Hermann, WaPost, 'Police in D.C., New York revise shooting policies in response to vehicle ramming attacks'

"William Terrill, a professor of criminal justice at Arizona State University who studies police use of force, said carefully written changes seem appropriate given threats of mass killings using vehicles. But he cautioned that they will have only an instant to judge a driver's intent."

From a tactical standpoint, in order to make any decision at all about the intent of a driver, the officer must be in front of the vehicle. Since a condition of imminent danger exists, there are no longer any 'rights' considerations and the officer is free to stop the danger anyway he can. The data in the article indicates that most such conditions have had the officer using lethal force (500 joules of kinetic energy) against the driver, but that doesn't necessarily stop the oncoming vehicle. For one thing, the normal pistol for police isn't powerful enough (450 joules) to stop a vehicle by shooting at the engine, although one or more bullets that entered the engine block would freeze the vehicle's ability to move regardless of the driver. Perhaps some experimenting could be done at Quantico on the tactical use of 5-shot 'backup' weapons that had magnum bullets (840 joules) that could stop a vehicle or a body-armored explosive vest.

You don't want the normal police weapons to be magnum because the bullets have enough energy to cause collateral damage some distance away, but a 'backup' that could stop an engine and transmission might have been appropriate in half the 193 instances of fatal encounters. Such a magnum round might even be appropriate for chases of stolen cars, although at high speeds, a frozen engine might cause the more collateral damage than bullets. There are things like 2-shot 44 magnum (1150 joules) derringers that at close range would stop a truck engine the same as 50 caliber weapons (17000 joules, very tough) used in AfPak and Iraq, so perhaps some experimentation on domestic imminent danger stoppers is appropriate.

2018.05.04:07:44 |LI|<1|TR|<3|WB|<1=|GW|n?

Scarborough in WaPost, ' Rudy Giuliani goes from 'America's Mayor' to Trump's chump':

"Why do I choose today to excavate Giuliani's record as mayor?"

This is beginning to sound like the entire New York 6th Street Plaza 'tribe', of which the author is a member, has moved their incessant 20-year long squabbles to Pennsylvania Avenue. The Plaza tribe with its media headquarters, billionaires, city government intrigues and glitz was a closed social club in New York that didn't relate to any problem outside its 5-block 'turf'. Do you suppose they have transplanted their 'turf' wars to the Nation? If so, it could be worse than the Curse of the Bambino.

2018.05.05:10:36 |OP|n?

Pallab Ghosh, BBC, 'Prof Stephen Hawking's multiverse finale':

"The laws of physics that we test in our labs did not exist forever. They crystallised after the Big Bang when the universe expanded and cooled. The kind of laws that emerge depends very much on the physical conditions at the Big Bang. By studying these we aim to get a deeper understanding of where our physical theories come from, how they arise, and whether they are unique."

If you start with a string theory estimate of multiple universes of different 'laws', such as a universe that consists entirely of 'dark' energy, then the math calculations of THIS universe might be unique. If the multiple universe concept is correct, it would be just as easy to theorize that the Big Bang happened because of a point-collision of two or three other universes in which a 'black hole' entity poured some form of combined phenomena through it to create THIS universe, and gravitational acceleration is simply one of the effects of the universes colliding. Of course, measurement of this theory would require a conscious being that could exist in both 'universes' on Hawking's arrow of time that was 20 billion years long.

2018.05.06:22:26 |WB|>?⋈ |GW|>3⋈ |CD|<1 |LI|<3⋈|JU|>1 ≈ |OP|>2

Leonnig, Harris, and Dawsey in WaPost, 'Gina Haspel, nominee to head CIA, sought to withdraw over questions about her role in agency interrogation program":

"Some White House officials were concerned by material being raised in questions from Congress, information they were just learning about, according to the U.S. officials. Those officials said the material was not revelations that have been unearthed in recent months, but the White House wanted to hear Haspel's explanation of it.'

What does that mean? If Congressional Intel Committees are examining everything about the lady, the interrogation episode (maybe 3000 man-hours out of 33 man-years) almost certainly isn't the only thing she was doing, especially after she acquired command authority as DDCI. Are there roque operatives running around that have leaked something because they are looking for a fall-girl? Or has something overseas come up where her command authority caused an operation to exceed any constitutional authority involving personnel use? Lots of people wondering around out there in the cold. The real issue doesn't change; was she acting to defend against attacks on the integrity of the Constitution as her Oath states?

I know, we can get a dozen books out of this.....

2018.05.07:09:48 |CD|>1 ≈|OP|>2 Ξ[WB]<1+|JU|>2 ⋈ |GW|>2

Sparkman, ex-Agency, in TheHill, 'In the CIA, Gina Haspel found her calling: protecting our country and freedoms':

"Whether in the CIA, the military, or Foreign Service, one of the most important days in one's career — arguably the most important — is when you hold up your right hand and pledge on your honor to uphold and defend the Constitution of the United States of America."

Very true, especially if the Oath is carried out through a lawful order from officers directly appointed and representing that Constitution. Anyone who has taken that Oath and has been given such orders don't change with seasons. As a test, did she at any time remove a subordinate for violating his oath and was the removal inside or outside the territorial jurisdiction of the Constitution? The Intel Committees might look at that test during their inquiries, not a singular operation of less than a thousand man-hours.

2018.05.07:22:20 |OP| ≈∑ |CD|>3[TR|>3 |LI|<2 ⋈ |JU|>1....|GW|>2

Ignatius, WaPost, 'Gina Haspel is tainted by her torture involvement. But she understands Russia.':

That's reassuring, in a way: Haspel's strength has been sheer competence — a calm, no-drama approach to managing complex spy operations.

and

"She has a Ph.D. in the FSB, SVR and GRU," jokes Dan Hoffman, a former Moscow station chief who worked closely with Haspel, referring to the initials of the three main Russian intelligence agencies. "That gives her a gravitas within the building and with our foreign liaison partners."

Multitasking many domain sets of complex 'systems' requires a special IQ. Even with substantial talent in all 12 of the Agency Mission Centers and 6 of the 8 operational directorates, someone viewing all of them would need perceptional IQs over and above the enhanced memory IQ of the Ph.D. types, ours or theirs. As for theirs, a study of why certain DNA haplogroups have lingered in the Moscow Oblast for such a suspiciously long time as 25,000 years might explain some things. And since she is an operations analyst on the Achilles Heels of the Muscovite Oblast totalitarians like the GRU, can we assume that those who are adamantly or fanatically opposed to her making analytical perceptions of Heels are themselves sympathetic to Leninist totalitarian influences?

2018.05.10:10:43 |CD|>3 ⋈ |GW|>1∪ |JU|<2|TR|<2 ≈ |OP|>3

Editorial Board, WaPost, 'Gina Haspel fails the test':

Similarly, Ms. Haspel's principal justification for saying that she would not allow the CIA to return to interrogations is that the agency is "not the right place to conduct interrogations. We don't have interrogators and we don't have interrogation expertise." That's true enough, but Ms. Haspel would have served herself better had she offered a principled argument, rather than a pragmatic excuse."

Lack of skilled interrogators was the principle reason the waterboarding occurred at all back then during an attack on We The People. This is like saying a policeman shouldn't shoot at an active wife-beater because the kids would be traumatized by the act in the future. In the absence of ANY mechanism for interrogation, wouldn't the principled argument be that you did what appeared necessary under the imminent danger circumstances? There are plenty of first responders, ambushed soldiers and triage doctors who had encounters that they wish they had back. Sorry, but you can't fail an ex post facto test because the Constitution prohibits everyone from making such a conditional.

TLO: in an existential threat to the constitution, Justice and Tranquility would have to suffer in terms of [OP]. There is no way around that, but the 'system' should be self correcting as the threat diminishes. To say that Justice and Liberty for the individual takes prescident over the General Welfare during an imminent threat is nonsense and displays a complete lack of understanding conceining predatory species.

2018.05.11:07:55 |CD|>1 ≈|OP|>2 Ξ |WB|<1+|JU|<2 ⋈ |GW|>3

Ignatius, WaPost, 'Tell us how this ends':

"But right now, the last thing the Middle East needs is another failed state [in Iran] — especially when it might widen the sectarian wars in Iraq, Syria, Yemen and Lebanon, like a zipper being ripped open."

Depends on how you define 'failed state'. If you have a hypocrite cult like the Pasdaran (leaders of the Iranian Revolutionary Guard) owning missile factories, oil wells, air fields and shipping vessels that are an economic 'state' engaged in terroristic activities all over the world, you might not have a choice about causing it to fail. The failure of the Pasdaran 'state' would be no different from the failure of the Nazi Schutstaffel (SS) cult within Germany. The same military ownership-for-profit of major resources by a minority 'state' cult also exists in Russia (GRU) and China (Minbing).

The failure of the Pasdaran 'state' in Iran would actually free the Iranian People to carry out a Republic as their constitution says they should, including a spiritual basis. Note that the American 'state' prohibits the intermixing of spiritual mechanisms and governance entities for the very reasons that the hypocrite Pasdaran 'state' tries to enforce by terror. In this case, the story only ends if there is a failed 'state' that frees a major people from hypocrite believers in a world Caliphate.

2018.05.13:23:17 |WB|>2 ⋈ [GW] +|CD| |TR|>3 |LI|<2 |JU|>2 ≈ |OP|>3

Editorial Board, WaPost, on another universal healthcare 'system':

"This is hardly the only option between sabotage and single-payer."

Extract from the Urban Institute study:

T H E H E A L T H Y A M E R I C A P R O G R A M TABLE 4

Health Reform Proposals Compared. Who is eligible for the new program?

Medicare-X (Kaine-Bennet): ACA Marketplace–eligible individuals and small groups

Consumer Health Insurance Protection Act (Warren): No new program; enhancements to existing programs

Healthy America (Urban Institute): All lawfully present people younger than 65

Medicare Part E (Hacker): All people lawfully present in the US

Medicare Extra (Center for American Progress): All people lawfully present in the US

Medicare for All (Sanders): All US residents

Note that the term 'citizen' is not used even though it is the U.S. citizens who must pick up the costs for any and all 'residents' healthcare in the proposals. Note also that none of the efforts (the need for a national, near universal health system is a given) describe a 'wellness' history record of each individual such as Electronic Health Records systems, which would be a pre-requisite for modern healthcare. A universal health card with lifelong diagnostics will just magically appear as the proposals gather steam. And note also that all of this comes under the authority of Article I, Section 8, clause 3, the interstate commerce clause, which one or two people might find morally offensive since the proposals concern enhancement of human life. Otherwise, the current attempts at universal care are carefully thought out.

2018.05.15:06:25 [WB]>1 ⋈ [GW] |TR| >3 |LI|<2 |JU|<2 ≈ |OP|<1

Armentano in TheHill, 'On marijuana and opioids — the DEA has no clue what it's talking about':

"One might expect the administrator of the nation's chief drug enforcement agency to be aware of at least some of this data [drug effects]. But Patterson's testimony proved otherwise."

From the DEA website:

"What is its legal status in the United States?

Marijuana is a Schedule I substance under the Controlled Substances Act, meaning that it has a high potential for abuse, no currently accepted medical use in treatment in the United States, and a lack of accepted safety for use under medical supervision. Although some states within the United States have allowed the use of marijuana for medicinal purpose, it is the U.S. Food and rug Administration that has the federal authority to approve drugs for medicinal use in the U.S. To date, the FDA has not approved a marketing application for any marijuana product for any clinical indication. Consistent therewith, the FDA and DEA have concluded that marijuana has no federally approved medical use for treatment in the U.S. and thus it remains as a Schedule I controlled substance under federal law.

Marinol, a synthetic version of THC, the active ingredient found in the marijuana plant, can be prescribed for the control f nausea and vomiting caused by chemotherapeutic agents used in the treatment of cancer and to stimulate appetite in AIDS patients. Marinol is a Schedule III substance under the Controlled Substances Act. "

Why would the author, who has vested interests in the economics of the substance, expect the DEA to know about the research? Note that the DEA does not define the use of marijuana, the Congress and the FDA as the administrative agency does. Change the laws so that Marijuana or the THC active ingredients (Marijuana, or synthetics, have several more medically beneficial ingredients) reflect the healthcare usages accurately. It isn't up to the DEA to enforce a lawful condition that doesn't exist.

What would it take to reclassify all THC related ingredients to a class III controlled substance as the research clearly indicates it is?

2018.05.16:08:08 GW|>1-[JU|>2+|LI|<3≈|OP|>3

Anapol, TheHll, 'Obama ethics chief accuses Trump of violating emoluments clause: 'See you in court Mr. Trump':

"Eisen on Monday tweeted in response to a recent report that a major development project linked to Trump in Indonesia is expected to be supported by $500 million from the Chinese government."

Article I, Section 9 of the Constitution:

"No Title of Nobility shall be granted by the United States: And no Person holding any Office of Profit or Trust under them, shall, without the Consent of the Congress, accept of any present, Emolument, Office, or Title, of any kind whatever, from any King, Prince, or foreign State."

Applying Section 9 can be pretty shaky against a president. The clause is in Article I, authorities and responsibilities of the Congress, not Article II authorities and responsibilities of the president. Further, the clause was intended to prevent direct payments to Americans by members of foreign states as a payment for services rendered. Note DIRECT payment, not remote corporate 'credit' transfers. The so-called 'injured party' in the United States must show that they were injured in a commercial activity before they could invoke constitutional conditions on a foreign economic activity. But show a DIRECT 'swamp' payment?

All this amounts to is another attempt to use 'rule of lawyers' in Washington, New York and San Francisco to carry out political harassment of office holders. The conservatives, (that is, non-constitutional conservatives), did the same thing in 2016 when they tied up 70 DOJ employees with FOIA requests for information about the Clintons and other political figures. The total cost of those legal activities, including court costs with no results, approached $300 million of which $40 million was picked up by the taxpayers. These emolument litigations(s) are almost in the same cost-benefit category; another $100 million for nothing gained?

2018.05.20:06:30 |OP|n $\approx \sum$ |TR|>3 [LI|<3⋈|JU|>1....|GW|>2+|CD|>2

Emile Bruneau in WaPost, 'Why it matters when the president calls people, even violent gang members, 'animals':

"In empirical studies on five continents involving tens of thousands of participants, my colleague Nour Kteily and I have used a provocative way to measure dehumanization: We show people the popular "ascent of man" diagram inspired by Charles Darwin, and we list groups below the diagram and ask people to place those groups along the "ascent of man" scale, from ape to advanced human, to indicate how "evolved and civilized" they judge each group to be."

The problem with the 'Ascent' diagram as a perceptional criteria is that about 70,000 years ago a series of drastic cognitive and mobility adaptions occurred that make current Homo Sapiens genetically different from all forms of the Homo Erectus species prior to that 70K years ago. It is not possible for large numbers of people to become Homo Erectus 'animals', so using the 'ascent' image might be a false dehumanization criteria.

Speculation:

From an Epigenetic (actual DNA changes in modern humans) standpoint, it might be more useful to define Homo Sapiens in terms of their predatory aggression toward other humans because there just might be 'junk' DNA in individuals that cause them to attack any humans around them. A Predator Index can indicate a lack of 'normal' Homo Sapien empathy that all 'humans' have towards each other. Lack of the genetic DNA sequences for empathy or cooperation might indicate something less than 'human'. Virtually no one equates a serial murderer as 'human' (as in MS-13?) and everyone equates altruistic acts helping others as very 'human'. Suppose you had measured people against the 11 conditions of Crimes against Humanity and used them as criteria for measuring the 'animal' characteristics of modern Homo Sapiens? Would you get much more accurate perception data from many people even if they can't see the DNA involved?

2018.05.24:08:58 |GW|<2 |CD|<3 |TR|<4 |LI|>4 |JU|>3 ≈ |OP|<1

Jenny Beth Martin in TheHill, 'Jim Jordan as Speaker is change America needs to move forward':

"Leaders, by definition, are those who succeed at getting others to follow. Great leaders envision bold possibilities, understand how to describe their vision, and are guided by steadfast principles. People gladly follow great leaders."

That assumes that a leader has 'steadfast principles' that are not based on a 19th century perception of the Constitution. If you have one group of 'leaders' who adhere to an economic 'freedom' model such as Milton Friedman envisioned AND one group of 'leaders' that adhere to the Marxist/Keynesian model of massive governance, you are NOT going to get the Preamble's remarkable balance of Common Defense and General Welfare with Justice and Liberty components. The 'steadfast principles' of the 1800s people now pray to are the problem in this century, not part of the solution.

2018.05.27:09:00 |CD|<3 ⋈ |GW|>2-|JU|<4|TR|<2 ≈ |WB|<4

Weiner, WaPost, 'Ex-spy accused of selling secrets to China claims he was trying to help the United States':

"He also spent years in the intelligence world, working as a covert case officer for the CIA from 1990 to 1996, for the Defense Intelligence Agency from 2007 to 2010, and at various government agencies and defense contractors in between. Since 2012 he has run his own consulting business.

Prosecutors say that business was failing, though, and Mallory's only income in 2017 was the $25,000 he was paid by the Chinese spies."

Timeline: Active Military 1977-1987 (age 21), Reserves 1987-2011 (age 31-40), CIA 1990-1996 (age 33-39) , Wounded 2005 (age 48), DIA 2007- 2010 (age 50-53).

Not really long enough to have a pension at any given workplace and he is pre-social security, even with a wound. One might say that is an Intelligence Community 'cheap out' since they were keeping him in a 'probationary work zone' since 1990 no matter who he worked for. A person wondering about the intelligence world without any long-term arrangements could be tempted to do lots of things, but what does that say about the Intel Communities' Human Resources 'system'?

If a person knew he had no possible long-term arrangement in a stressful, dangerous occupation, why would he go near it or would he try to make a 'score' while he could? How many more cases of mis-handled Human Resource operations are out there that need a 'Justice' fix? Is America really becoming a find 'em, field 'em, forget 'em society?

TLO: Own IC experiences affecting perception? Individuals don't count, except when the ripple effects of poor treatment affect [OP]?

TL Opservationis 2018.06

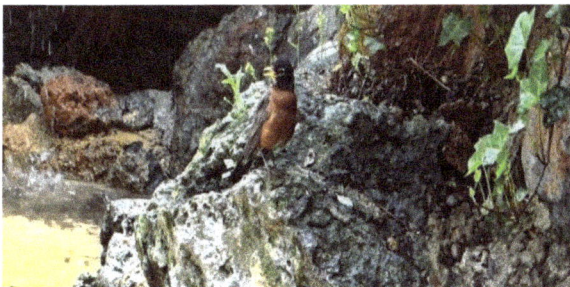

2018.06.01:06:28 |WB|<2⋈ |GW|>2⋈ |TR|>1 |LI|<3⋈|JU|<3 ≈ |OP|<2

Wax-Thibdeaux, WaPost, 'Arkansas abortion pill restriction seen as both protecting women and a major rights setback':

"The woman, now 27, said that the pill option instead of a surgical abortion seemed "less traumatic during an already emotionally traumatic time."

She said she thought about giving the child up for adoption, but the man, whom she described as "sexually abusive," said he would not sign over parental rights.

She said she didn't "want to bring a child into that situation."

Males or females who are 'sexually abusive' are usually prone to turning a partner into some form of involuntary servitude rather than having a genuinely empathic relationship. There are vast numbers of instances in which children are created for the simple purpose of enhancing the 'servitude' relationship rather than creating better life. Many of the children that appear on the borders as 'anchor' babies are there because of a cynical, morally depraved attempt to use them as commercial slaves by men and women 'owners'.

But note the 13th Amendment: "Neither slavery nor involuntary servitude, except as a punishment for crime whereof the party shall have been duly convicted, shall exist within the United States, or any place subject to their jurisdiction."

That should mean that ANY act that compels a form of servitude in another human qualifies as enslavement, including the process of forced pregnancy in a woman. Doesn't that mean that ANY process or law that enhances a condition of involuntary servitude through abuse of fetuses or children is unconstitutional according to the wording of the 13th Amendment? A law that allows the possibility of child or fetus enslavement, such as an anti-abortion pill law or parental rights laws to an anchor baby, should be unconstitutional in an 'enlightened' interpretation of using sex as a form of indenture rather than actual life enhancement.

2018.06.01:14:00 |CD|<4?

Timberg, WaPost, 'Signs of sophisticated cellphone spying found near White House, U.S. officials say':

"The same May 22 letter revealed that DHS was aware of reports that a global cellular network messaging system, called SS7, was being used to spy on Americans through their cellphones. Such surveillance, which can intercept calls and locate cellphones from anywhere in the world, are sometimes used in conjunction with IMSI catchers."

Russian Proverb:

Не бойся собаки, что лает, а бойся той, что молчит и хвостом виляет.

Don't be afraid of the dog who barks, but be afraid of the one who is silent and wags its tail.

2018.06.02:06:21 $|OP|n \approx \sum |TR|>3 |LI|>3 \bowtie |JU|>1 |CD|>2....|GW|>2$

Will, WaPost , 'The president we didn't know we always wanted':

The only president to have reached the Oval Office without first appearing on a ballot for either vice president or president, Ford became vice president (under the 25th Amendment) when scandals forced Richard Nixon's vice president, Spiro Agnew, to resign. Ford became president when Nixon resigned. Had Ford been assassinated, his vice president, Nelson Rockefeller (also confirmed by Congress under the 25th Amendment), would have become president."

The 25th Amendment was only 7 years old in 1974 and was largely the result of succession problems after the Kennedy assassinations. Or was there a sense in the 1960s that included the Constitution's Preamble concept 'secure the Blessings of Liberty to ourselves and our Posterity'? The Founders were noticeably interested in the Posterity covenant of the Preamble and there was some of this 'future view' in all of the Amendments after. Does that future view still exist or is living for the moment as media events all that's left?

2018.06.04:21:51 $|WB|>2 \bowtie |GW|>3 \bowtie |CD|<1 |TR|<1 |LI|<3 \bowtie |JU|>1 |OP|>2$

Whittington in TheHill, 'Not everyone is thrilled that Jeff Bezos wants to go back to the moon':

"Ozimek artfully leaves out what the quality of life might be for between 11 billion to 12 billion people packed in dense urban jungles, consigned to Earth without access to the boundless resources that space has to offer."

Anyone who has studied the DNA maps of human demographics on earth can easily postulate that Malthusian Population Traps would gradually sink humanity into a perpetual system of survival economics in which 'cleansing' WMD on other populations would be the only way to obtain the resources for a technological civilization. Once those resources are consumed by perpetual genocide conflict to get those very same resources, there won't be enough people or material left to even explore space. Five billion more people on a warming earth is not really an evolutionary advance.

Rather than just go to the moon with thousands of intelligent droids who can dig up the landscape (humans won't be able to survive that....), it might be better to consider Wernher Von Braun's 1950s 'wheel' space station with ion drive engines on it so it could actually go into several planetary orbits and even mine the extensive metals in the Astroid Belt or gas giant moons. The rotating wheel concept would allow a gravitational ability inside the 'wheel' space ship/station, something that might keep the human DNA from mutating drastically. Recent international space station long-period occupancy has shown human DNA undergoes subtle changes that might become permanent, so some of the humans going to the moon or elsewhere might not return as 'humans'. But planting humans on other planets as 'colonists' instead of a resource exploration vehicle? Why do that if you aren't evolving life on earth first?

2018.06.08:17:40 [JU]|[LI]|[TR]|⋈|[WB]≈ [OP|n

Krauthammer, WaPost, 'A note to readers':

"I believe that the pursuit of truth and right ideas through honest debate and rigorous argument is a noble undertaking. I am grateful to have played a small role in the conversations that have helped guide this extraordinary nation's destiny."

As always, thanks for your help on this and good luck.

2018.06.11:07:18 [CD]|<3 ⋈ [GW]>1-[JU]>2|TR|<2 ≈| WB|n |OP|<2

Juan Williams, TheHill, 'Trump's immigration outrage':

"The administration may claim its policy of separating families at the border is aimed at discouraging illegal immigration, but the number of border crossings has risen since the policy was implemented.

Also, the New York Times reported last week that many of the families being detained "enter at official border crossings and request asylum, which is not an illegal entry."

Why would a rational 'family' risk permanent separation, a lawful requirement in most states for parental disfunction or child endangerment, by bringing babies a thousand miles to a closed border? The author's two statements together imply that a political or economic agenda south of the closed border is at work and that the children are being used as marketable 'slaves' for that agenda. Are you freeing 'slaves' by removing them from their 'parents' or 'owners'? The issue is: why are they there to begin with, not what happens as a later reaction to their presence.

That suspicion of enslavement comes from one who has personally verified the need for nearly one million new 'citizens' a year, including next generation children. Current population growth in the U.S. is less than one percent and this isn't enough to sustain the economy even with the addition of 800,000 robotic jobs per year. Those robotic jobs, by the way, replace the unskilled work that might be done by those on the border. Somebody, somewhere, is gaining economically from this child misery and it isn't Americans.

The American mistake is exactly what the author says: failure to have a rational immigration policy. EXCEPT that the failure is 30 years long. Some avenue for citizenship is clearly needed, especially for healthcare eligibility at taxpayer expense, and that is a very clearly defined authority of the Congress in the Naturalization Clause. It is NOT the responsibility of the six Executives for the past 30 years, with endless yoyo effects on enforcement.

2018.06.13:23:25 [WB]n?

Phillips, WaPost, 'Albert Einstein decried racism in America. His diaries reveal a xenophobic, misogynistic side'

"I'm not apologizing for him or anything. … I still feel that the unpleasant remarks are quite shocking, but they do reveal that we all have this darker side to our attitudes and prejudices," he said."

Einstein's comment in these diaries sound suspiciously like quotes from his philosophical mentor in the 1880s, Immanuel Kant, who was known to maintain, and helped create, a prevalent view of Europe's Social Darwinism in many of his writings. Einstein was well aware of both Kant and Darwin by the 1920s when the voyages took place. The precise quotes by Albert also were made in a context of Asian dock areas in seaports. Anyone who has sailed around the world and visited harbor dock areas is going to have a certain view of the 'locals' inhabiting those docks and it is hardly xenophobic.

This commentary of 'The Travel Diaries of Albert Einstein' sounds suspiciously like an ex post facto perception based on modern intellectual stereotypes of 'race'. The term 'xenophobic' didn't even exist in the Social Darwinism era of Einstein and the concept of 'xenophilia' or the neurological programming of inherited fear of others certainly didn't exist before this century.

2018.06.15:00:00 |CD|<3 ⋈ |GW|<2-|JU|>2|TR|<2 ≈ |OP|<?

CRS InFocus, IF10906, 'CIA Ethics Education: Background and Perspectives':

"CIA officers also receive extensive ethics training specific to intelligence, which includes case studies of ethically challenging operational scenarios, to prepare them for the operational side of their jobs. This training includes familiarization with the legal authorities for the conduct of intelligence activities, principally Executive Order 12333, The Intelligence Community, as amended, and CIA's AR 2-2, Law and Policy Governing the Conduct of Intelligence Activities. However, while these baseline references spell out dos and don'ts from a legal standpoint, there is little mention of ethics per se. Section 2.1, of E.O. 12333, for example, merely requires intelligence collection be done in a manner that is "respectful of the principles upon which the United States was founded."

TLO:

How would they contribute to a Second Convention protective screen against foreign IC groups attempting to influence its deliberations.? First Convention in 1787 didn't have that problem. Could they have a 'detention' authority where habeas corpus didn't apply during the period of the Convention? How would their 'international' ethics prevent them from interfering with such deliberations for their own interests? Note the effect of the Pasdaran on the Iranian Guardian Council and the GRU influence on the Federation Council.

2016.06.19:11:13 |TR|<2=∑ |LI|>1WB|<2 ⋈ |GW|>1-|JU|>2….|OP|>3

Daley and Vaughan in WaPost, 'the only people who can fix gerrymandering now are voters':

"Just last week in Husted v. A. Philip Randolph Institute, the Supreme Court upheld Ohio's policies of purging voters from the rolls after not participating in three federal elections (and not responding to official notices mailed to their homes)."

In other words, people who were deceased or moved from a given federal District were removed from voter registration BECAUSE they were no longer a citizen in that District. The author is suggesting that any person who occupies space in America has a 1st Amendment 'right' to vote. That would include the 22 million KNOWN alien visitors who have established residency without citizenship, 3 million of whom appear as tourists in the months before an election in the United States. It may even include the 800,000 non-citizens who acquire registration 'rights' in urban areas like Miami, NYC and LA and then send in absentee ballots from the Riviera or Macao casino hotels.

Speculation: Technically, a person must prove citizenship in order to vote, see 15th Amendment, Section 1, and the Voting Rights Act General Provisions defined the conditions for defining that. Technically, if a defined citizen does not carry out his responsibility to vote, and that doesn't mean he gets a limousine to take him to a polling place, he can be 'taxed'. The prohibited poll tax only applies to citizens who are voting, not to those who negligently skip from one cycle to the next. In fact, if the citizen moves from one place to another without voting, he should be paying the 'citizenship negligence' tax in each location.

But non-citizens having voting rights simply because they have occupied space in America? NOT.

2018.06.21:07:21 |CD|<1 |LI|>3 ≈ |OP|>1 Ξ [WB]<1+|JU|<2 ⋈ [GW]>2

Editorial Board, WaPost, on current immigration:

"In fact, immigration rates are not soaring. In fact, dangerous criminals are not streaming in from the Middle East. In fact, immigrants — legal and illegal — commit crime at a lower rate than native-born Americans. In fact, most immigrants are doing what they have always done: helping to build up America and secure a better life for their children."

That 'lower rate' study involves only six counties in Texas, not the Nation, but the studies on the need for immigrants improving the Nation will hold up. Unfortunately, the article re-creates and enhances the original immigration problem that has existed for the last half century; that there is a 'right' to come to the United States and live regardless of the rule of law. Equating legal and illegal occupation of American space as 'normal' is itself a usurpation of the rule of law if not the Article I, Section 8 authorities of the Constitution. A person simply DOES NOT have a right to enter the country without a lawful invitation and the left/right dogmas that prevented reasonable 'invitations' by legislation are the problem.

2018.06.22:05:26 [WB]<3⋈ [GW]>3⋈ |CD|<2 ≈ |TR|>1 |LI|<3 ⋈ |JU|<4

Scarborough in WaPost, 'The most damning element of this tragic American tale':

"If nothing else, such a shift would recognize military reality. Now 2,300 kids are held in unknown locations with unknown individuals inside and absolutely no outside observation."

2300 kids could not have shown up on the border without a well organized political entity arranging it; the logistics of that many people require funding and structure. Describing the injustice of U.S. detention by the media and various political opportunists is carefully avoiding any description of the cause of the problem. That is, who committed the act of a crime against humanity by trafficking those children over a thousand miles? The cartels that run provincial governments in Central America or who? Find the cause, not wallow in the costly ripple effects of it.

2018.06.22:08:08 |CD|<3 ≈ |OP|>1 Ξ|WB|>1+[JU]<2 ⋈ |GW|<2

The Editors, BloombergView, 'Trump's 'Space Force' Is No Joke. It Might Even Work':"If nothing else, such a shift would recognize military reality. Space is an increasingly critical battlefield. Across its five branches, the U.S. military uses space-based technology for navigation, reconnaissance, weather forecasting, intelligence collection, communications, command and control, precision targeting, and much else. Its reliance on satellite-guided munitions has increased with each new conflict in recent years.

From the Diplomat, 2014.09.10, 'China's Military Creates New Space Force':

"Notably, the Yomiuri Shimbun article mentions the new Aerospace Force unit as an afterthought in a larger article about the new Joint Operations Command Center the PLA has established as a way to strengthen joint operations between different military services. This is significant because joint operations and space capabilities were both emphasized as central features of the Chinese military doctrine of winning "local wars under modern, high-tech conditions" (later changed to "local wars under informationized conditions").

Of course, China has been steadily expanding the PLA's space capabilities, including conducting an anti-satellite test (ASAT) earlier this year as well as last year. It also conducted an ASAT test in 2007 that destroyed a defunct Chinese weather satellite."

Note the Diplomat article date, 2014.09.10. Only a matter of time before some totalitarian system tries to 'occupy' the space between the earth and the moon in order to win 'local wars' on Earth. Oddly enough, a new American space force could be immediately tasked with operating droids in near space that removes the several million tons of precision alloy 'junk' orbiting the Earth. Such Space Force droid/drones might even be able to dissipate methane layers in the atmosphere, which are a large contributor of global warming acceleration. Reducing methane layers by 30% might cause a full one degree drop in the global average temperature, quite significant for human life.

But getting totalitarian space forces to do something useful like methane reduction? Not likely if you are imperialistic oligarchies. That, in turn, puts a new Space Force easily within the Common Defense AND General Welfare prime directives of the Constitution.

2018.06.23:06:09 [OP]n

In WaPost, in memory of Charles Krauthammer:

Charles is widely quoted in a series of books about Washington's Constitutional processes called the 'Chronicles of the Kwedaki Dikep' because he could range over a wide variety of those Constitution related subjects. Here are some of the extracts from his Post opinions in 2014. Hopefully, the Washington Post will keep his opinion archive set available for further inspection in spite of totalitarian suppression agendas. The bracket symbols reference the constitutional sets he was looking at. He will be remembered in this book as a strong contributor.

2014.02.06:21:26, [GW] [WB] [TR]:

Krauthammer, WaPost, about medical debacles: "moreover, other antioxidants, folic acid and B vitamins, and multivitamin and mineral supplements are ineffective for preventing mortality or morbidity due to major chronic diseases."

2014.02.29:00:00, [GW] [CD] [TR] [LI] [JU] [OP] :

Krauthammer, WaPost, on the latest version of Russian imperialism: "Sure, Obama is sympathetic to democracy. But it must arise organically, from internal developments. "These democratic movements will be more sustainable if they are seen as . . . coming from within these societies," says deputy national security adviser Benjamin Rhodes. Democracy must not be imposed by outside intervention but develop on its own."

2018.06.25:11:21 [TR]<2 = ∑ [LI]>1WB]<2 ⋈ [GW]>1-[JU]<2....[OP]<1

Rappaport and Veomett in TheHill, 'The silver lining in the Supreme Court gerrymandering decision':

"These are all valid [outlier model] maps, in that they satisfy widely accepted parameters for what a districting plan should look like, with contiguous geography and compact shape, among other measures. For each of these maps, the analysis determines how many districts each party would have won using past election data. Most voting maps generate roughly comparable numbers of Republican and Democratic representatives getting seats in Congress."

This mapping technique would not satisfy the Republic form of representation guaranteed by Article V, Section 4 of the Constitution, the originating authority for Supreme Court inspection of 'harm' to a given Electoral District population. The only mathematics model that could truly define a Electoral District, or a state Senate seat, is one in which at least 51 percent of the eligible citizens were taken into account in some form that did not 'harm' their vote. The math model would have to have an independent category as well as a eligible non-voter category (somebody who missed an election, but was in the census as an adult citizen).

That would mean that the outlier model had any combination of Republican, Democratic, Independent, and No-Confidence voters that made up 51 percent based on the census count (which may have an unconstitutional 'race' rather than 'citizen' measure in its accounting forms) and not the previous vote records which might be less than 30 percent of a District population. The Constitutional 'harm' is automatic if the represented voters in a given District do not SUM into a 51 percent majority regardless of affiliation.

2018.06.26:11:21 |OP|n ≈∑ |TR|>3 |LI|>3⋈|JU|>1....|GW|>2

Patton, WaPost, 'Charleston's apology for slavery is just empty symbolism':

"On social media, some people are saying there should be no apology for slavery because no one alive today should be held responsible for those past wrongs."

Article I, Section 9, U.S. Constitution:

No Bill of Attainder or ex post facto Law [a law that is enforced retroactively in the CURRENT timeline] shall be passed.

While that is generally applied to the authorities of the Congress to make laws, it can also mean that an individual citizen should not hold a mindset that is ex post facto or seeks reparation from the nearest available body for some past injustice. In this century, with a strong national DNA or genomic diversity existing, ANY mind-set involving racial injustice of three centuries ago (importation of slaves into Charleston was formally made criminal on 1 January 1808, not 1865, by the Congress) applied now would violate the intent of the Constitution. Basing laws on a previous injustice is a disservice to the meaning of the Constitution; try removing the mutually degrading xenophilia found in ALL skin tones instead.

2018.06.28:12:23 ∑ |LI|>3|TR|<2|WB|<2+| ξ |<n? ⋈ |GW|>1-|JU|<2 ≈ |OP|>

Ashley Baker in TheHill, 'Gorsuch's dissent in 'Carpenter' case has implications for the future of privacy':

"Rather than focus on the reasonable expectation of privacy analysis typically engaged in by the court in recent decades, Gorsuch's dissent argues that the court should follow a property rights-based theory of the Fourth Amendment. Under that theory, Carpenter had a property interest in his cell phone data. Gorsuch's decision to file a dissent may send a message to future defendants that without inclusion of a property-based argument his concurrence cannot be counted on."

Fourth Amendment, BOR:

"The right of the people to be secure in their persons, houses, papers, and effects, against unreasonable searches and seizures, shall not be violated, and no Warrants shall issue, but upon probable cause, supported by Oath or affirmation, and particularly describing the place to be searched, and the persons or things ..."

Note the 'and' between the two clauses. If one was an Originalist, the 'and' would mean that the 'to be secure in their effects' was a right in its own context and not dependent on the following clause involving government or judiciary warrants describing the 'effect'. As a stand alone human right, ANY seizure of a person's effects (ie, property) by ANY party would be an abuse of the right. Since information about a person is created in real time by that person, it should be his property under copyright law at least, not ANY third party who may hold it and definitely not someone who reproduces it for his own use. That would be a clear violation of the individual's intellectual property rights and might even be extended to include his DNA structure since he is continually recreating it with new DNA cells in his body. Wither the DNA was originally created by the parents and might belong to them is another matter.

In this instance of Court analysis, the 'effects' right of electronic data might supercede any other persons right to the data, including governmental, so the Carpenter opinion might be perfectly correct.

Question: If the 'effect' information in a mobile device involved a probable cause that it would cause harm to others as an imminent threat, such as a cell phone triggering an IED or nerve gas canister, would the individual right still stand? In virtually any case of even suspected imminent danger to others, the individual rights are suspended and that too is perfectly correct from a Constitutional point. How would the Court interpret an imminent danger threat VS rights in a molecular (EMR, electronic, binary, DNA, etc.) property context?

OVERVIEW 2018.07 to .10

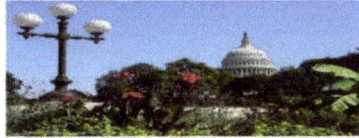

TIME LINE 2018.07.nn

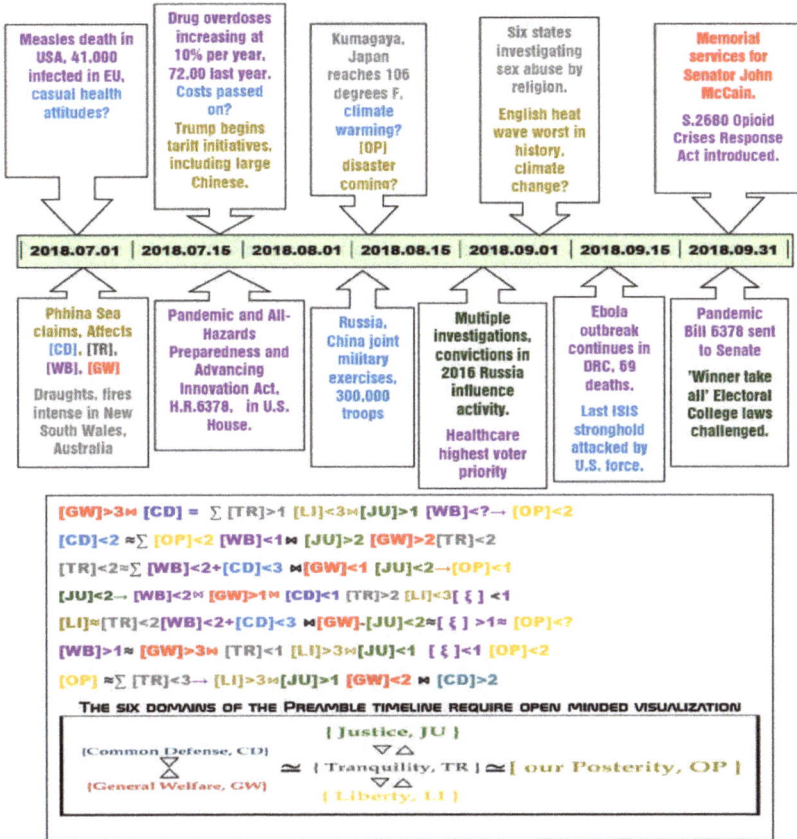

| Measles death in USA, 41,000 infected in EU, casual health attitudes? | Drug overdoses increasing at 10% per year, 72.00 last year. Costs passed on? Trump begins tariff initiatives, including large Chinese. | Kumagaya, Japan reaches 106 degrees F. climate warming? [OP] disaster coming? | | Six states investigating sex abuse by religion. English heat wave worst in history. climate change? | | Memorial services for Senator John McCain. S.2680 Opioid Crises Response Act introduced. |

| 2018.07.01 | 2018.07.15 | 2018.08.01 | 2018.08.15 | 2018.09.01 | 2018.09.15 | 2018.09.31 |

| Phhina Sea claims, Affects [CD], [TR], [WB], [GW] Draughts, fires intense in New South Wales, Australia | Pandemic and All-Hazards Preparedness and Advancing Innovation Act, H.R.6378, in U.S. House. | Russia, China joint military exercises, 300,000 troops | Multiple investigations, convictions in 2016 Russia influence activity. Healthcare highest voter priority | Ebola outbreak continues in DRC, 69 deaths. Last ISIS stronghold attacked by U.S. force. | Pandemic Bill 6378 sent to Senate 'Winner take all' Electoral College laws challenged. |

[GW]>3⋈ [CD] = ∑ [TR]>1 [LI]<3⋈[JU]>1 [WB]<?→ [OP]<2

[CD]<2 ≈∑ [OP]<2 [WB]<1⋈ [JU]>2 [GW]>2[TR]<2

[TR]<2≈∑ [WB]<2÷[CD]<3 ⋈[GW]<1 [JU]<2→[OP]<1

[JU]<2→ [WB]<2⋈ [GW]>1⋈ [CD]<1 [TR]>2 [LI]<3[ξ] <1

[LI]≈[TR]<2[WB]<2÷[CD]<3 ⋈[GW]-[JU]<2≈[ξ] >1≈ [OP]<?

[WB]>1≈ [GW]>3⋈ [TR]<1 [LI]>3⋈[JU]<1 [ξ]<1 [OP]<2

[OP] ≈∑ [TR]<3→ [LI]>3⋈[JU]>1 [GW]<2 ⋈ [CD]>2

THE SIX DOMAINS OF THE PREAMBLE TIMELINE REQUIRE OPEN MINDED VISUALIZATION

[Common Defense, CD] ⟨Justice, JU ⟩
         ▽△
      ⋈ ⟨ Tranquility, TR ⟩ ≅ [our Posterity, OP]
         ▽△
[General Welfare, GW] ⟨ Liberty, LI ⟩

Figure 10.   Overview 2018.07

TL Opservationis 2018.07

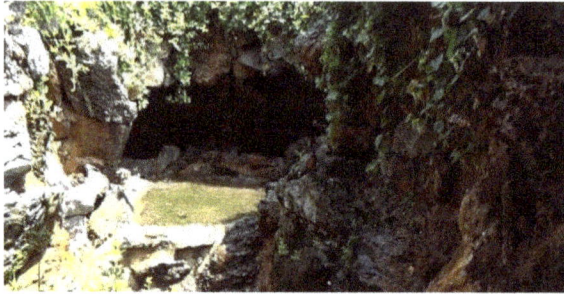

2018.07.01:07:06 [LI|>5 ≈ |TR|<2[WB|<2-[JU|>2|OP|<1

Sarah Turberville and Anthony Marcum in WaPost, 'Those 5-to-4 decisions on the Supreme Court? 9 to 0 is far more common.':

"The ratio is staggering. According to the Supreme Court Database, since 2000 a unanimous decision has been more likely than any other result — averaging 36 percent of all decisions. Even when the court did not reach a unanimous judgment, the justices often secured overwhelming majorities, with 7-to-2 or 8-to-1 judgments making up about 15 percent of decisions. The 5-to-4 decisions, by comparison, occurred in 19 percent of cases."

If one tracks that SC database over several years and monitors those 9-0 decisions, he will find that one of the major themes of those unanimous decisions concerned 'rights' VS the Constitution. In a very large number of instances, someone somewhere decided that whatever he was doing at the time was somehow his 'right' to do it and challenged the 'authorities' about his 'right'. The SC consensus almost always said that the Constitution superceded a narcissistic belief that anything a person did was automatically a 'god given' right to do it.

Bottom line: If you want to live in the United States, your instinctive, inherited desires to do whatever you want, including harming others, are not guaranteed as inalienable rights that you have made supreme instead of the Constitution.

2018.07.05:07:01 [LI|>3| ≈ TR|<2[WB|<2+|CD|>3 ⋈[GW|>1-[JU|<2⋈ |OP|>3

Bruenig, WaPost, 'Conservatives will always call socialists hypocrites. Ignore them.':

"it's only the white-collar world, collegiate life and its professional aftermath that prepare one for the kind of slick self-promotion and brand packaging that translate into skill with donors and voters.

This isn't inherent. Anyone can learn it — you just have to be given the opportunity, and only the relatively well-to-do generally are."

This assumes that the 'collegiate life' doesn't create the hypocrisy or narcissism inherent in both the Leninist red shirts and the Friedmanist brown shirts, depending on the 'school' one attends. The hypocrisy of both lies in their belief that the earned, note self-earned, wealth of citizens in general is an extractable property that both are free to manipulate through Constitutional systems of 'law'. Tax rates are adjusted according to the hypocrisy of one faction of partisans and are reversed by the hypocrisy of another faction a few years later without any regard to the Common Defense and General Welfare prime directives of the Constitution. Healthcare is 'lawfully' treated by both partisan factions as a form of interstate commerce rather than an altruistic enhancement of life. From a national operations research view, which comes first, the partisan hypocrisy or citizen voter attempts to correct for its damages?

From a purely practical standpoint, an individual who engages in politics does require a self discipline about managing wealth and time but is it 'collegiate'? Modern politics requires the ability to create and/or manage a continual net-worth of nearly a million dollars, as many in Congress with more than one term can attest, regardless of political belief. Even a truck driver coming into the 'system' would have to do that with a one million minimum, and hopefully he would extend that wealth management to other citizens. Without the hypocrisy.

2018.07.07:13:03 |OP|n?= |LI|<1|TR|<2|WB|<3?

Schneider, WaPost, 'Jefferson's powerful last public letter reminds us what Independence Day is all about':

Looney wrote in announcing the discovery, : "the later note speaks to something else: "the private Jefferson who to the last could not deny himself imported luxury goods for which he could not pay."

That is a very unwarranted assumption. Note the condition Jefferson was in:

"Worst of all, Jefferson suffered terrible health problems. He had chronic diarrhea and difficulty urinating, possibly from prostate cancer. His doctor prescribed the opiate laudanum."

It is very unlikely anyone with the age and intestinal problems of Jefferson could consume acidic wines. It is more likely he was trying to maintain things for any remaining guests who might wonder in. The comment that he had mismanaged Monticello might be unwarranted too; it could be the Estate was falling apart because Jefferson did not believe in slavery enough to use force on the few remaining slaves there, force which may have been required by the laws of a radical Richmond oligarchy, not him.

2018.07.10:09:32 |TR|>2 = |LI|>2 -|JU|<2....|OP|>3 + |CD|<1 ◄ |GW|>2

Sunstein, BloombergOpinion, 'The Test for Judge Kavanaugh; It is worth figuring out whether a Supreme Court nominee believes in judicial restraint.:

"Whether it comes from the left or the right, judicial restraint is honorable, especially if it operates in a nonpartisan manner. But movement conservatism – like its left-wing sibling – is a major threat to democratic ideals. It is well worth figuring out whether any Supreme Court nominee, including Judge Kavanaugh, subscribes to it."

Judicial restraint in a nonpartisan manner has plenty of room to work within the Constitutional intent as stated in the Preamble. Its six covenants are Justice (individual and for all), Tranquility (between states and between people), Common Defense,

General Welfare, Liberty (freedom to live without material indenture by others), and our, note OUR, Posterity.

Nonpartisan or even bipartisan inspection of conditions within a context of Article III, Section 2, Judicial Power has considerable leeway when Posterity (Justices are appointed for life, so Posterity is their domain) is applied to the other covenants, especially in cases of Justice for all vs Justice for each. Perceptions by the Court are Posterity oriented regardless of the other covenant combinations they examine and Justices can shift as needed in those six covenants without being 'labeled' by partisan dogmas.

2018.07.14:07:22 CD|<3 ⋈ |GW|<1 - |JU|<2|TR|<2 ≈ |OP|<1

Nakashima and Harris, WaPost, 'How the Russians hacked the DNC and passed its emails to WikiLeaks':

"The hackers worked for the spy agency called the Main Intelligence Directorate of the General Staff, or GRU, the indictment said.

They also allegedly targeted a state election board, identified by U.S. officials as Illinois. The Russians stole information about 500,000 voters, including names, addresses, partial Social Security numbers, dates of birth and driver's license numbers, according to the indictment."

Andrei Sakharov, oppressed Russian scientist of the Stalinist era:

"Our country, like every modern state, needs profound democratic reforms. It needs political and ideological pluralism, a mixed economy and protection of human rights and the opening up of society."

The Main Intelligence Directorate has shown how Sakharov's idea can work in Russia. But will it be Chinese from the East or Europeans from the West that 'opens up society' to democratic reforms? The only thing that is certain is the GRU oligarchy can't.

Further:

Item 1 has straw man conditionals. No one has suggested the GRU did that. They did gain 'dossiers' on most of the American Republican and Democrat partisans in a manner that they could control the funding of individual candidates from proxy accounts. This gives direct, influencing control of both parties to Mikhail Lesin in the Moskva Oblast . Remember the GRU objective, even since 1917, has been to undermine the concept of democracy and favor the Russian 'Nobility' system. Item 3 is false because the American 'security' services have been defending the constitutional concept of democracy since 1917.

2018.07.15:08:06 CD|<3 ⋈ |GW|>1-|JU|>2|TR|<2≈|OP|>3

Turley, TheHill, 'Ignore the spin — still no evidence of Trump collusion':

"Not long ago, our hacking of our own allies, including German Chancellor Angela Merkel, was revealed. Many nations regularly try to influence elections and this is nothing new for the United States, either as the culprit or as the target of such efforts.

In other words, if there were a real hunt for election witches, we would find ourselves at the head of the line to the pillory.

Does that mean that the Mueller investigation is somehow invalid? Of course not. This remains an attack on our system, there is still work to be done, and we should all want the FBI to continue that work unimpeded."

The issue might be whether the activity was carried out as an attempt to undermine the constitutional basis of a society. American siding with a partisan entity in a country is not the same as activities carried out as a military operation of imperialism. The GRU is the Main Intelligence Directorate of the GENERAL STAFF of the Russian Army, responsible for imperialist aggression against other states. One could say that the CIA usurped the Iranian secular constitution when Mossadegh was overthrown in 1952 unless one realized that the autocratic, totalitarian authorities Mossadegh had acquired in spite of the constitution were through the efforts of the GRU from the largest Soviet embassy in the world in Tehran. Sound familiar, Mr Erdogan next door in Ankara?

The issue is whether a MILITARY attack is underway in a country, not a political 'agent of change' activity that may or may not benefit the 'people' in a country. There can be no sociological gain from a totalitarian military activity. That's not their given orders.

2018.07.16:07:40 |CD|<3 ⋈ |GW|>3-[JU|<1|TR|>2 ≈ |OP|>1

Staniland in WaPost, 'The U.S. military is trying to manage foreign conflicts — not resolve them. Here's why.':

"As long as the U.S. government can limit the domestic costs of violence management overseas, few Americans will have incentives to pay attention to these low-level, far-flung wars."

Article I, Section 8, clause 11 gives the constitutional authority for declaring 'war' and virtually none of the current American military activities constitute a condition of 'war'. Violence management, as expressed in this article, would fall under clause 10, 'to define and punish Piracies and Felonies committed on the high Seas, and Offenses against the Laws of Nations.' That means pursuit and neutralization of cartel-level criminal attacks on humanity, which very few Americans object to, especially if they have been targeted by such criminal behavior.

Any police/military force engaged in violence management around the world that reduces the terroristic Offenses against the Laws of Nations (crimes against humanity) is a legitimate expression of American society, even if not directly authorized in each instance by the Congress. It is a well known academic misperception of the human race to regard all military force as an automatic act of 'war', which normally involves, according to Sun Tzu's 'Art of War', total destruction of the enemy society.

2018.07.24:22:58 |CD|<3? ≈ |OP|>2 Ξ|WB|<1+|JU|<2 ⋈ |GW|>2|LI|>3

Ignatius, WaPost, 'Trump can't win at foreign policy the way he wins at golf':

"The rest of the team has to know . . . what play you're calling. In golf, it's just between you and the ball. I think that's a major weakness. . . . The world is far too complicated for one person to control everything."

Scott Mautz, Inc. Magazine, 'Psychology and Neuroscience Blow-Up the Myth of Effective Multitasking':

"Earl Miller, a professor of neuroscience at MIT, says we simply can't focus on more than one thing at a time. Period. But what we can do is shift our focus from one thing to the next with astonishing speed.

Says Miller, "Switching from task to task, you think you're actually paying attention to everything around you at the same time. But you're actually not." The brain is forced to switch among multiple cognitive tasks as these tasks use the same part of the brain.

The catch here is that this task-switching, despite how fast it occurs, is incredibly unproductive in reality--I mean like Candy Crush unproductive.

In fact, research indicates up to 40 percent of productivity could be lost due to task-switching. It actually takes more time to complete the tasks you're switching between and you make more errors than when you focus on doing one task at a time in order."

A homosapien, neurologically advanced or otherwise, has no chance of operating a major complex entity with 3500 varying conditions per month like a head of state gets handed to him. That has become the major reason the long-lived oligarchic committee 'rulers' around the world have had more success at political power than nations who rely on pure democracy 'systems' with their constant trivia multi-tasking.

2018.07.25:08:50 |CD|>3 ⋈ |GW|>1-|JU|>2|TR|<2 ≈ |OP|>3

Representative Lesko, AZ-8, in TheHill, 'Congress must provide for the common defense':

"Thankfully, this year's National Defense Authorization Act, or NDAA, focuses on rebuilding our military and reinvesting in our national defense so America can remain the land of the free.

Years of reduced funding, sequestration, and the threat of Base Relocations and Closures have decimated our military and hampered our readiness and capabilities as threats arise."

Noticeably absent from this NDAA 2019 are provisions for the creation of a new 'trainer' aircraft and acquisition of pilots using such aircraft. It would take very little effort to start reproducing the multi-national defense aircraft known as the F-5 with new 5th generation sensors and navigation. F-5 type aircraft, even as trainers, cost about one third what a full fighter or bomber platform costs to operate. That would make it an ideal training or ground support aircraft as well as a possible theater ABM/drone patrol aircraft. The only provision needed then would be acquiring1000 pilots who have the cognitive dexterity for everything except B-1 and F-35 multi-tasking. A 'training' fleet of 400 doesn't appear to have been addressed in NDAAs 2019 or 2020.

2018.07.26:09:05 |TR|>2 = ∑ |LI|>1WB|<2 ⋈ |GW|>1-|JU|>3....|OP|>3

Kuperberg and Nugent, Rutgers University, in WaPost: ' An obscure British parliamentary rule was broken. Here's why it's a big deal.':

"This [reducing votes by absentee pairing] is informal practice, and the House of Commons does not officially recognize paired voting. Instead, MPs or party whips make these arrangements at the party level, as needed. For pairs to function as intended, both whips and politicians must honestly adhere to agreed arrangements. The legislatures of Canada, Australia and the United States all use versions of paired voting procedures."

Pairing might not meet the representation requirement of a legislature if the number of actual votes are reduced arbitrarily. This process involving absentee voting or other influences on legislative 'rules' might be more significant if it is detected as a mechanism by which a legislature can be 'dysfunction-ed' in an emergency. Obviously, the representative Members would come zipping back into a quorum condition if summoned in an emergency, but suppose a hostile power was able to disrupt communications to the point that a legislature could not have a 'quorum feel' for something the hostile agents were plotting? Could the hostile power prevent the creation of an AUMF at a critical point in time while its own asymmetric forces were in motion? Totalitarians would just love that ability to interfere with representative democracy, especially in their cooperative defenses and interactive economies.

Perhaps a system of 'droid proxies' could be established in legislative Chambers where an elected Member leaves a set of pre-recorded votes on current legislation, including SCI conditions the Member may be responsible for through Committees. A little droid box at the Member's chamber desk or seat that contained his yea or nay on designated issues that could only be accessed by the Member OR the Sargent at Arms would satisfy both the absentee needs of the Member AND the need for full representation on legislation. Modern AI systems could easily create a specialized, encrypted emergency 'Representative' for absentee voting. Subject to Chamber Rules override, of course.

2018.07.27:07:07   [CD]>3 ⋈ [GW]<4-[JU]<3[TR]<2 ≈ [OP]>3?

Weiner, WaPost, 'I don't feel that I'm any safer': Juror speaks out against 40- year sentence for drug dealer he helped convict':

"Attorney General Jeff Sessions himself said in 2015, when he served in the Senate, that "the stacking issue is a problem." But as head of the Justice Department, he has told prosecutors to charge "the most serious, readily provable offense." Exceptions must be defended and approved by supervisors."

If one applied the combination of the Common Defense and Justice covenants of the Constitution to this situation, which is purely Federal and not state, the 'gunstacking' could be considered a clear injustice. But the Common Defense could consider serial meth distribution a terroristic use of a weapon of mass destruction in which the individual would do it again and ANY sentence that permanently removes such danger makes everyone safer. But only if the process is serial, not singular instances.

Question: does a Presidential pardon authority, which also says 'reprieves' in the Article II, Section 2, apply to SINGULAR convictions within a 'stack' of convictions or is he bound as Commander in Chief to permanently remove the serial WMD distributor from society?

2018.07.27:08:39   [CD]<3 ⋈ [GW]>1-[JU]>1[TR]<2

Ignatius, WaPost, 'This is not your grandfather's KGB':

"When Butina was photographed near the U.S. Capitol on Inauguration Day, her alleged Russian handler messaged approvingly, "You're a daredevil girl," according to court papers. Three months later, when Butina's American contacts were outed in the media, her alleged handler wrote: "How are you faring there in the rays of the new fame? Are your admirers asking for your autographs yet?"

Sounds like her GRU handlers considered her expendable as a war 'grunt'. Definitely not like those 'agents' with cushy dachas in Zvenigorod.

2018.07.30:09:20 |WB|<2 ⋈ |GW|>2⋈ |CD|<3 |TR|>1 |LI|<3⋈|JU|<3 ≈ |OP|>2

Brnbaum, TheHill, 'Bernie Sanders's 'Medicare for all' would cost $32.6 trillion: study':

"All U.S. residents would be covered by the proposed health-care policy without copays or deductibles."

That 'residents' number would include 41 million 'non-citizens' in all categories who wonder about the United States. At the current healthcare cost per person of $11,000 per year, that would mean a cost of $4.51 trillion a year just for 'aliens'. Add in another 34 million citizens who have engaged in 'negligent health' (drugs, alcohol, sugar obesity, CO_2 toxins, etc) and you add another $3.74 trillion. Neither of these groups contribute substantially to the national or state revenues (true even if you had a 'tourist health bond' of $1, 000), so you would have a net loss of perhaps $7 trillion a year that MUST be made up by other societal mechanisms such as taxes, insurance and fees.

As for the remaining citizen 'residents' of 260 million at $11,000, you have a cost of $28.6 trillion per year. That is 1.5 times the POSSIBLE national GDP and there is no possible combination of revenues that could pay for this. Even an 8 percent sales tax added to income tax would increase the available revenue by only $400 billion of that $28.6 trillion.

Bottom line: Universal health care is physically impossible even if swarms of aliens AND health-negligent citizens are eliminated from the program. The best scenario might be to guarantee healthcare to all newly conceived life in the United States (900,000 at $11,000 per year) and for the first 18 months of life (individual ego generation point) which would be 1.5 million at $11,000 . Guaranteed pre and post natal care, even mandatory for citizens, would be perhaps $50 billion a year but, in this century only, might save $125 billion each year in future health care costs because the health effect is curative, not treatment, oriented.

Note: multi-year figures are 'ballpark'. Actual figures change every month.

2018.07.31:08:35 |TR|>2 = ∑ |LI|>1|WB|>2 ⋈ |GW|>1-|JU|<2....|OP|>1

Isaac Stanley-Becker in WaPost, '$8.8 million 'alienation of affection' penalty: Another reason not to have an affair in North Carolina':

"Alienation of affection and criminal conversation are common law torts widely viewed as outdated. "Conversation" is an old word for sexual intercourse, obsolete but for this usage.

Experts have warned about exorbitant rewards as well as to the possibility of blackmail. They also say this cause of action has failed to prevent adultery or promote marriage. "

Deliberate and pre-meditated 'Alienation of affection' in an existing empathetic pair of humans probably should be treated as a serious destructive process by a judge. But maybe not at a $6.6 million punitive damage level. Empathetic pairing between a man and a woman (aka, a loving relationship) is a well established evolutionary process that lets the pair safely create life over an extended timeline, usually about 10 years. Pre-meditated destruction of other peoples' loving relationship for any reason could easily come under the category of sociopathic narcissism or cruelty and should be treated as a 'violent' predatory attack on others.

This is especially true because empathetic pair-bonding can exist regardless of the promiscuity imperatives of the man and woman. Seeking alternate sexual partners (carried out by 60% of the males and 50% of the females in the homosapien species) is normal and doesn't necessarily involve the loving pair-bonding of the original couple. That is why the 'first-love' somehow stays permanent; it actually is not promiscuity as much as pair-bonding for procreation. Many amiable divorces even continue the love-bond, especially with children involved, and shouldn't be punitive or possessive at all.

Speculation:

North Carolina might have had the right idea, but it should have been in a context of a mandatory pre-nuptial agreement the expressly differentiates an empathic life-creation process from a random but normal promiscuity mating process. Adultery penalties should be confined to deliberate breaking of the love-bond of a pair, not normal one day attractions.

TL Opservationis 2018.08

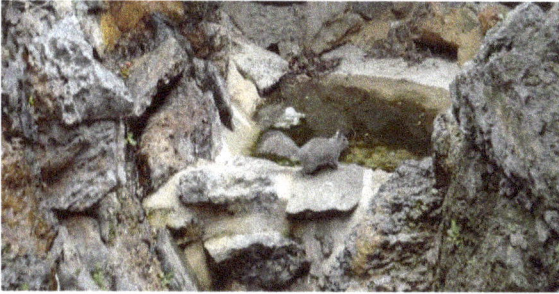

2018.08.05:07:34 |WB|<2 ⋈ |GW|>3⋈ |CD|>1 ≈ |TR|<1 |LI|<3 ⋈ |JU|>1 |OP|>2

Casey Burgat in WaPost, 'Congressional staff turnover isn't usually a problem. But when it is, it's bad.':

"Despite all the cautions from observers [about inexperienced staffers making policy], House turnover rates remained remarkably stable during the period I studied. On average, 18.5 percent of House staffers vacate their office in a given year, with very little deviation or differences by political party. This stability is supported by evidence that staffer tenures are getting a bit longer for a few positions and remaining steady for most, though the average number of years served is still strikingly low."

Many staff members come with the Member from their District and go home with him when he leaves for whatever reason. That would include relations who are nepotically hired because they are going to be on the Hill anyway. But the data also indicates a multi-partisan commitment to not just the power of District representation offices, but a commitment to national service and that is very laudable.

The turnover is as serious a problem for staffers as it is for Congressmen. The idea of limiting a congressmen to one or two terms of two years is proposed by those who DO NOT want a functioning legislature because the temporary status of staffers requires very expensive lobbyists to produce the wording of legislation, not the Congressmen and their 'limited' staffs. It might take the entire first year in Congress just to learn the complex nature of modern legislation. That might leave only six weeks of the term in which the staff and Member can interact with the actual process of Representation, a serious democracy functionality issue.

Speculation:

It might be worth considering a constitutional amendment that gives Members and staffs a more 'efficient' future by adding two years to each term. That would be four-year terms for Representatives, eight year terms for Senators and six year terms for Presidents and Vice Presidents, but THEN limited to two terms in that political context. That would save maybe $400 million in voting costs and allow functional representation by staffs and Members.

2018.08.10:08:03 **|CD|>1** ≈ **|OP|>2** Ξ **|WB|<1|LI|<3+|JU|>2** ⋈ **|GW|>1**

Ignatius, WaPost, 'How Mike Pompeo is succeeding where Rex Tillerson failed': "Pompeo said from his first day that he wanted to bolster a demoralized foreign service, and he sought advice from a wide circle of former State officials, including some who had been very critical of President Trump. Where Tillerson had left key positions unfilled, Pompeo has used his clout with the White House and Congress to clear appointments. More than a dozen major posts are likely to be confirmed next week, perhaps including four high-level "career ambassadors."

If one took the six covenants of Constitution (Justice, Tranquility, Common Defense, General Welfare, Liberty and Posterity) and applied them to the State Department, one might get the idea that the Department is too re-active to accomplish any of those covenants. The structure had, through several administrations, reversed its operating conditions in many countries as reactions to THEIR totalitarian agendas rather than as an expression of some combination of the six covenants. How do you apply Common Defense in a context of our Posterity if the people being put in place at State only react to THEIR Posterity?

Should trade negotiations be an expression of mutual General Welfare and mutual Posterity? Should arms control be a combination of General Welfare and Common Defense with international state Tranquility as an American objective? Should 'phased approach' in Korea mean that denuclearization of the North has Justice and Liberty as components for all of the parties involved? Would Common Defense for Americans involve retaliatory closing of the Hormuz Strait to Iranian shipping because their Pasdaran cult regard all of the Persian Gulf nations as private property?

The State Department needs to be more than just a structure for the individual 'players' at any time; it needs to be a consistent expression of the five covenants in some form as well if Posterity is the objective.

2018.08.13:00:00 **|CD|<4|LI|>3** ≈ **|WB|>2+|JU|>2** ⋈ **|GW|>1**

Brown and Lindsay, CRS-R41981, 'CRS-Congressional Primer on Responding to Major Disasters and Emergencies':

> Summary
>
> The principles of disaster management assume a leadership role by the local, state, and tribal governments affected by the incident. The federal government provides coordinated supplemental resources and assistance, only if requested and approved. The immediate response to a disaster is guided by the National Response Framework (NRF), which details roles and responsibilities at various levels of government, along with cooperation from the private and nonprofit sectors, for differing incidents and support functions. A possible declaration of a major disaster or emergency under the authority of the Robert T. Stafford Disaster Relief and Emergency Assistance Act (the
>
> Stafford Act, P.L. 93-288, as amended) must, in almost all cases, be requested by the governor of a state or the chief executive of an affected Indian tribal government, who at that point has declared that the situation is beyond the capacity of the state or tribe to

respond. The governor/chief also determines for which parts of the state/tribal territory assistance will be requested and suggests the types of assistance programs that may be needed. The President considers the request, in consultation with officials of the Federal Emergency Management Agency (FEMA), within the Department of Homeland Security (DHS), and makes the initial   decisions on the areas to be included as well as the programs that are implemented.

The majority of federal financial disaster assistance is made available from FEMA under the authority of the Stafford Act. In addition to that assistance, other disaster aid may be available through programs of the Small Business Administration, the U.S. Department of Agriculture (USDA), the U.S. Army Corps of Engineers, the Department of Transportation (DOT), and the Department of Housing and Urban Development (HUD), among other federal programs.

While the disaster response and recovery process is fundamentally a relationship between the federal government and the requesting state or tribal government, there are roles for congressional offices. **For instance, congressional offices may help provide information to survivors on available federal and nonfederal assistance, oversee the coordination of federal efforts in their respective states and districts, and consider legislation to provide supplemental disaster assistance or authorities.** Congressional offices also serve as a valuable source of accurate and timely information to their constituents on response and relief efforts.

Congressman direct help might be only feasible in Maryland and Virginia. Coordination with Washington's partisan systems would require a House and Senate secure network for EACH Member. No real control of funding distributions during disasters.   Link to FirstNet, CRS-R45179, somehow?

2018.08.15:10:27 |OP|? ≈ ∑ |TR|<3 |LI|<3◁|JU|<2....|GW|<2 [WB]<2 - [ξ]<?

Editorial Board, WaPost, 'We can't ignore this brutal cleansing in China':

"The truth is far grimmer. Hundreds of thousands of ethnic Uighurs, along with Kazakhs and other Muslim minorities, have been sequestered in the camps, which now number more than 1,000, according to outside experts. An estimated 2 million other people have been forced to undergo indoctrination sessions without formal detention. Those detained include Uighur intellectuals and relatives of journalists who have reported on the campaign, including those of U.S.-sponsored Radio Free Asia. Ms. McDougall said more than 100 Uighur students returning from abroad had disappeared and some had died."

Humanity has a long history of ethnics based 'relocation' of small cultures. Arabs forced the relocation and purging of Hebrews, Conquistadores in Latin and South America introduced the forced removal of Indians and Negros into slave pens, Slavs of the Moscow region forced the re-location of millions into gulags, Venezuelan and Cuban socialists forced the removal of the political 'impure' as refugees, etc. This process has occurred almost everywhere at one history point or another and perhaps there is a more underlying reason for the forced re-locations.

Could it be the 'national' socialists, as in the current Venezuela, force this type of relocation simply because the property previously occupied by the 'impure' then becomes something that can be owned by those who make 'laws'? Is forced relocation of those without 'rights' simply a way of acquiring property wealth for free, just as it has been done since the last ice age by this species?

2018.08.17:09:18 |LI|>3|TR|<2|WB|<2 ⋈ |GW|<2-[JU|<2 ≈ |OP|>3 | ξ| >2

Saba Ali in WaPost, 'I've worn a hijab for decades. Here's why I took it off.':

"Often, I couldn't argue back, even if I felt like it, because I had more questions than answers myself, especially about the sometimes unnecessary emphasis Muslims place on the headscarf. The Koran does instruct women to cover our bodies out of modesty, and the sayings of the prophet Muhammad specify that we cover our hair and, some say, our faces, too. However, modesty is a moving target, and men often define its parameters."

'Men often define its parameters' implies the decade of the 620s environment around Medina was a consideration concerning dress codes. Some of those non-Quranic sayings about living might even have been made by the Companions of the Prophet and not by him. That would make things like wearing the hijab a purely human governance process in the Medina Community of 627, not a spiritual process at all. As a human governance process, forced conduct by a theocracy, such as dress and education, would be a contradiction of the Quran's advocacy of enhancement through growth of holy spirit (Ruh, or jihad e akbar).

From a purely American standpoint, a theocratic imposition of 'law' is prohibited by the Constitution, so the wearing of specific dress intended for advocating theocracy is prohibited and is not protected by free speech. The key is that advocating religion, or its intolerance, as a government lawful policy is not free speech protected.

2018.08.19:10:37 |CD|<3 ⋈ |GW|<1-[[LI|<4JU|<3|TR|<2≈|OP|<1

Dan Baiz, WaPost, 'Former intelligence officials bite back after Trump goes after Brennan's clearance':

"The signers disagreed on whether Brennan's criticisms of the president were appropriate, in terms of his language, his harshness and whether he was crossing partisan lines. What they agreed upon is what constitutes proper presidential behavior and leadership. They concluded that the president was wrong to retaliate by pulling Brennan's clearance, saying the president was attempting to "stifle free speech." They called the action "inappropriate and deeply regrettable.""

All of the 'signers' were in positions over 20 years that accessed and approved operations of a covert, sensitive nature. The president is in a position of learning about these past operations through requests on the PDB (Presidential Daily Brief). Is it possible that the 'signers' are aware of something that is only parallel to the Mueller Russian GRU investigation, and the president has just began to learn of it? The dot connects show too many knowledgeable people being unhappy about a NSC process that may have little to do with that investigation but a lot to do with long-range 'deep state' processes in the Nation. Dot connects indicate more to this than the obvious political hostility.

Lots of Constitutional caution required by all parties if their oaths to protect it are coming into question.

Chronicles of the Kwedake Dikep

2018.08.20:18:54   TR|<3 = ∑ |LI|<2 -|JU|<2 |WB|<3

Moyer, WaPost, Southbound lanes of I-95 reopened in Prince William:

Having been caught in this [tractor-trailer accident], I had time to do the operations research on the ripple effects of one flipped tractor-trailer. Since the traffic southbound is backed up almost to the Pentagon, 20 miles, it means that 3 lanes have a 'parked' capacity of about 570 cars per mile, or 11,400 in all. If the individuals stuck there waste one gallon each while idling, that's $29,640. If each person loses one hour in wasted time at $40.00 per hour, that's $456,000. Add half that back to the Wilson Bridge and again to the Legion bridge on I495 west. The total losses might amount to a million dollars an hour, all for one tractor-trailer that is perilously close to a tanker on a major highway.

2018.08.21:08:39 |TR|<3 ⋈ GW|>2 ≈ |LI|<2 -|JU|<2 |WB|<3

Lazo, WaPost, 'More shared scooters are coming to the District's streets':

"But the personal travel devices have added a level of complexity to Washington's grid. Roads have become more perilous to navigate as people on scooters travel on general lanes and bike lanes, joining scores of bike commuters in a city dominated by cars."

Complexity? The scooters are adding a level of traffic danger that even the bikes cannot do. It is virtually an hourly occurrence in the Federal Triangle where a scooter with no lights or safety equipment at 15 mph will ignore a red light and scoot through an intersection because the operator somehow believes (or has been told) that the normal vehicle rules of the road don't apply to rental motorized vehicles. At dawn or dusk, it is virtually impossible to see such a person moving at 15 miles an hour, which is considerably more dangerous than a pedestrian stepping into a crosswalk when the light is against him. Nor can such a scooter be maneuvered among pedestrian on the National Mall walk (note WALK) ways without tapping someone, including children.

How about a District low-speed driver license with a scooter competency ID card that must be inserted into the vehicle before it will turn on? Entire new safety system at $5.00 per person that can be obtained easily by a tourist? GPS tracking of the vehicle while in operation? Why is ANY motorized device exempt from District and State traffic laws?

2018.08.23:09:10 |OP|>3 ≈∑ |TR|>2 |LI|>3⋈|JU|>1....|GW|>2

Emba, WaPost, 'Is the Internet evil? We will decide.':

"In the 20 years since Postman — who died in 2003 — gave his remarks, technology has rendered the world altogether different. Yet some crucial things remain the same: The things we create are still ours , for one. We still have the power to change them."

The technology of the internet as a human infrastructure is roughly equivalent to the previous dramatic changes the Homosapiens have gone through. The first, about 70,000 years ago gave homosapiens some cognitive abilities in their DNA that other sapien species like the Neanderthal and Denisovan didn't have. This led to the gradual ability to control food and energy regardless of environment which peaked in the formation of clan societies about 10,000 years ago. That in turn became the basis for written communication or universal memory, a very major evolutionary change, about 5,000 years ago. The modern creation of the Internet, or universal communication (you can translate any knowledge in any language to any other), is easily within that evolutionary 'event' sequence. The internet that effects homosapiens so strongly, however, is only part of the real evolutionary event: control of molecular energy that allows any current molecular form to be altered by homosapiens into any other. That includes his own DNA as a molecular form and the editing mechanisms for that, known as CRISPR, are only 10 years old.

All of Postman's five concepts will still hold for the Epigenetic evolution of this century, but who will decide how they turn out? Totalitarian oligarchies in ivory towers or We the People referendums based on universal communications around the world?

2018.08.23:16:29 |TR|<2 = ∑ |LI|<1WB|<1 ⋈ [GW]>1-|JU|<2....|OP|<2|CD|<3

Nakashima, WaPost, 'DNC says suspected hack attempt turned out to be a security test':

"The false alarm raised fears that the DNC was being targeted again by a malicious foreign government, as it came two years after Russian spies hacked its computers and released thousands of emails online, throwing the party into disarray in the midst of a presidential election. Election security is a hot topic, and the Trump administration is facing criticism that it has not done enough to safeguard the November midterm vote.

Those tests are probably fine, even if the DNC or RNC headquarters don't know the cyber warfare tests are underway. But it might not be the 'remote' attack that needs to be a concern. Anyone who has wondered around Capitol Hill will at one point or another notice that those HQs are quite open in the rear. All it would take is for someone who is VERY tech savvy to walk along the tracks behind DNC headquarters, walk inside like he belonged there and plant one of the new J-45 pass-thru couplers into any one of the DNC routers and he is going to have instant outside access to the databases. The same is true up the street at RNC headquarters with nearly open access from the rear Ramsey Court or local apartments.

Now it is assumed that both have taken precautions against physical access with cameras and reasonable lock systems, but you might not guess that from walking by the installations and seeing the comings and goings. That is especially true when members of both parties have displayed a casual attitude toward wi-fi cybersecurity on and off their trips to Capitol Hill.

2018.08.25:10:41 |CD|<3 ⋈ [GW]>1-|JU|<3|TR|<2 ≈ |OP|<2 WB|<2

Ryan, WaPost, 'U.S.-backed coalition in Yemen has cleared itself repeatedly in civilian deaths, analysis finds':

"After completing almost 80 investigations, the Saudi-led coalition's Joint Incidents Assessment Team (JIAT), formed with U.S. assistance in 2016, acknowledged problems with only 11 cases and found just one in which forces affiliated with the coalition had violated rules of engagement, Human Rights Watch said."

At least there exists such an organization as JIAT, which is not true of any Houthi tribal factions. The Houthi factions of Sanaa, called 'Popular Committees' carry flags with a motto that is identical to the motto of the Iranian cult known as the Pasdaran. These factions also use 'population control' tactics that are widely known Pasdaran doctrines in which arms, jail chambers and Popular Committee militia are quartered in densely populated sections of cities so that attempts to remove them will automatically kill many civilians. It is a Pasdaran cult doctrine tactic used in Sadr City, Iraq, Mosul, Aleppo and Homes in Syria and Gaza in Palestine. The doctrine of population expendability, which is listed as a crime against humanity in international law, is a common policy of virtually all totalitarian apparats and the existence if the Coalition JIAT is itself proof that such crimes are not the intent of the Coalition.

The Houthi have been targeting Sunni populations in Taizz, Al Bayda and Adan with a new Pasdaran mortar, the Razm, which they have imported from Iran through the Al Hudaydah port. The Razm has an untraceable, accurate range of 10 kilometers and uses a 120mm explosive, which has a killing radius of 20 meters. It's damage in urban areas is almost identical to that of a small 'smart bomb' launched by an aircraft. In at least one instance in Taizz, a Razm launched from outside the city killed a dozen civilians.

Further:

Perhaps more discussion is needed concerning the crimes against humanity doctrines maintained by state supported militias who now are being given weapons of mass destruction in pickup trucks as well as this discussion of air strike use on militia targets forcibly embedded in communities.

2018.08.27:08:42 |CD|<3 ⋈ |GW|>1 ≈ |OP|>1

Ignatius, WaPost, 'John McCain understood that the Republican Party was selling its soul. He refused.':

"But with his passing on Saturday, McCain's human qualities only bolster his stature as a real and enduring leader. Of all the politicians on the landscape during this generation, I suspect McCain may be among those who stand out most clearly in historical memory, not because he succeeded in bending the country toward the good values he embodied, but because he tried so hard and failed."

We the People oath of a Commissioned Officer in the Uniformed Services and of a Member of the Congress:

I, [name], do solemnly swear (or affirm) that I will support and defend the Constitution of the United States against all enemies, foreign and domestic; that I will bear true faith and allegiance to the same; that I take this obligation freely, without any mental reservation or purpose of evasion; and that I will well and faithfully discharge the duties of the office on which I am about to enter. So help me God.

No failure in either case of the Oaths. Wasn't conservative or liberal enough to fail on this oath taking, perhaps?

2018.08.27:16:01 |CD|<2 ⋈ |GW|>3-|JU|>2|TR|<2≈|OP|>1

Mathew Heiman, TheHill, 'Trump Iraq policy shows he's learned from past US mistakes':

"An Iraq that stands independent of Iran and that has a stable, participatory form of government are goals that benefit both Iraq and the U.S. Achieving these shared goals requires a continued military presence in Iraq, and the Trump administration should stay the course."

The 'withdrawal' problems with Iraq and the Gulf States is well known and accurately documented here. But lacking a new AUMF that allowed American forces to engage ANY cult, clan, tribe, or city-state in the prevention of crimes against humanity (an activity that is automatically within the Justice, Common Defense and Tranquility covenants of the Constitution), there is not much justification for maintaining large combat forces in the region.

What might be more useful is to establish engineering bases along both the Euphrates and Tigris Rivers that are recycling centers for all the 100 million tons of metals left since the first Gulf War. These centers could pay Iraqis, Kurds and Syrians, regardless of politics, to bring any metal parts found in Iraq and Syria to the centers where they could be cut up and sent for world recycle. The metals centers might even use a barter system, in which a ton of metal was traded for a knapsack of hospital supplies, food bars, or school supplies rather than cash. Might be a surprise how fast kids respond to such centers. This would require engineering troops guarded by a combination of Iraqi and American special forces units at the centers. Costs over a long time certainly would be less than 'surges' at $100 billion per.

The only ones who would object to this arrangement would be Iranian hypocrites and imperialists. Remember, Baghdad was not only a Persian province (6 times) but a Mongol province (twice). For them, it still is.

2018.08.30:00:00 |LI|>2 -|JU|<2....|OP|>3+|WB|<2 ⋈ |GW|>2

Allen Brownatein, TheHill, 'Originalism is at war with America':

"Non-originalists believe that the American people have worked with constitutional law for over two centuries. We learned a lot. We struggled to create constitutional doctrine that reflects who we actually are as a people, not some ideologically manipulated picture of who a few judges think we once were."

That 'a few judges think' works both ways. A number of judges around the United States have made sweeping decisions about health, environment, wealth and minority privilege that had no devolved Constitutional basis at all. Their 'thinking' process was not even based on the Article III, Section 2 authority 'Power shall extend---to Controversies to which the United States (ie, We the People) shall be a Party', let alone the other Section 2 conditions OR the Justice covenant of the Preamble. They were reacting, in many cases, to one of the twin abominations the Founders originally (sic) tried to prevent: mob rule OR individual ownership of power.

As for 'Constitutional law', that should mean that a valid law was devolved from some wording within the Constitution's Articles, Bill of Rights, OR other Amendments. There was nothing originally (sic) in the Constitution or subsequent Amendments that gave minority privilege to individual human body parts such as procreative organs, skin tone, organ dysfunctionality, OR neural structures of the brain that governed greed (dopamine addiction as in individual estate taxes?), hate (insula cortex or xenophilia?) , or mutated libidos (genetically reversed hypothalamus?) . And yet, many consider these 'rights' for body parts rather than the whole being OR We the People Justice to be significant enough to be ideologically manipulable in court. Needs work for 'our Posterity', as the original Preamble puts it. Second Constitutional Convention?

TL Opservationis 2018.09

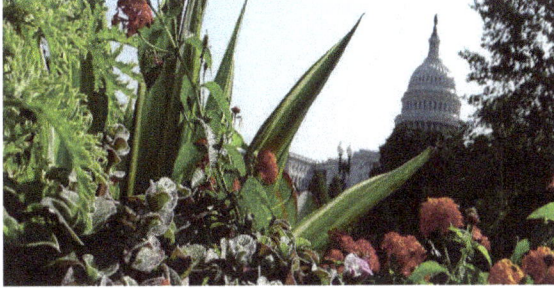

2018.09.02:09:07 |CD|<3 ⋈ |GW|>1-[JU|<2|TR|<2 ≈ |OP|<2

Axelrod, TheHill, 'Doctors, scientists say microwave strikes may have caused mysterious ailments of US embassy workers: report':

The Nanjing Research Institute in central China could easily have come up with a version of the YLC-15 microwave system with a tight beam antenna operating at 2.4 GHz and 1 megawatt. It is well known such gigahertz frequencies at high intensities can seriously degrade unshielded neural activity of the brain. It wouldn't take much for the Nanjing Institute to custom fit a standard delivery van with the components and include a thin plastic door on the back so the the antenna can be pointed and remain unseen. Even a 1 megawatt generator wouldn't take more room than a van's third seat row. Only needs 40 minutes of exposure to wreck somebody, but might not be useful against troops with metalized Kevlar helmets. Might be able to ship the component 'kit' anywhere in the world and have local sympathizers outfit a local vehicle with the kit. Welcome to the century of the new totalitarian empires.

2018.09.03:10:28 |LI|>2 -[JU|<2....|WB|<2 ⋈ |GW|>2 ≈ |OP|>3

Brockwell, WaPost, 'George Washington's Supreme Court nominees were confirmed in two days. Only half showed up to work on time.':

"Within two days, all of the nominees — John Blair Jr. of Virginia, William Cushing of Massachusetts, Robert Harrison of Maryland, John Jay of New York, John Rutledge of South Carolina and James Wilson of Pennsylvania — were confirmed by voice vote in the Senate."

Note the geographical representation that Washington preferred in his nominations. If you were going to add six more Justices to make 15 total, perhaps they should ONLY be nominated if one each represented a rotating sequence from the 11 Court of Appeals regional systems. This would allow an experienced nominee to 'represent' a given population of the country (noting that the huge western 9th district would need splitting into three Districts to be representative) and this would fulfill the Article I, Article II and Article IV requirements for a representative government in two of the three branches.

2018.09.08:10:03 |CD|<3 ⋈ |GW|>1-|JU|>2|TR|<2≈|OP|<3

Nikki Haley, U.N. ambassador in WaPost, 'When I challenge the president, I do it directly. My anonymous colleague should have, too.':

"By making sweeping, but mostly unspecific, anonymous claims, the author creates many problems. Taking this course sows mistrust among the thousands of government workers who do their jobs honestly every day. It unfairly casts doubt on the president in a way that cannot be directly refuted because the anonymous accuser's credibility and knowledge cannot be judged. It encourages U.S. adversaries to promote their hostile claims about the stability of our government.

What's more, by throwing gas on a fire of endless distraction, the author and the frenzied media reaction to the op-ed have hurt all of us trying to do our jobs for the country."

This assumes the op-ed was actually written within the EOP. The syntax stream of the op-ed is nearly identical to foreign attempts to usurp the credibility of the EOP and not just the current president. Similar 'office' related syntax's can be found in planted material in global media, including Wikileaks. Some of the syntax clauses can be drawn directly for NYTimes, LATimes and Guardian 'news items' that are unsourced.

'It encourages U.S. adversaries to promote their hostile claims about the stability of our government.' Very definitely and might have no other purpose. Op-ed really from the EOP?

2018.09.09:06:50 |LI|>1|TR|<2|WB|<2+|CD|>3 ⋈ |GW|>1-|JU|<2 ≈ |OP|>2

Shafer in Wapost's Retropolis, 'The thin-skinned president who made it illegal to criticize his office':

"Just one decade after adoption of the U.S. Constitution, the United States had survived its first constitutional crisis."

Odd that the convictions weren't challenged through the 1st and 4th Amendments in the Bill of Rights, which would have been automatic after 1870. It might be remembered that the national atmosphere in Adam's administration was that the anti-federalists who did not want a federal or state constitution at all were actually gaining strength. Many of the anti-federalists were 'libertarians' in a primitive, instinctive manner where they could not abide ANY authority other than themselves (as slave owners?) and much of their criticism was exceptionally vile against 'authority' figures for this reason.

The Alien and Sedition act as worded would not have passed eventual Supreme Court scrutiny even with a 'packed' Court of anti-Federalists and Jefferson wisely let it die of its own injustice. But in the modern era, malicious disinformation has become an art form by people who are dedicated to authoritarian and totalitarian ownership of power in a manner that would make Caligula, Ivan the Terrible, Tamerlane, and Hussein look like novices. There is little doubt that modern defamation is intended to undermine trust in democracy and the mechanisms it employs for checks and balances against absolute power. Their idea of 'limited government' means usurpation of any government that opposes totalitarianism as legitimate. Do we need some form of defense, such as a 'contempt of constitution' law, that makes support of totalitarianism a high crime or misdemeanor?

2018.09.10:08:48 **|TR|>2 = ∑ |LI|>1WB|<2 ⋈ |GW|>1-|JU|<2….|OP|>1**

Flynn, WaPost, 'How 'The Caine Mutiny' and the paranoid Capt. Queeg influenced the 25th Amendment's drafters, making it harder to sideline a president':

"It would be a mistake to say that the 25th Amendment is an easy remedy to deal with a president who might be unpopular," Feerick said. "It wasn't intended to deal with policy differences or unpopularity. You're looking at the wrong place if you're looking to the 25th Amendment to solve the differences."

Unfortunately, a large number of people, citizens and otherwise, in the U.S. think that a president is automatically insane and should be removed BECAUSE the president is not following that person's world view and orders. In this century, you could not define mental incapacity without an MRI scan for molecular or quantum level degeneration and that might have nothing whatever to do with the accumulated holistic memories that are interpreted by the two frontal lobes or cortex. Incapacity isn't real unless the lobes themselves were damaged, as in the case of a Representative Gifford but not in the case of a Senator McCain. Both removed themselves from active Article I processes, but not from their offices. No presidents have done so because the diagnostic mechanisms didn't exist in their time. But the MRI scan showing actual damaged molecules in the brain (320 known possibles) should be the only criteria for removal from office under the 25th and who decides that unelecteds with a personal narcissist agenda and an LCD screen of some type?

2018.09.14:07:38 **|CD|>1 ≈ |OP|<2 Ξ |WB|<1+|JU|<2 ⋈ |GW|>1**

Bert Ely in TheHill, 'Tariffs already starting to bruise US consumers, businesses': "The United States clearly runs a trade deficit only partially offset by the positive balance of services U.S. firms sell to the rest of the world. Consequently, the United States has become the world's largest debtor nation.

While that status has allowed the country to reap the benefits of the low interest rates of recent years, arguably, the United States would be stronger economically if it was less of a debtor nation. Tariffs, though, are not the answer."

Tariffs could very easily be part of the answer for not being a debtor We the People. Advocating an unending Friedmanist non-intervention dogma in any economic thing is the reason We the People are a debtor nation. Advocating a Ricardo trade 'system' that is continually manipulated by a Communist monopoly on trade with the U.S. means the U.S. will always be supplying to China $31 billion a month in subsidized trade goods, $2.2 billion a month in U.S. Treasury interest and $3.7 billion a month in third party imports like illegal drugs (fentanyl, opioids, supplements, etc) or counterfeit electronics and clothing.

The tariffs amount to a sales tax on 'cartel' style economics and could be used as capital for a re-industrialization of goods in the United States. Such local consumer industries make the American people far more independent in the long run and immune to interdiction by foreign navies(note 1813 and 1917), whose rapid growth is actually being financed by the monopoly profits of sales to the United States. Milton Friedman's dogmas on global economic manipulations as 'freedom' don't count if it effects the survival of your society. A sales tax on imports, subject to the definition of 'luxury', would not hurt this country as much as some think, but it doesn't have to be done with arbitrary tariffs.

2018.09.15:09:56 | ξ| >2 |WB|>??

Zapotosky, WaPost, 'A solar observatory in New Mexico is evacuated for a week and the FBI is investigating. No one will say why.':

"He said the researchers did not spot anything in the sun to necessitate them leaving, nor were they aware of any scientific reason — such as an anomaly in the data they were collecting — for doing so."

The sun has ended its 11-year 'hot' cycle and there hasn't been a single solar flair in two weeks. Because there is nothing to do, someone thought up an excuse for a 'leave' that doesn't count vacation days. Besides, it is known the aliens had moved further into the Mescalero Reservation near Kenney Peak to be closer to the airport.

2018.09.15:11:35 |OP| ≈∑ |TR|<3|GW|<2⋈ |CD|<1

Pry in TheHil:' On wealth, war and peace':

"What to do about modern predator states Russia, China, North Korea and Iran?

Do not assume World War III will replay World War II, that the U.S. will have time to mobilize its economic wealth to prevail. In our age of nuclear missiles and cyber-warfare, the first blows are likely to be decisive."

Mao Tse Tung:

" We Communists never conceal our political views. Definitely and beyond all doubt, our future or maximum program is to carry China forward to socialism and communism. Both the name of our Party and our Marxist world outlook unequivocally point to this supreme ideal of the future, a future of incomparable brightness and splendor."

Brightness and splendor for who? Certainly not Russian and Korean provinces of a communist empire that are already feeling the consequences of being proxy armies of the empire.

2018.09.18:17:21 |LI|<3 -|JU|<2....|OP|<1+|WB|<2 ⋈ |GW|<2

Rubin, WaPost, 'Trump is violating his oath, again':

"Trump's actions constitute such a grave violation of his oath to "take care" that laws are faithfully executed, his decision raises constitutional concerns."

Article II, Section 1, clause 8, U.S. Constitution:

Before he enter on the Execution of his Office, he shall take the following Oath or Affirmation:—"I do solemnly swear (or affirm) that I will faithfully execute the Office of President of the United States, and will to the best of my Ability, preserve, protect and defend the Constitution of the United States."

Where is the phrase 'take care' in this presidential oath? Protecting the Constitution might have a higher bar than the 'accusations' described here. 'best of my ability' can have many interpretations in a context of 'high crimes and misdemeanors', but what happened to protections of the 6th Amendment about having a right to face the witnesses against him? Only applies to criminal trials, not public media?

Note that release of information about people that is taken through a FISA warrant OR through 'publication' of protected data is a violation of the 4th Amendment protections against unreasonable search and seizure unless the presiding judge or his constitutional replacement authorizes it. The harm to individuals by release of 'raw' computer data such as that done by Drake, Sterling, Manning, Wolfe, and Snowden, all of whom took a nearly identical oath, can be a serious violation of the 'unreasonable seizure' clause of the 4th and is more than enough for prosecution if there is harm to others.

2018.09.22:12:48 |TR|<2 = $\sum$ |LI|>1 WB|<2 ⋈ |GW|>1-|JU|<2....|OP|<3 |CD|<3

Hassan Rouhani, Iran President in WaPost, 'Iran is keeping its nuclear commitments — despite Trump':

"It is on the record that during the negotiations on the nuclear dossier, our supreme leader said that the other side's honesty would pave the way for further talks on issues of mutual interest. Washington's insincere approach toward the implementation of the deal, from day one all the way through its ultimate illegal exit, is indicative of the lack of honesty in the implementation of its international obligations."

The Persian taggiyah philosophy makes any 'dossier' that is not on the level of Sharia law a tool of deception intended for non-believers of Shia dogma. A treaty would have had to be approved by a legitimate representation of the Iranian people. Not just the Pasdaran cult.

2018.09.23:07:40 |OP| $\approx\sum$ |TR|>3 |LI|>3⋈|JU|>1....|GW|>2

Kat Imhoff in TheHill, 'The Constitution at 231: What does 'We the People' really mean?':

"The results [of a survey on Constitutional relevance] quantify and ground what many of us understand at a gut level: ethnicity, gender, and socio-economic status strongly influence perceived stability of constitutional rights and protections."

Note that Madison's research ideas on 'rights' as they appeared in the Bill of Rights prior to the Constitutional Convention of 1787 were not included in the Constitution itself and were added to the Constitution after state and community referendums about them approved. The interaction of 'rights' with ethnicity (which largely involves the body part called 'skin tone'), gender (which largely involves the procreative body parts) and socio-economic status (which largely involves functionality of brain parts) is a modern, this century only process involving instincts of We the People, but why body parts as constitutionally important? Assigning specific privileges to various human components might not have been what Madison and other Founders were considering during the Convention.

But they clearly intended that the Bill of Rights would eventually apply to all who could be defined as 'citizens' (see Article I, Sections 9 and 10) and then left that definition out of the Constitution as one of the items to be decided as history progressed. Sorry, originalists; they DID intend for the Constitution to work as the Nation progressed. There was also no doubt in the Bill of Rights referendums that We the People wanted protections against predatory abuses of power by other 'citizens' but, strangely, it wasn't until 1925 that the Bill of Rights was made universal in the states as well as the federal government. Now, it is in the interests of We the People to extend Madison's idea of protections against inherited primate instincts to all citizens by a universal protection of a 'right' to health.

Want to clarify the 'rights' of citizen's body parts in modern health terms? Try a Second Convention, preferably one that is free of the instinctive trivia ideas about body parts having a rights status instead of a complete human being needing to be fit and healthy.

Comment on above:

Since we know that the U.S. Constitution is the world's oldest existing written constitution, and was crafted as a compromise among delegates assembled under the false pretense that their purpose was to amend the Articles of Confederation, it seems reasonable to contemplate what might be the result if there were a serious effort to revamp it. Parsing the constitution line by line reveals large chunks of it which make no sense in modern times, but removing or replacing these chunks runs the risk of unintended consequences. Maybe it's wiser for the Supreme Court to issue interpretations of it that better serve "we the people" and our modern policy needs than we now experience.

Reply Avatar

 dmh • 5 minutes ago

Revision of the Articles of Confederation actually was the intent of delegates sent there by various legislatures and they very quickly determined that some 12 clauses of the Articles had no functional purpose. They voted to go from there, with the Federalists taking the lead in July, 1787.

The problem with the Supreme Court being 'activist' in its interpretations is that they are not elected representatives and according to the original method, only representatives of referendums could 'create' a valid human right for all. Government entities cannot create rights; only a form of We the People can. You need only look around the modern world and see what happens when government employees define 'rights'.

A Second Convention that was empowered to ADD things to the the original wording might be a better way of doing things, but even then a 'right' would need a specific referendum approval.

2018.09.24:08:32 CD|<4|TR|<1 |LI|<3 ⋈ |GW|>3⋈ |JU|>1 + |OP|>2?

Applebaum, WaPost, 'Putin's war is transforming Ukraine':

"Russian cultural influence, once all-powerful, is also disappearing, partly thanks to official decisions."

When the Russian State employees routinely ignore virtually every Article in Chapter 2 of the 1993 Constitution, no one who speaks Russian would allow the 'cultural influence' of such employees to enter their lives. Such members of the State appear to recognize only Chapter 3, Article 55 as legitimate:

'Human and civil rights and freedoms may be restricted by the federal law only to the extent required for the protection of the fundamentals of the constitutional system [not Chapter 2], morality, health, rights and lawful interests of the persons, for ensuring the defence of the country and the security of the state."

Why would anyone accept the word of a State employee or sympathizer who can overturn any human right at will? On the other hand, adherence to that entire Constitutional infrastructure would place the Rus peoples from Primorskaya to the Leningradskaya oblast in the position of an advanced human society/state that had finally removed the cultural influences and degradations of the Czars and Tatar Khanates.

From the basis of the American 1789 Constitution and the Russsian multi-national Constitution of 1993, the Americans and Russians should have a very high level of cultural affinity and political/economic coordination. Odd that the 'imperial' influences of both societies have prevented that mutual respect and security cooperation. Tatar love of absolute power still too strong a 'cultural influence', perhaps?

2018.09.26:22:14 |CD|<1 ⋈ |GW|>3-|JU|>2|TR|>4≈|OP|>3

Ajit Pai in WaPost, '5G is in reach. But only if we set the right policies.':

"And we're working with other federal agencies to free up spectrum held by the federal government (which has held a majority of the airwaves for some time). These auctions not only provide more wireless capabilities to more consumers, but they also raise billions of dollars in non-tax revenue for our nation."

This can very quickly be overdone. Some of that 5G bandwidth needs to be reserved and allocated for emergencies on a national level, not be subject to operations by local communications companies that may or may not be secretly owned by foreign interests or 'shareholders'. At least one full gigahertz (600mhz to 800mhz and somewhere between 3.0 to 4.0?) of bandwidth should be allocated entirely to the first responder emergency system known as FirstNet. This would allow instantaneous transfer of catastrophe damage information to control centers and allow EMRs to consult with medical staffs on injuries during disaster events. All such imagery consumes bandwidth and it might be ten times what a 4G system can handle in an emergency. Katrina and Maria were good examples.

The idea of 'local', low power repeaters is fine and would have been enormously helpful during Sandy and even during the man-made shooter disaster in Las Vegas. Such a fibre optic 5G infrastructure for national defense purposes is easily within the

Common Defense and General Welfare prime directives of the Federal government and should not be casually assigned to under capitalized local consumer technology groups without 'federal regulation', regardless of the ideologies involved in current politics.

2018.09.27:16:31 |TR|<2 = ∑ |LI|>3WB|<2 ⋈ |GW|>3-|JU|<2

Janes, WaPost, 'The Nationals were better....:

"Perhaps the difference lies on the bases and in the field, both places where the Nationals have made more mistakes than they should have this season — both places where they conceded enough runs to make a difference in the 24 one-run games they lost. Had they won even half of those, they would be comfortably leading the National League East."

In the Land of the Swamp, from the ancient Canal along the Potomac to the Basin with its nearby arenas and to the Anacostia shores with its nearby stadiums, the teams falter with little errors and missteps at critical moments in their seasons. Mistakes that are sudden deficits of skill or talent that normally would not possess these trained athletes appear in the air. Yet the trickle of deficits that Ben Franklin always warned about pursues those of the Swamp just as the Curse of the Bambino pursued the athletes of Boston and Curse of Wahoota did in Cleveland and the Olympia Curse did in Atlanta. The symptoms are the same, unseen dearth's of talent and motive, in these Curses but that of Ben is more pervasive because the cause of deficits is so much larger in the nation's Capital.

When Ben Franklin wrote his letter approving the newly conceived Constitution of We the People with its Congress that could tax and spend without restraint of reason, thus causing an endless tyrant of deficit, he added into the letter this Curse:

"There is no form of Government but what may be a blessing to the people if well administered, and believe farther that this governance is likely to be well administered for course of years, and can only end in Despotism, as other forms have done before it, when the people shall become so corrupted as to need despotic Government, being incapable of any other."

Further:

Only the wording of legislation appears to alleviate the Curse of Ben as its foggy, corrupting mists role across the river marshes and reflecting Pools, causing many to see only the green of the dollar and not its waste. But what wording would be the exact addition to the Constitution that would truly drive out the Curse's malevolent Despotism of greed and stress from deficits? There are so few examples…

OVERVIEW 2018.10 to .01

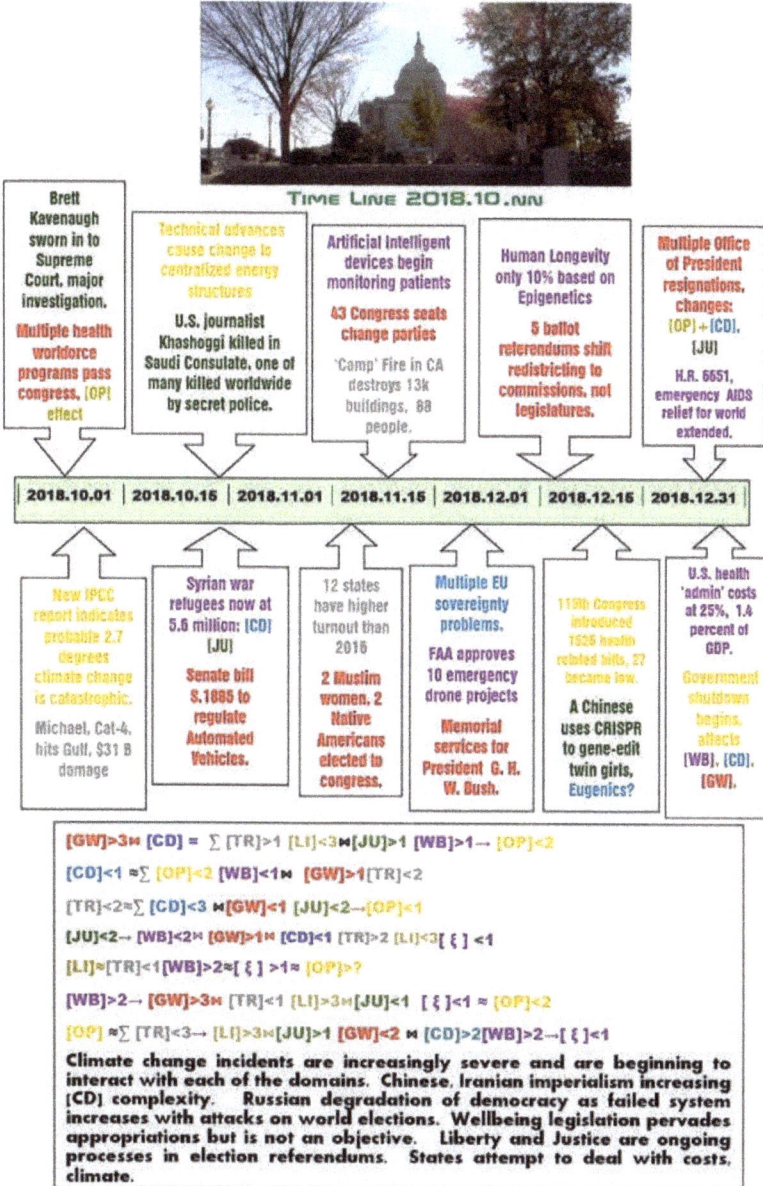

TIME LINE 2018.10.nn

Brett Kavenaugh sworn in to Supreme Court, major investigation.	Technical advances cause change to centralized energy structures	Artificial Intelligent devices begin monitoring patients	Human Longevity only 10% based on Epigenetics	Multiple Office of President resignations, changes: [OP] + [CD], [JU]
Multiple health workforce programs pass congress, [OP] effect	U.S. journalist Khashoggi killed in Saudi Consulate, one of many killed worldwide by secret police.	43 Congress seats change parties	5 ballot referendums shift redistricting to commissions, not legislatures.	H.R. 6651, emergency AIDS relief for world extended.
		'Camp' Fire in CA destroys 13k buildings, 88 people.		

2018.10.01	2018.10.15	2018.11.01	2018.11.15	2018.12.01	2018.12.15	2018.12.31

New IPCC report indicates probable 2.7 degrees climate change is catastrophic.	Syrian war refugees now at 5.6 million; [CD] [JU]	12 states have higher turnout than 2016	Multiple EU sovereignty problems.	115th Congress introduced 7625 health related bills, 27 became law.	U.S. health 'admin' costs at 25%, 1.4 percent of GDP.
Michael, Cat-4, hits Gulf, $31 B damage	Senate bill S.1885 to regulate Automated Vehicles.	2 Muslim women, 2 Native Americans elected to congress.	FAA approves 10 emergency drone projects	A Chinese uses CRISPR to gene-edit twin girls, Eugenics?	Government shutdown begins, affects [WB], [CD], [GW].
			Memorial services for President G. H. W. Bush.		

[GW]>3⋈ [CD] = ∑ [TR]>1 [LI]<3⋈[JU]>1 [WB]>1→ [OP]<2

[CD]<1 ≈∑ [OP]<2 [WB]<1⋈ [GW]>1[TR]<2

[TR]<2≈∑ [CD]<3 ⋈[GW]<1 [JU]<2→[OP]<1

[JU]<2→ [WB]<2⋈ [GW]>1⋈ [CD]<1 [TR]>2 [LI]<3[ξ] <1

[LI]≈[TR]<1[WB]>2≈[ξ] >1≈ [OP]>?

[WB]>2→ [GW]>3⋈ [TR]<1 [LI]>3⋈[JU]<1 [ξ]<1 ≈ [OP]<2

[OP] ≈∑ [TR]<3→ [LI]>3⋈[JU]>1 [GW]<2 ⋈ [CD]>2[WB]>2→[ξ]<1

Climate change incidents are increasingly severe and are beginning to interact with each of the domains. Chinese, Iranian imperialism increasing [CD] complexity. Russian degradation of democracy as failed system increases with attacks on world elections. Wellbeing legislation pervades appropriations but is not an objective. Liberty and Justice are ongoing processes in election referendums. States attempt to deal with costs, climate.

Figure 11. Overview 2018.10

TL Opservationis 2018.10

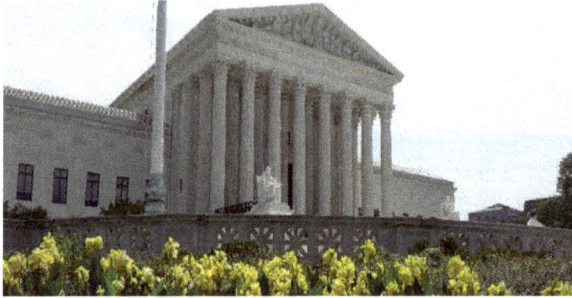

2018.10.01:09:51 CD|<3 ✉ [GW]>2-|JU|>2|TR|>2≈|OP|>1

Sen. Warner in WaPost, 'I voted against an assault weapons ban. Here's why I changed my mind.:

"And let's agree that modifications such as binary triggers and bump stocks, which skirt the law to effectively turn semiautomatic rifles into fully automatic weapons, should never have been on the streets in the first place."

The Congress might find more difficulty on agreeing about 'modifications' than anyone realizes. There is a $400 trigger assembly 'drop-in' that makes an AR-15 fire more accurately and faster than the military version. There is another trigger assembly that flips a 'safety' on for each shot, requiring the user to press a latch whenever he pulls the trigger. While that slows the AR-15 down to about three times the speed of a bolt action hunting rifle, it drops the firing out of the assault category. How would Congress word the legislation that makes it OK for the same rifle slow version but not for the Simple Weapon of Mass Destruction (SWMD) modification in the other version?

Many of the legislative efforts on writing constitutional 'well regulated militia' text for weapons have invariably wound up with obscure syntax that can be applied to a wide range of devices whether they qualify as SWMD or not. This same vague wording process is the reason most referendum initiatives are overturned by equal numbers of people in the left, right and independent categories. Since a Bill of Rights item is involved in 'regulation' of weapons, the wording of the legislation on SWMD modifications should have not just bi-partisan consensus, but the syntax needs to have a true referendum-level agreement from the entire spectrum, not some minority intellectual faction who doesn't know where the trigger is. The Constitutional objective should be to make SWMD difficult to use, nothing else.

2018.10.04:08:03 [JU]<2|LI|>4|TR|✉|WB|<2≈?

Kevin Cokley in TheHill, 'There should not be a litmus test for patriotism':

"Whatever her reason, Landry does not believe that the flag represents "liberty and justice for all." Regardless of whether someone agrees with Landry, is punishment how we should treat students who peacefully exercise their First Amendment right to freedom of speech?"

"I pledge allegiance to my Flag and the Republic for which it stands, one nation, indivisible, with liberty and justice for all"

Note the Preamble to the Constitution: We the People of the United States, in Order to form a more perfect Union,

1. establish Justice,

2. insure domestic Tranquility,

3. provide for the common defence,

4. promote the general Welfare, and

5. secure the Blessings of Liberty to ourselves

6. and our Posterity,

do ordain and establish this Constitution for the United States of America.

Not pledging allegiance to a flag might be considered an expression of the first Amendment, but is renouncing the intent of the Constitution as expressed in the Preamble free speech? Could the student involved have passed a civics exam as a condition of graduation that determined whether that person was entitled to citizenship according to the Constitution itself? Note that the wording in the Preamble predates the Bill of Rights and therefore supersedes the right itself, so allegiance to the Preamble 'intent' of America may be a citizenship responsibility, not a matter of 'rights'.

Would it be Constitutional to require a student to swear allegiance to the Constitution itself as a function of citizenship rather than to a 'flag'? If the student is unwilling to validate a belief in the Constitutional basis of society, why would he or she be entitled to the benefits of citizenship?

2018.10.06:08:26   CD|>2 ⋈ [GW|>1-|JU|<2|TR|<2 ≈ |OP|>1

Nakashima, WaPost, 'Former NSA deputy is Mattis's leading choice to head the spy service if it splits from Cyber Command':

"If the two organizations split, Nakasone is expected to continue to lead Cybercom, which recently was elevated to full combatant command status on a par with U.S. Central Command, which oversees military operations in the Middle East, and others with purview of the Pentagon's missions worldwide. He, too, is highly regarded, and no matter what happens, officials have said, the NSA and Cybercom will continue to work closely with one another."

Tough call. If the two organizations are to maintain the standard security compartmentalization require for all strategic security day-to-day operations after their command separation, they will inevitably 'drift' in their coordination. They might not even coordinate with other Agencies either, a process that in the past has cost the U.S. dearly. Perhaps some consideration might be to have the DEPUTY directors of each organization be dual-hat and physically relocate into each other's position every six months of so. The 'chief of operations' might be more critical to interaction between compartmentalized groups than the actual constitutional appointee who is running the administration and logistics of the group as well as command approval authorizations.

Most operations research analysts look at the internal operating officers as much as the 'shareholder' Chairman when they look for DMAIC 'satisficing' , but do you gain more than you lose by rotating sensitive operations facilitators between corporate divisions?

2018.10.08:07:17 |TR|<2 = ∑ |LI|>1|CD|<2 ⋈ |GW|>1-|JU|<2....|OP|<3

Fifield and Denyer, WaPost, 'China tells Trump administration to stop its 'misguided' actions and allegations':

"We urge the U.S. to stop such misguided activities," Wang told Pompeo at the start of a meeting, citing the "escalation" of trade friction, actions towards Taiwan and "criticizing China's internal and external policies."

"We believe that we need to keep our relationship on the right track," a stern-faced Wang told his American counterpart.

A 'foreign' minister in Beijing said that? Such comments sound more like the words of an Interior minister of the Ming Dynasty talking to a sheng xunfu or a coordinator in a remote Ming Empire province. Is this the new imperial 'order' of Beijing to prevent world chaos, to treat all those outside its borders as errant or autonomous provinces of the central world imperial State?

2018.10.10:08:21 |TR|>3 = ∑ |LI|>2|OP|>3+|WB|<2 ⋈ |GW|>2

Jamison, WaPost, 'Climate bill would move D.C. to 100% renewable energy by 2032':

" About 20 percent of the money generated from those fees would be used to provide financial assistance to low-income ratepayers, while the rest would fund other local sustainability initiatives."

It might be better to utilize this funding, and others, for the direct support of the local installation of ethanol power generators like the nifty conversion that GE did with its LM6000 turbine generators in Brazil. The Benning facility in NE is ideal for sliding a half dozen LM6000 units that burn ethanol OR natural gas into the Washington power grid. If you wanted to do renewal energy right, do it at the power generator level itself. The ethanol LM6000s have about half the NOX emissions of diesel or coal generators and the only problem would be the continuous supply of ethanol, but not natural gas.

Could local Maryland and Virginia corn farmers with their own 'stills' create the necessary 100,000 liters of ethanol a year to give true renewable fuel to the District, with its increasing use of electric vehicles?

2018.10.11:09:25 |CD|<3 ⋈ |GW|<2-|JU|>2|TR|<2 ≈ |OP|<3|WB|<5

Adalja in TheHill, 'Clusters of polio-like illness in the US is not a cause for panic':

"It is also important for the medical and public health communities to thoroughly investigate the causes of the AFM cases, cataloging the various viruses that are responsible."

Adalja et al, Center for Health Security, 'The Characteristics of Pandemic Pathogens, Executive Summary':

"Preparedness against GCBR-level threats should first be focused on those pathogens with the characteristics that are most likely to result in GCBRs. But the work should be flexible enough to encompass new knowledge of pathogens and

resist focusing entirely on lists of specific proscribed potential microbial agents. The most probable naturally occurring GCBR-level threat that humans face is from a respiratory-borne RNA virus, and so this class of microbes should be a preparedness priority. However, because other classes of microbes (viral and other) still possess some ability to incite a GCBR-level event, they will continue to merit significant study and appropriate preparedness efforts."

GCBR means 'Global Catastrophic Biological Risks' and people need to regard this term in the same manner they would regard the term 'Nuclear War'. The modern societies in most developed nations can actually communicate such viral infections much more effectively, but a world wide computer management system for such reporting wouldn't hurt at all in this century. Little outbursts of air-borne enterovirus D71 (EV-D71) type cases can be something that might be spread by transportation contact and the sooner the 'cluster' is detected in an automated system, the sooner containment processes can be effective.

One might even consider that any government employee who suggests they don't have to comply with biological reporting processes because of their nation's 'sovereignty' might be considered a suspect in a crime against humanity. 'Global Catastrophic' does mean everyone everywhere.

2018.10.13:09:43 | ξ|<2 |WB|<1 ✉ |GW|<1 ✉ |TR|<1 |LI<>3✉|JU|<1 ≈ |OP|<?

Ignatius, WaPost, 'Jamal Khashoggi's long road to the doors of the Saudi Consulate':

"He told her that night that he had decided to seek refuge in the United States, and he moved here a few weeks later. He texted Rubin in September about MBS: "This kid is dangerous, I'm under pressure . . . to be 'wise' and stay silent. I think I should speak wisely." But in the end, he couldn't censor himself."

Speculation:

If he was 'under pressure' in London, it would have meant that he was under the surveillance of the Saudi prince even then in 2017. But the surveillance would have been by the secret police apparatus of another country at the request of the 'prince' in power. Nothing new. You have a man who is the personal enemy of a 'prince' in Russia who is dosed with a toxin, you have an Interpol officer who is investigating the activities of 'princes' in Beijing who suddenly disappears through a state apparatus. And you have a Korean 'prince' who casually orders the death of a family rival in a third country. A long, totalitarian road there.

Only in a literate democracy would it be difficult to carry out a personal vendetta using government resources against someone who threatens you and men like Jamal create that difficulty. The 'princes' of the world seeking life and death powers over their enemies go back to the Shang Emperors and Pharaohs. Does abuse by government security forces for personal hates disqualify a person from legitimacy in a government?

Has nothing really changed as a new generation of 'princes' evolves with modern surveillance and lethal technologies?

2018.10.15:12:13 |OP|<3 ≈ ∑ |TR|<3 |CD|<4|LI|>3⋈|JU|>1….|GW|<2

Samuelson, WaPost, 'We're on mission impossible to solve global warming':

The emissions increases are almost certainly because of global industrialization, of which Americans are now, note now, only one of the contributors. Humans, by the way, emit CO_2 as they breath to the amount of 6 billion tons per year, or 6 gigatons (GT). Their industries are emitting something like 40 GT per year, more than enough to overwhelm the earth's global cycle of absorbing 27 GT of CO_2 per year. Note that the earth measures CO_2 in gigatons of matter, so the totals are colossal. The oceans have almost 40,000 gigatons stored and the earth surfaces, largely in trees, has another 3,200 gigatons, with about 750 GT floating in the atmosphere. The problem lies in the unabsorbed industrial GTs.

The key to lowering global warming is to reduce the industrial emission below 20 GT so that the natural absorption can actually work the other 20 GT. This is very tough to do because the amount of energy needed to do the sequestration of 20 GT of CO_2 would produce more CO_2 than it absorbs. It is not quite a lost cause if some technologies that convert CO_2 into its component carbon and oxygen atoms are developed using hydro or nuclear energy, which don't have a carbon footprint. But the scales involved are large. A single tree absorbs and stores 50 pounds of CO_2 a year, so absorbing one GT would require 40 billion new trees world wide. Not impossible, and beneficial for other reasons, but such a planting would require a commitment by ALL human societies. Good luck, considering human history.

Both reducing the waste of carbon based fuels (waste emissions by humanity at 3 GT?) by some form of carbon tax along with increasing the carbon capture by various means (4 GT?) could slow the future warming be perhaps 2 degrees F and avert the truly catastrophic effects warming causes of not having food growing lands for 9 billion people in 2070.

TLO: No posterity win at all unless a form of free energy sequestration is found and massively introduced world-wide.

2018.10.15:17:49 [ξ]>2 [WB]<2 ∪ [GW]>3⋈ [LI]>3 ⋈ [JU]<1

Wagner, WaPost, 'Warren releases DNA test suggesting distant Native American ancestor':

"The nearly six-minute video also tackles claims that Warren represented herself as a minority to advance as a law professor, a notion that White House press secretary Sarah Huckabee Sanders, among others, have advanced.

The video shows Sanders making that claim from the White House briefing room and then shows interviews with several law professors who deny that Warren's Native American heritage played a role in her hiring or advancement. Her colleagues also tout Warren's skills as a teacher."

Speculation:

Her DNA tests would also have mapped the linage of her M253 haplogroup as well as her 'Cherokee' M173 haplogroup. The M253 linage would almost certainly have placed her in one of the most oppressed minorities in modern North America, that of the lingering tribes found in cultural pockets of what is now called New England. In those modern scholastic environments, she almost certainly would want to hide the ultimate degradation of being in the haplogroup M253, because that is the one for the White Anglo Saxon Protestant or WASP.

2018.10.16:10:54 |CD|<3 |TR|>1 |LI|<3⋈|JU|<3 ≈ |OP|<1

Ignatius, WaPost, MBS's rampaging anger will not silence questions about Jamal Khashoggi':

"This breakdown was evident immediately after Khashoggi's disappearance, when official Saudi statements were all happy talk. Behind the scenes, says one knowledgeable source, "MBS went into a funk for several days after learning of Khashoggi's death before re-emerging on a rampage of anger around what happened and trying to figure out a response."

Speculation, pure type:

That sounds a lot like someone who agreed to 'something' a satrap underling suggested and it didn't come out anywhere near what the 'something' agreed to was supposed to be. It is just a little bit of a stretch to believe that someone who had been around Middle Eastern power struggles for 20 years would agree to an execution in a third country of someone who was not an existential threat to his authority, as the Huthie/Iranian alliance in Yemen was. Sometimes giving a command order doesn't materialize as expected.

2018.10.18:07:54 | ξ| >2 |WB|<2 ∪ |GW|>3⋈ |LI|>3 ⋈ |JU|<1≈ |OP|>2

Fact Checker, WaPost, 'Just about everything you've read on the Warren DNA test is wrong':

"Warren's Native American DNA, as identified in the test, may not be large, but it's wrong to say it's as little as 1/1024th or that it's less than the average European American."

All the test really proved was that she was about 98% WASP with a haplogroup of M253. What is noticeably absent from the discussion is whether the tests also indicated the degree to which she had the DNA sequences known as Human Accelerated Regions or HARs. The 'Accelerated' regions, all 49 of the principal ones, are what makes a person different from his ape ancestors. No one wants to know the degree to which these sequences are present in an individual because it might have indicated a lack of genuine human empathy, especially if the coding of HAR21 is distorted.

Speculation:

In the future, would there be a requirement for any public figure, elected or appointed, to show whether he has ALL of the Accelerated Regions in a high percentage? Never mind this candidate selection process based on tribal origins or such minor DNA sequences as skin-tone or sexual orientation. The true measure of a man or women should be an identification with humanity itself and that requires possession of all of the HARs given to, or created by, humanity.

2018.10.18:21:53 |CD|<3 ⋈ |GW|>1-|JU|>2|TR|<2≈|OP|>3

Ignatius, WaPost, 'What did U.S. spy agencies know about threats on Khashoggi — and when?':

"Saudi sources tell me that those who oppose MBS are quietly rallying around Prince Ahmed bin Abdulaziz, the last remaining son of the founding King Abdul Aziz ibn Saud. Have U.S. intelligence agencies provided the White House any assessments about Ahmed's views and political prospects? Would he stabilize the kingdom after the MBS earthquake, or produce greater instability?"

Careful what you wish for in the Middle East. MBS may be doing things with an apparent look-the-other-way attitude by the NATO countries, just as they did when Hussein invaded Iran (1980) and Assad begin his massacres of Sunni Muslims in Syria (2010). He may have decided, as a 33 year old absolute leader, that he had a free hand in dealing with enemies.

And some of those enemies are very real; the Shia majority in Tehran, Iran would like nothing better than to use its Shia allies in Syria, Gaza, Yemen and Qatar to take over rule of the Holy Cities of Mecca and Medina. You would see a bloodbath in all of the Middle East similar to the one in Basra and Sadr City, Iraq after Shia militias took over there. Tehran in Control of Mecca would coincidentally give them the ability to fix the world oil price at $120 a barrel and support a true world caliphate.

But a 'prince' in the 21st century who thinks he has god powers of life and death on planet earth that justify him being a genocider like some of those around him in recent history? Replace him with what?

2018.10.19:00:00 |CD|>3 ≈|OP|>2 Ξ [WB]<1+|JU|>2 ⋈ |GW|>2|TR|<3

Morgan Gstatler in TheHill, 'Trump administration to tell Russia that US will pull out of key arms control treaty':

"The 1987 pact bans all land-based missile with ranges of 310 to 3,420 miles and includes missiles carrying both nuclear and conventional warheads. The original ban between Moscow and Washington resulted in 2,692 missiles being destroyed."

Things have changed so drastically in the last 30 years that the INF treaty is almost meaningless now. The only totalitarian oligarchy who is a signatory is Russia and that has put them in an state of automatic violation with not only the Iskander cruise missile (range: 2000 miles) but with the AA S-500 (range: 450 miles). The S-500 is similar to the one being given to the Pasdaran cult of Iran, which has developed its own Qiam-2 (range: 600 miles), which is based on the North Korean Nodong system (range: 800 miles). None of these are as sophisticated as the Chinese DongFen-26 (range: 1900 miles) now being deployed along their borders and in their new bases in the Sea of Asia. This may force Sea of Asia countries like Japan, Vietnam, Indonesia, Philippines and Singapore to acquire American or European HIMAR mobile launchers with x-52B hypersonic rockets (range: 500 miles in 12 seconds). No end to this escalation.

The technologies for mass killing are becoming so common that no unilateral treaty between two nations means anything at all. The Chinese, North Koreans and Iranians, because they have a 'Mandate of Heaven' for their sovereignty, have no intention of reducing ANY missile program that enhances their ability to carry out warfare. It is not in their nature or dogmas, so such treaties are meaningless and our society should not be limited in our own defenses unless every 'Great Leader' in oligarchies does the same.

2018.10.21:07:56 [OP|n ≈∑ |TR|>3 |LI|<3⋈|JU|<1....|GW|>2 ⋈ |CD|<3

Kagan, WaPost, 'The myth of the modernizing dictator':

"Yet we do [expect a dictator to 'liberalize'], and for a variety of reasons. Some are simply racist. Much like the racial imperialists during the 19th century, we just assume that some people aren't ready for democracy, or that their religious or historical traditions did not prepare them for democracy. Another reason springs from dissatisfaction with the messiness of our own democracy. There is a certain palpable yearning for the strongman who can cut through all the political nonsense and just get things done — a yearning that our current president plays to very effectively."

At the time of Huntington's expertise, the 1950s to the 1970s, most of the world's societies were still very much feudalistic in culture and structure. That included socialist Russia and China, along with all of the Middle East, Africa and South America. Socialist Russia, China, Korea, and Vietnam, outside of a few cities, had land-bound 'serf' populations working their agriculture, the same as the 'imperial' societies they claimed to replace. Many dictators of that period were, in fact, transitional in nature and were genuinely attempting to create modern communication, water, food and industrial infrastructures through a dictatorship system, which coincidentally made their families wealthier .

But as the author says, personal ownership of power is only useful to the family and kin of the person in power, the same as it had been for the last 6000 years. But the dictators also start protecting that 'clan' interest when they discover that at least two dozen other 'clans' are always seeking the power they possess, BECAUSE DESIRE FOR POWER IS A NATURAL, DNA-BASED, GENETIC IMPERATIVE OF HUMANS. True, regardless of the power structure in existence.

The only way to circumvent that power addiction is with political checks and balances as found in representative republics and democracies that have imposed restrictions on the 'liberal' majority power desire as well as totalitarian power desire because they are both primate instincts with carefully arranged dogmas rather than conscious societal problem solving mechanisms.

2018.10.24:21:17 [WB|<2 ⋈ [GW|>2⋈ |TR|>1 |LI|<3⋈ |JU|<3 ≈ [OP|<2

Senators Durbin and Grassley in WaPost, 'An essential step to give Americans a break at the pharmacy counter':

"Each year, the pharmaceutical industry spends more than $6 billion in direct-to-consumer prescription drug advertising. Every hour on television, an average of 80 prescription drug ads are aired, and the ordinary American sees more than nine such ads every day."

$6 billion? Which is passed on to the patients at the counter. 80 advertisements per hour would mean that a drug might be advertised once every hour for weeks at a time. A person, not counting kids, might see that at least once per day during normal viewing but is then 'required' to watch the same thing 5 or 6 more times per day when he no longer has any functional need to watch it. Doesn't the ad become a 'luxury expression' not protected by the 1st Amendment after some three broadcasts a day? If the advertisement itself is a 'luxury' airing of a commercial product, rather than the nominal educational or news item, why wouldn't it be subject to a federal excise tax on publicly licensed media? An excise tax of two percent on unnecessary repetitions after three a day ($200 billion industry expenditure) would generate $10 billion in federal revenue AFTER the number of drug ads per day had dropped in half. Interesting…

2018.10.25:21:16 |LI|<3|TR|<2|WB|<2+|CD|<3 ⋈|GW|>1-|JU|<2

Ignatius, WaPost, 'Why was MBS so afraid of Jamal Khashoggi?':

"My guess is that Khashoggi was seen as dangerous for the simple reason that he couldn't be intimidated or controlled. He was an uncensored mind. He didn't observe the kingdom's "red lines." He was an insistent, defiant journalist."

There isn't a totalitarian anywhere on the planet that isn't afraid of an uncensored mind on the loose. A person thinking for himself is an insult to the existence of a 'control freak', regardless of the freak's place in society. The first thing an invading force's 'public relations team' does is attempt to eliminate any freethinkers in their path. The same is attempted in any organization; elimination of critical minds can be made by newsroom propagandists with an agenda, a corporate clique, or a political cult in control of something. Jamal somehow just wasn't expecting the standard totalitarian reaction to his activities to show up where it did, and it cost him. But the author has the right idea: pick up where he left off.

2018.10.31:08:02 |WB|n ⋈ |CD|<2…..|LI|<3|TR|>3-|JU| + |GW|>1 = |OP|>3?

George T. Conway III and Neal Katyal in WaPost, 'Trump's proposal to end birthright citizenship is unconstitutional':

"Congress has specific powers over immigration in Article I; the president, none whatsoever, except as Congress has given to him by statute. And Congress has already spoken. In 1952, Congress declared, "The following shall be nationals and citizens of the United States at birth … a person born in the United States, and subject to the jurisdiction thereof.""

This Article I authority expressed in 1952 has never been challenged because it is also clearly enumerated in Article I, Section 8 as the Naturalization Clause. Under this clause, the Congress could establish a legal definition of the terms 'national' and 'citizen' (neither is currently defined under modern DNA Genome conditions of birth). The Congress could establish, under its Naturalization authority, that a person was not born under the jurisdiction of the United States unless at least one parent had the genetic profile of a 'U.S. National' that had previously been born in the United States.

Speculation:

Without the prior genetic evidence, a person would therefore be a 'U.S. National' at birth and the Congress could require a test of citizenship at age 14 that THEN, and only THEN, established him as being within the Citizenship jurisdiction of the United States. A National is, of course, protected by the Bill of Rights, but is not a citizen. A person would remain a National, such as Native Americans on reservations do now, with appropriate green card, until such time after age 14 he demonstrated his citizenship right through acts of loyalty to the States of the Nation. Unfortunately, such a law of verified loyalty to a constitution for representative democracy would also apply to people born in the United States as a test for voting citizenship rights.

TL Opservationis 2018.11

2018.11.01:07:52 |TR|>3 = ∑ [LI]<1 -[JU]<2....|OP|>1+|WB|<2 ⋈ [GW]<2

Mallaby in WaPost, 'Why Britain should vote on Brexit again':

"Two years after Britain voted to leave the European Union, there is a clear case for a second referendum. It's not just that yanking Britain out of its most important trading relationship will be costly. It's that yanking Britain out won't deliver the promise of "taking back control" that Brexit supporters cherish. The deal now emerging is likely to require Britain to continue to abide by at least some European rules."

The original reason for the Brexit referendum was that the EU Council was arbitrarily imposing the socio-economic rights of first generation transients from areas with climate related turmoil. Such economic rights, as opposed to universal civil rights, were being imposed at the perceived and actual usurpation of the 'locals' who had established their 'rights' for many generations. This is demonstrated by the distribution of the 3 million 'leave' majority votes during the referendum. The first generation economic rights were clearly being given precedence by the EU Commission and had caused a number of Malthusian Populations Traps in Brittania cities which could only get worst due to climate migrations. Such imposed rights might not qualify as constitutional.

A second referendum might be legitimate if the 'remain' option contained a provision for local, non-EU, arbitration of socio-economic rights, including health, along with the total Brexit option and the negotiated option. Note that the Treaty of Lisbon that incorporated the socio-economic rights of first generations was never submitted to referendum within the UK or even EU and is therefore illegitimate as a human right system given by humans to all other humans. The American Bill of Rights was, of course, confirmed by popular and/or designated electoral referendums and there is no reason other rights, such as socio-economic, should not have the same test.

Very complex set of operations research domains. Maybe too complex to solve?

TLO: U.S. ripple effect [CD]<3

2018.11.09:09:08 |OP|>n ≈∑ |TR|>3 [LI]>3⋈|JU|<3....|GW|<2 ⋈ |CD|<3

Markovits and Ayres in WaPost, 'The U.S. is in a state of perpetual minority rule':

"Look behind the midterm elections' outcomes — and the distortions produced by small states in the Senate and by gerrymandering in the House — to focus directly on the votes that constitute democratic bedrock, and a very different picture comes in to focus. The partisan balance of power — even the new balance, including a Democratic House — subjects the United States to undemocratic minority rule."

Votes that constitute democratic bedrock? This appears to be a perversion of the originating concept in the Constitution that expressly states in Article IV, Section 4 that a 'republic form of government is guaranteed'. The Articles of the Constitution do not at all suggest that voting should be done by proportionate allocation, as was necessary to have some semblance of democracy in the 735 tribal cultures of Europe. Brexit and the failed Russian Commonwealth are indicators of the reaction to imposed 'pure' democracy. They dissolve back into little democracy enclaves that can be victimized by a central oligarchic 'nobility'.

The concept of pure population democracy is not in the Constitution because such a majority rule at any given time dissolves into an unaccountable 'committee rule' system. That is the purpose of Constitutional checks and balances inherent in three branches in a large area; to protect minorities of ANY kind against the arbitrary rule of a remote 'committee'.

A popular democracy rule in America is currently unconstitutional and therefore morally unjust. If you want to change that, have 38 states vote to change the Constitution's Article IV. The most hated thing in America right now is gerrymandering with a 71% vote against it. That is very close to the 38 state requirement. If you want a mass, proportionate democracy to be geographically real, and it doesn't yet exist anywhere above a city-state size, have 38 states create it in the Constitution.

2018.11.16:08:13 [WB]<3|CD|<3 ⋈ |GW|>1-[JU]<2|TR|<2 ≈ |OP|>3

Joshua Kuriantzick in WaPost, 'Unfixable: Several nations have tried to restore democracy after populist strongmen. It was never the same.':

"But autocratic populists erode faith in democracy itself — a faith already damaged in many countries by the failures of democratic politicians to deal with issues like inequality, migration and weak worker protections. "

Which democracy form is being discussed here? There is an implication that socialist, cosmopolitan democracy is automatically the only 'rational' form of democracy that can exist. It implies that socialist democracy with integrated economic, political and ethnic 'values' and a world universality of these conditions is so logical that it can be imposed in the name of Justice and Welfare. But, in fact, there are other forms of legitimate democracy or expressions of popular will, including authoritarian, that are still representative democracies. Authoritarianism is usually a reaction to the 'logic' of socialist democracy that cannot solve problems in a crises because of its anarchic distribution of power.

With modern mass communication, a totalitarian system like Nazi Europe or Maoist Asia would be very difficult to maintain because the inherent, genetically induced sixth sense of Justice Homosapiens have would eventually alter its tyrant structure after a generation or two. But it would not necessarily come out as a progressive or socialist 'democracy' because the effects of that inability to solve a crisis might last for several generations. In this century, if you start adding in global heating, you might need an authoritarian democracy to deal with the human situations global climate cycles create.

It might be a coincidence that a severe drop in global temperatures, after a long warming cycle, began just before the Mongols of Asia became united in1206 CE with their democratically chosen leader Ghengis Khan. Guess what happens when half a million cold and hungry Mongols go on the march…

In a recent poll from Axios and Survey Monkey, for instance, only half of American respondents said they had confidence in democracy as a political system. Similar declines in faith in democracy can be seen in several hotbeds of autocratic populism.

2018.11.16:20:36 [TR]>3 = ∑ [LI]>2 -[JU]<1....[OP]>3+[WB]<1 ⋈ [GW]>2

J.J. McCullough in WaPost, 'Why are Canadian politicians obsessed with changing the voting system?'

"Getting rid of so-called first-past-the-post-style (FPTP) elections, in which parliamentarians are elected based on whoever gets the most votes, even if that's not an absolute majority, has been one of the great failed crusades of modern Canadian politics."

There is one good reason why the FPTP holds up in Canada: demographics. Canada has a population of 36 million citizens, not counting 2 million first generation 'residents', and this works out to a population density of less than 4 people per square kilometer (England: 255/sqkm, Poland: 122/sqkm, Austria: 100/sqkm) and with huge areas governed by small numbers of people. In order to have democratic representation of all communities with such densities, it might be a matter of someone in an area being 'picked' by a national party that by definition operates in the entire society rather than just some local cultural enclave. European style proportionate representation would be almost meaningless with less than a hundred people per square kilometer. Such forced representation would eventually create two dozen city-states with their own cultures and 'rights' that can be picked apart by totalitarians who are already actively engaged in such things in North America.

As far as a powerful premier beholden to a given FPTP party victory, the easiest fix would be a direct, national vote for premier with a 'no confidence' voting option on the ballot in case the election candidates are deemed unrepresentative in some way by We the People (Canadians are too, even in this country). That should leave the 'electoral college' parliament with the task of appropriation and law making, along with its own 'no confidence' authority.

2018.11.18:10:04 [CD]>3 ⋈ [GW]<1-[JU]>2[TR]>3 ≈[OP]>2

Rebecca Kheel, TheHill, 'Trump and Congress on collision course with military spending':

"The National Defense Strategy Commission, a 12-member panel created by Congress to study and make recommendations on the U.S. defense strategy, recently released its final report.

The commission concluded that U.S. military superiority "has eroded to a dangerous degree" because of political, financial and international issues. Its report warned there will be "grave and lasting" consequences if Washington doesn't act quickly to reverse the damage and adequately fund the Pentagon."

Providing for the Common Defense, The Assessment and Recommendations of the Nation Defense Strategy Commission, November 2018:

Pentagon Reform: Necessary but Not Sufficient

> "Resourcing a strategy is not only an issue of providing reliable, adequate, and timely funding. It also entails ensuring that the available dollars are spent as efficiently and effectively as possible. This is more than a matter of treating taxpayer dollars with respect, as vitally important as that is. It is equally a matter of sharpening the

U.S. military's ability to compete with its rivals by wringing maximum value out of the resources at hand.

This being the case, the NDS is correct to argue that the Pentagon's culture and way of doing business must change. Sustained reforms, implemented across every aspect of the Department's activities, are sorely need to bring one of the world's largest bureaucracies into line with 21st century business practices. This will be critical to fostering innovation, improving responsiveness and agility, enhancing the speed at which capabilities are developed and fielded, and improving the efficiency, effectiveness, and accountability with which the Department expends limited funds. Every recent Secretary of Defense has recognized these 60 imperatives, which has only become more pressing as America's competitive edge has eroded."

The Commission Report talks about the 'Pentagon's culture and way of doing business must change' but also notes that any massive attempt at fiscal responsibility by cutting the total budget won't work. That is an accurate assessment from DOD in that the Congress cannot operate on its two-year electoral cycle (even though Defense appropriations are Constitutionally mandated at two years) because that in itself causes enormous waste in DOD. What might be more useful is for the Congress to fund and law-up a new AI auditing system that operates parallel to each DOD department that makes purchases BUT reports through the IG offices instead of the local department's management. Modern AI accounting computers can flag many waste and fraud debits no matter how well the local 'slyde drool' manipulates the department expenses data.

The military may already have the 'system' for doing such real-time auditing regardless of where the DOD department is physically located. DARPA has several projects under way to upgrade military BARS type computers to 32 core capabilities. The transferable real time auditing software already available might fit nicely in such a mobile, plug-in system. 75 DOD abuse dollars saved for each dollar invested in BARS auditing computers?

2018.11.19:14:55 |CD|<4 ⋈ [GW]>1|JU|>2|TR|<4 ≈ |OP|<3

Judd Gregg, TheHill, 'Not your father's cold war:'

"China has no significant history of expansion beyond what it deems its historic borders."

Someone needs a history lesson. While Kublai Khan was considered a Mongol, he operated out of Beijing with the full aid of the Han Chinese bureaucracy in his invasions of Korea, Russia, Vietnam and Indonesia. There are clear indicators that one Zheng He ,as a Chinese admiral in the early 1400s, laid claim to coastal areas of east Africa and the North American west coast.

What is of interest in this century is that Chinese bases established around the world are quite systematic (Pakistan, Panama Canal, Greece, etc) and designed for just one purpose; control of world energy supplies.

Gregg (and Li Keqiang agrees):

" There is no likelihood that China will economically self-destruct. Its people, at least those that have input, have made a bargain in which they accept the loss of individual liberties in return for stability and economic opportunity."

1 kilogram of oil is equal to 11.63 kwh of energy, industrialized countries need about 6000 kg of oil equivalent energy per person per year. The energy requirements of China will, by 2030 with 1.5 billion people, be about 84 billion kg of equivalent energy. That is more than the entire world produces and six times that which China is capable of producing within its 'borders'.

Do the math on 'expansionism'.

2018.11.21:00:00 |CD|<3 ◪ |OP|<4 ≈ |WB|<4?+|JU|<3 ◪ |GW|<2

CRS report, CRS-R45392, 'U.S. Ground Forces Robotics and Autonomous

Systems (RAS) and Artificial Intelligence (AI): Considerations for Congress':

Summary

The nexus of robotics and autonomous systems (RAS) and artificial intelligence (AI) has the potential to change the nature of warfare. RAS offers the possibility of a wide range of platforms—not just weapon systems—that can perform "dull, dangerous, and dirty" tasks— potentially reducing the risks to soldiers and Marines and possibly resulting in a generation of less expensive ground systems. **Other nations, notably peer competitors Russia and China, are aggressively pursuing RAS and AI for a variety of military uses,** raising considerations about the U.S. military's response— to include lethal autonomous weapons systems (LAWS)—that could be used against U.S. forces.

The adoption of RAS and AI by U.S. ground forces carries with it a number of possible

implications, including potentially improved performance and reduced risk to soldiers and Marines; potential new force designs; better institutional support to combat forces; potential new operational concepts; and possible new models for recruiting and retaining soldiers and Marines. The Army and Marines have developed and are executing RAS and AI strategies that articulate near-, mid-, and long-term priorities. Both services have a number of RAS and AI efforts underway and are cooperating in a number of areas. A fully manned, capable, and well-trained workforce is a key component of military readiness. The integration of RAS and AI into military units raises a number of personnel-related issues that may be of interest to Congress, including unit manning changes, recruiting and retention of those with advanced technical skills, training, and career paths.

RAS and AI are anticipated to be incorporated into a variety of military applications, ranging from logistics and maintenance, personnel management, intelligence, and planning to name but a few. In this regard, most consider it unlikely that appreciable legal and ethical objections to their use by the military will be raised. The most provocative question concerning the military application of RAS and AI being actively debated by academics, legal scholars, policymakers, and military officials is that of "killer robots" (i.e., **should autonomous robotic weapon systems be permitted to take human life?).**

Potential issues for Congress include the following:

1. Would an assessment of foreign military RAS and AI efforts and the potential

impact on U.S. ground forces benefit policymakers?

2. Should the United States develop fully autonomous weapon systems for ground

forces?

3. How will U.S. ground forces counter foreign RAS and AI capabilities?

4. How should the Department of Defense (DOD) and the Services engage with the private sector?

5. What are some of the personnel-related concerns associated with RAS and AI?

6. What role should Congress play in the legal and ethical debate on LAWS?

7. What role should the United States play in potential efforts to regulate LAWS?

TLO: Items 6 and 7 might set the stage for many ethical processes around the world, but dependent on Item 1? Fire 'em and forget 'em could have ominous ripple effects on future humans if DNA destruction/modification is used in the RAS devices.

2018.11.20:08:17 | ξ| >2 |WB|>1⋈ |GW|>3⋈ |TR|<1 |LI|>3 ⋈ |JU|<2 ≈ |OP|>2

Rampell, WaPost, 'Arkansas's Medicaid experiment has proved disastrous':

"This was predictable. A Hamilton Project report found that the preponderance of evidence suggests Medicaid has little or positive effects on labor-force supply. For many families, safety-net services support work, rather than discourage it."

From the Hamilton Project Report:

"We find that the majority of SNAP and Medicaid participants who would be exposed to work requirements are attached to the labor force, but that a substantial share would fail to consistently meet a 20 hours per week–threshold. Among persistent labor force nonparticipants, health issues are the predominant reason given for not working."

This is a classic 'damned if you do, damned if you don't' process. Many low-income or part-time or seasonal workers need various medications in order to effectively work (also the primary reason that people over 65 are barred from working by most HR departments) and can't possibly pay for them without 'organizational' help. 20 hours of work a week in Arkansas might also mean 10 hours of logistics time per person, which would leave 42 daylight hours a week free of work commitments. Double that if night time hour access to the 'system' were available, which isn't likely in a rural state where most live in towns of less than 30,000, with maybe 300 'low-income' per town.

Under those demographics, the state Medicaid and/or SNAPs systems might not be physically able to cover the territory as a safety net for the 20,000 in the category. Even the Feds with a single payer system wouldn't be able to cover the health needs of potential part time workers in this category even if its medical aid did improve the potential for working citizens. Incremental improvements of the infrastructure might be all that can be done at this stage, especially since the safety net is not itself a Constitutionally based 'right'.

2018.11.21:19:35 |OP|>?

Michael S. Rosenwald in WaPost, 'Ben Franklin didn't champion turkeys. In fact, they never survived encounters with him.':

"Franklin, Thomas Jefferson and John Adams were on a committee that was supposed to come up with a national seal. The founders were many things, but not artistic.

In letter to his wife, Abigail, Adams wrote, "Dr. F. proposes a Device for a Seal. Moses lifting up his Wand, and dividing the Red Sea, and Pharaoh, in his Chariot overwhelmed with the Waters." Jefferson proposed "the Children of Israel in the Wilderness, led by a Cloud by day." As for Adams, "I proposed the Choice of Hercules," he wrote, "as engraved by Gribeline in some Editions of Lord Shaftsburys Works."

There was no mention of turkeys or bald eagles. There was also no winning design."

At least these three Founders didn't propose anything like some societies in the 1700s. Some societies were representing their 'prowess' with emblems of a flying, fire breathing dragon, which oddly had drawings and paintings in nearly every human society dating back to the Chin, Babylon, and Maurya empires. There is, of course, no such thing and there weren't any exposed skeletons of the 100 million year old, 40 foot Azhdarchidae to give ANY humans a reference. The Founders were more practical in their compromises. Hint, Hint.

2018.11.22:06:27 |CD|>3 ≈ |OP|>2 [WB]<1+[JU]<3 ⋈ [GW]>2 [LI]<3

Fred Ryan, WaPost, 'Trump's dangerous message to tyrants: Flash money and get away with murder':

"Instead, it [The Congress] should use its investigative and subpoena powers to press for an independent, thorough inquiry — no matter where it leads. It should use its power of the purse and authority to regulate foreign commerce to impose effective penalties on Khashoggi's murderers and suspend the sale of U.S.-made weapons to the Saudis."

Treating an entire culture as criminal because of the acts of some totalitarians in positions of control in that culture is a serious perceptional mistake under the American Constitutional Preamble's covenants of Justice, Tranquility, Common Defense, General Welfare, Liberty and our Posterity. You would have to treat the entire Chinese culture as criminal for the high ranking order to 'detain' the former head of Interpol, or the Russian society for the activities of its GRU head. Under Justice for all, you might even vilify a culture that has allowed several of its GRU members to die under mysterious circumstances.

Using non-constitutional economic leverage on an entire society for the identifiable criminal activities of some of its members is not within the framework of the American three branches. You could easily be better off bringing the 'perps' to some place like Guantanamo where they don't have human rights until they can prove they acted as 'humans' with appropriate genetic codes. Targeting one culture for political reasons while leaving other oligarchic structures immune is a form of hypocrisy that devalues the Constitution itself.

2018.11.23:07:23 [LI]>1|TR|<2[WB]<2+[CD]<1 ⋈ [GW]>1-[JU]<2≈|OP|>?

Dana Hedgpeth, WaPost, 'A Native American tribe once called D.C. home. It's had no living members for centuries.':

"One village was east of what is now the U.S. Capitol, where they grew corn, beans and squash on plots where the Supreme Court and Library of Congress buildings now sit. Historians at the American Indian museum say tribe members could look down from what's now Capitol Hill and see ducks and geese flying over what's now the Mall."

The Nacotchtank tribe or their descendants are also described in the series of books called the "Chronicles of the Kwedake Dikep, a timeline of the Indian Spring on the Hill". Just to the west of the Capitol building is a odd brick structure called the 'Summer House' built over a natural spring by the Capitol architect Frederick Olmstead in 1880. In the 1600s, this spring was one of several used by tribes crossing through the Nacotchtank region, including Cherokees from the south and Iroquois from the north. The language generally used by the tribes of the area was from the Iroquois basic language which was very widespread in the 1600s and the term Kwedake Dikep means the 'Spring on the Hill' in Algonquin-Iroquoi languages.

The book series Kwedake Dikep is about the modern day political dynamics of the Constitution and how the three branches operate on the Hill in this century, so the name is a bit misleading. Although the Iraquois and Cherokee met with local tribes in the area, it was not always a pleasant outcome as both needed warriors for their 'Nations' and Anacostia was between the two cultures with much smaller tribal groups. But even in the 1600s, The Kwedake Dikep was occasionally a conference area and the Summer House actually did that later while people watered both themselves and their horses there in the 1800s. It is now a pleasant little rest area with a pipe-fed grotto and pool for various plants and birds.

2018.11.23:20:05 | ξ| >? |WB|>?

Bowden, TheHill, 'Former Bush CIA chief Hayden hospitalized after stroke':

"He is receiving expert medical care for which the family is grateful," the center said in a statement.

"As General Hayden begins the healing process, the family requests that their privacy be respected. The General and his family greatly appreciate the warm wishes and prayers of his friends, colleagues, and supporters."

Sometimes these go with the age 73 patriot territory. Hope it is just Ischemic and best wishes.

2018.11.25:18:43 ≈ |OP|>1....|GW|>2WB|<2+|JU|<3 |TR|<3|LI|>3

Representative Connolly, et al:

Please note the following 2020 census considerations in your efforts.

Honorable Gerry Connolly (D-VA11) quoted in WaPost concerning 2020 census:

"I worry a lot about the reaction of many of these households to a census with this question," Connolly said in a recent interview. "I want them to be able to comply with the census with no fear that someone will get them because of their answers. That fear is real and palpable."

Civil Rights Act, Title II, SEC. 202:

All persons shall be entitled to be free, at any establishment or place, from discrimination or segregation of any kind on the ground of race, color, religion, or national origin, if such discrimination or segregation is or purports to be required by any law, statute, ordinance, regulation, rule, or order of a State or any agency or political subdivision thereof.

In order to avoid Title II, Sec. 202 forms of discrimination devolved from the 2020 Census, wouldn't it be necessary to eliminate Questions 8 and 9 on the Census D-91 form? While the protection of Census original information is legally quite strong, in this age of cyber break-ins, even the Question 4 telephone number might be a hazard. It might be more suitable to replace Question 4 with the location data of the current congressional District and the USPS zip code. This is because the Census forms should reflect the Constitutional requirement for the Census (Article I, Sec. 2) AND the guarantee of a representative republic (Article IV, Sec. 4). The District number and zip code combine to establish the geographical location regardless of computerized gerrymandering. The modern computation mechanisms have made some Districts a clear violation of Article IV, Sec. 4 in that the election might represent less than 10% of a given Census population.

As for citizenship questions, only citizens are lawful voters according to the Article IV guarantee regardless of the mix between citizens and nationals in a District. How is it that a Representative or a Senator can engage in CRA types of discrimination if he takes an oath of office to the Constitution? Is he, by the oath, automatically representing a majority of the Census defined population of a District or a State?

Speculation:

While 200 million Americans have the DNA haplogroup R1a or R1b, the astonishing diversity of the Nation only appears when a 'Census' of the existing haplogroups is made. This is a sample:

Four states, KS, ME, NH, and WV are most strongly just R1b (West European – English, German and Italian-French). The largest number of states, 12, the historic south, plus MO, are primarily R1b and secondarily E. Six states are also strong in R1b and E, but also in R1a, eastern Europe, IN, MD,MI, OH, NY (also has Hispanic and Jewish), and PA. Somewhat similar are IL and NJ (notice that many of these are contiguous), with R1b, E, and R1bh. HI is unique as the only state with a dominant O, Asian, group, and the District of Columbia as the only area dominated by E (African origin).

From an Affordable Care Act or a universal single payer health viewpoint, the haplogroups would be a much better method of defining political districts since they do not discriminate according to skin-tone (a minor DNA pair sequence) and predict the possible health problems of the entire population. That might be included in a citizen's health data card in the future as well as an automatic voter registration system, but how would you differentiate between a 'citizen' and a visiting 'national' if the haplogroup data is correct?

Please consider the need for care in defining a District population because although non-citizen Nationals must be taken into account by the Congress, it is the local citizens who define a District in the Census.

2018.11.28:09:05 |OP| ⋈ |CD|<3 ≈ |TR|<3 [LI|<3⋈|JU|<1 |GW|<2

Ignatius, WaPost, 'The Khashoggi killing had roots in a cutthroat Saudi family feud':

"The brutal paranoia of MBS's royal court in Riyadh recalls Baghdad in the days of Saddam Hussein. The spotlight cast by Khashoggi's killing gives Saudi Arabia, and the United States, a last chance to check a slide toward Hussein-like despotism from overwhelming the region."

The personalization or ownership of state power by using 'intelligence' personnel as a death squad isn't limited to Saudi Arabia. There is a dozen such 'ownership' oligarchic families around the world using security 'teams', with at least one on each continent and some in possession of WMD. Since they don't represent a threat to North American checks and balances on power, it would be hard to interdict them with an AUMF style expression of the Constitution. Even the President's CinC authority in Article II might not have enough authorization to isolate a hit squad at some place like Guantanamo even if their ripple effects reach inside the U.S. The Chinese Ministry of State Security didn't quite know how to handle oligarchic politics even in Shanghai and they have the most experience with 'Tongs' or imperial power struggles, so this type of WMD equipped group (note the aircraft used) might be a serious world problem at some future point.

The author's event timeline is so detailed that it might qualify as a world politics short story except that it is a very believable reality of life on Earth. Welcome to the third century BC.

TL Opservationis 2018.12

2018.12.02:07:28 |OP| ≈ ∑ |TR|>3 |LI|>3⋈|JU|>1| ξ] >2 |WB|>1

Editorial Board, WaPost, 'George H.W. Bush had no grand dreams. His competence and restraint were enough.':

"What Mr. Bush did was handle a series of historic crises with competence and restraint, while dealing with the everyday conflicts and compromises of legislating and budgeting in a responsible and reasonable way. Mr. Bush did well while holding office. His most unattractive acts came in the seeking of it."

Psalm 15:1-3:

Lord, who may dwell in your sacred tent?   Who may live on your holy mountain?

The one whose walk is blameless, who does what is righteous, who speaks the truth from their heart;

whose tongue utters no slander, who does no wrong to a neighbor, and casts no slur on others;

Speculation: More like this person wouldn't hurt the Nation at all.

2018.12.06:07:42 |OP|n ≈ ∑ |WB|<3+|CD|<2 |TR|<3 |LI|<1 ⋈ |JU|<1|GW|<2

Eileen Hunt Botting in WaPost, 'A Chinese scientist says he edited babies' genes. What are the rights of the genetically modified child?':

"Regardless of whether the claim of gene-edited twins in China proves true, we can expect to see many more genetically modified children whose DNA has been heritably altered through CRISPR-Cas9 and other biotechnologies."

Many more genetically modified children? In a world that will be increasingly overpopulated because of global warming related turmoil such as Yemen, Philippines, and Venezuela, why isn't the 'right' of the individual to procreate 'mutated' human embryos a bioethics question for societies? Is the author suggesting that ANY procreative activity, such as creation of spare body parts, should automatically be protected by the current 'rights of the child' conventions? From a modern, post-Darwin/Mendel bio-ethical standpoint, why isn't the act of procreation itself subject to the Article 7, Section k crimes against humanity:

(k) Other inhumane acts of a similar character intentionally causing great suffering, or serious injury to body or to mental or physical health.

The researcher in China operated in secret at an obscure state funded laboratory. How many more such laboratories for profit exist or will exist for the procreation of 'mutated' embryos that those with the normal DNA of 'Human Accelerated Regions' will need to make economic and ethical sacrifices for?

TLO: Does liberty to do research have to be completely suppressed for humanity's safety?

2018.12.08:07:45 $\Sigma \mid \xi \mid >n=\Sigma \mid OP \mid n$

Albert Einstein, letter to Gutkind, 1954, a year before his passing:

"The word God is for me nothing more than the expression and product of human weaknesses, the Bible a collection of honorable but still primitive legends," he wrote.

Christie's books and manuscripts specialist Peter Klarnet said the letter is notable for its bluntness.

"Here he is actually quite blunt in what he says," Klarnet said. "The word 'God' is a product of human weakness."

Perceptional weakness, perhaps? Taken together in the letter, Albert was talking about the era of 200 years before and after 0001 AD when the bible was written and the term was used in that context. He is correct; the people who acted out the Bible at that time were in fact 'primitive legends' and should be regarded as such when chronicling the Bible or Torah. They could no more have understood the meaning of spirituality or Parakletos than they could have understood Newton's 'primitive' concept of gravity or time. Note that Albert's many writings carefully avoided a description of a 'holy spirit' or a spiritual form of energy, which both he and Newton suspected was a parallel 'universe'.

2018.12.09:09:04 $|CD|>3$ ⋈ $|GW|>2|JU|>2|TR|>2 \approx |OP|>3$

Prime Minister Imran Khan in WaPost, 'Pakistani leader to the U.S.: We're not your 'hired gun' anymore':

"From the mid-1980s onwards, we were hit with growing corruption. Corruption goes into megaprojects which have mega-kickbacks. When your political leadership makes money, it cannot park the money in the country because it will be visible. [Past leaders] took that money out of the country, which means the country ends up getting short of foreign exchange. Once your leadership starts making money, it goes right down to every level."

Perhaps that pervasive corruption was the reason that Fazlur Malik's concept of the al-Jihad al-asghar in Pakistan was so ruthlessly suppressed by the hypocrites in the government and political structure of Islamabad. Malik on many occasions equated use of public funds for personal wealth with a form of false jihad that lessened the Pakistani people's ability to bring about the spirituality of the 'inner jihad'. These government munafiq, especially in the 'security' services, were so busy transferring U.S. hundred-dollar bills to Qatar banks that they were blind to the spiritual needs of the many Pakistani cultures.

Note Quranic surah 8:39:

And fight the hypocrites until there is no more tumult or oppression, and there prevail justice and faith in Allah altogether and everywhere; but if they cease, verily Allah doth see all that they do.

American and NATO forces, but perhaps not Russian or Chinese forces, could fight in Afghanistan, Iran or in Pakistan with the permission of those who had renounced the hypocrisy of the al-jihad al-asghar but under no other banner. Removing hypocrite corruption from power is a universal value.

2018.12.09:09:06 |OP| ≈ ∑ |TR|>1 |LI|>3⋈|JU|>1....|GW|<4|CD|<1

Burke, TheHill, 'Top Dem: Illegal payments would 'certainly' be impeachable offenses if directed by Trump':

"Nadler added that Congress shouldn't "necessarily launch an impeachment against the president because he committed an impeachable offense."

It is only an impeachable offense AFTER the Article II, Section 1 Oath of Office is taken as president, where the Executive can be held to the 'high crimes and misdemeanor' standard.

TLO: to be an endless pogrom?

2018.12.10:06:19 |CD|<3 ⋈ |JU|<4....|GW|>1- |TR|<2 ≈ |OP|>2

Portnoy, WaPost, 'Kaine hopeful that senators will warm to new military force authorization after Yemen vote':

"The United States has used those early authorizations in 37 instances to send forces to 14 nations, including Libya, Turkey, Georgia, Syria, Iraq, Afghanistan, Yemen, Eritrea, Ethiopia, Djibouti, Somalia, Kenya, the Philippines and Cuba, according to Kaine's office.

"The height of public immorality is to order troops into war without Congress having the guts to vote on it, and that has been my feeling for a very long time," Kaine said in a recent interview."

There is a persistent belief among many Senators and Representatives that use of force by military personnel in a foreign country is automatically a condition of 'war' under the Constitution's Article I, Section 8, clause 11. That is just not the case. Many of the described deployments were for humanitarian prevention of crimes against humanity and had little to do with the condition of declared war. The military operations were much more relevant to clause 10, not 11, concerning the 'Offenses against the Law of Nations', and crimes against humanity, all 13 categories, easily qualify as a national interest under the Constitution.

If they are going to rescind the current Authorizations, they need to specify the new ones are acting directly against crimes against humanity under clause 10 as 'police' activity, not war. These military operations do not come close to acts of 'war' and shouldn't be considered in that context.

2018.12.14:09:28 |WB|n+|CD|<1.....|LI||TR|>3[JU|+ |GW|>1=|OP|>n

Editorial Board, BloombergOpinion, 'The Science of Gene Editing Demands Caution and Consensus. News of a reckless experiment demonstrates the dangers.':

"True, the congressional ban — added as a rider to the omnibus spending bill, and since renewed — blocks irresponsible genetic engineering. But the FDA was in a position to block it anyway. This extra restriction is mistaken because it stops the FDA from engaging in any thoughtful regulation of embryonic gene-editing."

Question: Under exactly which Article I, Section 8 authority of the Congress was the 'irresponsible genetic engineering' blocked? Interstate commerce Clause 3? The necessary and proper Clause 18 as applied in an 'omnibus' appropriations bill?

Promote the 'Progress' of Sciences in Clause 8? There is really nothing in the Constitution, or in state constitutions, that gives the authority to control life creation by individuals engaged in CRISPR or molecular editing such as germline splicing.

If a person wants her children to have a neutral green skin with blue eyes as opposed to a mandatory yellow or black skin, by what authority does the government have to prevent this if she can buy the gene-editing kits on the open international market and carries out the editing in the privacy of her own home?

Molecular modification of human life needs some serious bio-ethical evaluation throughout the society and most world governments are still trying to get past social Darwinism ideologies and dogmas of the 1800s.

2018.12.15:09:42 [LI|>1|TR|<2|WB|<2+|CD|<3 ⋈ |GW|>1-|JU|<2≈|OP|?

Wheeler, TheHill, 'Mueller probe has cost more than $25M so far':

"The bulk of those costs came from personnel compensation and benefits, which totaled about $2.9 million. Another $580,000 was spent on travel and transportation, and $942,787 was spent on rent, communications and utilities."

In 2015 and 2016, the Justice Department had to allocate some 40 high ranking legal personnel to respond to FOIA requests by conservative legal PACs seeking documents on Secretary Clinton and her associates in the State Department. This eventually rounded out as a taxpayer expense of $70 million over two years created by people who were themselves earning $600 per hour for initiating the requests. Their pay might have been three times what the taxpayer costs were, even though the requests found virtually nothing of a 'high crimes and misdemeanor' nature.

The Mueller investigation has resulted in indictments of 33 people related to anti-constitutional processes, or $750,000 per person. That doesn't include court costs in the name of Justice or penal costs later at $36,000 per year per person. We needn't even go into the media costs in man hours of describing these events.

All this because of a systemic attack by a foreign mercenary oligarchy on the idea of Democracy with Justice for all?

2018.12.16:08:17 |TR|>2 = ∑ |LI|>1WB|<2 ⋈ |GW|>3-|JU|<2....|OP|<3

Editorial Board, WaPost, 'The Democratic House is taking on ethics reform first. We need it.':

"The plan will be finalized over the coming weeks, but the outlines are becoming clear. Democrats will make the biggest push to fight money in politics......"

One of the proposals would allow matching funds for small donations that are six times the donation. All this does is throw more money into an election system where there is too much money already. A bipartisan solution might be a 'luxury' tax on advertising that becomes an endless repetition rather than a form of political or educational comment necessary for democracies. You only need to see data once or twice a day to be informed, not once every ten minutes in the media, so anything expressed beyond the once or twice a day is not covered by 1st Amendment press protections and therefore qualifies as a 'luxury' purchase by the advertiser. This might even slow down the meaningless false news processes of foreign totalitarians intent on undermining all democracies.

One of the other ethics problems that has existed since the 2nd Congress of 1791 is that of Representatives being beholden to the wealth of their home districts to support them in representing a population in an Electoral District. That usually meant getting the equivalent of two year's expenses from a local 'banker'. It might be worth while for the Congress to allow a successful candidate to allocate campaign small 'donations' for first year re-location expenses equivalent to a year's congressional salary of $174,000. Who would a newly elected be beholden to then?

As for voter registration 'rights', there MUST be tests of citizenship in this century, not mere proof of residency where anyone getting off an airplane, rich private ones included, can say he is a 'voter'. A test of citizenship means that a person is willing to go a distance to perform a citizenship duty like voting and that distance might mean a guaranteed proof of citizenship, not residency.

2018.12.16:11:43 |CD|>4|TR|>2 ≈|OP|>2 ....|WB|<4+|JU|>3 ⋈ |GW|>2|LI|<4

Editorial Board, WaPost, 'Mexico has a plan to reduce the migrant flow from Central America. Trump should embrace it.':"If Mr. Trump signs on to Mr. López Obrador's vision for reviving Central America with an ambitious aid plan — one that would also serve U.S. interest as a means to "disincentivize" migration — that could be just the sweetener Mr. López Obrador needs to go along with Mr. Trump's asylum plan."

Mexico's own problems with feeding and keeping healthy an extensive population is shown in the table below. Mexico may have Malthusian problems of their own that virtually require them to seek aid from less dense societies to the north (U.S. is 33 people per sq/km, Canada is 4 people per sq/km). Everyone knows what climate related disasters do to a population. Katrina in New Orleans, and Maria in Puerto Rico caused major population shifts. The same is going on in Central America as arable land disappears in the new heat and cartels fight over what's left.

Demographics in the Central American and Caribbean region.

'Dens' is people per sq/km, 'AL' is Arable land for crops

Puerto Rico	Dens: 385	AL: 22%	People: 3.1 M
El Salvador	Dens: 306	AL: 77%	People: 6.7M
Jamaica	Dens: 266	AL: 41%	People: 3.1M
Trinidad and Tobago	Dens: 266	AL: 10%	People: 1.4M
Dominican Republic	Dens: 220	AL: 44%	People: 11.3
Guatemala	Dens: 155	AL: 32%	People: 18M
Cuba	Dens: 110	AL: 60%	People: 12.1M

Costa Rica	Dens: 95	AL: 35%	People: 5.2M
Honduras	Dens: 81	AL: 29%	People: 9.7M
Mexico	Dens: 66	AL: 12%	People: 138M
Panama	Dens: 54	AL: 30%	People: 4.3M
Nicaragua	Dens: 51	AL: 42%	People: 6.5M
Belize	Dens: 16	AL: 7%	People: 385K

You can be as compassionate as you want but at some point, the human density-to-food problems have to stay home rather than be transplanted somewhere else. Perhaps the Mexican president has the right idea, but is throwing money at a region when it might wind up in a Caribbean bank as the Panama Papers indicated really the solution?

Evolutionary rule? If you have no hope of feeding We the People, do you still create them?

2018.12.17:18:52 |CD|<2 ≈|OP|>1 Ξ|WB|<1+|JU|>2 ⋈ |GW|<2

Michael McFaul in WaPost, 'Why Vladimir Putin is a terrible strategist':

"In the short run, Putin has won several tactical victories. In the long run, however, these same wins have planted the seeds of long-term isolation and weakness for Russia on the world stage. Nearly every single short-term Putin achievement has undermined a long-term Putin objective."

These 'tactical' victories, initiated by a military-industrial complex led by the GRU, would make perfect sense if they were intended to keep Europeans, Middle Eastern and North American peoples in a state of continuous internal conflict. But that would be an idea from Mao Zedong's 'On Protracted War' concept where subordinate 'provinces' keep enemies of the Beijing government occupied while it gathers overwhelming strength and wealth to itself.

Does someone in this century consider the Moskva Oblast a western province as they have in the past, with Bogatyr leaders doing his bidding once again?

2018.12.17:06:49 |OP|>1 ≈∑ |CD|<2 ⋈ |GW|>2 |TR|>3 |LI|<1⋈|JU|>1

Devine, CRS, 'Congressional Oversight of Intelligence: Background and Selected Options for Further Reform':

Potential Questions for Congress

• Is current congressional oversight of the IC "dysfunctional" as the 9/11 Commission alleged in 2004? What criteria would so indicate?

• Could oversight of intelligence be further improved such that the IC would, as a result, be more effective in support of national security? Would enhancements in oversight enable Congress to measure the IC's effectiveness more effectively?

• To what extent have oversight reform measures been effective in promoting (1) an apolitical IC; (2) committee experience; (3) committee capacity to handle workload; and/or (4) relations with the IC?

• Is the JCAE model an appropriate analogy for consideration of a joint congressional intelligence committee as some have maintained?

• Should Congress hire additional professional staff to serve on the select intelligence committees?

• Would parallel intelligence structures in each chamber be conducive to improved oversight? Should the HPSCI abolish term limits and adopt the model of ensuring the majority party not exceed the minority party's representation by more than one?

• Would a consolidation of authorizations and appropriations authority in the congressional intelligence committees consolidate too much authority or enhance congressional oversight?

Direct political responsibility for IC activities? More than one way that can come out.

2018.12.20:22:22 |OP| ≈∑ |WB|<1+|CD|>3 |TR|>3 |LI|<1✉|JU|<1|GW|>2

Here is the full text of Mattis' resignation letter, as released by the Defense Department:

Dear Mr. President:

I have been privileged to serve as our country's 26th Secretary of Defense which has allowed me to serve alongside our men and women of the Department in defense of our citizens and our ideals.

I am proud of the progress that has been made over the past two years on some of the key goals articulated in our National Defense Strategy: putting the Department on a more sound budgetary footing, improving readiness and lethality in our forces, and reforming the Department's business practices for greater performance. Our troops continue to provide the capabilities needed to prevail in conflict and sustain strong U.S. global influence.

One core belief I have always held is that our strength as a nation is inextricably linked to the strength of our unique and comprehensive system of alliances and partnerships. While the US remains the indispensable nation in the free world, we cannot protect our interests or serve that role effectively without maintaining strong alliances and showing respect to those allies. Like you, I have said from the beginning that the armed forces of the United States should not be the policeman of the world. Instead, we must use all tools of American power to provide for the common defense, including providing effective leadership to our alliances. NATO's 29 democracies demonstrated that strength in their commitment to fighting alongside us following the 9-11 attack on America. The Defeat-ISIS coalition of 74 nations is further proof.

Similarly, I believe we must be resolute and unambiguous in our approach to those countries whose strategic interests are increasingly in tension with ours. It is clear that China and Russia, for example, want to shape a world consistent with their authoritarian model — gaining veto authority over other nations' economic, diplomatic, and security decisions — to promote their own interests at the expense of their neighbors, America and our allies. That is why we must use all the tools of American power to provide for the common defense.

My views on treating allies with respect and also being clear-eyed about both malign actors and strategic competitors are strongly held and informed by over four decades of immersion in these issues. We must do everything possible to advance an international order that is most conducive to our security, prosperity and values, and we are strengthened in this effort by the solidarity of our alliances.

Because you have the right to have a Secretary of Defense whose views are better aligned with yours on these and other subjects, I believe it is right for me to step down from my position. The end date for my tenure is February 28, 2019, a date that should allow sufficient time for a successor to be nominated and confirmed as well as to make sure the Department's interests are properly articulated and protected at upcoming events to include Congressional posture hearings and the NATO Defense Ministerial meeting in February. Further, that a full transition to a new Secretary of Defense occurs well in advance of the transition of Chairman of the Joint Chiefs of Staff in September in order to ensure stability within the Department.

I pledge my full effort to a smooth transition that ensures the needs and interests of the 2.15 million Service Members and 732,079 DoD civilians receive undistracted attention of the Department at all times so that they can fulfill their critical, round-the-clock mission to protect the American people.

I very much appreciate this opportunity to serve the nation and our men and women in uniform.

Jim N. Mattis

2018.12.22:07:33 |TR|<2 = ∑ |LI|>1WB|<2 ⋈ |GW|>1-|JU|<2....|OP|<3

Applebaum, WaPost, 'The lure of chaos is leading Britain straight into the abyss':

"Millions of British citizens living in Europe, and millions of E.U. citizens living in Britain, will be in legal limbo."

Wasn't that the original problem to begin with? Most of the pro-Brexit votes came from the shires of England, not Wales or Scotland and if one checks the demographics carefully, the votes were in direct proportion to the population density of the shires and urban districts in the south eastern third of the land areas. Those are also the areas that most of the unlimited immigration foolishness imposed by the EU takes place. That is, the areas were becoming too densely populated to sustain life in a reasonable, unchaotic form. The stresses of population density is something all 'revolutionaries' from the Marxist-Leninist left and Locke-Keynes right exploit without being able to do anything about it.

The real problem is the unsustainable population growth that, oddly enough, was considerably slowed by the mass killing of young males in World War I and II. This may have led to the prosperity of the 20th century that was working until the EU forced new immigrations and caused the increasing 'tavern idleness' of the southern Brits as the labor hours became shared with more and more immigrants. Any politician promising a 20-hour work week around London? But if you don't produce enough food, clothing, health, and shelter without massive imports what good is 'idleness'?

"In theory, generic markets should be the Walmart of the health-care world, where everything is dirt cheap and readily available.........Lots of drugs, especially those used by only a smaller number of patients, have at best a handful of firms producing them."

Can't have it both ways in the private sector ONLY. If you only have 1,000 patients with a particular bio-molecular problem, NO company is going to set up shop to make the relevant medication because it would take a hundred years to see an ROI without national infrastructure help. Some drug fabrication facilities, not counting meth and crack, require extreme isolation, 'clean-room' facilities that would look like the inside of Fort Knox. There are at least two facilities in the U.S. that cost $300 million each to build in order to create one safe production line for a drug and that was after they had waivers for many of the fed regulations for such facilities.

Speculation:

Some secret police organizations have began to use addictive medications (and radioactive isotopes) as a form of warfare and to suggest that less regulation of chemicals in shipments around the U.S. is a good idea is nonsense. Iran transships Afghan and Pakistani opioids around the world for profit. Venezuela was doing the same with Colombian and Bolivian drugs. Fentanyl is manufactured in farm communities near Chinese cities and shipped out.

It might be much better to treat drug manufacture as a non-profit, MILITARY defense process in which separate manufacturing facilities are distributed as a defense infrastructure around the U.S. This might prevent drugs from being used the way Fentanyl is along with bringing down the costs. The private sector then becomes not-for-profit contractors that are under extreme biohazard regulation on or near military facilities. Capitalization is rewarded for the research and development of drugs instead of the 'market' related production.

But if medical 'rights' are involved, so are constitutional additions involved.

2018.12.24:07:15 |CD|<3 ⋈ |GW|>1-|JU|>2|TR|<2 ≈ |OP|.2

Samuelson, WaPost, 'Wake up. America's military isn't invincible.':

"This is not a call for war. It is a call for stopping many self-inflicted wounds. We need to stop underfunding the military, especially on research and cyberwarfare, even if that means less welfare."

You can blame the current situation on one Milton Friedman's dogmatic concepts in 'Capitalism and Freedom' in which Common Defense in the Constitution meant defense of a completely free economic 'system', world-wide or otherwise. At the time of its writing in 1962, the wealthy elite in the United States (and they were largely American citizens) were approving but disliking their 70% income tax rate that was creating a nearly invincible protective screen around the United States and allies.

The point is the wealthy of the United States were willing to infuse the Defense with Cold War levels of taxation and are no longer willing to do this even as they are the 'usury' beneficiaries of the American security and economic umbrellas. The military withdrawals from around the world are a dot-connected effect to the lack of willingness by the top tiers of income to expend revenues necessary to maintain world countermeasures to ancient totalitarian imperial and primal impulses.

About the only way you could improve the 'strategic' security umbrellas of the Capitalist economies (and freedoms) around the world is through a combined infusion of wealth into the mechanisms for defense. That would mean an incremental income tax increase of perhaps one percent per bracket every three years for the next 15, possibly with dedicated funding of Defense and Medicare processes. Neither political party, or their wealth contributors, are willing to do this because of the Friedmanist dogmas concerning relations between government and a 'world', not 'American', economy. Cutting their own throat on everybody else's time, perhaps?

2018.12.27:12:41 |CD|>3 ⋈ |GW|>1|JU|<3|TR|<2≈|OP|>1

Alexander Bolton, TheHill, 'Border wall impasse awaits senators returning to Washington':

"The House last week passed a measure that would provide $5.7 billion in border security and wall funding and $8.7 billion in disaster relief. But that bill is considered dead on arrival in the Senate, with Democrats and the White House remaining at odds over funding for President Trump's border wall."

Really odd where these cost estimates in the appropriations are coming from. A common highway concrete slab sound barrier at 16 feet high costs about $700,000 per mile and you only need such barriers on about 500 miles of the unprotected 1100 miles that remain. That works out to about $350 million. The rest, about 1200 miles, only need intense surveillance and drone interdiction 'walls' at about $130,000 per mile. That's $156 million and might even be considered 'disaster relief funding' since the all-spectrum surveillance with drones might prevent the 200 bodies a year that show up near the borders that have 110-degree deserts on both sides.

But where do the Executive's $5 billion and the Congress's $1.3 billion estimates come from ? The sample border walls shown in the media are almost identical to the sound barrier walls being installed on U.S. highways. Most of the surveillance 'gear' and outpost sensor poles are off-the-shelf military equipment found in recon detachments already deployed around the world. $8 billion in disaster relief or border support over how long a period? Really need a combination of $8 billion and $5 billion for this?

2018.12.28:07:33 |CD|<3 ⋈ |GW|<3|JU|<3|TR|<2≈|OP|<3

Sheridan, WaPost, 'While Washington focuses on the wall, Mexico fears its own border crisis':

"We didn't come all this way to stay here," said Jonatan Orantes, 27, a moto-taxi driver who said he fled Guatemala because gangs tried to extort money from him. "Mexico isn't safe."

Unfortunately, Guatemalan organized gang or cartel crimes of violence such as rape, extortion or enslavement, and multiple murders don't meet the International Criminal Court's definition of 'systemic' attack against a civilian population. They are individual acts of violence against civilians, not a 'program' of genocide such as that carried out by the Iran, Iraq, Syrian and Venezuelan government entities. There is no UN justification for international forces to bring martial law and order to Guatemala like it would have in Iraq and Syria. As a consequence, the U.S. Congress could not create a Guatemala Use of Force Authorization for American soldiers to prevent crimes against humanity in that country under Article I, Section 8, clause 10 'offenses against the laws of nations'.

Very unfortunate because bringing martial law to Guatemala by sending American and Mexican Marines there would be cheaper over a ten-year period than dealing with mass displacement of humans in the border states and provinces. One billion a year instead of fourteen billion a year, not counting misery indexes, perhaps?

2018.12.30:08:33 [OP]>n?

David Anderson in WaPost, 'How TV shows use serious archaeology to promote bogus history':

"During the episode, Fox tells viewers that legends "contain legitimate historical information" and suggests that if the Trojan War really happened, it "could mean that there might be truth in other Greek gods and legends." She thus enacts the adage that all myths have an element of truth."

Homer's version of the Trojan War may have had some 'legends' of its own, because Heinrich Schliemann's examination of the 'ruins' indicated about eight distinct levels of an inhabited fortress. That included a couple of bronze age levels that predates Homer's War. Even some of the really ancient Egyptian, Indus River and Han River societies had scripts that could be interpreted as 'speculative fiction' or sci-fi renderings of local facts. These can sometime lead to completely wrong timeline interpretations such as the Mayan 2012 Calendar.

The same could be said of something like the current 'The Expanse' series of the 2800s with its hi-def images of a human-occupied solar system. What would happen if a species ten thousand years from now with VERY advanced Human Accelerated Regions of DNA (HARs) dug up a DVD copy of the 'The Expanse' episodes and interpreted them to mean humans were engaged in Homeric quests all over the solar system?

How would such a species visualize a pre-quantum society, let alone bronze-age, at all unless it had accurate event records of societies the way archaeologists try and fail to find in dig sites around the world? Even modern Chinese and Russian media with its systemic distortion of facts could contribute to a false interpretation of current history. Good luck, archaeologists.

2018.12.31:06:54 [OP]? ≈∑ [WB]<3+[CD]>2 [TR]<3 [LI]<1 ✉ [JU]<1[GW]>2

Dionne, WaPost, 'There is much to fear about nationalism. But liberals need to address it the right way.':

"Globalism, Judis argues, "subordinates nations and national governments to market forces or to the priorities of multinational corporations." Internationalism, on the other hand, accepts that nations may sometimes have to "cede part of their sovereignty to international or regional bodies to address problems they could not adequately address on their own."

Judis, and this author, also assume that urbanized social democracy is the only legitimate form a 'human' society can be allowed to take and therefore any 'internationalism' that enforces social democracy is legitimate. They imply that some international oligarchy operating a controlled market force through governmental 'law and order' in order to extract wealth from unprotected populations, AKA Asian Hegemony, has legitimacy because it opposes 'nationalism' in America.

They apply the mistaken ideological dogmas of a century ago when nationalism did produce fascism, democide (mass murder for ethnic, economic, political, or religious reasons by governmental entities) and genocide (systemic extermination of a culture by another culture) as an expression of totalitarianism to the modern American social system. Not a reality perception. That 'progressive' mentality doesn't fit no matter how many neurotic labels are used to define American society because the nationalism is simply a reaction to globalist AND internationalist economic aggression against western cultures.

Wars and Democides are created by self-centric urban elites as much as by anything else, because their paranoia about fascism and genetically undefinable 'racism' won't allow a society to protect itself against globalism OR manipulative internationalism. The ideology of the 'liberal' democracy itself, not nationalism, is suspect if a society is under economic and physical attack by offshore monopolies.

Constitutional Summary,   Timeline of 2018

The summery is intended to give a timeline progression of the 2018 election year as it relates to the six existing covenants of the Preamble as national interactive domains. While there has developed during the previous Chronicles are reluctance to break down or categorize the Six into further subsets because it involves an inability to 'sense' the direction of the domains as a group. The idea of a constitutional perception is to SUM the domains in some order that can show a progression in time.

We the People of the United States, in Order to form a more perfect Union,
(1) establish Justice [JU] ,
(2) insure domestic Tranquility [TR],
(3) provide for the common defence [CD],
(4) promote the general Welfare [GW], and
(5) secure the Blessings of Liberty [LI] to ourselves
(6) and our Posterity [OP],
do ordain and establish this Constitution for the United States of America.

The SUM of the constitutional domains might be sensed as:

$$\Sigma|CD|\text{-}/\text{+}n,\ \ |GW|\text{-}/\text{+}n \rightarrow |TR|\text{+}/\text{-}n,\ \ |JU|\text{+}/\text{-}n,\ \ |LI|\text{+}/\text{-}n \ \rightarrow [WB]>nn \ \rightarrow [OP]>?$$

The [WB] domain is currently imbedded in all of the six domains, not a separate one, and is shown here as a sensed addition. But what happens when you run into an 'ethnic diversity' map showing the placement of peoples in the United States? The colors in the ethnic image represent Americans with a majority density in a given county, not the spectrum of the domains, but from a constitutional standpoint how do you represent that much ethnic diversity as 'Common' and 'General' found in the Constitution, especially when the Bill of Rights and the 14th Amendment says you *must*?

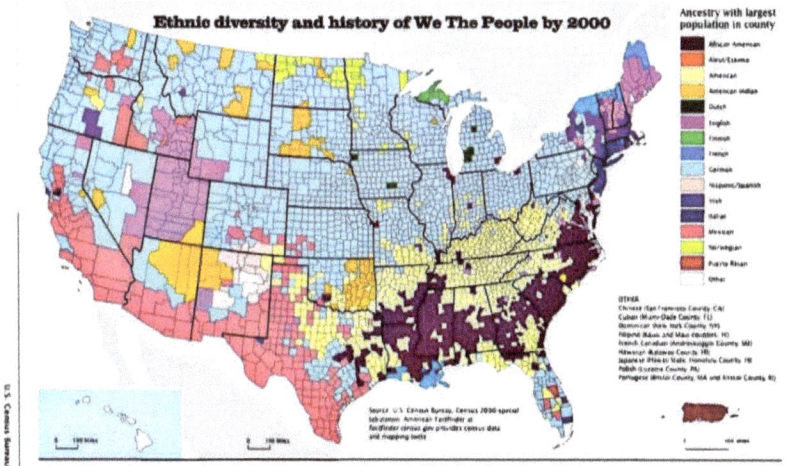

Figure 12.   U.S. ethnic diversity

You cannot break the visualization formula into ethnic {subsets} because that is exactly what the Constitution was designed to prevent, noting that ethnicity is a genetic inheritance process with many hundreds of DNA variances. Overcoming such a deeply rooted ethnicity of primate tribal societies is a complexity issue all its own and some societies have solved it by elimination of all other ethnicities they come across.

That tribal xenophobia that is expressed by all cultures and has led to many wars and atrocities is continually reborn in newer cultures. A very complex problem to resolve as an optimization within the Posterity domain. Even a modern mapping of the Congress Districts will show a 'natural' tribal ethnicity of Americans because of a desire to socialize and politize with 'similar' people. The practice of political or ethnic gerrymandering for what ever purpose is also outside the established boundaries of Article IV representation in most cases and is routinely defined as such by the Supreme Court. In 2018, the Supreme Court declined to rule on gerrymandering as the number of cases involving it increased dramatically. They had determined many cases of 'ethnic' gerrymandering were unconstitutional in the past and held to that, while political division of Districts was more of a state issue. It was considered more of a [TR] issue than a [OP] concern. But how would you define gerrymandering in terms of {subsets} that had an effect of [TR] → [OP]>? By each district or each political faction or by each ethnic faction?

Gerrymander index scores, 113th Congress

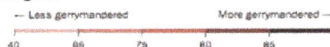

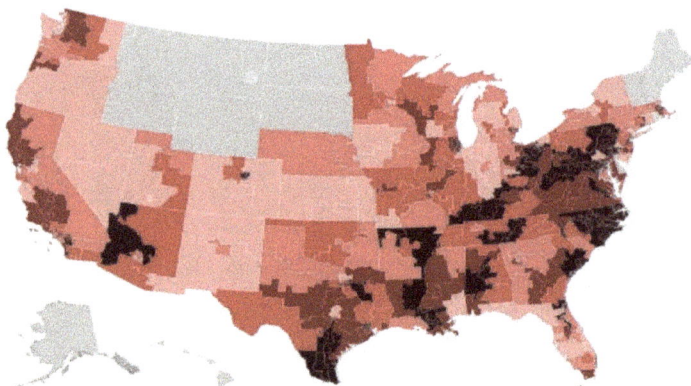

← Less gerrymandered   More gerrymandered →

40   86   75   80   85

In ethnicity, the concept of scientific reduction becomes more of an exercise in motivational reasoning in which the ethnic values of the individual or tribe become the reason for political activity, with a possible [JU] value the most dominate. In many cases that would be correct use of the Constitution; correcting ethnic injustices is inherent. But gerrymandering politics can become a form of tribal dominance of a territory and other tribes, which is a purely primate instinct, not reductionism toward a goal.

The complexity of a {set} of Constitution values being applied to any population is further multiplied when the base, We the People, do not effectively participate in the 'system'. This can be shown by the very wide voter turn-out variations in the 2018 elections, not a presidential election, shown in the following image. If one compares the ethnicity map with the gerrymander map and the turnout map, some general sense of what is going on appears, but reductionism would lead almost anywhere. Why would an ethnic area like Louisiana have such high gerrymandered counties along with a low turnout of voters? Why would a nearly 'pure' ethnic society like Ohio have a high turnout with 'gerrymandering' that shouldn't exist because of ethnicity? Is voting in an off year more about personalities in Representation than constitution related issues?

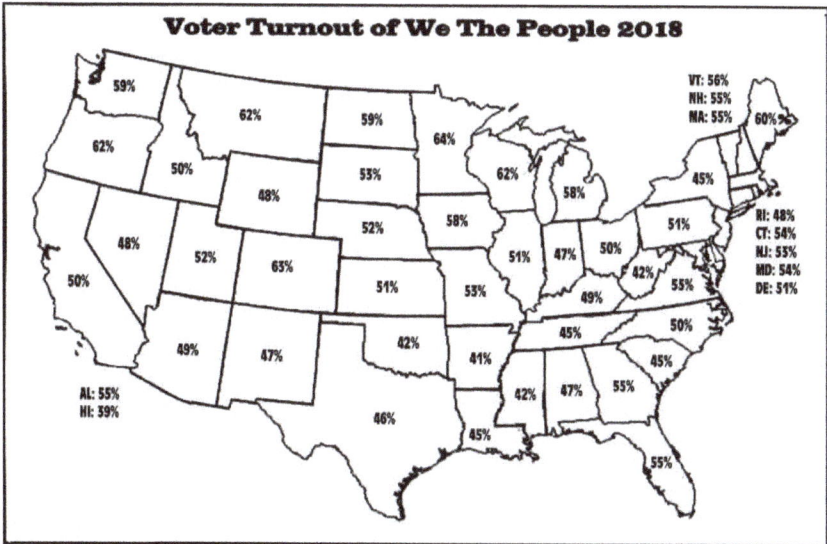

Voter Turnout of We The People 2018

If We the People are voting local political processes rather than national issues, would it show up in a exmining the {subsets} of the federal government? Note again the 'sense' of progression:

Σ[CD]-/+n, [GW]-/+n → [TR]+/-n, [JU]+/-n, [LI]+/-n → [WB]>nn → |OP|>?

Here the five domains are summed into a [WB] domain and then into a [OP] superset. But each of these has a U.S. Budget component and [CD] is shown as:

Table 3.2 - OUTLAYS BY FUNCTION AND SUBFUNCTION: 1962 - 2023
(in millions of dollars)

[CD] Common Defense {DOD}, {State}

Function and Subfunction	2011	2012	2013	2014	2015	2016	2017	2018	2019	2020 estimate
050 National Defense:										
051 Department of Defense-Military:										
Military Personnel	160,866	152,266	150,825	148,922	143,596	147,905	144,301	145,837	156,267	162,286
Operation and Maintenance	290,693	282,297	259,660	244,481	247,239	245,190	243,184	256,657	271,699	283,609
Procurement	128,003	124,712	114,902	107,481	101,842	102,656	104,127	112,869	124,699	135,097
Research, Development, Test, and Evaluation	74,871	70,394	66,892	64,920	64,524	64,873	48,137	76,976	89,230	97,318
Military Construction	19,391	14,550	12,518	9,823	8,153	8,677	6,671	6,706	7,412	8,600
Family Housing	3,402	3,341	1,829	1,354	1,366	1,304	3,207	1,153	1,568	1,373
Other	603	4,298	1,357	903	4,342	-1,345	-2,121	491	3,463	1,721
051 Subtotal, Department of Defense-Military	678,044	650,816	601,705	577,697	562,499	565,379	561,806	600,683	653,966	688,300
053 Atomic energy defense activities	20,600	19,286	17,034	17,416	18,692	19,183	20,482	20,916	22,383	21,486
054 Defense-related activities	3,000	7,710	8,017	8,344	8,468	8,615	9,344	9,526	9,256	9,381
Total, National Defense	701,554	677,812	631,488	603,453	589,659	593,378	591,735	631,100	684,900	724,800
150 International Affairs:										
151 International development and humanitarian assistance	23,552	21,882	21,551	23,554	24,007	24,128	24,342	23,162	26,376	28,286
152 International security assistance	12,642	11,464	9,954	11,381	12,000	11,305	12,240	11,417	11,227	14,882
153 Conduct of foreign affairs	12,686	13,546	13,038	13,819	13,566	13,874	13,884	13,058	12,644	14,866
154 Foreign information and exchange activities	1,577	1,936	1,519	1,464	1,531	1,548	1,595	1,641	1,611	1,600
155 International financial programs	-1,873	-11,646	-599	-2,156	269	-3,546	-4,956	-1,122	923	-1,536

The [CD] domain has any number of significant subsets and many are interactive with both General Welfare and Wellbeing. International Affairs are described as a [CD] component even when much of its activities are both [GW] and [WB]. A 'sensing' might indicate that quadrupling and optimizing the costs of International Affairs relations might eliminate some overseas contingency funding of 'operations' at $256 billion but not personnel at $145 billion. Strictly a Commander in Chief and Congressional committee 'sensing' process, which might not show up in the detail numbers. [CD]>3, optimization, won't look well if the subsets develop as

$$[CD]>3 \approx \Sigma \{WB\}<3 + \Sigma \{GW\}>2 + \Sigma\{CD\}>2 + \Sigma\{JU\}<2$$

especially if Justice in the form of the Uniform Code of Military Justice has a form such as that of [JU]. That is actually the case for some 2 million Americans, as is the [subset] for Veterans Administration, which has a cost/benefit system that is now a percentage of the GDP.

Note that the 'administration' of Justice both in [CD] and [GW] does not calculate the appalling effects lack of Justice, [JU]<3, has on human capital under the Constitution. The effects usually show up as wellbeing costs to those near the injustice incident such as predatory violence or parasitic attachment of generated wealth. Example: a serial murderer using an automobile as a terrorist weapon might destroy the lives of a dozen people before Justice intercepts him. The loss of human capital for a dozen lives, plus ripple effects on those directly associated, might run into the millions of 'dollars', all because an individual has a defective frontal lope or cortex disability. At what point does an individual affect Common Defense or General Welfare (or wellbeing) and does societies' Justice system have a right to intervene?

What the effect of these 'system dynamics' is might appear vague, and people can draw their own conclusions as 'sensing'. In many 'laid back' communities, the more 'tribal' cohesion, the easier it is to solve local problems. But as the representation starts to add up at the state and national level, this problem solving begins to be pre-empted by special interests not represented by votes. The classic corruption of governance systems of systems. In many intense urban Districts, this corruption of non-representation can occur with half of one percent of the 'voters' after an election. You could not guarantee the 'the fifth' (Article, that is) under such conditions, much less a Convention, as the presidential platforms every four years indicate.

This 'effect' on [OP] shows up as appropriation manipulations by various special interests at the *national level,* leaving many local communities bewildered by why some entities exist in the federal government agencies. But the General Welfare and

Common Defense authorities of the Constitution are very broad and sometimes the systemic increases in outlays are very much within its domain boundaries, possibly the only exception being when only one of the domains is considered at the entire expense of the other . That is, a generational imbalance occurs the requires enormous effort by the entire political spectrum to re-balance. Sometimes only a consented authoritarian 'system' can correct it, as was the case during World War II. Even a glance at the federal budget by function can sense the domain imbalance.

Table 3.1—OUTLAYS BY SUPERFUNCTION AND FUNCTION: 1940–2018—Continued

Superfunction and Function		2011	2012	2013 estimate	2014 estimate	2015 estimate	2016 estimate	2017 estimate	2018 estimate
		In millions of dollars							
National Defense	[CD]	705,557	677,856	660,037	626,755	612,305	589,214	589,735	592,021
Human resources	[GW]	2,414,742	2,348,587	2,488,727	2,658,304	2,772,781	2,931,955	3,027,315	3,130,789
Education, Training, Employment and Social Services	[OP]	101,233	90,823	84,556	129,041	106,476	106,327	113,166	120,176
Health	[WB]	372,504	346,742	371,664	442,697	514,058	556,393	579,448	596,784
Medicare	[WB]	485,653	471,793	510,544	530,893	543,359	585,387	594,544	614,728
Income Security	[OP] [GW]	597,352	541,344	563,994	541,816	534,499	544,171	543,054	541,965
Social Security		730,811	773,290	818,403	865,635	916,734	970,122	1,026,781	1,085,694
(On-budget)		(101,933)	(140,387)	(56,251)	(26,839)	(32,562)	(36,011)	(39,614)	(43,281)
(Off-budget)		(628,878)	(632,903)	(762,151)	(836,796)	(884,172)	(934,111)	(987,167)	(1,042,413)
Veterans Benefits and Services	--[CD] [GW]	127,189	124,595	139,568	148,222	157,055	169,555	170,322	171,422
Physical resources		161,920	215,459	202,975	161,212	160,348	156,534	150,001	156,575
Energy	[CD]	12,174	14,857	15,101	12,680	10,725	8,001	5,415	6,632
Natural Resources and Environment	[TR]	45,470	41,628	37,660	40,156	40,767	41,411	41,385	41,346
Commerce and Housing Credit	[GW]	-12,573	40,823	17,730	-30,126	-40,793	-32,105	-26,720	-19,927
(On-budget)		(-13,381)	(38,153)	(18,094)	(-25,289)	(-41,054)	(-38,084)	(-26,992)	(-19,904)
(Off-budget)		(808)	(2,670)	(-364)	(-4,837)	(261)	(5,979)	(272)	(277)
Transportation	[GW] [CD]	92,966	93,019	94,486	103,839	115,804	111,782	109,880	111,804
Community and Regional Development	[TR] [OP]	23,883	25,132	37,998	34,663	33,846	27,445	20,041	16,420
Net interest		229,962	220,408	222,750	222,887	253,580	300,114	373,408	461,487
(On-budget)		(345,943)	(332,801)	(328,328)	(322,927)	(349,205)	(392,128)	(464,134)	(550,341)
(Off-budget)		(-115,981)	(-112,393)	(-105,578)	(-100,040)	(-95,645)	(-92,014)	(-90,725)	(-89,354)
Other functions		179,345	178,353	205,584	201,263	207,957	218,554	214,456	212,658
International Affairs	[CD]	45,685	47,189	56,929	55,883	53,361	52,834	52,485	51,940
General Science, Space and Technology	[OP]	29,466	29,060	30,734	30,157	30,604	31,162	31,613	32,056
Agriculture	[GW]	20,662	17,791	27,049	23,454	16,565	18,281	16,892	17,044
Administration of Justice	[JU]	56,056	56,277	60,580	58,737	58,981	59,848	58,999	60,131
General Government	[GW]	27,476	28,036	30,469	28,949	29,889	32,956	34,446	37,978
Allowances				-177	4,083	17,957	23,473	20,021	14,410
Undistributed offsetting receipts		-88,467	-103,536	-95,126	-82,614	-98,795	-106,535	-107,468	-104,291
(On-budget)		(-73,368)	(-87,944)	(-78,948)	(-75,810)	(-81,139)	(-87,898)	(-88,043)	(-84,040)
(Off-budget)		(-15,099)	(-15,592)	(-16,178)	(-16,804)	(-17,656)	(-18,637)	(-19,425)	(-20,251)
Total, Federal outlays		3,603,059	3,537,127	3,684,947	3,777,807	3,908,157	4,089,836	4,247,448	4,448,240
(On-budget)		(3,104,453)	(3,029,539)	(3,044,916)	(3,062,692)	(3,137,025)	(3,260,397)	(3,370,159)	(3,516,155)
(Off-budget)		(498,606)	(507,588)	(640,031)	(715,115)	(771,132)	(829,439)	(877,289)	(933,085)

Figure 13. [domains] in U.S. budget

Excerpt from 2016 Chronicle, further speculation here:

Look at the [domain's sets] again:

How does one view the [sets] interacting with each other so that there is a Posterity improvement of some kind? Pure speculation, with arbitrary constants from 1 to 6 used to measure each covenant and project it toward a model of a Constitutional Convention.

Would the left Convention agenda score look like?

[JU]:+5. [CD]:-5 [GW]:+3, [LI]:-3, [TR]:-1→ [OP]: +

resulting in a minority representation of 22% plus 9% offshore representation?

With the conservative interest agenda score as:

[CD]:+4, [LI]: +3, [TR]:+3, [GW]:-3, [JU]:-4→ [OP]:+2

resulting in a representation of 24% plus 6% offshore representation?

But would an open-minded referendum consensus score as in 2030:

Σ[TR]: +5, [CD]:-2, [JU]:-3, [GW]:+2, [LI]:-1, $\rightarrow$ [WB]:< 3 + [OP]:+?

resulting in establishment of a health right that won't have an effect for a generation?

In this speculation, remember generations are involved. An Article addition under current stress conitions on [GW] and [CD] would take political will that seperated out the entire process of a Convention for adding an Article on Wellbeing from virtually all of the political agendas underway during the 2016 election year. You simply could not attach many of the [GW] values to either a purely Justice or Liberty set and come up with a better future. The same applies with a world in which assymetric warfare is causing security pressures on [JU], [LI], and the entire [CD] domain set. Any combination of forces , whether from the left or right or international special interests, would make consideration of a Wellbeing genetic security system very difficult, {Ki_ξ} being more of a major subset than in previous timelines.

Then there is the little matter of Bonini's Paradox which states:

"As a model of a complex system becomes more complete, it becomes less understandable. Alternatively, as a model grows more realistic, it also becomes just as difficult to understand as the real-world processes it represents"

and this easily applies to a modern citizenry attempting to understand what is going on in their world. Many of those elected in the previous two cycles were elected with an order from citizens to 'do nothing' because what ever they did might be worse than what already existed. People have become justly apprehensive about the future in 2018 and if the Bonini Paradox applies to EACH of the Preamble Six covenants, adding another complexity will make all of them worse. This was essentially the great fear concerning the Affordable Care Act or Obamacare where many of the subsets were so complex that they couldn't get people to subscribe even when it was very much in their benefit to do so. That, by the way, involves another Paradox which closely resembles a gem called the 'Prisoner's Delema' in which one must aid others in order to aid oneself. You don't have to be in a prison for that one, merely a voter with unreadable options on a ballot.

This summery of the Pramble Six effects for the year is describing that complexity of systems with added observations on what might be necessary for adding anything to the Constitution while seperating out the process of referendum from the 'normal' politics of America. A completely open-minded problem solving 'consciousness is attempted for this, deliberately excluding items of even reasonably high priority such as assymetric warfare around the world and wealth degradation within the Nation.

A government description of national activities again shows the inter-relations of the Preamble Six covenants, although the graphic 'Outlays by function' is only about half of the subfunctions described as the Federal government . It is notable that many of the functions are directly related to Wellbeing even though embedded in other Preamble domains. The most worrisome parts are whether [CD] imperatives will overwhelm other domains AND the little problem of interest on the debt reaching $700 billion a year in the near future. It doesn't take much TimeLine Observation to see that the interest level and income security and national security would combine to make health care extremely difficult without reducing the need for, not the ripple effects of, healthcare.

The Preamble Six are taken in order in this Summery, with an evaluation of Wellbeing and Article VIII speculation added toward the end.

Justice [JU]

While the Department of Justice is in the Executive Branch where laws are protected and administered, Justice is usually an expression of the Judiciary Branch where the courts are administered starting or ending with interpretations of the Supreme Court. The Judiciary branch summery of activity is usually defined by the Term that starts in October and ends in June of the following year.   Under Article III and various acts of the Congress, which sets the laws and appropriations for [JU] and the Office of the Executive, who administers their decisions of [JU], a look at the 'Stat Pack' for the Supreme Court gives its overall activity for the Term. But the real effects of the Court are summarized in its decisions, which are shown as the Merit Opinions with an attachment of the possible effects on the Preamble Six. Some items show the wide disparity of {agents} affecting Justice, but not a coherent 'perception' of the multiple layers involved. The layers of Justice in some ways qualify as {agent} fields that interact with each other the way a 'tensor' would with more than three dimensions.

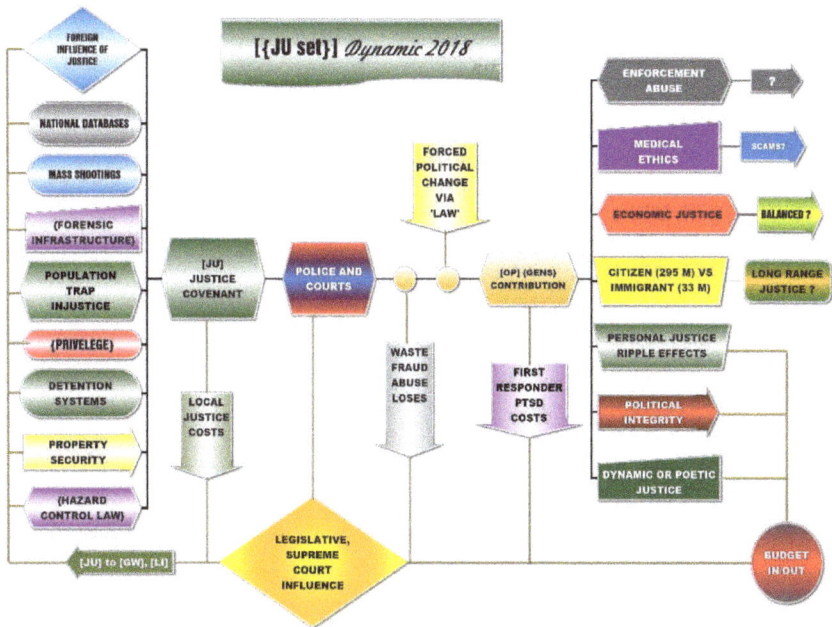

Figure 14. Justice [JU] dynamic set

Types of justice

- {1} Distributive justice: reasonable or equitable use of resources
- {2} Environmental justice: Reaction to climate change
- {3} Injustice: absence of fairness, empathy
- {4} Occupational injustice: lack of wellbeing opportunity

{5} Open justice: No police state courts

{6} Organizational justice: Fairness within groups

{7} Poetic justice: Divine intervention?

{8} Social justice: Privileged minorities

{9} Spatial justice: population density causation

But no {10} Molecular Justice?

This group of [JU]{sets} is directly related to the inherent 'fairness gene' that most people have. This has led to the 'get even' mentality that is so pervasive among humans that it alone has caused wars and atrocities defeating the original perceived injustice act. Humans have used the motivational reasoning process of injustice to carry out equal injustice of their own. This is usually a combination of the Wiki sets {3}, {5}, {6} and {8} above, but how do you account for a 6-month old baby being able to perceive an injustice as well? Not in the uneducated environment the baby is in, but it is clearly there, even if inaccurately sensed.

In the analysis here, these nine sets are distributed into the activities in society as determined by the activities of the Justice Department, the Supreme Court and various polled [JU] concerns of people such as immigration justice or fairness, civil rights, states rights and economic 'fairness', which is not a right. But neither is molecular health of the mind and body even when it shows as a Justice component in all five of the other covenants.

The executive branch Justice Department appears in the functions of the 2018 budget as:

Table 3.2 - OUTLAYS BY FUNCTION AND SUBFUNCTION: 1962 - 2025
(in millions of dollars)

[JU] Justice {crime}, {admin}

Function and Subfunction	2011	2012	2013	2014	2015	2016	2017	2018	2019	2020 estimate
750 Administration of Justice:										
751 Federal law enforcement activities	29,802	28,977	27,295	26,106	26,937	28,886	29,818	31,333	34,156	39,555
752 Federal litigative and judicial activities	15,076	16,211	14,764	14,224	14,717	14,892	15,105	16,974	17,279	19,889
753 Federal correctional activities	6,546	6,753	6,761	6,751	7,049	6,952	6,977	6,821	7,091	7,415
754 Criminal justice assistance	4,632	4,336	3,781	3,376	3,203	5,038	6,044	5,290	7,214	12,711
Total, Administration of Justice	56,056	56,277	52,601	50,457	51,906	55,768	57,944	60,418	65,740	79,570

With much of the other 'fairness' components of Justice in both [CD] and [GW], but especially in the hypothetical Wellbeing component.

{1} General Opservationis

2018.02.16:13:02 |JU|<4 ≈ |LI|<3 |CD|<3 ⋈ |TR|<1|GW|>1 |OP<?

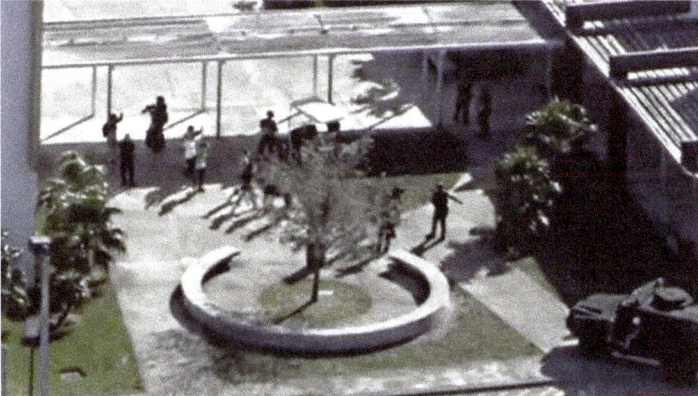

**Parkland FL, 2018.02.14:15:18, mass shooting with
17 dead, 14 wounded, 1200 (?) direct life PTSD
ripple effects. Justice for all and each?**

Killer was a possible PTSD carrier himself, but carefully planned massacre over several months? Genetic ripple effects rather than environmental? How many more?

2018.04.03:21:02 [LI]<1 [CD]<3 ⋈[GW]>1-[JU]>2 ≈ [OP<

Ignatius, WaPost, "How the courts — not Congress — could protect Mueller's investigation':

"The judicial branch's power to appoint prosecutors is clearly established in cases involving contempt of court, argues Peter Shane, a professor of constitutional law at Ohio State University. He cites Rule 42 of the Federal Rules of Criminal Procedure, which specifies that in contempt cases, if the government refuses to prosecute, "the court must appoint another attorney to prosecute the contempt."

In a case of a presidential contempt, as in firing a prosecutor or his investigators, a serious Pandora's Box would be opened up. The implication is that the court could try and convict a president for contempt of THAT court independently of a Congressional impeachment and a Supreme Court trial for removal from office. On the other hand, if the court makes a report of the compelling evidence of contempt to the Chief Justice, what do his options include? Does he then send the report to the Congress with a recommendation for impeachment or can the Supreme Court begin a trial of its own under its Article III, Section 2, judicial powers? If the Congress receives the report but then fails to begin impeachment, are Congressmen then in contempt of the original court as well as the Supreme Court and can they be tried for conspiracy to usurp the constitution itself? This scenario has Made-in-Asia all over it the way things having been going with deliberate undermining of democracies.

Further:

The Court can intercede, but according to Article II (The Article of presidential authorities) impeachment is sufficient for removal from office and Article I, Section 3 says only the Senate can impeach. But Article II also says 'impeachment for and conviction of' which are two different activities. Can the Court do the trial to convict if only contempt is involved? No conclusions on the matter have been drawn.

2018.07.08:18:04 [JU]<2...|OP|>3 ≈ |WB|<2⋈ [GW|>1⋈ [CD]<1 [TR|>2 [LI]<3

Sullivan, WaPost, 'A journalist's conscience leads her to reveal her source to the FBI. Here's why.':

"In their reporting, journalists talk to criminals all the time and don't turn them in. Reporters aren't an arm of law enforcement. They properly resist subpoenas and fight like hell not to share their notes or what they know because doing so would compromise their independence and their ability to do their work in the future."

That is perfectly correct and laudable within a context of Justice. But in this case, a process was under way in the secure, closed hearing rooms of the Senate. The appearance of even the least 'probable cause' of an act that brings imminent threat to the integrity of the Constitution, as classified information transfer does automatically, should be reason enough for any citizen to carry out his protective obligations. That imminent threat obligation should hold regardless of whether an oath to defend and protect the Constitution had been taken. The security breach 'perp' certainly had taken such an oath.

Other conditions of journalistic non-disclosure where Justice for all is required as part of the silence or whistle blowing is perfectly acceptable, but not on a Constitutional corruption level.

2018.07.20:21:27 |LI|>3[TR|>2|WB|>1+|CD|<3 ⋈|GW|>1-[JU|<2≈|OP|>2

Elizabeth Wydra in WaPost, 'Those who deny birthright citizenship get the Constitution wrong':

"Meanwhile, if undocumented immigrants or their children commit a crime in the United States, they can be and are punished under U.S. law. In other words, they are — obviously! — subject to the jurisdiction of the United States. If born on American soil, they are also citizens of the United States."

That doesn't quite make sense. If they [the non-citizens] are within the physical domains of the Constitution, that would include ANY primates who are occupying space anywhere within the United States' lands. It doesn't matter whether they are citizens or not, but whether their existence in the United States represents some form of imminent danger to the actual citizens already within the authority of the Constitution. The equal Justice clause of the 14th also means that ANY primate born in the United States is entitled to equality, but not necessarily others who are not. It does not matter whether the people are citizens or not; they are still subject to the 'jurisdiction' of the Constitution. That means that the Article I, Section 8, clause 4 authority 'to establish a uniform Rule of Naturalization' is not superseded by the 14th Amendment, so any rule of law governing Naturalization can define citizenship.

As for a person born in the United States being a citizen, fine, but that could easily mean that the child must automatically be removed from the parents who have committed a Naturalization crime that makes them unfit as parents under the 13th Amendment, which slightly preceded the 14th. That is technically true; that the newly born citizen, however naturalized, must be protected against various dangers including parental abuse and greed.

Further:

We needn't go into the long history of why a 'uniform Rule of Naturalization' has NEVER come into existence through the power of the current political parties, which might have prevented the current 'asylum' migrations. But indenture through immigration trafficking does violate the 13th Amendment as well as nearly the entire Bill of Rights. Much more serious than currently realized.

TLO: This isn't clear. If the individual 'occupier' is not a citizen and has no intention of becoming one, as in 'tourist', he is under the jurisdiction of the Judiciary as a 'ward', not the jurisdiction of the Constitution and perhaps not under the jurisdiction of the Bill of Rights. Physical occupation does not automatically mean a person is 'subject to the jurisdiction thereof' because of the 'and' starting the phrase in the 14th.

Remember that the [JU] set includes activities within the Bill of Rights although the set also includes {entities} concerning Crimes against Humanity in the international system, economic contract activity, and criminal behavior. Note that criminal behavior is the normal definition for violating the rights of others, with Crimes Against Humanity the largest expression of that.

TLO: These cases of merit Opinions were deemed those most interactive with Americans, as defined under Article III, Section 2.

Other Justice {sets} of interactive note:

Criaghum justice: Worldwide is [CD]+2, [WB]-4. U.S. might be [JU]+4.

Voter, state justice:

Rights Justice:

Human Trafficking: too normal to be criminal?

Congressional Research Service, Domestic Human Trafficking Legislation in the 113th Congress, R43555, Alison Siskin, Coordinator, 2018.05.19:

> For more than a decade, Congress has been actively engaged in anti-human-trafficking efforts within the United States. Through the Trafficking Victims Protection Act of 2000 (TVPA, Division A of P.L. 106-386) and its four reauthorizations (TVPRAs),12 Congress has aimed to eliminate human trafficking within the United States by creating domestic grant programs for both victims and law enforcement, creating new criminal laws, and conducting oversight on the effectiveness and implications of U.S. anti-TIP policy. Most recently, in March 2013, the TVPA's grant programs were reauthorized through FY2017 in the Violence Against Women Reauthorization Act of 2013 (Title XII, P.L. 113-4).

TLO: Compensation of victims or creating a safe infrastructure for victims of essentially a violation of the 13th Amendment, prohibition of slavery, might require a stronger [CD] + [WB] response against the perpetrator who has shown an abnormal desire to control others. Note abnormal or extreme desire, not to be confused with routine control of others in order to operate as a team and accomplish a goal. Cooperation with a leader for a purpose is a normal human evolutionary process somewhere around [OP] +4.

2018.07.03:10:29 |WB|>1⋈ |GW|>3⋈ |TR|<2 |LI|>3⋈|JU|>3 ≈ |OP|>2|CD}<1

Hugh Hewitt in WaPost, 'Here's who Trump should pick for the Supreme Court':

"So the first question [for an Associate Justice] is: Has the nominee ruled steadily in a fashion consistent with the original intent of the Constitution and its amendments and faithful to the statutes passed by the executive and legislative branches?"

That is A question concerning Originalist interpretations of Article III, Judicial Powers. Article III also suggests very strongly in Section 2 that ITS original interpretation as applied to 'Controversies to which the United States shall be a Party' involved assessments in CURRENT terms or conditions. One of the major conditions of this century is the discoveries involving Epigenetic manipulations of DNA and cellular life, which has ripple effects all over the United States in terms of molecular health. The 'ripple effects' involve Epigenetic curative processes involving one fifth of the American GDP. The Supreme Court has no authority on this matter other than assuming human life is based on the Article I Congressional authorities for interstate commerce. That is, human life is a commercial activity in this century, the same as it was when the idea led to the Civil War?

None of the current Justices or the current candidates, Originalist or otherwise, have any understanding of the bio-ethics of Epigenetic related law processes even though their ripple effects are beginning to effect major components of the health, education, wealth and tranquility of the entire citizenship and 22 million visitors. Originalism does NOT mean living in the 1790s when vaccinations against disease had just been discovered. It is the 21st century and the entire Human Genome has been mapped, not just Social Darwinist misconceptions of it that the Court has attempted to deal with in the past.

Need someone with a modern but history-based bioethical law background on the Court?

{2} Supreme Court activity:

In June, the Supreme Court upheld President Obama's health care plan in a five-to-four ruling. Chief Justice John Roberts cast the deciding vote.

It wasn't just the fact that the justices in a bitter 5-4 ruling upheld the federal health care law. It was the unusually dramatic way in which they did it, with Chief Justice John Roberts reportedly switching his vote to save the law. There will be many more legal battles ahead over the Care Act-- indeed, the justices already have welcomed another challenge to it-- but the case's most profound legacy, apart from the bad feelings it apparently created among the justices, may be the Court's cramped new interpretation of the Commerce Clause, which traditionally has been a source of federal economic power and authority.

For example, predictive policing was a huge success in Santa Cruz, Calif., this year. Through the use of advanced analytics and predictive technology, the Santa Cruz Police Department reported a 19 percent reduction in property theft in the first six months of 2016 compared to the same time period in 2011. No changes were made in the department during that time, except for the use of data-driven prediction methods. Some experts believe big data will expand beyond statistics into behavioral practices, leading to further success in anticipating crime through technology.

Contempt of Constitution: Congressional Research Service, *Congress's Contempt Power, a Sketch*, RL34114, 2018.04.10:

> Congress's contempt power is the means by which Congress responds to certain acts that in its view obstruct the legislative process. Contempt may be used either to coerce compliance, punish the contemnor, and/or to remove the obstruction. Although arguably any action that directly obstructs the effort of Congress to exercise its constitutional powers may constitute a contempt, in recent times the contempt power has most often been employed in response to non-compliance with a duly issued congressional subpoena— whether in the form of a refusal to appear before a committee for purposes of providing testimony or a refusal to produce requested documents.

TLO: Should contempt of Constitution be made into an Amendment process for a [JU] of +4? This would be like the original Sedition Act of 1798.07.14 except that it would involve a contempt violation of individual rights by any other citizen (not just the government), such as in DNA theft, induced narcotic addiction, tax info manipulation, tampering with evidence after introduction to court, foreign identity theft, and so on. Would such a contempt prohibition create a [JU] +4 condition that feeds back into an [OP] covenant?

2018.04.03:15:10 [LI]>1|TR]>3[WB]>1+|CD|<1 ⋈ [GW]>3[JU]>1 ≈ |OP|>3

Lane, WaPost, 'This solution to gerrymandering is worse than the problem':

"A certain irreducible constitutional ambiguity may be sustainable when courts deal with words and images, but not if they get into distributing political power between our mutually antagonistic parties.

Sandra Day O'Connor was right: The Supreme Court should leave partisan politics to the partisan politicians."

In fact, if you take into account Article IV, Section 4 guarantee of representative governance, the Supreme Court could create a test like the Rule of Fives that says no congressional district can be 'representative' if it has consecutive elections from just one political faction. Bell curve distributions of people just don't work that way. The Rule of Fives divides a District into five societal factors like two major parties, independents, unaffiliated write-ins AND a 'no confidence' category.

In order for a candidate to be elected legitimately, the Supreme Court could say that the District, however gerrymandered by a state legislature, is not legitimate unless all five categories of representation are on the ballot for national elections. Under this criteria, a district candidate MUST acquire a majority vote of the five categories, not just one party. If there is a 51 percent 'no confidence' vote for a candidate that eliminates him from office, true representation is achieved. The Supreme Court might not even have to defer to or test state legislation on re-redistricting all over the country when deciding that a district was not truly Article IV, section 4 representative under the Rule of Fives.

2018.09.08:20:03 |CD|<3 ⋈ |GW|>1-|JU|>3|TR|<2≈|OP|>3

John McLaughlin in WaPost, 'Why so many former intelligence officers are speaking out':

"Meanwhile, we should take care, as we would in foreign intelligence assessments, to limit our comments to what the facts can reasonably support in the minds of most Americans — what we can all indisputably see, hear and document."

We can be reasonably sure that the ones who know somebody with a black star on a foyer marble wall in Langley did not create the directorate dogma of 'hear no evil, speak no evil, see no evil of ourselves', but who did? Such a person would make a mockery of the oath to the Constitution if even one instance of contempt for it was allowed to stand without checks and balances. But that problem is internal, not a concern with hearing, speaking and seeing 'foreign intelligence assessments.

USA today, 2018.01.00

2018.03.27:08:05 |OP|>1 ≈ ∑ |TR|>3 |LI|>3⋈|JU|<1....|GW|>2

Schmidt, WaPost, 'California sues Trump administration over decision to add citizenship question to census':

" Lowenthal said. "Between evidence that the administration is manipulating the census for political gain, and fear that the administration will use the census to harm immigrants, confidence in the integrity of the count could plummet. And the census is only as good as the public's willingness to participate."

This is not an accurate consideration. The current laws say that the information put on a census form cannot identify the individual contributor for 72 YEARS. Most bigdata analysts cry in their martinis over this law because they cannot make accurate demographic models from one census to the next. It might even be an impeachable or termination offense to attempt such access.

The census 'enumeration' clause in Article I, § 2. states: 'The actual Enumeration shall be made within three Years after the first Meeting of the Congress of the United States, and within every subsequent Term of ten Years, in such Manner as they shall by Law direct.'

Note the clarity of 'in such manner as they (the Congress) shall by law direct'. That might easily mean that a state cannot even sue the Executive for carrying out a Congressional enumeration law, only appeal to the Supreme Court because of the Article IV, Section 4 guarantee of a representative 'form' of governance. However, it is generally held by the Court that the enumeration clause meant everybody, not just citizens. But it is entirely up to the Congress under its naturalization authority to determine what qualifies as a voting citizen, and that would not include 'residents' of states who might be included in the census (estimated to be 43 million in 2018), only voters.

Being included in some population form in a census DOES NOT AUTOMATICALLY qualify a person with a citizen's voting rights and NO state authority can change that any more than access an individual's census data.

{3} Immigration:

Jennings v. Rodriguez, Decided Feb. 27, 2018, 5-3

The court ruled that immigrants held in detention facilities have no rights under a federal law to periodic hearings to decide whether they may be released on bail.

Sessions v. Dimaya, Decided Feb. 27, 2018, 5-4

The court struck down a law that allowed the government to deport

Is Trump's travel ban against five predominantly Muslim countries legal and constitutional? That question has lingered for 15 months as federal courts from Maryland to Hawaii have blocked it on both grounds. The high court's conservative majority appears poised to overturn those rulings.

Trump v. Hawaii, Decided June 26, 2018, 5-4. The court ruled that President Trump had the legal authority to restrict travel from several mostly Muslim countries.

2018.07.21:08:08 |LI|>3|TR|>2|WB|>4+|CD|<3 ⋈ |GW|>1-|JU|<2≈|OP|>4

Elizabeth Wydra in WaPost, 'Those who deny birthright citizenship get the Constitution wrong':

"Meanwhile, if undocumented immigrants or their children commit a crime in the United States, they can be and are punished under U.S. law. In other words, they are — obviously! — subject to the jurisdiction of the United States. If born on American soil, they are also citizens of the United States."

From Wikipedia:

Human accelerated regions (HARs), first described in August 2006,[1][2] are a set of 49 segments of the human genome that are conserved throughout vertebrate evolution but are strikingly different in humans. They are named according to their degree of difference between humans and chimpanzees (HAR1 showing the largest degree of human-chimpanzee differences). Found by scanning through genomic databases of multiple species, some of these highly mutated areas may contribute to human-specific traits. Others may represent loss of functional mutations, possibly due to the action of biased gene conversion [2][3] rather than adaptive evolution.

Question: If an ambulatory primate (not a tree dweller) does not have the newly defined HARs in its DNA sequences, would it still be entitled to human rights? Race, by the way, is defined by less than one tenth of one percent of the Human Genome, while HARs might constitute a full two percent of the Genome. The genetic difference between a primate and a homosapien is also about two percent, not counting the so-called 'junk' DNA sequences.

The Constitution and its devolved rule of law could not have handled this modern definition of life, let alone the modern distortions of what 'race' means. How does the Justice covenant in the Preamble determine Justice for each when Justice for all isn't defined by the Constitution?

reply:

The proposal is not to do away with birthright citizenship but to replace one type of birthright citizenship with another. We should replace jus soli—right of the soil—birthright citizenship with jus sanguinis—right of blood—birthright citizenship. Instead of granting birthright citizenship to anyone born on U.S. soil, we would grant birthright citizenship only to those born to a parent or parents or who are U.S. citizens.

(I think we should add anyone born to permanent legal residents.) The switch wouldn't be retroactive. No one currently a citizen would lose citizenship as a result of the change.

comments:

As the author points out, some argue that the change could be made by a reinterpretation of the Citizenship Clause by the federal courts. However, a constitutional amendment could also make the change, which would align U.S. citizenship policy with the citizenship laws of most developed countries. The Constitution isn't that difficult to amend. There have been six amendments in my lifetime.

34 minutes ago

But why would this "right of blood" be an improvement? Would we be better off if we denied citizenship to people who were born and raised in the US? I don't think so and I can't think of a single rational argument for that position.

29 minutes ago

: Anyone convicted of a felony is essentially denied citizenship, but on a Federal level, citizenship is defined by the Naturalization Clause, not the 14th Amendment. That kicks in immediately after birth as a citizen and can be removed by law.

5 minutes ago

Those damn felonious newborns, I tell ya

5 minutes ago

Not true.

26 minutes ago

Your reply to my comment is non-sensical.

5 minutes ago

Check it out. Virtually every state denies voting rights, gun rights, mobility rights, and other Bill of Rights conditions of citizenship after conviction of a felony, Constitutional authority for doing that is well established.

7 minutes ago

It makes immigration laws easier to enforce. Children born to illegal immigrants within the United States would not be citizens. It would do away with so-called "anchor babies."

reply:

It would also shut down birthright tourism, in which foreign tourists vacation in the United States during the final stages of their pregnancy so they babies will be born U.S. citizens. This defeats the purpose of immigration quotas.

5 minutes ago

'The Constitution isn't that difficult to amend. There have been six amendments in my lifetime.'

Nothing wrong with the idea, but the last Amendment ratified was in 1972. Congress won't touch the Amendment process in Article V because of 'special interest' interference. The Russian and Chinese, along with their American internationalist friends, would just love to get their hands on a constitutional change process.

5 minutes ago

Terrible idea. Try thinking of doing things not motivated by your sadism.

10 minutes ago

This is just more disguised anti-DACA nationalism, and, as such, is a way to legalize xenophobia.

14 minutes ago

birthright citizenship with jus sanguinis—right of blood—birthright citizenship' could also mean citizenship according to DNA. That would put most people in Northern Mexico, Canada, the Caribbean, West Africa, Europe and Siberia in a condition of being an American 'National' eligible for immediate citizenship regardless of ignorance of the Constitution. Might be a better interpretation of citizenship than the 14th, but who decides, Congress or a national referendum?

6 minutes ago

No. To obtain citizenship, one would have to prove his or her parents were U.S. citizens. DNA testing alone would not prove a person's parents were U.S. citizen,

1 hour ago

Thank you for saying what needed to be said to yet a new generation of racists.

It is amazing that some people don't recognize in themselves, today, the evil parties of the historical debate. Nasty people. With no shame.

48 minutes ago

Always racism in the speech of the haters. Europeans do it too. You are the racist to assume it only happens to non whites.

38 minutes ago

It's blatantly obvious who it's aimed at.

25 minutes ago

It would apply equally to all racial and ethnic groups.

5 minutes ago

Your target, whether you admit it or not, is brown people.

12 minutes ago

What do you think is racist about jus sanguinis citizens? It would make anyone born to U.S. parents a citizen, regardless of race or ethnicity. It would apply to children of naturalized citizens as well as children of native-born citizens. Do you just charge racism whenever you disagree with an idea?

1 hour ago

From Wikipedia: Human Accelerated Regions (HARs), first described in August 2006,[1][2] are a set of 49 segments of the human genome that are conserved throughout vertebrate evolution but are strikingly different in humans. They are named according to their degree of difference between humans and chimpanzees (HAR1 showing the largest degree of human-chimpanzee differences). Found by scanning through genomic databases of multiple species, some of these highly mutated areas may contribute to human-specific traits. Others may represent loss of functional mutations, possibly due to the action of biased gene conversion [2][3] rather than adaptive evolution.

Question: If an ambulatory primate (not a tree dweller) does not have the newly defined HARs in its DNA sequences, would it still be entitled to human rights? Race, by the way, is defined by less than one tenth of one percent of the Human Genome, while HARs might constitute a full two percent of the Genome. The genetic difference between a primate and a homosapien is also about two percent, not counting the so-called 'junk' DNA sequences.

The Constitution and its devolved rule of law, including the 14th, could not have handled this modern definition of life, let alone the modern simplistic distortions of what 'race' means. How does the Justice covenant in the Preamble determine Justice for each when Justice for all isn't defined by the Constitution?

27 minutes ago

comments:

The proposal is not to do away with birthright citizenship but to replace one type of birthright citizenship with another. We should replace jus soli—right of the soil—birthright citizenship with jus sanguinis—right of blood—birthright citizenship. Instead of granting birthright citizenship to anyone born on U.S. soil, we would grant birthright citizenship only to those born to a parent or parents or who are U.S. citizens. (I think we should add anyone born to permanent legal residents.) The switch wouldn't be retroactive. No one currently a citizen would lose citizenship as a result of the change.

As the author points out, some argue that the change could be made by a reinterpretation of the Citizenship Clause by the federal courts. However, a constitutional amendment could also make the change, which would align U.S. citizenship policy with the citizenship laws of most developed countries. The Constitution isn't that difficult to amend. There have been six amendments in my lifetime.

{4} Civil Rights conditions:

Masterpiece Cakeshop v. Colorado Civil Rights Commission, Decided June 4, 2018, 7-2

The court said the baker had been mistreated by a state civil rights commission based on remarks of one of its members indicating hostility to religion.

2018.06.07:09:03 | ξ| >2 |WB|>1⋈ |GW|>3⋈ |TR|<1 |LI|>3⋈|JU|<1 ≈ |OP|>2

Lawrence Friedman in TheHill, 'In weighing religion versus equality, the Supreme Court takes the cake':

"But the court did no such thing [completely resolved the issue]. Rather, Justice Anthony Kennedy, writing for the majority, concluded that, because the Colorado Civil Rights Commission's consideration of a same-sex couple's challenge to a baker's refusal to make them a wedding cake reflected a bias against religious freedom, the ruling against the baker could not be upheld."

What an unelected, politically appointed Commission did was attempt to impose their declared bias against the existence of spirituality in a person and not just a specific 'religion' dogma. The Constitution's First Amendment prohibits Congress, note federal Congress, from making any law prohibiting 'religious' exercise. The Court determined that the Commission had violated this specific exercise clause while adhering to equality of all citizens later in the text as read by the Court. The narrow ruling that the free exercise of spirituality had been violated by an imposed outside value was correct.

Speculation: Religion in general, but not specific material object expressions of it, is a form of 'spirituality' or whole-mind integration held in common by Christianity (Parakletos or Holy Spirit), Islam (Ruh or Holy Spirit), Buddhist (Satori or Holy Enlightenment). This spiritual expression is held in common in virtually all 'religions', including animist, Hindu and even atheists who don't believe in a paranormal 'god'. The spirituality is why the Founders specifically prohibited a religious test of people in Article VI; you could not tell in the Nation how spirituality might form. But a Commission allowed to impose a concept that religious spirituality doesn't exist at all because of THEIR beliefs?

As far as modern Constitutional interpretations of 'religion' by a Supreme Court, it might have to take into consideration what neurological scientists have known for some time; the amount of quantum energy in a human brain does not match the energy generated by individual sums of the brain molecules; the total energy is larger than the parts. How is it that a brain part that determines sexual orientation, the peanut-sized hypothalamus, has more 'rights' than a whole-brain parts entity like spiritual energy or 'religion'?

Jesner v. Arab Bank, Decided April 24, 2018, 5-4. The court ruled that foreign corporations may not be sued in American courts for complicity in human rights abuses abroad.

Epic Systems Corp. v. Lewis, Decided May 21, 2018, 5-4. The court ruled that employers can require workers to pursue claims for wage theft and other workplace issues in individual arbitrations.

Husted v. A. Philip Randolph Institute, Decided June 11, 2018, 5-4. The court upheld Ohio's aggressive program to purge its voting rolls.

Carpenter v. United States, Decided June 22, 2018, 5-4. The court ruled that the government generally needs a warrant to collect troves of location data about the customers of cellphone companies. A series of armed robberies in Michigan led police to obtain 127 days of the suspect's cellphone records

2018.12.01:07:50 |TR|>2 = |LI|>3WB|<2 ⋈ |GW|>1-|JU|<2

Lillis, TheHill, 'Dems vow quick action to bolster voting rights upon taking power':

"Democrats, and a number of Republicans, have a decidedly different view [of the new Civil Rights Commission report], pointing to a long list of states that have adopted higher hurdles to voting since the 2013 ruling took effect, including photo-ID requirements, shorter windows of early voting and the elimination of same-day registration."

Adopted higher hurdles to voting? Or are the states requiring a minimum level of proof of citizenship with 11 million 'aliens', 14 million 'U.S. Nationals' and 3 million 'tourists' wondering about the country? Virtually all voting rights and civil rights legislation have accepted the process that only Constitutionally validated (Article I, Section 8, clause 4) CITIZEN can vote in a federal election. Sorry about that, Mr. Goodlatte, but a Federal election IS federal. With so many categories of non-citizens, another issue, any Federal Electoral District can have 20% of its population wave a 'residency' paper at a Registrar and say he has a right to vote. That doesn't mean the U.S. Nationals aren't entitled to Civil Rights Act protections; it means that modern ID card proof of citizenship, possibly even through advanced DNA mapping as 14th Amendment proof of birth rights, is the barest minimum necessary to establish a CITIZENSHIP ONLY voting right in a District.

Re-establishing the 'ancient' 1900s standards for voting rights may even be a violation of Article IV, Section 4 guarantees, as the Supreme Court decisions(s) implies.

{5} States Rights:

Benisek v. Lamone, June 18, 2018,. The court ruled in an unsigned opinion against Republican voters who had challenged the congressional map drawn by Democratic lawmakers in Maryland.

Gill v. Whitford, June 18, 2018. The court sent back the challenge to Wisconsin's legislative map to the lower courts.

2018.06.18:08:00 [TR]<2 = ∑ [LI]>1WB]<2 ⋈ [GW]>1-[JU]<2....|OP]>3

Wheeler, TheHill, 'Supreme Court faces major decision on partisan gerrymandering': "However, Levitt said he believes that the justices are more likely to create a basic principle that it is unconstitutional to intentionally disadvantage one party and say there are a number of ways it can be proven."

The issues in all cases of 'gerrymandering' for the advantage of a state-level party is whether the Court has the authority to intervene in constituted state legislative processes and whether the process involved is a valid expression of 'representative form' as guaranteed by Article IV, Section 4. The intervention in state affairs is expressed in Article III, Section 2 'judicial Power shall extend to Controversies to which the United States shall be a Party;- to Controversies between two or more States'. Any activity involving the election of a Federal candidate, who must move across a state boundary, should automatically fall to the Court's decision making and possibly no other. Article IV states that a 'Republic' (although it says 'Republican') form of governance is guaranteed by ALL branches of the Federal system and the term means a 'representative vote system' then and now. Combining the two Constitutional authorities should mean that ONLY the Supreme Court can decide if a Federal congressional district is representative according to the mandated census every ten years. If the district fails a representation test, it (the election instance) should be held unconstitutional.

That would mean that a district in which a 10 percent vote by citizens in a primary (14 districts in 2016) that selected an uncontested candidate could not possibly be representative of the 600,000 or so in the district mandated by the census. The only way it could represent a majority 51 percent is if the citizens had the choice of a 'no-confidence' vote on the uncontested ballot. Either that or a bell curve distribution in which independent write-ins must be included on the ballot and the total equals 51 percent of the eligible citizens of the district, not just the 30 per cent who normally voted. Republic representation means exactly that: at least half of a district population is represented at the election.

How partisan can state legislatures be when drawing election districts for Congress and statehouses without violating voters' constitutional rights? The justices heard a Wisconsin case in October and a Maryland case in March, when they appeared baffled by imperfect solutions. They also must rule on election maps in Texas that challengers say discriminate against racial and ethnic minorities.

South Dakota v. Wayfair, Decided June 21, 2018, 5-4. The court ruled that states can require internet retailers to collect sales taxes in states where they have no physical presence. Can states require online retailers to collect and remit sales taxes in states where they have no physical presence? South Dakota's challenge to Supreme Court precedents dating back 50 years would be a boon for state coffers, but it's a threat to smaller sellers who would have to navigate state and local sales tax systems.

Janus v. American Federation of State, County and Municipal Employees, Decided June 27, 2018, 5-4. The court ruled that government workers who choose not to join unions may not be required to help pay for collective bargaining.

2018.02.01:08:30 [WB]>2 ⋈ [GW] +|CD| |TR|>2 ≈ |OP|>2

Bershidsky, BloombergView, 'How Amazon & Co. Could Fix Health Care':

"Lower pay than in the rest of the U.S. health care economy would be justified by having to do zero insurance paperwork -- something that forces U.S. doctors to hire extra staff and waste precious time. The companies would merely set pay levels based on tasks performed -- something that, in much of Europe, falls to health care providers' unions to negotiate with the government or with payer pools. That's the system the joint venture would ultimately end up with. Amazon's tech could help track the tasks in real time."

This combination of corporate entities also has the ability to automate the HC system to the point that not only puts doctors in a 'pay- per-cure' (as opposed to pay-per-service) process, it can automate many diagnostic processes to the point that employees and families can engage in very positive pre-emptive self-health. It helps to have employees who are young and healthy to start with, as nearly all of the million employees involved would be, but allowing them to have full mind-body scan diagnostic rooms in the work place (instead of going to offshore hospitals?) would create a national infrastructure model that employees were responsible for their own health as much as the HC system. Preemptive, droid administered health systems might cut overall costs by half and the model might be cloned into a national self-care system that actually was profitable.

National Institute of Family and Life Advocates v. Becerra, Decided June 26, 2018, 5-4. The court blocked a California law that required "crisis pregnancy centers" to provide information about abortion.

2018.07.15:07:16 |LI|<3|TR|<2|WB|<2+|CD|<3 ⋈|GW|>1-|JU|<2≈|OP|<1

Julie Burkhart in TheHill, 'The terror of a future without Roe':

"Among other restrictions, Kansas has laws on the books requiring women to receive state mandated anti-choice materials that are purposely meant to discourage her from having an abortion, and then wait 24 hours before the procedure. Minors seeking an abortion must obtain dual parental consent, and women must be offered to view the ultrasound image of their fetus before obtaining an abortion."

This sounds a bit like someone reading a person their 'rights' during a pre-trial process. If the woman doesn't understand that she is creating life with her womb, how is she competent to make a choice that respects human life? Some women aren't even aware they 'accidently' created life until the second trimester. If the life being created has any of the 1400 birth 'anomalies' (Fragile X Syndrome, Downs Syndrome, Encephalopathy, diabetes, heart defects, etc) already detected by Genomic DNA mapping, it is almost certainly going to be an 'undue burden' to the citizens around the birth mother who is unaware of what she is creating.

Question: If a woman was designed by evolution to create life and she has a 'human right' to do exactly that, what are her 'citizenship' responsibilities in creating an entity that is certain to be a burden, spiritual, economic, or temporal, to others? Abortion is only a part of the procreation 'right', not an end value. If a woman has the 'right', what are the responsibilities within a human society that might carry the burden of the right? What is the real terror involved?

Note that the question couldn't be asked when Row v. Wade was considered, only after the DNA mapping was completed in this century.

Murphy v. National Collegiate Athletic Association, Decided May 14, 2018, 7-2.

The court struck down a federal law that effectively banned commercial sports betting in most states, clearing the way for legal wagering.

A 1992 law says so, but New Jersey's challenge to the Professional and Amateur Sports Protection Act could act as a springboard to legalized sports betting in other states as well.

2018.09.22:07:31 |JU|>3 ≈ CD|>2 |TR|<3 |LI|<3

George Will, WaPost, 'The Supreme Court was America's least damaged institution — until now':

"All [recent Justices] were eminently qualified, but none were more so than Merrick Garland, the shabby treatment of whom was supposedly justified by a terrible and profoundly anti-constitutional idea that fuels today's conflagration. It is the idea that the selection of justices should be tethered to our never-ending political campaigns so that the court will reflect voters' shifting constitutional preferences."

A 'tethering' that defeats the purpose of creating an intellectually independent group of nine. If the Court follows its Article III authorities without control of the 'purse' or the 'sword', it should generally evaluate conditions in the Nation according to a 'secure the blessings of Liberty for ourselves and our Posterity' context as the Preamble defines the intent of the Nation. That Posterity component would not necessarily mean the Court decides according to the economics of the Mob or Power Broker and many times it has not.

But should candidates in this Supreme category of Posterity judgement meet the same criteria of a citizen who must pass the polygraph requirement of a high-level security clearance? The candidate passes most of the background investigation requirements for a TS/SCI clearance except the polygraph verification, but should the Hart Building hearing room have one of the room 216 upstairs press alcoves converted to a 21st century biometric analysis installation to carry out the 'final' citizenship test with very modern polygraphic sensors? Might determine a 'fact' in a half hour instead of spending another $2 million in tax dollars to analyze the endless media events associated with candidates.

2018.07.21:13:40 |GW|>2↔ |TR|>4 |LI|<1 ⋈ |JU|>3 ≈ |WB|<2 ⋈|OP|>2

Alex Kaplan in TheHill, 'Pack the center: How Democrats and Republicans can fix the Supreme Court, together':

"New ideas for fixing the Court are needed. Depending on your point of view, this one may seem either fresh or naive, but it isn't quite new. The Constitution says that the President shall appoint justices with the "Advice and Consent of the Senate." Now is high time to fulfill its text. To pull back from the brink and save our country, we need both parties to pack the Supreme Court, together."

If you were going to 'pack' the Supreme Court (already tried by both parties, btw), the only Constitutional process available would be one in which the guarantee of representative democracy AND the guarantee of checks and balances were fulfilled. That should mean that any additional Justices, whether 4 or 6 or 8, would be drawn from the federal Judiciary Districts through an elective process. It would mean that an elected Justice from one District, who might represent an interstate population of 30 million, would have term limits of 16 or 20 years and the same District could not nominate a new Justice consecutively. This would rotate several Justices as population 'representatives' along with those appointed by the parties of President or Senate (they can 'appoint' since their advice is crucial to the process). That 'packing' doesn't require an Amendment, only agreement by the three branches and satisfies checks and balances by representative election.

2018.07.21:13:40 |GW|>n⋈ |CD|<n |TR|>4 |LI|<1 ⋈ |JU|>3 ≈ |WB|<2 ⋈ |OP|>2

CRS, R45129, 2018.03.15, 'Modes of Constitutional Interpretation'[by Supreme Court 'sensing']:

"It is possible to categorize the various methods that have been employed when interpreting the Constitution.[22] This report broadly describes the most common modes of constitutional interpretation; discusses examples of Supreme Court decisions that demonstrate the application of these methods; and provides a general overview of the various arguments in support of, and in opposition to, the use of such methods by the Court. The modes discussed in detail in this report are (1) textualism; (2) original meaning; (3) judicial precedent; (4) pragmatism; (5) moral reasoning; (6) national identity (or "ethos"); (7) structuralism; and (8) historical practices."

Article III, Section 2 authority involves 'controversies to which the United States is a Party'. So, would the 8 modes all work within the domains?

Could [OP] be interpreted by a combination of (1), (2), (5) and (8) ?

The [CD] would be seen as (2), (4), and (6), with [GW] as (1), (3), (5) and (7).

But how would [WB{n}] be interpreted? It has major [GW] components and some [CD] components. (4), (5), (6) only or also a (1) with 'sunset' text.?

[JU] 2018 Conclusions:

The mixture of rights and justice is a major condition of We the people and 2018 is no different from other periods. Many Supreme court decisions were made in this context , along with some decisions of the Constitutionality of healthcare. Attempts to remove the Affordable Care Act from law failed both in the Congress and the Court.

Immigration problems posed serious Court and Justice [JU] movement as border 'asylum' seekers reach high (and unsustainable) levels.   The issue of habeas corpus 'rights' for non-citizens who were affecting Justice [{}} at a rate of $200,000 per year per person was approaching a [CD] level of significance. It was no longer a [LI] or even [WB] priority.

The levels of complexity involved in Justice per person and for all were both putting strains on the economic system. Fairness values in voting, representation, health and

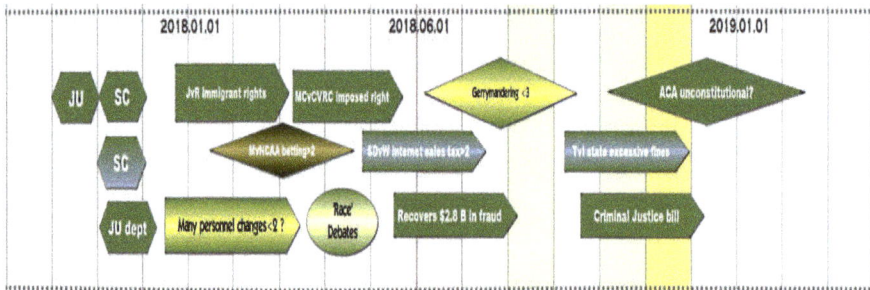

state governance, along with 'gun' rights and civil rights were all increasing. during 2018.

A sensing of the qualia involved showed that population movement and demands along with an increasing 'smaller government' administrative process was causing negative ripple effects in other domains besides Justice.

Tranquility [TR]

The Constitution gives the Preamble intent or domain as 'insure domestic Tranquility' and originally in 1787, this would mean peace between the states. Any Founder who had witnessed the 'States' of Europe and Africa would know that the constant strife between them was to be avoided. They meant that all of the interactions between States would be 'mitigated' or 'mediated' under law by a federal authority that was absolute with in a context of state sovereignty. But as the Nation grew, it also came to mean peace between city-states and individuals migrating about. About the time of the Civil War, notably in the 14th Amendment, the idea of Tranquility was also extended to individuals within a community within a State. By the 1870 census, there were 38 States with 25 communities over 50,000, with the city of New York gaining 200,000 immigrants per decade. What does that do for Population Traps?

By 2010, Tranquility was being extended to 50 States with over 100 cities at more than 200,000 people and very many cities with populations under that acquiring immigrants coming from climate--related strife areas. Population densities were becoming a [CD] and [GW] issue nationally and not just in cities. These population pressures were appearing as shared problems in all of the States by 2018 and this was reasonably clear in the 'sensing' for Tranquility.

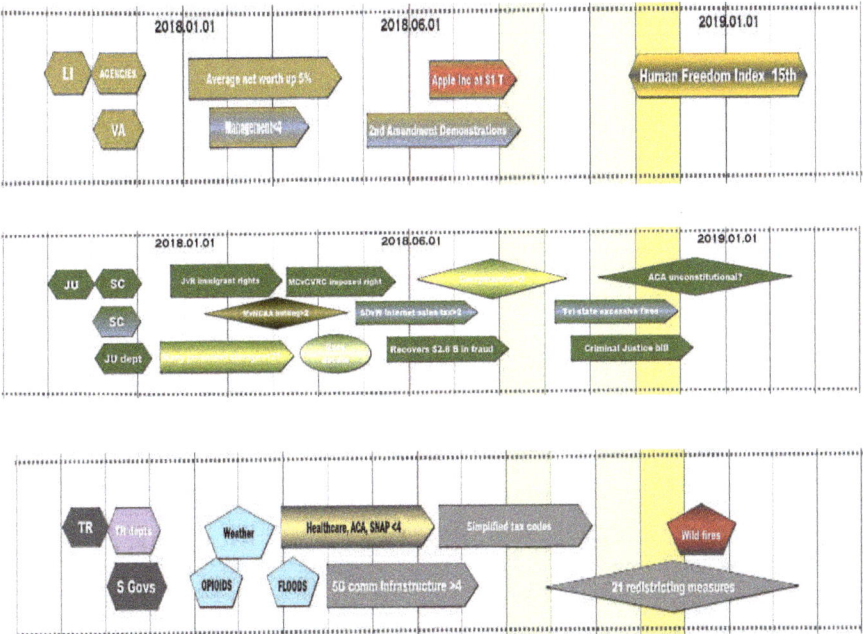

Items like federal tax reform and downsizing were affecting Tranquility from the State to the family and individual. A serious chemical abuse problem has also began to take its toll on the Justice and Liberties (you are not free if addicted to someone else's chemical property) domains. This alone was making wellbeing progress very difficult to administer at the community level. Education and health infrastructures were also being affected by the chemical abuse in many states, with Colorado's legal usage had not turned out ot be a tax benefit to the State and might have led to a serious increase in related injuries. A sampling of 'Tanguility' domain {subsets} follows. .

2018.07.23:06:58 |TR|>3 = ∑ |LI|<3WB|>2 ✉ |GW|<1-|JU|>2....|OP|>3|CD|<1

Sepulveda and Ghosh in WaPost, 'California's privacy law a commendable step toward national standard':

"But Congress needs to act because the California law does not incorporate some key ideas that have been presented in prior deliberations. For example, the OECD privacy principles and prior efforts at legislation in the United States, including the bipartisan Kerry-McCain Commercial Privacy Bill of Rights Act of 2011 and the Obama administration's Consumer Privacy Bill of Rights, are all useful guides for constructing new law and building on the California benchmark."

What is noticeably absent from these law systems, national and state, on cyber-privacy is a modern version of protection under the 4th Amendment that applies to all interstate personal information USAGE, not just storage. The information collected by cyber-droids about an individual's commercial or search habits doesn't mean much unless it is accessed by a human somewhere. There is nothing in these current privacy laws that penalize individual abuse of the data, which could become a 4th Amendment 'unreasonable seizure of effects' if that individual uses the stored data to 'stalk' a person in real-time. The simplest version of that is continuous calling of an individual's communication device by auto-dialing.

But there are worse forms, including sociopathic harassment of humans, political candidates and otherwise, by communication means that are being used by cyber-terrorists that can be addressed as abuses of an individual's 4th Amendment protections. The 4th Amendment has been used to prevent government unreasonable seizures, but it actually doesn't say that. It says that ALL instances of unreasonable seizure of 'effects' (personal data) violate a person's rights. It is this form of data abuse for cyber-stalking that needs to be criminalized in privacy laws along with the other provisions.

2018.09.17:08:24 |TR|>3 = ∑ |LI|>1 ✉ |GW|>1-|JU|>2|OP|>3 ✉ |CD|<2

Lindsey Stroud in TheHill, 'This Constitution Day, states should finally unwrap the gift of Article V':

"As Americans celebrate the signing of the Constitution, all policymakers should adhere to the principles of the Constitution. Furthermore, state legislators must hold the federal government accountable — and they can do so through Article V. As the deficit and debt continue to spiral out of control, federal lawmakers' ambivalence is shocking. Fortunately, the founding fathers anticipated the likelihood of a tyrannical, spend-thrift central government — it is for incumbent state legislators to utilize the power granted to them under Article V to put the nation back on a fiscally sustainable path."

It might be easier, under the Constitution's prime directives of Common Defense and General Welfare, to actually create an infrastructure that reduces the costs of the 'system' itself. The only reason for seeking a BBA is because it works in state Constitutions THAT TRANSFERRED ALL COMMON DEFENSE FUNCTIONS TO

THE FEDERALS and therefore have only half the costs of the Feds. A BBA through a Second Constitutional Convention or Article V voting process simply will not work when the 'barbarians' are knocking on the gates with 21st century economic and military weapons.

As for a Second Convention not being a run-away, the author states the reason the Convention **would be** a run-away: "However, these fears are unfounded. Constitutional law scholar Rob Natelson argues there are "redundant protections against a runaway convention," including political factors, provisions in states' applications, possible lawsuits, and "the potential for more judicial challenge, at every step of the process."

The very fact that the Convention is subject to continuous 'lawsuits', 'political factors', and 'states applications' will guarantee its failure. The only way a Second Convention can convene and be effective is if it is through a politically (and sociologically) independent Electoral College mechanism where state legislatures have defined what the Electors can be elected to do. The Idea is to use the Electoral College constitutional purpose as a check and balance on the CURRENT political structure because that partisan entity had become destructively inoperative and the Convention had become absolutely necessary in not transferring the current inabilities to the Constitution itself, including those certain manipulations of foreign oligarchies. In 1787, the European czars and emperors did not even become aware of the Convention until it was nearly over, so intellectual and physical isolation of the Electors, once convened, would be necessary for optimization of the issue under consideration. Note that the state legislatures or the Congress under Article V can designate multiple issues to be considered.

It would be more the duty of the existing three branches to guarantee the security and independence of the convened Electoral College in a Second Convention rather than directly have their Members interact with it, since that would defeat the purpose of the society-initiated problem solving EC.

{1} Redistricting

According to Ballotpedia, no less than one-eighth of state lawmakers who will be orchestrating that post-2020 Census redistricting were elected in November.

Democrats, after suffering state-level losses across the nation since 2010 before the last Census redistricting, dominated the process in the 1970s and 1980s. Republicans have since taken that advantage, "gerrymandering" districts in a way that benefits them.

Redistricting rules vary by state, but state legislators are responsible for the process in 37 states. Seven of the least populated states — Alaska, Delaware, Montana, North Dakota, South Dakota, Vermont, Wyoming — do not need to redistrict.

Redistricting will not generate many bills in state legislatures in 2019, but it will be a pervasive undercurrent in committee appointments and bureaucratic structure within newly configured chambers and gubernatorial administrations.

2018.11.10:21:07 [TR|>3 = ∑ |LI|>3WB|<2 ⋈ [GW]>1-|JU|<2....|OP|>2

Lane,WaPost, 'Voters took on gerrymandering. The Supreme Court doesn't need to.':

"The stakes are too small to justify the risks of involving federal courts in this sordid political business.

America's partisan gerrymandering problem is real, but it's on its way to being cured, with no need for federal judicial intervention. And if that intervention is not necessary, it's probably not proper."

This is not an accurate conclusion. The Article III, Section 2, of the Constitution specifically authorizes the Supreme Court to have Judicial Power over 'Controversies to which the United States [more than one] shall be a Party' and the specific question for the States is in Article IV, Section 4 where the Constitution federal government will guarantee a representative form of government in all states. The implication is that ONLY the Supreme Court could decide if a given Congressional District or a Senate seat was elected through a 'representative' method and gerrymandering by AI droids almost certainly would not meet the test under state controls. The poor history of gerrymandering involves both parties over 10 censuses, so it is a clear Supreme Court issue.

They can decide that a representative District is created by a census in which a mathematical 'center point' in each state's population of 710,767 (the 2010 census of population per District). That is, in order to be representative, the state would have to divide the itself into EQUAL 710K person (0ne million per seat in 2020?) demographic areas regardless of party or citizenship. Such demographics would arrange for a center point of the population (also done by AI droids) so that no citizen would be represented at the other end of a large state.

But determining the mathematical definition of a Constitutionally representative District or State is, in fact, a Supreme Court process and not that of a state oriented subordinate court or legislature.

Obviously a small population state might just split itself in half to be representative, but you wouldn't have one District representing just a city and no one else.

2018.08.02:13:09 |TR|>3 |LI|>2 |JU|<2 ≈ |OP|>?+|WB|>1 ⋈ |GW|>2

Will, WaPost, 'A California election that might actually matter':

"Tuck is a Democrat, as is his opponent, Tony Thurmond, a state legislator. Thurmond finished a close second to Tuck in California's primary system, wherein candidates of both parties appear on the same ballot and the top two meet in the general election. Thurmond, who knows who butters his bread, says, "I am not trying to cultivate Republican votes."

California may be 'representative' in who appears on the ballot provided some combination of registered citizens reaches a 51 percent population threshold. But in some districts ONLY Democrats OR Republicans can be elected. It is well known that both parties in 2018 are adhering to the 19th century dogmas of Marx, Keynes, and Friedman. That adherence to ancient dogmas defines both parties as intellectually incapable of solving modern social, economic or bioethical problems of Californians. Since only the Independent Peoples of America have the intellectual and moral fortitude capable of saving California, how could they do it without falling into the money trap of being a dogmatic political party? By definition, you cannot be an

Independent problem solver AND a member of a political organization, as recent world history has shown everywhere.

2018.07.09:07:04 |TR|>3 = ∑ |LI|>2 -|JU|<2....|OP|>31+|WB|<2 ◒ |GW|>2

Grofman in WaPost, 'This might be the way to prove partisan gerrymandering, according to the new Supreme Court standard':

"Many experts, including me, had hoped the Supreme Court would declare a standard for finding districts had been unconstitutionally gerrymandered for partisan advantage that looked at effects statewide. A district-specific standard is the next best thing, and completely manageable, if we adapt tools from the cases described above."

It might be more Article IV, Section 4 (representative form of government guarantee) correct to view each District individually than by state. Correcting a single representative District against statistical outliers, either political or national origin, would automatically shift neighboring District representation conditions and in many states, that means affecting the ENTIRE set of state's Districts. Gerrymandering on a state level might not be important so long as the single District representation of 600,000 is guaranteed.

But representation means that a statistical majority of the 600,000 (as determined by 10-year census) MUST be reflected in the winning candidate in order for the District to be Constitutionally acceptable. Even with all outlier anomalies accounted for by statistical distribution based on a District's geographic population 'center point' reference, a 'no-confidence' and 'Independent write-in' conditional would need to be on all ballots. A legitimate 51 percent majority can only be some combination of a political spectrum, not some pre-determined 10 percent minority vote in a primary.

Further:

Race, of course, might be a completely illegitimate District representation consideration since the DNA sequences for determining 'race' are composed of less than one tenth of one percent of the homosapien DNA pairs and could not possibly meet the Constitutionally defined 'citizen' who votes.

2018.08.13:07:32 |OP|>3 ≈ ∑ |TR|>3 |LI|<3 |JU|>1↔|GW|>2 [ξ| >2 |WB|>2

Editorial Board, WaPost, 'An assault on minority voting continues in North Carolina': "Voting laws, including for felons, vary enormously across the country. In some states the right to vote is restored automatically when people leave prison; in others, including North Carolina, felons are required to complete their sentences, including serving probation or paying fines, before their rights are restored. Elsewhere, ex-felons face waits of several years before they can regain voting rights. In two states, felons may vote even while incarcerated."

The issue for a Federally related election is whether the person attempting to vote actually has the status of a citizen. Restoration of citizenship rights such as voting, driving, bearing arms, or mobility (ankle-bracelet, breathalyzer) should be conditional on proving that citizenship itself has been re-acquired, a federal Naturalization Clause activity, not a local regulatory process. That is, there is nothing that says the Naturalization Clause cannot require all persons convicted of high crimes and misdemeanors to take a verifiable citizenship test while attached to a biometric analyzer (aka polygraph, but more modern and accurate). This citizenship bio-test could even be a requirement for parole from an institution regardless of state and it is purely within federal jurisdiction.

The idea is that a person who violates the 'rights' of others by predatory aggression (robbery, fraud, misuse of lethal devices like drugs and guns, political defamation, etc) losses his own in proportion and these have to be re-earned by self-education with biotesting. That would also eliminate the easily abused skin tone test now common in the world by accurately taking the measure of a being's citizenship or empathy toward humans.

Further:

21 minutes ago:

Or how about you act like a civilized nation and take seriously the "inalienable" before "rights"? If you commit a crime, you will lose your freedom for a time. But voting rights should be irrevocable. What about the wrongfully convicted? Will they get to retroactively vote in all the elections they weren't allowed to participate in? One person, one vote - whether that person is a billionaire, a store clerk or a convict; whether they live in a rural town or a major city.

22 minutes ago:

So, are you saying people lose their citizenship if they commit a crime and get put in jail? Or should? "biotest" for parole to answer what question? What will we require of those committing white collar crimes? The same citizenship test? Or, is this all about immigration for you?

14 minutes ago:

They actually do lose their citizenship 'rights' if they go to prison in most states, even though 'citizenship' is strictly a federal process. The biotest would mean answering all of the questions in a naturalization citizenship test (currently 100 or so) while under biometric measure. 'fraud' was included in the comment for crimes, normally a white collar activity. Immigration is only part of the citizenship problem, since demographic distribution of anti-social behavior is the same for citizens and the 22 million non-citizens who occupy U.S. space.

3 minutes ago:

I don't see why they should have to take any citizenship test. Their rights should be reinstated when their time is up. Period.

1 minute ago:

I think everyone who registers Republican should take a citizenship test before being allowed to vote.

59 seconds ago:

I don't trust you... AT ALL.

11 minutes ago:

 you forgot to talk about the brand on the forehead, that indicates current citizenship status.

5 minutes ago:

Actually, that is now done with a GPS implant under the skin, which any South American drug cartel boss can tell you how to insert them in their 'citizens'.

{2} Interstate Commerce, infrastructure.

2018.02.22:07:10 |TR|>2 ≈ **WB|>1+|CD|<1** ⋈ **|GW|>3-|JU|>2**

McCartney, WaPost, Metro financing:

"The House bill in Richmond would shrink the 16-member Metro board to a "reform board" of four or five members at first, and later create an eight-member board. It also calls for limiting the agency's annual growth in operating costs to 2 percent and adopting a "right-to-work" provision for any Metro projects solely within Virginia."

From an operations research standpoint, the main problem with the Metro system over the last 20 years was the 'mission creep' labor costs that instantly absorbed all fare and government revenue increases. This labor cost increase in turn did not leave enough funding for effective, note cost effective, safety and infrastructure improvements. A corporation or even a military unit simply would not survive if its labor costs exceeded its functional value due to mission creep. Having the two state government infrastructures contribute to their original 1789 federal District contribution of land for the U.S. Capitol with proportionate revenues now is fine as long as there are provisions to limit the 'creep', such as the 2 percent limit on cost increases.

But the Federal contribution should be a no-brainer in that transport infrastructure 'facilities' is directly authorized by Section 8 authorities of the Congress. It might even be proportionate to the number of federal employees within the total Metro region that could benefit from the system. It could also have a provision that said the 'hardware system' would get a substantial 'bonus' in revenues after every three years of neutral cost increases. Again, the idea would be to prevent 'creep' by rewarding efficient use of revenues.

2018.09.21:06:20 |TR|>3 = ∑ **|LI|>1|WB|<2** ⋈ **|GW|>1-|JU|<2....|OP|>2**

Mellnik and Williams, WaPost, 'Is Canada 'ripping' us off'? Or is it the best U.S. trade partner?':

"For Trump to impose the 25 percent auto tariff, the U.S. Commerce Department must find that auto and parts imports threaten national security. ....."A car put together with American-made parts is not a national security threat," Toyota spokesman Ed Lewis said."

The trade between local industrial organizations only becomes a national security issue if any one of the manufacturing 'entities' in the North American Economic Union (Greenland, Canada, U.S.A., Mexico, Caribbean, Central America, Polynesia) becomes dependent on non-Union energy and materials in order to stay in business. If the auto parts sub components like the plastic coverings, touch screens or piston ring alloys are made outside the NAE Union and shipped in, they become dependent on the political and economic motivations of a hostile power. It would be more cost effective to have ALL of the components of a given product made within a 1000 kilometers of the assembly plant itself and that would apply to all industrial processes within the Union (4 million total jobs?). The Lexus engine graphic in the article doesn't show a hidden transportation cost of perhaps $50 per engine because of the multiple assemblies. It might be better to have each of the locations shown as a 'final' assembly with the parts being made within a 1000 km of those assembly points.

The same rule might apply to medical and sport health equipment manufacturers, provided raw materials are available within the Union. Some things, like ethanol, might be regionally dependent and only be cost effective to produce in sunny regions of the Union like the Caribbean. They might qualify as an energy reserve area when the oil and shale deposits of Canada, Mexico and the U.S. are consumed in this century.

Further:

The idea for the big three of the Union is to build a common manufacturing distributed infrastructure that is independent of anything else over the next century and quibbling over 25% of a $10.00 item within the economic borders of such a Union might be counter-productive in the long run. But not if the sub-component materials can be shut off by a cartel some where on a moments notice. Canada and Mexico can 'rip us off' at a 4 or 5 per cent level any time and it won't matter in the slightest unless they are doing it by bootlicking some totalitarian economic interest somewhere.

2018.06.06:07:48 |LI|<1|TR|>2|WB|>1+|CD|<3 ⋈|GW|>1-|JU|>2≈|OP|>1

Ignatius, WaPost, 'Trump's tariffs give Democrats a big opportunity':

"Or they can try to frame a genuinely progressive stance on trade, one that focuses on industries that are growing rather than shrinking."

Unfortunately, a 'progressive stance' on trade has meant a strategic give-away of what is known as OEM or Original Equipment Manufacturer ability to state subsidized entities. In China's case, not only was the OEM ability transferred, but the intellectual property of OEMs as well was forcibly taken with it by the Chinese socialist monopoly state. There are dozens of OEM conditions in which American strategic defenses MUST go to foreign resources to get a finished product. The infamous purchase of American military uniform components, electronics and even arms parts from Asia being a simple example.

'Protectionism', but not Mckinley type, should mean maintaining, even with Federal subsidies, industries that are not only critical but also just OEM extensions of strategic resources. That does NOT mean tariffs on consumer goods that are operating in a competitive but free trade environment. Consumer related goods in which items in one country are traded for other goods in a second country as a perfect 'Ricardo' model with mutual benefit. But that is not the same as protecting OEM products used in a strategic defense of the country, such as raw materials, agricultural products or healthcare equipment (as examples) that the Nation needs to maintain independently of other sources. Foreign nations who appear to have state run computer models that target strategic resources like uranium, steel, aluminum and rare earths in America are not 'Ricardo model' oriented.

Targeting OEM units in America by subsidized undercutting is not the same as free trade that is mutually beneficial to both societies. Unilateral trade sometimes means mutually beneficial, but economic targeting is just another form of warfare.

Realchoices:

That is an argument used by those favoring central planning. The wonderful and virtuous state, underwritten by the taxpayers must prop up industries deemed "vital" by politicians. It often turns inefficient industries into white elephants that become a perpetual drain on the public coffers. No thanks.

That can happen. China does it all the time. But if they control all lithium deposits on the planet, as they are carefully arranging, where would you go to get a battery for your military or first responder radio?

2018.03.26:07:14 |LI|>1|TR|>2|WB|>2

Hiatt, WaPost, 'This is a story about American democracy working':

"The exact funding mechanisms may not be ideal. Metro still will have plenty of problems. But politicians will have done the right thing. The system will have worked."

Anyone in operations research could identify the Washington Metro as a cycling dysfunctional system five years ago. Any organization that absorbs any revenue given it with inflated operating costs like an 80% labor budget is dysfunctional in an extreme. Making an organization progressively functional is always a success story.

While 'post' roads as defined by the Constitution's Article I, Section 8 in the modern since are electronic as wells as physical, it is clear that the federal government has the authority to build infrastructures within its jurisdiction and that should include a Metro system for the District and other cities with a federal administrative enclave. But that doesn't mean it feeds the daily operating costs of a transit system in the U.S. It more accurately has the authority to appropriate funding for the 'hardware' of a transport infrastructure on a multi year basis. That would mean that the feds can appropriate funds for new equipment and parts of the infrastructure IF, and only if, the organization has shown effective control of its operating expenses and a man-hour savings to the local population like alleviating congestion (at minimum wage, DC metro area congestion losses are around $70 million a day).

The DC Metro has very much met those conditions and is entitled to a federal hardware infrastructure bonus of $400 million every three years.

2018.07.06:22:23 [TR]>2 = |LI|>1WB|>2 ⋈ [GW|>1-|JU|<2

Siddiqui, WaPost, 'With ridership falling, Metro will spend $2.2 mllion to study bus business model':

"In his widely anticipated Metro overhaul analysis, former U.S. transportation secretary Ray LaHood called for Metro to overhaul its bus routes and "offer service that matches actual demand," meaning service reductions. He also called for a fare increase of $2.10 from $2."

Anyone who has watched Metrobus operations from the National Mall can see that the only time the buses, which are 40 feet long and carry a maximum of 60 passengers, are cost effective is during rush hours when full of incoming passengers. These hybrid-electric vehicles are pretty comfortable and energy efficient, but run 40 foot long monsters with 4 riders in the off-hours? They roam the streets as traffic lane-barriers when they are not operating at capacity. For extended routes to the 'burbs' and within the District, Metro might consider 20 passenger mini-buses, noting that the operator might not be cost effective at 10 passengers, which can maneuver on almost any District street even without stop stations.

If one checks out the Wikipedia website on mini-buses,

  https://en.wikipedia.org/wiki/Minibus,

it becomes almost immediately obvious that minibus conversions of the Ford Transit or Chevrolet Express could create an entire made-in-USA, 20 passenger fleet that doesn't have the overhead of the Metro Monsters. One might even add luxury features of the American custom mini-coach makers and still get a 500 unit fleet that cost less to operate than the Hybrid 40 footer fleet carrying less than 10 passengers. The minibuses could also be used as MetroAccess emergency units and rented out to private transit groups for conventions after identity conversion features. Minibus routes are worth a cost-benefit study at least.

2018.04.16:00:00 |TR|<1 = |LI|>3 ⋈ GW|>2-|JU|<2↔|OP|<1

S.A. Miller, WaTimes Special Sections, *Infrastructures 2018,* ' Disputes over spending, permitting dog infrastructure plan':

"We can't toll our way out of this problem," Sen. Bill Nelson, the ranking member on the Senate Commerce, Science and Transportation Committee, said at recent hearing on the proposal. The Florida Democrat was ripping Mr. Trump's plan to use public-private partnerships or P3s to finance some projects, one of several options to help state and local governments pick up more of the tab. With financing options and other incentives, Mr. Trump wants $200 billion in federal spending to leverage a total investment of $1.5 trillion over 10 years. "The president's plan calls for $200 billion but has no clear way to pay for it," said Mr. Nelson. "At the same time, the administration's budget cuts critical infrastructure programs. We can't cut our way to prosperity. "He echoed criticism of the vast majority of Capitol Hill Democrats, who want $1 trillion of direct federal spending to rebuild American's crumbing highways, bridges and airports. Democrats balked at Mr. Trump's plan to cut regulations, including environmental regulations, to streamline the Byzantine federal approval process."

TLO: Not exactly cherry-picking of the previous seven plans on re-building the infrastructure. Classic partisan erasure of the other parties' programs rather than a planned 10-year concept.   Not in this Congress or Executive....

2018.08.29:08:18 |TR|>3 = ∑ |LI|>3 |WB|<2 ⋈ GW|>1-|JU|<2....|OP|

Schneider, WaPost, 'In Virginia, governor and appointees at odds over gas pipelines':

"That project will carry natural gas 600 miles from West Virginia through the central part of Virginia and into North Carolina……

The Union Hill compressor station faces a key state air-quality permit hearing on Sept. 11, and the advisory council recommended that Northam suspend that process to give it deeper review."

It might be useful to ensure that a 'deeper review' of all the environmental conditions of new gas pipelines is carried out in mid-construction. Lots of little details pop up during any major infrastructure activity. But an inspection of a east coast pipeline article on the internet shows a 'strategic' value of such a pipeline. See:

http://www.virginiaplaces.org/transportation/gaspipeline.html

It is very noticeable that southern Virginia and North Carolina are being energy-serviced by a couple of gas pipelines that MUST use propane style trucks (gasoline burning?) to reach large areas because of a lack of local pipelines. Much of the gas for the region comes up a single Transco pipeline from the Gulf Coast, which has a major connection station in the Virginia suburbs of Washington DC (any complaints there?). Re-distribution of gas from the Appalachians to coastal mid Atlantic communities appears to be a logical choice if it is going to be used in new power generation systems that allow availability of electric cars in the future. What might even be needed is more local storage facilities in the region as well as local pipelines that make the energy supply in the District, Maryland, Virginia and Carolina more independent of Gulf and Canadian systems.

There is a future need in the region that is a General Welfare and state 'Tranquility' Constitutional process rather than an individual lifestyle process. If the 'deeper review' of the infrastructure environmental conditions are satisfied, the process should be expedited by the governmental organizations involved.

2018.08.07:08:37 [CD]<3 ⋈ [GW]>1-[JU]<2[TR]>1≈[OP]>1

Eldib and Spencer in TheHill, 'Investing in understanding cities is investing in national security':

"Cities have also become vulnerable to political violence. While governments struggle to govern and secure today's rapidly growing and complex urban environments, insurgent and terrorist organizations have learned the advantages they can gain, negating the advanced technologies and weapons of military forces by fighting among the dense populations and structures of cities. This is most recently demonstrated by the fierce urban battles against ISIS in cities across Iraq and Syria."

What the Russians and Syrians have demonstrated in the past six years was their own 'urban warfare' development stages and that unfortunately appears to involve various methods of wiping out entire urban neighborhoods with WMD in order to remove individual 'enemies of the state'.

An urban warfare center in the DOD that has expertise access to ASU or Columbia or the Santa Fe Institute wouldn't hurt at all, especially if such a combination were able to devise mechanisms for preventing the Malthusian Populations Traps (MPTs) that appeared when even minor disturbances of urban life support logistics occurred. Places such as Gaza, Aleppo and Mosul have MPTs that caused a social collapse when even 10 percent of the safety nets were destroyed by armed force. Such a Urban Security Center with serious demographic modelling from universities might prevent the 'collateral' slaughter that was inflicted by totalitarians in Iraq, Iran, and Syria by advising field operations of local density problems. This was actually done during the Mosul campaign against ISIS but not well enough that the data allowed quick rebuilding of the urban support structures.

Question: Could a DOD Urban Security Center have aided the aftermath in Louisiana after hurricane Katrina, which was almost instantly turned into a MPT?

TLO: While disaster MPTs are an international [CD] issue in most cases because of their association with asymmetric warfare, they also can crop up in ANY American State region, making them a [TR] {consideration} . That is especially true in drastic climate change states like Florida, Louisiana, Texas and California.

{3} Higher Education

The Wikipedia website at

https://en.wikipedia.org/wiki/Higher_education_in_the_United_States on education in the United States shows why the states consider this a major priority under [TR] and actually understand it to be a Posterity issue much more than those who decide policy in Washington D.C.   The two maps on the site show that a large concentration of advanced degrees is in the New York **and** the Washington D/C. metro areas, with Colorado a close second. A mountain state with a population density of 52 people per square mile has a high concentration of advanced education?   Might be worth a research thesis all by itself.

2018.06.25:07:24 [LI|<1|TR|>2|WB|<2

Mathews, WaPost, 'Harvard alum reflects on his experiences interviewing Asian American applicants for admission':

"The most interesting statistic I saw in the analysis compiled by the Asian American plaintiffs — and sharply criticized by Harvard — was that alumni interviewers like me gave Asian Americans personal ratings comparable to those for whites. But the professional admissions officers at Harvard gave them the worst personal scores of any ethnic group."

Speculation: Harvard's 'culture' makes it statistically difficult for the school(s) to discriminate as a policy or even from an individual 'good old boy' level, except possibly at the Business School across the Charles. It is possible that admissions officers are convinced Asian-Americans belong down Mass Ave at MIT because of their inherent Asian math skills and there really isn't any skin-tone discrimination among the officers, just practical reality.

2018.09.01:06:25   [TR|>3 = ∑ [LI|>3 -[JU|<2....|OP|>1+|WB|>2 ⋈ [GW|>2

Timothy S. Huebner in TheHill, 'Teach the Constitution':

"Second, improving civic literacy will elevate and enrich our public discussion. The Constitution, after all, is a set of rules by which we all agree to play. Knowing the rules — and knowing how American ideas and institutions based on those roles have developed over time — is the key to sustaining civic engagement, civil debate, and health of the republic."

You could go a step further and add a Constitutional Amendment that says as a condition of citizenship (never defined in the Constitution, by the way), a senior in High School, or a GED candidate or even a GRE candidate must be able to pass a civics exam based on knowing 66 of 100 questions about Constitutional history of Americans (not America). The 66 is two thirds, the same as it took to ratify the Bill of Rights. If the test, which actually would be similar to the one taken by citizenship candidates now, is based on 500 possible questions, the 'graduating' person would have to know what is taught in most dormitory basements about modern Constitutional dynamics as civics courses.

But does that mean an employer is obligated to only hire persons who have a 'certificate of expertise' on Constitutional dynamics along with other knowledge base degrees?

Always an exhaustive realm for state lawmakers, but with the Every Student Succeeds Act (ESSA) rolling back federal involvement in education policy and administration, this component of federal deregulation will remain an intensive emphasis in state legislatures in 2019.

4PolicyMatters45tuition and non-tuition charges can occupy a greater share of family income. There has been progress on affordability through state-level free college plans. The extent to which these state proposals expand—or are even maintained—in 2018 will depend on available state budget revenue. Rhode Island, for example, approved a free college program in 2017, but had to scale back the original proposal due to state budget considerations. Likewise, the administrators of Oregon's free tuition program rationed their program in 2017, due to a lack of revenue. New York approved a highly touted free college plan in 2017, but it comes with numerous requirements that narrow the number of eligible participants. A few other states have unveiled free tuition programs in recent years, but limited eligibility to those enrolled in certificate and associate degree programs leading to jobs in select high-demand fields.

{4} Economic and Workforce Development.

Technical illiteracy has been a serious problem since the advent of video media, which some studies indicate might be a prohibitor of technical mental 'focus'. This has become a serious issue as successive 'recession' waves have disrupted the American ability to have a stable workforce, although there is a suspicion that the waves are orchestrated to remove workforce pressures from corporate profit entities. Technical workers normally need a mind-set for nearly any technical operation, even at the level of an automotive, medical, or building technician. This technical focus mind-set tends to disappear in a prolonged media intensive environment such as a recession lay-off. Many, after a year outside of the corporate technical environment, must be completely re-trained and this combination is a serious Tranquility issue for nearly every state. One of the principal functions of community education facilities, usually with state help, was to re-intensify this technology awareness as the 'hardware systems' changed with time and scientific research. At some point in a time line, failure to do this leads to both [CD] and [GW] problems because of a lack of a genuinely literate citizenry.

{5} Healthcare, chemical abuse

November's elections essentially determined if the Trump Administration would have a Congress it could – in its fourth attempt – repeal the Affordable Care Act (ACA) with.

At the state level, expanding, adjusting, and capping Medicaid financing will remain a 2019 issue of legislative emphasis, regardless of party configuration, although the proposed solutions could change in some chambers after November's elections.

Among concerns will be Trump Administration rules shortening enrollment periods for federally run exchanges, significantly cutting funds for enrollment assistance/outreach, ending cost-sharing subsidies to insurance companies, and rolling back requirements for employers to include birth control coverage in health insurance plans.

Marijuana: Bills relating to the legalization of medical and/or recreational marijuana have been introduced in every state in one form or another and will continue to be a hot topic of legislative discussion in 2019.

2018.03.04:07:23 [LI]>3|TR]<2|WB]<2+|CD]<3 ⋈|GW]>1-[JU]<2≈|OP|<2

Minter, BloombergView, 'Killing Junkies Doesn't Work in Asia Either':

"The most compelling evidence that executions have failed as an anti-drug strategy is the fact that many Asian governments have begun to retreat from them. The trend can take modest form, such as Singapore's 2012 decision to reduce the number of drug crimes eligible for mandatory executions, or China's quiet, decade-long effort to open methadone clinics and voluntary rehabilitation facilities."

1998 Rome Statute on the definition of a crime against humanity (criaghum):

For the purpose of this Statute, 'crime against humanity' means any of the following acts when committed as part of a widespread or systematic attack directed against any civilian population, with knowledge of the attack:

(1)(k) Other inhumane acts of a similar character intentionally causing great suffering, or serious injury to body or to mental or physical health.

(2)(a) 'Attack directed against any civilian population' means a course of conduct involving the multiple commission of acts referred to in paragraph 1 against any civilian population, pursuant to or in furtherance of a State or organizational policy to commit such attack.

Organized production and distribution of molecular combinations such as Opioids, Fentanyl, meth, nanothermites, Botulium, Cobalt-60 (DNA destroyer), and radium-226, meet the entire criteria of item (k) as a crime against humanity. Note that criaghum means an attack against one is an attack against all, and therefore the profit from such an attack in itself qualifies as sub-human predatory criaghum against people everywhere. Use of a simple weapon of mass destruction for a crime against humanity simply cannot be tolerated by normal humans. It is not a matter of unjustly removing a person who is the victim of molecular criaghum as much as it is the permanent removal of the attacker AND his capital supporters.

The human DNA structures, especially the 49 Human Accelerated Regions, have made people the most adaptable entity on the planet and to have a sub-species of predators feed off that adaptability with neurotoxin molecular combinations cannot be allowed by any governing entity intent on protecting its humans. It doesn't matter if the drug or toxin profiteer engaged in criaghum is replaced after he is eliminated from human contact; the criaghum is the manufacture and distribution of the toxin and should be eliminated under all circumstances, including circumstances where justice is temporarily, note temporarily, set aside. Humanity cannot allow such a predator to walk down a street or carry the toxins off an aircraft or have the toxins in a sanctuary.

Eight states and the District of Columbia have legalized marijuana for adult recreational use, while 29 states, D.C., Guam, and Puerto Rico, have legalized medical marijuana. Forty-six states have legalized access to some low-THC cannabis products.

More than 75 million Americans are enrolled in Medicaid. Since the 2012 U.S. Supreme Court ruling that confirmed each state's right to opt out of the ACA, debates on expanding Medicaid have occupied many State House sessions.

Only 14 states have not expanded their Medicaid programs to one degree or another under the ACA. Of the four states with Medicaid expansion proposals on the ballot in the November 2018 elections – Nebraska, Idaho, Utah, and Montana – only Montana failed to pass the proposal.

2018.10.26:22:30 [WB]<4 ⋈ [GW]>2⋈ [CD]<3 [TR]>3 [JU]<3 ≈ [OP]<2

Dr. Marion Mass in TheHill, 'Medicare for All' will never work, so let's stop pushing it':

"Consider: The number of health-care administrators — many drawing salaries well into the six figures — has risen by 3,200 percent between 1975 and 2010. (The number of physicians grew by 150 percent over the same timeframe.) This bureaucratic bloat diverts precious resources away from treating patients and inflates the cost of care. Reversing this administrative growth to all but the most critical positions could allow for a dollar-for-dollar offset in health-care costs.

Meanwhile, the clerical burden on doctors continues to grow. Doctors now report spending two-thirds of their time on paperwork."

This doesn't make sense. If there are 3200 percent more administrators, many of whom are in doctors' offices AND in the private insurance sector, how is it that a provider can wind up doing paperwork two-thirds of the time? Anyone who is familiar with the medical disease classification system known as ICD-10 knows that it lists a required classification of some 14,000 problems, along with an optional 70,000 insurance related codes that medical offices must deal with. This results to some degree in a national health cost of 'undiagnosed problems' of $270 billion a year, much higher than #2, heart disease treatments. Interpret as administrative costs for the 3200 percent increase in administrators, perhaps?

The 'market' solutions listed here will not work because modern communications will allow for pricing adjustments industry-wide on a given ICD-10 disease condition. This in turn guarantees that the costs per ICD-10 item will increase at a 6 or 7 percent level rather than the inflation level of 2%. There is no gain for Americans by just this process, but neither would a universal Medicare at an additional $4.0 trillion a year because there is still no attempt to remove the 'admin' costs from the system. You would be better off manufacturing 800,000 AI med-bots that record everything they see in a health environment, including mistakes, and make up the ICD-10 (or ICD-15 in 2025) reports for both the private sector and the government HHS agencies. Would intelligent med-bots with 500 terabyte memories drop $200 billion a year off the costs?

{6} **Election Security**

2018.06.20:06:54 [LI|>1|TR|>2|WB|<2 ⋈ |GW|>1-|JU|<2 ≈ |OP|<1

Drehle, WaPost, on voter fraud:

"She ruled, after a lengthy trial, that Kobach, Kansas's secretary of state, produced no credible support for his theory that large numbers of noncitizens are **illegally** voting in American elections. Thus, the Kobach-inspired law requiring Kansas voters to provide documentary proof of citizenship is unconstitutional because it imposes the burden without a reasonable justification."

The judge only inspected Kansas state records, so how did she conclude something about American elections in general? Kansas demographics indicate it has nearly 3 million people with nearly one million in 4 cities. Its 82,000 square miles (35 people per) also has some 6,000 'ghost' towns with dwindling populations, so the statistical probability of finding a non-citizen in the State rapidly approaches zero outside four downtown concentrated neighborhoods. That would make the judge's Kansas conclusion correct; there is no Constitutional danger of non-citizen distortion or harm of voter rights. The 'defendant' probably should be held in contempt on Kansas non-citizen issues.

But 'provide documentary proof of citizenship' is unconstitutional? The 15th Amendment specifically says the right of a **citizen** to vote shall not be denied by any state and that only the Congress is empowered to create 'appropriate legislation' to enforce that. Various Amendments and voting rights laws have defined this and requiring proof of citizenship to register cannot possibly be unconstitutional no matter who claims it.

While a good number of **non-citizens might be voting legally in U.S.** elections, such is in Metro New York City, that does not mean such voting is constitutional. New York's spectacular diversity (nothing wrong with that from a Human Genome reference) has 36 percent foreign born out of a density of 27,000 per square mile, so there might be half a million non-citizen voters. That doesn't make it a constitutional model for the nation.

As election audits become more widespread, so will paper-based voting. About a month before its general election in 2017, Virginia abruptly decertified its paperless voting machines over cybersecurity concerns; Georgia is piloting paper ballots for the same reason. And Delaware put out a bid for machines that used paper. About a quarter of the nation's voters still live in election districts with paperless voting machines, but after Virginia's announcement last fall, that number is sure to shrink.

The cooperation came about last year after Homeland Security notified 21 states that Russian hackers had targeted their voter registration files or websites. No evidence suggests hackers actually tampered with voting machines or vote counts, but the federal agency still moved to designate election systems as "critical infrastructure." Under the designation, states and localities should have an easier time getting federal assistance to protect voting machines, storage facilities and voter registration databases.

{7} **Interstate disasters.**

2018.01.06:13:10 [TR]|<1 + [WB]|<2→ [GW]|<2 ⋈ [CD]|<1

Resnick, Vox, 'Winter storm 2018: almost the entire East Coast is covered in snow':

"This week is ending with almost the entire East Coast being covered in a sheet of snow. A large, rapidly intensifying winter storm that began on Wednesday dumped over a foot of snow in New England, but also brought with it damaging winds, and dangerous, icy, coastal flooding.

The city of Boston, according to the National Weather Service, also broke a record for its high tide, the result of the storm's winds pushing an already high tide further onshore. "

Intense storm with eye. Climate related and more to come?

2018.08.22:09:09 [CD]|<? ≈ [OP]|<?

"Hurricane Lane strengthened to a powerful Category 5 storm late Tuesday as it made its way to a dangerously close encounter with the Hawaiian Islands in the coming days."

Speculation:

It could be that Lono, the Hawaiian god of water and weather, is gathering energy from the hurricane just as his sister Pele, goddess of fire, has been gathering energy from the intense plasma eruptions of Kilauea. As they are my personal guardian angels from having lived in Kona, I always take an interest in their paranormal energy activities.

Could it be that Pele and Lono are about to bring their combined energy of fire and water to the mainland Kahicki election period? Already, there are many fires and floods from the 'global warming' 1000-year cycle, but have Pele, who is quick to anger, and Lono, who usually brings water just for life growth, become unhappy with the politics of the mainland and will move to alter their fire and water degeneration in this election?

Mere speculation, of course…..

2018.09.08:11:34 [WB]|<3⋈ [GW]|<3⋈ [CD]|<1 |TR]|<1 |LI]|<3 ≈ [JU]|>1 |OP]|<2

Louissant in TheHill, 'What Puerto Rico's death toll really tells us':

Milken Institute study, 'c) Assessment of Crisis and Mortality Communications and the Information Environment':

"Puerto Rico Government personnel and key leader interview respondents indicated that communication contingency plans were not in place to anticipate multiple cascading failures of critical infrastructure and key resource sectors. Consequently, the central government was not prepared to use alternative communication channels for health-related and mortality surveillance, public health information dissemination and coordination with communities, including radio and interpersonal communication. This contributed to delayed information availability, gaps in information and the dissemination of inconsistent information to the public. Furthermore, there were gaps in the information provided by the Government of Puerto Rico, including limited explanation of the death certification process, distinguishing between direct and indirect deaths, or explanations of barriers to timely mortality reporting."

Speculation:

In a hurricane climatic zone with a population existing in a classic Malthusian Population Trap of 3.327 million residents?

The modern Malthusian Trap interpretation, not Malthus original 1700s version, involves the inadequate resource infrastructure to sustain human life and is a combination of structures for food, shelter, health and energy that can sustain a population for extended periods. The Puerto Rican government for 30 years had failed its responsibilities for creating an adequate resource structure by siphoning off the $100 billion in investment wealth to individualized use. This created a lessening of the four 'needs' availability for many years and a sudden catastrophe like a hurricane (see Andrews, Katrina, Taiwan Nina of 1975, etc.) or prolonged draught (see Mayans, Oklahomans, Egyptians, etc.) accelerated this to such an extent that the existing support infrastructure itself fell apart.

As such a health, energy and nutrition infrastructure (along with common security and rights infrastructure) is a Constitutional requirement of a democracy or a republic, its failure is a form of direct constitutional neglect and usurpation. As a U.S. Territory, the region's political parties, which have received some $300,000 per member from various investment and tax sources, can be held as too incompetent to govern and should be disbanded in favor of PROMESA style oversight until the island 'recovers' to a level above a Malthusian Trap.

2018.05.08:17:05 [LI|<1|TR|>2|WB|<1+|GW<1

Kilgore, WaPost, 'Capitals' win puts a dagger in the D.C. sports 'curse':

It earned the label "D.C. Sports Curse," because karma provided order where logic could offer none. It turned regular-season joyrides into postseason gut-punches. It got coaches fired, tainted players' reputations and made fans question their sanity. And now, it is dead.

"It's almost embarrassing it's taken this long for us to get past it," Capitals and Wizards Owner Ted Leonsis said Monday night, smiling in the victorious visitors' locker room.

Poor, innocent lambs. The 'sports curse' is only a side effect of the famous 'Curse of the Ben' that Franklin wrote into his concurrence speech on the formation of the Constitution in 1787. He entered that Curse on all who would disavow rational spending by the Federal government in favor of endless deficits and it is no coincidence that the Curse re-appeared in 1998 at the same time the District sports teams began fumbling away their attempts to enter the final playoffs. 1998 was the year of the last surplus that made a slight dent in the corruptive evil of deficit spending. Just as Ben predicted, that evil of relentless spending without chance of future revenue had taken hold in the Keynesian and Friedmanist debaucheries, causing the endless chaos of Capitol Hill.

The evil chaos of deficit corruption spreads the Curse in many forms, including sports. It's dark, un-dead mists flow down the Hill into the streets of the District, even touching an athlete here or there so that he losses wealth at a fast-changing light. But the mists of Ben's Curse cannot be satisfied, whether flowing through the streets, into the subways or across the benches of the stadium or the rink; they will cause the inevitable famine of luck or skill .

Yet, in May, it is no coincidence that a team passed the 1998 barriers of malediction into higher victory at the same time prayers for rational spending were allowed to resume on the Hill.

Further: Or flowing over a lobbyist there until he shimmers with the gold of other folks' deficits or passing by an optimistic coach with a deficit of six-footers. [??]

2018.08.02:11:34 |TR|<2 + |WB|<3→ |GW|<2⋈ |CD|<1 |LI|<3 → |OP|<n?

"Schleuss, Kim, Krishnakumar, LATimes, 'Here's where the Carr fire destroyed homes in Northern California':

The Carr fire started on July 23 after a vehicle malfunctioned on California Highway 299. The fire quickly exploded in size, destroying 1,564 buildings, scorching more than 121,000 acres and killing six. By late Wednesday it was 35% contained.

The fire penetrated the city of Redding, which has about 91,000 residents. More than 280 buildings were destroyed, many of them homes in the Land Park and Stanford Hills neighborhoods. The Lake Redding and Mora Court subdivisions lost at least 68 buildings."

Strictly climate warming effects in populated areas. See :

https://en.wikipedia.org/wiki/2018_California_wildfires

Not just California, although the state has the most combustible fuel. Costs to We the People: $3.5 billion direct, human capital ripple effects including 103 deaths and 18,000 structures, both business and home, near $10 billion.   Other states proportionate in human capital costs. Serious [WB] ripple effects.

Speculation: With no Santa Ana wind, would burn-off of excess dead foliage prevent 'resident' damage? Where are the Army surplus MRAP vehicles when you need them domestically? Need an MRAP type vehicle in each community fire station by 2028?

→ [GW]<2 ⋈ [CD]<1 [LI]<3 → [OP]<n? is significant enough so it is not just [TR] but affects the nation also as well as personal liberty through economic losses. Only a low Posterity effect unless the climate warming creates new acreage of unburned foliage in the west over a ten-year period.

2018.11.27:00:00 |TR|<2 + |WB|<3→ |GW|<2⋈ |CD|<1 |LI|<3 → |OP|<n?

CRS, R45819, 'The Disaster Recovery Reform Act of 2018 (DRRA): A Summary of Selected Statutory Provisions':

Summary [of the report itself, some 50 {sections}]

The Disaster Recovery Reform Act of 2018 (DRRA, Division D of P.L. 115-254) was enacted on October 5, 2018. DRRA is the most comprehensive reform of the Federal Emergency Management Agency's (FEMA's) disaster assistance programs since the passage of the Sandy Recovery Improvement Act of 2013 (SRIA, Division B of P.L. 113-2) and the Post-Katrina Emergency Management Reform Act of 2006 (PKEMRA, P.L. 109-295). DRRA focuses on improving pre-disaster planning and mitigation, response, and recovery, and increasing FEMA accountability. As such, it amends many sections of the Robert T. Stafford Disaster Relief and Emergency Assistance Act

(Stafford Act, P.L. 93-288, as amended; 42 U.S.C. §§5121 et seq.) and also includes new standalone authorities. In addition, DRRA requires reports to Congress, rulemaking, and other actions.

This report provides an overview of selected sections of DRRA that significantly change the provision of services or authorities under the Stafford Act, and includes:

an overview of programs as they existed prior to DRRA's enactment, and how they were modified following DRRA;

the context or rationale for program modifications or changes to disaster assistance policies following DRRA's enactment;

potential considerations and issues for Congress;

a table of amendments to the Stafford Act following DRRA's enactment; and

tables of deadlines associated with DRRA's reporting, rulemaking and regulations, and other implementation actions and requirements.

This report does not specifically address every section included in DRRA, nor does it address every subsection or paragraph of those DRRA sections which are addressed herein.

TLO: If a given Congressional District, 435 plus , is hit in the same time frame by natural disasters like extreme climate, then state dysfunction, societal breakdown AND pandemics conditions, is there provision for a martial law declaration by Congress and States that allows the destroyed District(s) area to be placed under a federal 'territory' jurisdiction for a generation? Territorial [OP] enhancement as objective.

{8} Gun regulation as a state issue.

Firearms-related legislation has been a huge issue in state legislatures for more than 20 years, but in 2018, the sustained nationwide trend in state lawmakers expanding gun-rights ended in the wake of the Valentine's Day school shooting in Parkland, Florida.

According to FiscalNote, 126 firearms-related bills were passed by state legislatures in 2018, which include banning bump stocks after October 2017's Las Vegas shooting, and "red flag" laws that allow police to temporarily seize guns from individuals showing signs of mental instability or violence.

Fourteen states with Republican governors and GOP-controlled legislatures adopted more than 50 new gun control laws, while eight states adopted laws expanding gun access, according to the NCSL.

2018.04.02:07:15 |LI|>3|TR|>2|WB|<1+|CD|<3

Phillips, WaPost, 'A disaster about to happen:' A student who bought rifles and showed odd behavior is arrested':

"Between late January and early February, authorities said Sun bought two weapons — a LWRC 300 Blackout rifle and a .308 Ruger Precision rifle — as well as a couple hundred rounds of ammunition."

and

"Beary, the police chief, said Sun had modified the rifle by adding a bipod and "very, very expensive optics.""

Any Afghan mountain sniper could tell you that you could not use that optical/bipod combination of weapon for hunting in the flat, grassland regions of Florida. The nearest hunting area for that 300 Blackout might be the Osceola lake region south of Orlando and the precision scope wouldn't help in swampy grasslands against deer or wild pigs. Plus, the area only allows hunting with 5-round magazines, which is perfectly sensible. Even with the absence of a stated threat, it is pretty obvious the weapons were intended as a SWMD or Simple Weapon of Mass Destruction on people.

2018.05.21:19:38 |GW|<2 ⋈ |CD|<1 ↔ |TR|>2 |LI|>3 ⋈ |JU|>1 |OP|>1

Baron in WaPost, 'Antonin Scalia was wrong about the meaning of 'bear arms':

"In his opinion in Heller, Justice Antonin Scalia, who said that we must understand the Constitution's words exactly as the framers understood them, disconnected the right to keep and bear arms from the need for a well-regulated militia, in part because he concluded that the phrase "bear arms" did not refer to military contexts in the founding era."

People should keep in mind what the environment was like in the mid-1700s through the end of the century when the Constitution began to take effect in the new States, as did Justice Scalia. If you do a Wikipedia search on 'minutemen', you will find a description of what life was like at the time and the idea of bearing arms becomes clearer. Basically, the 'minuteman' was a farmer or storekeeper or teacher living in a spread-out community like Lexington, Massachusetts or Cowpens, South Carolina. This meant that he kept arms in the home so that he could carry it or 'bear' it to an assembly of militia that had been called up to defend a community. Militias of minutemen were common in nearly all communities, but a person did not become 'military' until he had actually joined the unit somewhere. Until then, he would just 'bear arms' from his home and maybe pick off something to eat along the way.

A western 'Posse' was also a deputized militia, even in 1950, with the members carrying sidearms and rifles that they brought from home, but in many cases they were assembled for law enforcement purposes, not as soldiers.

Bottom line is that the Founders believed it was necessary for all citizens to be ready to bear arms in defense of their communities or Nation if called to do that. From an evolutionary standpoint, a modern minuteman would be able to handle any object he could use to defend his self, family, or community and that includes such things as autos, cell phones, first-aid kits, hazardous waste disposal kits, viruses cleaners and maybe in this century, simple WMD. A gun is just another object that needs bearing in an emergency that requires defense and an evolved person could do that.

2018.06.20:11:54 | ξ|<3 |WB|<2 ⋈ |GW|>3⋈ |TR|>2 |LI|<3⋈|JU|<1 ≈ |OP|>1

Berman, WaPost, 'Active shooters usually get their guns legally and then target specific victims, FBI says'

"Other research has similarly found tenuous links connecting shooting rampages and mental illness. In a 2015 study, Michael Stone, a clinical psychiatry professor at

Columbia University, examined 235 people who carried out or attempted to carry out mass killings, and he concluded that about 22 percent could be considered mentally ill. An article published the same year in the academic journal Annals of Epidemiology found that "the large majority of people with mental disorders do not engage in violence against others, and that most violent behavior is due to factors other than mental illness."

That probably means the FBI profilers are using the DSM IV rather than the DSM-V (Diagnostic and Statistical Manual for Mental Disorders) which contains much more detail about PTSD. Stress disorders do not necessarily mean mental illness in the neurological sense, although one can trigger the other. The conclusion by the profilers that nearly all of the perpetrators had some form of developing stress disorder is probably correct; many of the mass shootings were proceeded by careful planning, which true mental disorder might not allow. But that also means warning signs were ignored and that might not be something modern societies can afford, rights and justice for all being involved.

Curative treatment as a mandated health 'right' for PTSD might be the solution.

[TR] 2018 Conclusions:

General Opservationis

2018.02.02:18:20   **|LI|<1|TR|>2[WB]<3⋈|GW|>1-|JU|>2 ≈ |OP|>3**

Christine Emba, WaPost, 'White Americans, welcome to the club of being asked, 'Where are you really from?':

"This new census question upsets that thinking. Adding color to the binary definition of whiteness could push us all to come to terms with what being white really means...... And with so many distinctions and gradations newly visible, we may be able to focus on new conceptions of unity that can include us all."

This idea of measuring hominids by their skin tone is silly. The only genetic function of skin tone is through the variations of gene MC1R, which is primarily designed by evolution to protect hominids from excessive amounts of Ultra-Violet sunlight. That is why the equatorial humans have dark skin and this MC1R gene code becomes less significant the further from the equator. MC1R is one gene variation out of some 155 million gene variations and that makes it a silly indicator of being human or a genetic member of a 'race' and certainly not an indicator of American citizenship.

The only actual measure of a human 'citizen' would be the genome codes that clearly differentiate a homosapien from earlier forms of apes, especially the chimpanzee that has 97% of a human DNA. . The codes for this are the 49(only?) Human Accelerated Regions or HARs that brought about the different evolution, including consciousness, that true humans have experienced over the last 70, 000 years. The HARs started earlier, but 'accelerated' just that 70K years ago.

Having some percentage of each of the HARs is a much better census condition that should be included in the Constitutionally mandated 10-year census, not skin-tone or even geographic origin.

Forget trying to define a citizen by skin tone or national origin; from a Constitutional 'Blessings of Liberty to ourselves and our Posterity', the idea is meaningless. It takes 5 sequential censuses to define Our Posterity.

There are several books on DNA mapping including one entitled 'DNA USA' by Bryan Sykes which had some origination surprises in it, but might already be outdated by HAR data.

2018.04.04:22:06 |LI|<1|TR|>2 $\sum$ |WB|>1|CD|<1 ⋈ |GW|>1-|JU|>2 ≈ |OP|>3

Gopal Ratnam, RollCall, 'Facebook Case Highlights Possibility of New Privacy Laws':

"Instead of mandating every step of how companies communicate data-sharing practices with their users, a U.S. data privacy law could act as a legislative backstop guaranteeing basic transparency while allowing companies flexibility to try different approaches and offering incentives to go beyond the bare minimum, Jerome said."

The problem isn't just data in 'public' bigdata memory systems, but also 4th Amendment protections of the individual's 'papers and effects' in ALL cases. In order to insure that the Constitution's Bill of Rights is itself protected not only from government abuse but citizen abuse as well, it might be necessary to have a 9th Amendment extension of those protections with the addition of a 'contempt of constitution' law that specifically addresses misuse of individual data by ANY other entity, including artificially intelligent. The idea is that using information that a person has built up during his life to attack or harm the person would be a disregard of the Constitution itself and would be a criminal aggression from a misdemeanor level all the way to a crime against humanity level.

Such contempt of constitution laws through the authority of the 9th Amendment does not require further amendment to the Constitution but merely expresses data privacy (not required during the 1787 First Convention deliberations) as an enumerated right like the first eight. Such contempt for constitution laws could include conditions of privacy formed by other Representative Democracy constitutions, which the EU, Russia and China are not. But the 9th Amendment can have 'rights' laws added into it under the Congressional authority of Common Defense and General Welfare in Article I, Section 8, clause 1. A privacy right with penalties for abuse that apply to ANY individual , inside or outside the government, might give the necessary protection against bigdata entity attacks.

2018.05.08:09:55 |LI|<1|TR|>2|WB|<3+|CD|<1 ⋈|GW|>1-|JU|<2≈|OP|<1

TheHill article: Kanye West on TMZ, : "The reason why I brought up the 400 years point is because we can't be mentally imprisoned for another 400 years. We need free thought now. Even the statement was an example of free thought. It was just an idea. Once again I am being attacked for presenting new ideas."

The point on slavery might be quite accurate. Homosapiens are the most adaptive species ever on this planet (and maybe the Quadrant) with Human Advanced Regions of DNA code (HARs) that specifically allow them to adapt to whatever surroundings they find themselves in, including environments of cruelty, indenture and slavery that are seen as unimaginable by later 'civilizations'. They adapt to those surroundings over a period of generations as a survival 'choice' because that's where they are at any given time, although multiple generations can make erroneous DNA adaptive choices such as sugar, alcohol, rice starch and quite possibly in the future, marijuana, which currently is a 'choice' addiction by only 6 percent of any population. Forced enslavements to fentanyl or crack cocaine are not the same as 'choice' adaptions to an indentured environment. Some forms of enslavement are forced in order to satisfy the pleasures of a psychiatric disorder of the 'control freak', which itself might be a DNA-based Human Primitive Region of DNA evolution. HPRs would be the opposite of Advanced Regions that allow environmental survivability.

The point is that Homosapiens do, by 'choice', adapt to their surroundings even if such are intolerable to others. But there are also those who believe that a world of rulers and serfs is normal and that may not be a 'choice' adaption.

2018.07.08:18:04 |JU|<2....|OP|>3 ≈ |WB|<2⋈ |GW|>1⋈ |CD|<1 |TR|>2 |LI|<3

Sullivan, WaPost, 'A journalist's conscience leads her to reveal her source to the FBI. Here's why.':

"In their reporting, journalists talk to criminals all the time and don't turn them in. Reporters aren't an arm of law enforcement. They properly resist subpoenas and fight like hell not to share their notes or what they know because doing so would compromise their independence and their ability to do their work in the future."

That is perfectly correct and laudable within a context of Justice. But in this case, a process was under way in the secure, closed hearing rooms of the Senate. The appearance of even the least 'probable cause' of an act that brings imminent threat to the integrity of the Constitution, as classified information transfer does automatically, should be reason enough for any citizen to carry out his protective obligations. That imminent threat obligation should hold regardless of whether an oath to defend and protect the Constitution had been taken. The security breach 'perp' certainly had taken such an oath.

Other conditions of journalistic non-disclosure where Justice for all is required as part of the silence or whistle blowing is perfectly acceptable, but not on a Constitutional corruption level.

2018.08.20:16:31 |OP|>2 ≈∑ |TR|>3 |LI|>3⋈|JU|>1....|GW|>2⋈ |CD|<1

Michaels and Maue, TheHill, 'Trump's choice for science adviser should be confirmed':

"One criticism libertarians may have with Droegemeier is, like most, he believes that government funding of basic science is "critical for growing our economy." In fact, as noted by the likes of the OECD, American University's Walter Park, and our Cato colleague Terence Kealey, there's no clear relationship between government funding of basic science and economic growth. In fact, government funding of basic science crowds out that of the private sector. With rare exceptions, almost all U.S. science was non-governmentally funded until World War II—but it was in this era that the U.S. economy overtook those of the rest of the world."

The libertarians and anti-government anarchists in general may not have much sympathy for a governmental office like the OSTP, but such agencies are, in fact, very nearly a Constitutionally defined mandate under Article I, Section 8, Clause 8 authorities of the Congress and Executive. Clause 8 says 'To promote the Progress of Science and useful Arts' through protection of intellectual property.

However, in this century, there is a need to protect intellectual property of 'Science' by maintaining a central analytic office such as the OSTP that can sample and track the enormous explosion of molecular level manipulation going on all over the world. Many of these molecular combinations, especially Epigenetic and WMD, are so dangerous to the human species that they need to be monitored by an Executive Office of the President task force, if not within the National Security Council itself. Some WMD technologies, such as those under development by Syria and its allies, need to be in a perpetual classified SCI state under the direct tracking of the OSTP and special NSC data systems. There were a number of instances from just before 9/11 to the present where critical WMD technology awareness was not passed on in the memory banks of the Executive Office systems and this is a serious Common Defense issue.

These 21st century technologies under development are so massive that a Director could do little more than maintain Executive Summery timelines that were extracted from a sophisticated AI Common Alerting Protocol system in-house and available to the White House. But a meteorology-oriented person with a general background would certainly be in a position to refine the predictive algorithms found in the Protocol by adapting them to track dozens of science trends, just as it does in meteorology now.

For the purposes of 'sensing' the direction of the States and communities, some reductionist methods are needed at least to the 'major' impact of {subfunctions} These are some, others are: climate related disasters like hurricanes, floods, and wildfires, hazard control including vehicles and guns, and gerrymandering or vote security.

1. Opioid Epidemic (pandemic?) precludes wellbeing, [WB]{ξ}<3

2. Immigration Overhaul , State cost and civil rights, [JU]<2, [LI]>2?, [CD]<1

3. Deregulation of Federal Rules, un-systemic regulatory costs [GW]<2, [JU]<1,

4. Cybersecurity Threats   privacy and election breaches? [LI]<3, [JU], [CD]<1

5. Health Care ACA, SNAP, CHIPS, Medicaid reduced at Federal? [GW]+/-2

6. Education infrastructure, education loans, teacher quality [LI]<3, [GW]<1, {ξ}>3?

7. Federal marijuana , drug control, imposed on communities [LI]<1 [CD]>3

8. Autonomous Vehicles, AI automation blessings , ed technologies? [GW]>2

9. State energy regulation, revenues, low gas and oil prices? [GW]<1, [LI]>2,{ξ}>1?

10. Federal Tax Reform   Tax Cuts and Jobs Act effects [OP] >0<?

Many problems of the state governments were increased by the down-sizing efforts of the federal government and increasing costs of basic institutions. This translated into many population stresses involving Justice and Liberty including personal safety.

Figure 15.   Tranquility [TR] dynamic 2018

CRS, RL34680, 2018.12.10, 'Shutdown of the Federal Government: :Causes, Processes, and Effects':

Possible National Security Implications

A federal government shutdown could have possible negative security implications, **as some entities wishing to take actions harmful to U.S. interests may see the nation as physically, technologically, and politically vulnerable.** The Antideficiency Act is silent regarding which specific organizations would be excepted in whole or part from a government shutdown. The act's provisions and historical guidance from OMB, however, suggest that entities that perform a national security function may be allowed to continue many of their operations. Historically, individuals responsible for supporting the nation's global security activities, public safety efforts, and foreign relations pursuits have been excepted from furloughs that accompany a government shutdown. In FY2018, the Trump Administration issued specific guidance that states,

"cybersecurity functions are excepted functions as these functions are necessary to avoid imminent threat to Federal property."

The actions that are taken in anticipation of a government shutdown may lessen the negative effects of an incident of national security significance occurring during this period. How agencies and OMB prepare for a government shutdown may have short- and long-term consequences if an incident occurs during a period of reduction in government services or soon after a resumption of all government activities. Should federal government organizations traditionally not viewed as an excepted part of the security apparatus be shut down, and subsequently become needed during a crisis or emerging situation, the nation's ability to respond to an incident could be delayed. Such a situation could result in increased risk to the nation and a longer recovery time as services and support activities normally provided to nonfederal entities may not be available when needed. **Some security observers may offer concerns that the longer the duration of a government shutdown, the more at-risk the nation becomes as enemies of the United States may seek to exploit perceived vulnerabilities.**

If [CD]<2? ⋈ [GW]>1 ↔Σ [TR]<3[LI]>1|JU|<2 ≈ Σ [WB]<2{ξ}<1 [OP]<n??

Common Defense [CD]

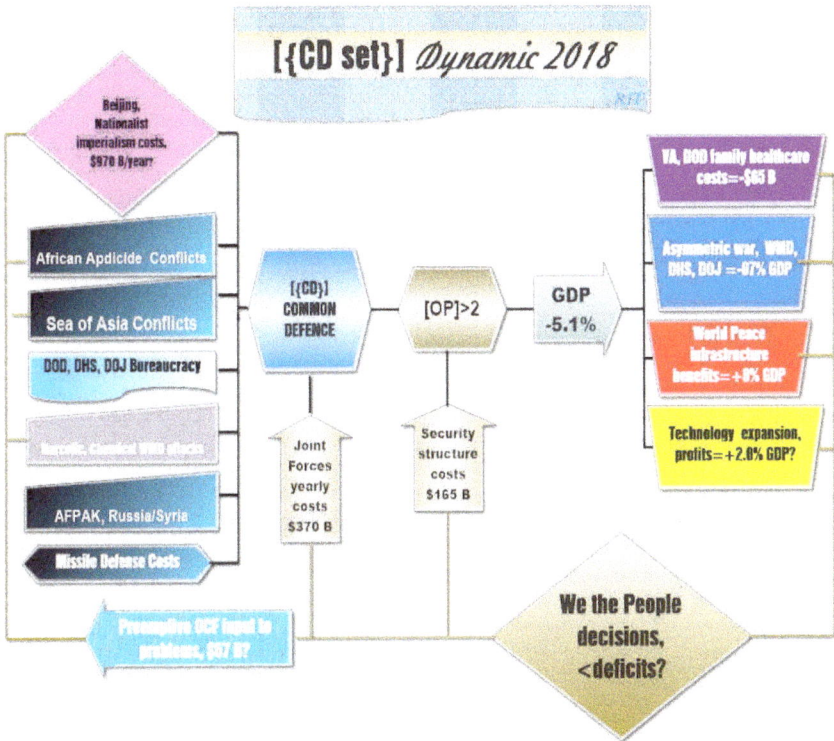

Figure 16.   Common Defense [CD] dynamic

2018.10.25:00:00 |CD|>2 ≈|OP|>2 Ξ [WB]<1+[JU]>2 ⋈ [GW]>2

National Defense Strategy Summery, 2018, Defense objectives include:

{1} Defending the homeland from attack;

{2} Sustaining Joint Force military advantages, both globally and in key regions;

{3} Deterring adversaries from aggression against our vital interests;

{4} Enabling U.S. interagency counterparts to advance U.S. influence and interests;

{5} Maintaining favorable regional balances of power in the Indo-Pacific, Europe, the Middle East, and the Western Hemisphere;

{6} Defending allies from military aggression and bolstering partners against coercion, and fairly sharing responsibilities for common defense;

{7} Dissuading, preventing, or deterring state adversaries and non-state actors from acquiring, proliferating, or using weapons of mass destruction;

{8} Preventing terrorists from directing or supporting external operations against the United States homeland and our citizens, allies, and partners overseas;

{9} Ensuring common domains remain open and free;

{10} Continuously delivering performance with affordability and speed as we change Departmental mindset, culture, and management systems;

{11} Establishing an unmatched twenty-first century National Security Innovation Base that effectively supports Department operations and sustains security and solvency.

2018.04.30:00:00 |CD|<2 ≈ |TR|<1+|JU|>2 + |OP|<2 ⋈ |GW|>1

Wong and Chan, South China Morning Post, 'China's first home-grown Type 001A aircraft carrier begins maiden sea trial':

"It took nearly six years for the Liaoning to become fully combat-ready after it entered service in 2012. But Song said that the experience gained would allow the new vessel to become combat-ready within about two years."

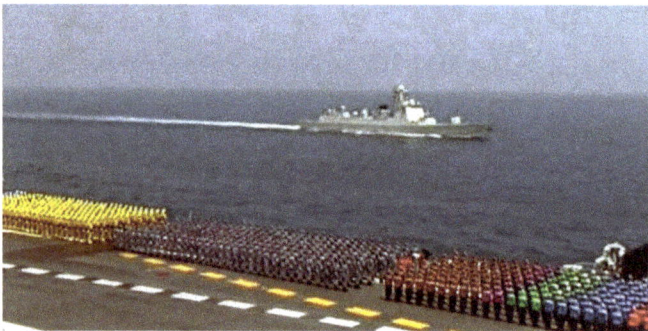

Crew of Chinese carrier Shandong during sea trials, 2018

Second carrier of six projected. It took four carriers to attack Pearl Harbor at the start of World War II. But since then, carriers have almost completely eliminated massive troop movements of imperialists around the world, except for their own troops. Were American carriers preventing imperialism or ,as their enemies say, protecting imperial interests?

2018.06.02:10:26 |CD|<1 ≈ |OP|>2 Ξ |TR|<1+|JU|>2 ⋈ |GW|>2

Harshaw, BloombergView, 'James Clapper Has Some Thoughts on Donald Trump':

"JRC: I guess the way I think about that [government overthrow] is that through our history, when we tried to manipulate or influence elections or even overturned governments, it was done with the best interests of the people in that country in mind – given the traditional reverence for human rights."

Probably an accurate statement. Some of those 'governments' gave all the appearance of being democratically or constitutionally elected leadership systems, but had secret one-party state agendas that would have began a systemic purge of liberal or progressive entities within the society. American 'interference' almost never involved attempting to overturn a democracy, even authoritarian, with voting institutions that had taken hold for a generation or two because the human rights had also become more pervasive in that type of society. American Intelligence Community organizations only became nervous or reactive when a single party structure somewhere attempted to become Orwellian in its population control.

What America lacked was a consistent Constitutional 'Authorization for the use of Force' against totalitarian entities who invariably threatened Republic forms of democratic institutions as authorize by Article IV, Section 4. Section 4 specifies States within the Union only, but from a crimes against humanity standpoint, ALL totalitarian entities are in the Union of humanity. The Intel Community has overlooked that 'rights' issue on occasion.

2018.06.29:12:32 |CD|>2 ≈|OP|>2 Ξ||LI|>2WB|<1+|JU|>2 ⋈ [GW]>2

Bever in WaPost, 'A plan to keep drug users from shooting up in public restrooms — and why it may be a bad idea':

"Jon D. Groussman, president of CAP Index Inc., a security consulting firm based in Exton, Pa., said that "in certain markets where you know you're having a problem, it's worth trying." But he added that closely monitoring public restrooms and sending employees to check on them periodically is typically "the best deterrent."

This problem might resolve itself in the near future. Some of the new bio-sensors for gas emissions are so sensitive that they can be incorporated into self-cleaning 'smoke detector' devices that can be place in bathrooms and detect ANY form of drug or hostile molecule arrangements. They may even be sensitive enough, with AI interpreters, to detect health problems by analyzing urine and feces gases in the bathroom.

Question: Since a person with chemical imbalances in his brain or organs almost always represents a misdemeanor imminent danger to others through various psychotic episodes, inability to drive devices, clumsiness, predatory de-inhibition, or sudden suicidal impulses, why would his expectation of privacy be true in ANY location?

2018.11.06:10:03 |CD|>2 ≈|OP|>2 ....|WB|<1+|JU|<3 ⋈ [GW]>2[LI]<4

Michael Morrell in WaPost, 'What Trump should be asking of the CIA on Khashoggi':

"And, importantly, what about deterrence? If we choose not to impose sanctions, will the Saudi regime — or others around the world — be emboldened to commit similar atrocities in the future? Would taking action against Riyadh deter other countries? Or, would it not make a difference?"

Deterrence might need to be very selective as far as the Agency authorities under Executive Orders go. Advising the EOP and Congress Committees on a 'sanction option' might need to include the effects of holding an entire governing regime responsible for the Democide (The intentional killing of an unarmed or disarmed person by government agents acting in their authoritative capacity and pursuant to government policy or high command) activity instead of the actual perpetrators. The actual 15-man 'hit' squad, as the Turks called them, engaged in Democide and might have been doing that for some time.

Deterring such people from carrying out independent acts around the world might be more useful than attempting to hold an entire regime responsible as the perpetrator. Iran is a good example; do you sanction the Iranian people for the acts of the Pasdaran murder cult headquartered within its borders? Or do you sanction the entire Syrian tribal system for the activities of the Baathist 'special units' building chemical barrel bombs for use in Democide? Or do you hold all of Mexico responsible for the Democide activities in Mexico carried out by El Chapo?

Perhaps the Congress should come up with an Authorization for the Use of Military or Police Force (AUMPF) in the case of the specific perpetrators of Democide which would give the Executive authority to act against them as a deterrence. That type of AUMPF might require some Agency analysis they don't want to talk about.

2018.11.06:10:03 |CD|>2 ≈|OP|>2 ....|WB|<1+|JU|<3 ⋈ |GW|>2[LI]<4

Michael Morrell in WaPost, 'What Trump should be asking of the CIA on Khashoggi':

 "And, importantly, what about deterrence? If we choose not to impose sanctions, will the Saudi regime — or others around the world — be emboldened to commit similar atrocities in the future? Would taking action against Riyadh deter other countries? Or, would it not make a difference?"

Deterrence might need to be very selective as far as the Agency authorities under Executive Orders go. Advising the EOP and Congress Committees on a 'sanction option' might need to include the effects of holding an entire governing regime responsible for the Democide (The intentional killing of an unarmed or disarmed person by government agents acting in their authoritative capacity and pursuant to government policy or high command) activity instead of the actual perpetrators. The actual 15-man 'hit' squad, as the Turks called them, engaged in Democide and might have been doing that for some time.

Deterring such people from carrying out independent acts around the world might be more useful than attempting to hold an entire regime responsible as the perpetrator. Iran is a good example; do you sanction the Iranian people for the acts of the Pasdaran murder cult headquartered within its borders? Or do you sanction the entire Syrian tribal system for the activities of the Baathist 'special units' building chemical barrel bombs for use in Democide? Or do you hold all of Mexico responsible for the Democide activities in Mexico carried out by El Chapo?

Perhaps the Congress should come up with an Authorization for the Use of Military or Police Force (AUMPF) in the case of the specific perpetrators of Democide which would give the Executive authority to act against them as a deterrence. That type of AUMPF might require some Agency analysis they don't want to talk about.

{1} Defending the homeland from attack;

2018.05.18:08:37 |CD|>2 ⋈ |OP|>2 ≈ |WB|>2+|JU|>2 ⋈ |GW|<3

Editorial Board, WaPost, 'A GOP senator stands up to pressure — and rebukes the House on Russian interference':

"Mr. Burr and Mr. Warner deserve credit for continuing to cooperate in the face of extreme partisan pressure. The president himself has leaned on the chairman and other Senate GOP leaders to end the legislative inquiry. The panel's findings reinforce a conclusion that, no matter how familiar by now, should remain stunning and unacceptable to all Americans: A hostile foreign power intervened on behalf of a particular presidential candidate, who is now in the White House, and that power likely intends to meddle again. Also stunning is that, in the face of this continuing national security threat, partisanship has led many Republicans to deny the obvious and smear patriotic intelligence officials."

As the Editors point out, the two Senators do deserve credit, as do several other members of the Committee(s). But in fact, they were simply following their Oaths of Office, something that narcissistic, purely narcissistic, Libertarians and Progressives apparently have trouble doing. You cannot put a self-serving ideological interest above the values of the Constitution and still adhere to 'support and defend' with 'true faith and allegiance'. Need 60 more in the Senate and 110 in the House who can really support and defend without checking their 401K.

2018.05.06:08:12 |CD|>4 ≈|OP|>2 Ξ|WB|<1+|CD| ⋈|GW|>2

Anderson, Brookings Institution, in TheHill, 'Why war powers need an expiration date':

"And while enemies may make more rhetorical use of a AUMF than this other legislation, allowing their messaging to drive U.S. policy would be ill-advised."

One of the problems with the 'sunset provisions' and 'reporting clause' combinations in the new AUMF is that an enemy proxy force through hostile state intelligence aid would be able to scatter (as the Taliban and ISIS small forces have done) and re-concentrate after the Authorization had terminated. That is a serious national security issue, since some of them could be 'concentrated' in a constitutional democracy as both Osama Bin Laden and Muammar Qaddafi managed. Remember, believers in the Quranically false Caliphate world ruler doctrine will invariably attack humans engaged in democracy, as will those who adhere to the Leninist world ruler concept. An absolute sunset and detailed reporting AUMF serves them both, not human, let alone American, security.

It would be better if the AUMF sunset clause had the wording 'except when an active, systemic crime against humanity is being perpetrated by members of the named hostile entities'. The new AUMF could also have a provision concerning the 48 hour reporting requirement that said the report of ongoing actions need only the approval of the House and Senate Committees involved along with the Speaker and Senate President. This would allow the ongoing actions concerning 'Offenses against the Laws of Nations' (as put in Article I, Section 8, Clause 10) to remain hidden for appropriate periods. These are criminal activities against humans, not necessarily 'war' activities under the ancient War Powers Act, even if hostile WMD is involved.

2018.05.16:09:00 |CD|>3 ≈∑ |OP|>2 Ξ|WB|<1⋈|LI|<2 ⋈ |JU|>2 ⋈ |GW|>2

Bloomberg Editorial Board, 'Follow the Constitution on Waging War':

"Congress, and only Congress, has the power to declare war; the president and his military advisers are responsible for waging it."

and

"The Corker-Kaine approach is right to want Congress back in the game, but wrong to go about it like this."

There are actually a half dozen AUMF proposals, including an October 2016 Obama request, that have evolved in the Congress, but largely centered around termination of the existing 2001 AUMFs and close adherence to the ancient 1970s War Powers Act. There is, however, nothing in the Constitution that says use of military force is AUTOMATICALLY a condition of 'war'. The Founders also inserted Article I, Section 8, clause 10 which address conditions that are 'Offenses against the Laws of Nations', under which modern AUMFs could be initiated. That has not occurred, largely because 'progressives' do not want ANY use of military force for 19th century ideological reasons and 'conservatives' do not want interference with the CinC to engage in instant retaliation for attacks, including economic or political, which also appear to be 19th century based ideologies.

One of the problems with the 'sunset provisions' and 'reporting clause' combinations in the new AUMF (April version) is that an enemy proxy force through hostile state intelligence aid would be able to scatter (as the Taliban and ISIS small forces have done) and re-concentrate after the Authorization had terminated. That is a serious national security issue, since some of them could be 'concentrated' in a constitutional democracy as both Osama Bin Laden and Muammar Qaddafi managed. Remember, believers in the Quranically false Caliphate world ruler doctrine will invariably attack humans engaged in democracy, as will those who adhere to the Leninist world ruler concept. An absolute sunset and detailed reporting AUMF serves them both, not human, let alone American, security.

It would be better if the AUMF sunset clause had the wording 'except when an active, systemic crime against humanity is being perpetrated by members of the named hostile entities'. The new AUMF could also have a provision concerning the 48-hour reporting requirement that said the report of ongoing actions need only the approval of the House and Senate Committees involved along with the Speaker and Senate President. This would allow the ongoing actions concerning 'Offenses against the Laws of Nations' (as put in Article I, Section 8, Clause 10) to remain hidden for appropriate periods. These are criminal activities against humans, not necessarily 'war' activities under the ancient War Powers Act, even if hostile WMD is involved.

Use of Force really needs a new conceptual basis in this century by all three Branches.

2018.06.27:07:58 |CD|>3 ≈ |TR|>3|OP|>2 Ξ |WB|<1+|JU|<2 ⋈ |GW|<2

Ignatius, WaPost, 'Now is the time for the Space Force. Trump just needs to get it right.':

"Two feasibility studies, mandated by Congress, are due later this year. The Pentagon hopes that will allow some thoughtful discussion of costs and benefits."

One of the feasibility studies on a Space Force, while acknowledging that most of the components for it already exist in the Air Force and Navy, goes into considerable detail on the Earth-space control doctrine of the People's Liberation Army and just a listing of the technologies they are implementing in their 'Study of Space Operations', 2016, indicates a very advanced force is being created for Chinese control of the world's space technologies and regions that have them in orbit.

Americans are creating 'feasibility' studies when they should be creating implementation Tables of Organization and Equipment based on a national defense doctrine like the National Security Strategy implies. While some Air Force objections about implementing another bureaucracy are legitimate, they are putting America in the same position the lack of an offensive Cyber Command put us in for the last ten years, which includes attacks on our banking, citizen ID and electoral media systems. Those feasibility studies should have been completed and presented to the Congress in 2015, not next year.

2018.08.18:00:00 |CD|<3 ⋈ |GW|>1-|JU|>2|TR|>3 ≈ |OP|>2

Congressional Research Service, CRS-IF10950, Toward the Creation of a U.S. "Space Force"

"It may conceivably be argued that congressional authority is limited to "land and naval forces," including "Armies" and "the Navy" as well as the "Militia" (i.e., the reserve components), and thus would not extend to a new armed force operating primarily in the realm of space. The President's **commander-in-chief** authority is similarly limited to the Army and Navy and activated reserve components. However, it is unclear whether a new Space Force would actually carry out functions in space or that its functions would be any different from those related to space operations already carried out by the various services. Given this uncertainty, it is possible that a Space Force would already constitute a land and naval force under the Constitution. Finally, it is of note that respective congressional and presidential authorities over the Air Force—which is not specifically mentioned in the Constitution—have not been historically called into question."

Article I, Section 8, clause 1 'common defence' authority would take precedence over a specific 'land or naval force' requirement to be Constitutional. Especially since Common Defense is specified as a universal intention in the Preamble. Murky in terms of the CinC authority, but the intent clearly implies ANY method of defense that protects the We the People concept, space warfare just being another aspect of an inherently imperialistic humanity.

2018.11.30:11:37 |CD|>3|LI|<5 ≈ |OP|<2 Ξ|WB|<1+|JU|<2 ⋈ |GW|>2|TR|>3

Kyl and Morell, WaPost, 'Why America needs low-yield nuclear warheads now':

"In this way, Russia is intent on exploiting what it perceives as a U.S. nuclear capability gap on the lower levels of the escalatory ladder. That is because a high-yield, long-range U.S. response to Russia's first, limited use of a low-yield nuclear weapon against a military target is not credible. The Russians believe we are not likely to risk a global thermonuclear war in response to a "tactical" nuclear attack by them."

This is a well-known tactical strategy conceived by Vladimir Putin some time ago and in advanced stages of development now. The GRU assessments that America would not use large-yield, city busters (1 megaton and up) if others are using local, non-nuclear WMD as in Syria and Chechnya is correct. A variable yield nuclear 'tochka' can deliver a 50 kiloton (4 times Hiroshima) explosion 200 km, but Russian militaries still consider that 'tactical'. A European, American or Indian 'Pluton' style device is about 10 kilotons, but a version can be as small as 1 kiloton, which is smaller than some chemical bombs and has a destruction radius of half a kilometer. However, the small tactical can also be used as an anti-missile device and that might be its only value, especially if mounted in a hypersonic vehicle.

Russia, unfortunately, must also contend with 15 Chinese mechanized divisions near their borders which are also being equipped with DF-15 medium devices. The Chinese 'territorial occupation' philosophy which all 15 divisions are capable of involves concentration of force between enemy forces and Russia has no defense against this tactic except tactical nukes.

{2} Sustaining Joint Force military advantages, both globally and in key regions.

2018.02.07:09:10 |CD|>≈|OP|<1 Ξ|WB|<3+|JU| ⋈|GW|≈|OP|<3

Ignatius, WaPost, 'Trump shouldn't take Jordan for granted':

"American support has been Jordan's backstop, thanks to bipartisan congressional backing and strong support at the CIA, Pentagon and State Department. That momentum will continue next week (Feb. 13), when the two countries are expected to sign a new "memorandum of understanding" extending U.S. financial aid for five years and perhaps increasing it to $1.5 billion annually from the current $1.275 billion."

This should be a Defense no-brainer, along with an additional $1.5 billion that is specifically intended for support of the Syrian and Iraqi refugees that are trying to establish an independent state free of Assad's genetic minority engaged in mass murder of Arabic peoples. The provinces of Hims, Ar Raqqah, Dayr Az Zawr, and Al Hasakah should be an independent country and merged as such with the Iraqi provinces next to Jordan and Saudi Arabia. Such a new nation could reflect the Jordanian form of 're-enforced' moderation that can only exist with external support from nations with representative republic experience. The Iranian Shiite model in Lebanon, Iraq, and Syria is a dismal failure as their continued use of chemical WMD on civilians indicates. A fully supported nation of moderates between Iran and the Syrian coastal hegemony would aid ALL of the peoples in the region.

Question: If a new form of AUMF includes protection of Arabic peoples subjected to genocide by various Shiite minorities and the AUMF is automatically authorized by the UN Charter to prevent crimes against humanity, how would it be worded in order to satisfy the 'offenses against the Laws of Nations' clause 11 in the Constitution?

2018.04.14:07:10 |CD|<3 ⋈ |GW|>1-|JU|>2|TR|>2 ≈ |OP|>1

Susan Hannah Allen and Carla Martinez-Machain in WaPost: 'The U.S. just bombed 3 sites in Syria. Here's what we know about why states choose airstrikes.':

"We looked at some popular expectations about why states would choose air power. Traditionally, there is the perception that democracies are more likely to use airstrikes

— and only airstrikes — because democratic leaders are too afraid to put boots on the ground and risk casualties.

Policymakers and even potential target states themselves have shared this perception. Since the U.S. withdrawal from Vietnam, numerous militarily weaker states have gambled on their ability to outlast American public acceptance of casualties."

That 'waiting them out' routine apparently no longer works as American 'boots' in Afghanistan and Iraq have shown. A WMD criminal intent on mass murder of local citizens OR remote Americans from a sanctuary region should be an automatic target of airstrikes under rules of engagement for crimes against humanity (systemic, terroristic murder). But equating the 'state' in such a region as being sovereign in the same sense as a representative, constitutional government is not viable in any research. A totalitarian entity represents only itself in its behaviors, not a population, so its mass destruction facilities are automatic targets of airstrikes regardless of military or police interdiction.

Note 'Airstrikes are more likely when the stakes for an intervener are low'. That is what you want when a localized criminal activity has been detected, not nuclear or carpet bombing of a city in order to remove the criminal facility. You don't demolish a six-block area of Garfield Park, Chicago when a SWAT team takes down a meth factory in the middle of it. Criminal behavior on a large scale is not a state vs state 'war' issue anywhere in the world anymore and it is time American 'researchers' and their Congressmen recognize that with appropriate definitions of force.

2018.06.29:12:32 |CD|>2 ≈|OP|>2 Ξ|[LI|>2WB|<1+|JU|>2 ⋈ [GW|>2

Bever in WaPost, 'A plan to keep drug users from shooting up in public restrooms — and why it may be a bad idea':

"Jon D. Groussman, president of CAP Index Inc., a security consulting firm based in Exton, Pa., said that "in certain markets where you know you're having a problem, it's worth trying." But he added that closely monitoring public restrooms and sending employees to check on them periodically is typically "the best deterrent.""

This problem might resolve itself in the near future. Some of the new bio-sensors for gas emissions are so sensitive that they can be incorporated into self-cleaning 'smoke detector' devices that can be place in bathrooms and detect ANY form of drug or hostile molecule arrangements. They may even be sensitive enough, with AI interpretors, to detect health problems by analyzing urine and feces gases in the bathroom.

Question: Since a person with chemical imbalances in his brain or organs almost always represents a misdemeanor imminent danger to others through various psychotic episodes, inability to drive devices, clumsiness, predatory de-inhibition, or sudden suicidal impulses, why would his expectation of privacy be true in ANY location?

2018.11.06:10:03 |CD|>2 ≈|OP|>2 ....|WB|<1+|JU|<3 ⋈ [GW|>2|LI|<4

Michael Morrell in WaPost, 'What Trump should be asking of the CIA on Khashoggi':

"And, importantly, what about deterrence? If we choose not to impose sanctions, will the Saudi regime — or others around the world — be emboldened to commit similar atrocities in the future? Would taking action against Riyadh deter other countries? Or, would it not make a difference?"

Deterrence might need to be very selective as far as the Agency authorities under Executive Orders go. Advising the EOP and Congress Committees on a 'sanction option' might need to include the effects of holding an entire governing regime responsible for the Democide (The intentional killing of an unarmed or disarmed person by government agents acting in their authoritative capacity and pursuant to government policy or high command) activity instead of the actual perpetrators. The actual 15-man 'hit' squad, as the Turks called them, engaged in Democide and might have been doing that for some time.

Deterring such people from carrying out independent acts around the world might be more useful than attempting to hold an entire regime responsible as the perpetrator. Iran is a good example; do you sanction the Iranian people for the acts of the Pasdaran murder cult headquartered within its borders? Or do you sanction the entire Syrian tribal system for the activities of the Baathist 'special units' building chemical barrel bombs for use in Democide? Or do you hold all of Mexico responsible for the Democide activities in Mexico carried out by El Chapo?

Perhaps the Congress should come up with an Authorization for the Use of Military or Police Force (AUMPF) in the case of the specific perpetrators of Democide which would give the Executive authority to act against them as a deterrent. That type of AUMPF might require some Agency analysis they don't want to talk about.

2018.11.07:07:37 |CD|>2 ≈ |OP|>3 +|JU|<2 |LI|<2◓ |GW|>2|TR|>3|WB|>1

Ignatius, WaPost, 'China's application of AI should be a Sputnik moment for the U.S. But will it be?':

"The United States is struggling to respond to this world-changing challenge. What's underway is frail and exists mostly on paper. Congress this year passed legislation calling for a national AI commission, but so far it's just a concept."

Extract of speech by Admiral Hyman Rickover, Columbia University, 1982:

> A good manager must have unshakeable determination and tenacity. Deciding what needs to be done is easy, getting it done is more difficult. Good ideas are not adopted automatically. They must be driven into practice with courageous impatience. Once implemented they can be easily overturned or subverted through apathy or lack of follow-up, so a continuous effort is required. Too often, important problems are recognized but no one is willing to sustain the effort needed to solve them.

> Nothing worthwhile can be accomplished without determination. In the early days of nuclear power, for example, getting approval to build the first nuclear submarine—the Nautilus—was almost as difficult as designing and building it. Many in the Navy opposed building a nuclear submarine.

Rickover's efforts and the tacit support of both the Congress and the CinC made a nuclear powered fleet possible and the result of 30 years probably saved the Nation from both encirclement and nuclear devastation by the totalitarians. It is odd that everyone wants AI droids in human shape, but they are much more useful in manufacturing and black box shapes. Losing an escalating technology war with robotic entities replacing 'mortal' human soldiers over the next 10 years (just 10…) would be equivalent to surrender to a tiny, hostile totalitarian force in control of droid swarms.

This article is accurate; the Nation needs another Rickover for AI development that can have spill-over ripple effects from Common Defense into healthcare, agriculture and human infrastructures.

TLO: AI and Qubit technology combinations easily qualify as both swords and plowshares.

2018.12.27:09:14 |OP| ≈∑ |WB|<3+|CD|>2 |TR|>3 |LI|<1 ⋈ |JU|<1|GW|<2

Binder, WaPost, 'five takeaways for 2018':

"Why doesn't unified party government endure? Call it the curse of overreach. Majorities exploit their newfound power to push hard on policy and procedure to advance their agendas. When they inevitably veer off-center to appeal to their base, the public acts as a "thermostat": When government activism increases, the public demands less, and vice versa."

Neither the 'curse of overreach' or the 'curse of gridlock' could exist if the American people started elected Independents who represented the majority in a given Electoral District. Many of the governance problems are created by people in both the Congress and Executive branches who are attempting to 'overreach' with their personal view of reality rather than serving a given District of Americans somewhere. That is the reason Americans keep trying to switch party control of the national direction; their choices of representation are limited to people who might represent 10 percent of a District or even a small economic oligarchy such as an international banking institution.

Speculation:

Would you have a perpetual condition of 'no-party' rule that formed and administered legislation in the interest of a non-polarized America if you had a substantial number of Independents in all three branches? If the extremes in both parties knew that they would have to deal with an Independent representative caucus that controlled just 20% of the votes in both Houses, would they be pulled toward a rational solution of a particular problem rather than always bowing to their minority sponsors? Would a 30% Independent caucus allow the Congress to actually plan taxation, regulation, and appropriation over a ten year cycle instead of the constant partisan destruction of the two year cycle?

Further:

Could ANY 'my way or the highway' agenda causing 20 years of gridlock exist if Americans were allowed to vote for someone with NO prior agenda, such as Independents profess and swear oaths to? Could ANY high ranking appointee in the Executive branch pass an 'advice and consent' review if Independents insisted on impeachment for administrative incompetence instead of for political affiliation?

2018.05.18:08:37 |CD|>2 ⋈ |OP|>2 ≈ |WB|>2+|JU|>2 ⋈ |GW|<3

Editorial Board, WaPost, 'A GOP senator stands up to pressure — and rebukes the House on Russian interference':

"Mr. Burr and Mr. Warner deserve credit for continuing to cooperate in the face of extreme partisan pressure. The president himself has leaned on the chairman and other Senate GOP leaders to end the legislative inquiry. The panel's findings reinforce a conclusion that, no matter how familiar by now, should remain stunning and unacceptable to all Americans: A hostile foreign power intervened on behalf of a particular presidential candidate, who is now in the White House, and that power likely intends to meddle again. Also stunning is that, in the face of this continuing national security threat, partisanship has led many Republicans to deny the obvious and smear patriotic intelligence officials."

As the Editors point out, the two Senators do deserve credit, as do several other members of the Committee(s). But in fact, they were simply following their Oaths of Office, something that narcissistic, purely narcissistic, Libertarians and Progressives apparently have trouble doing. You cannot put a self-serving ideological interest above the values of the Constitution and still adhere to 'support and defend' with 'true faith and allegiance'. Need 60 more in the Senate and 110 in the House who can really support and defend without checking their 401K.

2018.05.31:07:39 |WB|<3↔ |GW|<1⋈ |CD|<3 |LI|<3⋈|JU|<3 ≈|OP|<2

Nikki Haley, UN Ambassador, in WaPost, 'South Sudan has failed its children. We must not.'

"It is long past time the U.N. Security Council imposed an arms embargo on South Sudan. This concrete measure can save lives. Rather than continue to hold meetings, the United States is calling on our colleagues on the Security Council and our partners in the region to act."

An arms embargo might not be effective if all of the male citizens are in a tribal genocide mental state that requires perpetual self-defense just to walk down a street. The real evil is the climate of tribal mass murder between the 12 major tribal territories, the Dinka and Nuer tribes being the largest. Many of the massacres that have occurred are also attempts to acquire the cattle herds in areas as food from other tribes. A village killing of 50 might involve stealing 200 head of cattle in the village. If genocide has become a way of life, an arms embargo won't work and even certain retribution for murder might not work.

It might be more worthwhile, especially for the children, for the UN to set up 'nutrition health centers' where modern 4-ounce nutrition and protein bars can be distributed in such a massive number that the cattle stealing is pointless. The nutrition bars, costing 30 cents to mass produce, might even be enough to change the brain chemistry of people trying to survive in a hot, resource hostile environment. Is it possible that the intense hatred in the area are caused by nutritional deficiencies? The tribalism is so intense and universal that it qualifies as a 'pandemic' condition of a neural illness in that region. People who leave the region also drop out of the hate mindset, so perhaps there is some nutritional deficiency unique to the area, including in the cattle source of food itself.

Further:

Such UN nutritional facilities, with massive stores of food bars, would need UN military protection and just possibly might be locations of UN genocide courts where a person is assumed guilty unless he can prove through polygraph analysis that he isn't. At some point, drastic UN action to break up the tribal hate cycles with arms and food and perhaps contraceptives will be necessary. The $11 billion already sent there might have been better used in these mental health areas.

TLO: Ripple effects of tribalism have no positive gains anywhere, but no direct We the People interaction? No 'humanitarian' AUMF?

2018.06.29:12:32 |CD|>2 ≈|OP|>2 Ξ|[LI|>2WB|<1+|JU|>2 ⋈ [GW|>2

Bever in WaPost, 'A plan to keep drug users from shooting up in public restrooms — and why it may be a bad idea':

"Jon D. Groussman, president of CAP Index Inc., a security consulting firm based in Exton, Pa., said that "in certain markets where you know you're having a problem, it's worth trying." But he added that closely monitoring public restrooms and sending employees to check on them periodically is typically "the best deterrent.""

This problem might resolve itself in the near future. Some of the new bio-sensors for gas emissions are so sensitive that they can be incorporated into self-cleaning 'smoke detector' devices that can be place in bathrooms and detect ANY form of drug or hostile molecule arrangements. They may even be sensitive enough, with AI interpreters, to detect health problems by analyzing urine and feces gases in the bathroom.

Question: Since a person with chemical imbalances in his brain or organs almost always represents a misdemeanor imminent danger to others through various psychotic episodes, inability to drive devices, clumsiness, predatory de-inhibition, or sudden suicidal impulses, why would his expectation of privacy be true in ANY location?

2018.07.13:06:09 |CD|>3 ⋈ [GW|>2-|JU|<2|TR|<2 ≈ |OP|>3

Lamothe, WaPost, 'Army to unveil details about new Futures Command in biggest reorganization in 45 years':

"As part of Futures Command, the Army will create "cross-functional" teams focused on specific things the service wants to improve. Each team will include about 25 people, and be based in an area typically associated with the skill involved. For instance, the team focused on the Army's next-generation combat vehicle will call the automotive hub of Detroit home, and the team focusing on making individual soldiers more deadly will be based at Fort Benning, Ga., where the Army has a few schools focused on ground combat."

Those 'teams' could have all sorts of CAC security holes, especially if such teams are designed to look at Eastern Oligarchic technology enhancements described in the National Security Strategy or Estimates. Simple things like an individual E4 soldier controlling multiple 'drone sniper' technologies in the field or dealing with the new nerve toxin 'grenades' developed in Syria involve complex 'systems' that can be compromised over the next 10 years. Will Futures Command have an office at Fort Detrick or Cheyenne Mountain or Area 51 as well as 'cushy' locations like Austin and

Raleigh? $22 billion in abandoned technologies is hard to take by itself, but is Future Command able to control that in view of the WMD technologies the imperial Eastern Oligarchies are developing?

{3} Deterring adversaries from aggression against our vital interests.

2018.04.27:18:31 |CD|<3 ⋈ |GW|>1-|JU|<2|TR|<2≈|OP|<3

Witte and Gearan, WaPost, 'Trump- Merkel meeting is more business than pleasure for both leaders':

"Grenell shares Trump's deep skepticism about the Iran deal, calling it "a direct blow to the U.N.'s credibility" and the negotiations that led to it "a colossal and dangerous waste of time."

Macron emphasized the importance of keeping the deal during his meetings with Trump in Washington this week."

American and German relationships have traditionally been more business-like than social, nothing new. Most of the economic issues of two mutually beneficial integrated economies could probably be solved by a coin-toss between equal business partners.

The Iranian treaty, in which one side has many followers of the cult of Tagiyya among its Pasdaran leaders, is another international security issue altogether. One of the most obvious objections to the 'treaty' was the lack of IAEA inspector access to Pasdaran independent facilities that could have WMD construction components hidden inside. This happened in Libya, Sudan, Iraq, Pakistan, and Syria. The military installations can operate outside the sovereign authority of the Supreme Leader or the Guardian Council, as 'the Base' does on the Iraqi border. This is a serious international WMD danger to any society, Arabic, European, or North American.

The only way that this threat could be eliminated is by the IAEA inspectors having arrest authority for 'international obstruction of justice' by cultists attempting to hide evidence of WMD manufacture. The other objections can be set aside as the sovereign government of Iran adheres without Tagiyya deception to the treaty terms. It is only this one item that the international community should insist on; the ability of inspectors to appear at un-sovereign locations in a country with arrest authority for obstructionists at the specific location. Both Germany and America should be able to abide by the treaty except for that one item.

 Objections to treaty:

3. The inspectors have limited monitoring powers.

Trump has complained that the International Atomic Energy Agency, the U.N. organization responsible for inspecting Iran's facilities, does not have sufficient monitoring powers over the nuclear facilities. He and other critics say the inspectors have no access to closed military sites where any suspect work might be done in secrecy.

Actually, the agreement does make some provision for inspecting military sites. But in requesting access, the IAEA must show Iran the basis for its concern. Iranian officials have repeatedly said the military sites are off-limits to the IAEA.

 Further:

IAEA inspectors, with no arrest authority or personal security ability, are largely European experts. They were the ones who discovered the 2002 transfer of several tons of Polish insecticide neuro-toxins to the Iraqi secret police at an airbase in Ramadi, Iraq. There is no possible good reason for insecticide concentrates to be in the hands of a 'cult', then or now. As for hiding the stuff, just spray it into five acres of desert sand. You could, by the way, find 50 times that amount of biotoxins in American landfills if you looked for them and that isn't even a crime, let alone a crime against humanity.

{4} Enabling U.S. interagency counterparts to advance U.S. influence and interests.

2018.05.21:09:52 |OP|n ≈∑ |TR|<3 |LI|>3 ⋈ |JU|>1….|GW|>2+|CD|<3

Scarborough in WaPost, 'Trump isn't the first president to follow his gut into Mideast trouble':

"If the 21st century has taught Americans anything, it is that Middle East policy decisions demand that our presidents question their assumptions and challenge their ideological instincts. Following their "gut" always ends in disaster."

Got that right. That 'gut' stuff simply will not work in an area with as many conflicts and issues as the Middle East. Even attempting to apply the six covenants of the Preamble (Justice, Tranquility, Common Defense, General Welfare, Liberty and our Posterity) can get sidetracked when you add the ideas of a state theocracy (with a false Caliphate idea) to conditions of over-population (1.5 million in a Gaza that couldn't support 100,000) and energy greed ($900 billion in private Qatar accounts). These combinations have made American political electeds purely reactive, as in 'gut', to processes after the situations damage Americans.

No win in the Middle East unless there is a persistent 'Marshall Plan' view in the Congress and Executive branches that can be carried from one decade, not election cycle, to another.

2018.06.03:09:32 |CD|<3 ⋈ |GW|>1-|JU|>2|TR|<2≈|OP|>1

Yoav Fromer in WaPost, 'The Middle East doesn't lack democracy. It has too much.':

"Motivated by deeply rooted historical, economic, cultural and religious grievances, large majorities throughout the Middle East are hostile to the United States and Israel. Democracy and self-determination are, in most circumstances, salutary goals to be pursued and promoted. But in the Middle East right now, they are also catalysts for regional conflict. "

By definition, you cannot have a democracy or even a representative republic in a one-party socialist state. The mere fact that all revenue and means of livelihood are funneled through a singular political/economic entity (Iran, Iraq, Gaza, now Turkey, Qatar, etc) that in turn disseminates some of that wealth to a controlled public media system means the region is no longer a definable democracy. Such one-party states arrange not only the voting results by exclusionary ballot practices but arrange the 'democratic' opinions and polls seen by others AND the captive populations within the one-party state. The opinions are created through artificially creating 'enemies' that require the self-serving party to acquire resources to 'defend' against.

The existence of the unrepresentative, single party entity with access to the wealth of a population IS THE enemy of republic forms of governance and American policy should be based on aiding representative democracies, such as Israel, Kurdistan, Armenia, and free Syria. American traditions of spreading democracy only work when the local region's power addicts are unable to remove constitutional checks and balances, as the usurpation of checks and balances did occur in Egypt (3 times), Iran (4 times), Iraq (twice) and Lebanon (6 times).

The Middle Eastern one-party states cannot be democracies because they consider populations expendable serfs without constitutional representation and THAT is the problem facing American policy makers.

{5} Maintaining favorable regional balances of power in the Indo-Pacific, Europe, the Middle East, and the Western Hemisphere.

2018.04.14:07:10 |CD|<3 ⋈ |GW|>1-|JU|>2|TR|>2 ≈ |OP|>1

Susan Hannah Allen and Carla Martinez-Machain in WaPost: 'The U.S. just bombed 3 sites in Syria. Here's what we know about why states choose airstrikes.':

"We looked at some popular expectations about why states would choose air power. Traditionally, there is the perception that democracies are more likely to use airstrikes — and only airstrikes — because democratic leaders are too afraid to put boots on the ground and risk casualties.

Policymakers and even potential target states themselves have shared this perception. Since the U.S. withdrawal from Vietnam, numerous militarily weaker states have gambled on their ability to outlast American public acceptance of casualties."

That 'waiting them out' routine apparently no longer works as American 'boots' in Afghanistan and Iraq have shown. A WMD criminal intent on mass murder of local citizens OR remote Americans from a sanctuary region should be an automatic target of airstrikes under rules of engagement for crimes against humanity (systemic, terroristic murder). But equating the 'state' in such a region as being sovereign in the same sense as a representative, constitutional government is not viable in any research. A totalitarian entity represents only itself in its behaviors, not a population, so its mass destruction facilities are automatic targets of airstrikes regardless of military or police interdiction.

Note 'Airstrikes are more likely when the stakes for an intervener are low'. That is what you want when a localized criminal activity has been detected, not nuclear or carpet bombing of a city in order to remove the criminal facility. You don't demolish a six-block area of Garfield Park, Chicago when a SWAT team takes down a meth factory in the middle of it. Criminal behavior on a large scale is not a state vs state 'war' issue anywhere in the world anymore and it is time American 'researchers' and their Congressmen recognize that with appropriate definitions of force.

{6} Defending allies from military aggression and bolstering partners against coercion, and fairly sharing responsibilities for common defense.

2018.12.07:09:16 |TR|<2 + ∑ |CD|>3|LI|>1WB|<2 ✉ |GW|>1-|JU|>2 ≈ |OP|<3

Charles Edel in WaPost, 'How democracies slide into authoritarianism':

"Around the world, authoritarian rulers are on the march, waging a sustained assault on facts, reason and democracy. China, Russia, Saudi Arabia and other authoritarian states have worked to interfere with and suppress debate in other nations, just as they stifle dissent at home."

Many cases of authoritarianism are a reaction to the inevitable imperialist aggression of the totalitarians. Roosevelt in World War II is a good example. Israel, India, and the Philippines are other examples. Czeslaw Milosz wrote, through accurate observation, about the literate bourgeois of the world gradually accepting the authoritarian view of eternal conflict (which was of their making) and adapting to it in the form of an intellectual mercenary. You can see its final form in totalitarian 'adaptive' nations like Iran, Turkey, Cuba, North Korea and Kazakhstan, noting that none of these countries had populations with very long exposure to constitutional democracy.

But is democracy a 'luxury' that overpopulated societies cannot afford, regardless of what the local bourgeois say or do? Many areas of the world are becoming Malthusian Population Traps (MPTs) as the climate warms up and the population can no longer be sustained without massive drains on neighboring societies. Note Gaza with its 1.6 million people in a region that couldn't support 130,000 a century ago. Or North Korea, which has never been able to support 18 million people regardless of how totalitarian it becomes. Or Guatemala with 4 distinct MPTs and the climate reducing arable land.

Is democracy a bourgeois illusion in the face of endless environmental crisis? It certainly was in the mini-ice age of the 1500s and 1600s and in many ways led to the democracy checks and balances of the 1700s. But at what point does authoritarianism become necessary for survival of a society?

{7} Dissuading, preventing, or deterring state adversaries and non-state actors from acquiring, proliferating, or using weapons of mass destruction;

2018.04.13:08:24 ∑|CD|<3 ✉ |GW|<1|WB<3-|JU|>2 |TR|<2≈|OP|<2

Editorial Board, WaPost, 'A few cruise missiles from Trump won't stop Syria's war crimes':

"Mr. Trump does have an advantage that Mr. Obama lacked: Thanks to the capture by U.S. and allied forces of a large part of eastern Syria, the United States has the capacity to stabilize at least part of the country and has leverage in demanding an acceptable outcome to the war."

Syria maintains 11 major chemical facilities, including one at the Russian naval base at Latakia. A much larger complex had been built in the western foothills of Aleppo, but it appears to have been degraded by various asymmetric operations and might be little more than a buried VX storage facility. The other ones around Homs are still very active but appear to be focused on World War I style chlorine production, which is very dangerous but not in the same class as VX, which is lethal at 6 mcg. Only the facility near the 'friendly' embassies in Damascus appears to be experimenting with VX. The use of chlorine sometimes means the intent is not to kill, but to permanently 'punish' a human who might oppose the ruling oligarchy or tribe such as the Alawite in Syria. You can't get chlorine out of the lungs once it is breathed in.

If we had enough troops or allies, the only way to stop chemical crimes against humanity is the physical occupation with force of each chemical facility and the space within a radius of 5 miles. Otherwise, you would be telling the criminal elite that they are ALLOWED to and have a 'right' to create WMD facilities. Surrounding nations might not even need a Security Council resolution to use occupying force; under Article 51, preemptive closure of the facilities is automatic since crimes against humanity removes all sovereignty from the perpetrator.

2018.04.13:07:20 |WB|<2⋈ |GW|>2⋈ |CD|<3 |TR|>1 |LI|<3⋈|JU|<3 ≈ |OP|<2

Ignatius, WaPost,'Enough whiplash on Syria. Trump needs an actual strategy.':

"As with any use of military force, planners need to think carefully about "the day after." Would a U.S. strike trigger a widening conflict in a part of Syria where its leverage is limited?"

The American problem is not just the 'day after' ripple effects, but the 'decade after' ripple effects. The entire region from Baghdad to Damascus was illegally occupied by Baathist totalitarians after the British and French eliminated traces of the Ottoman Empire. According to the UN oversight, strong dictators with the ability to kill any dissidents was the only way to rule such a region with several thousand major tribal and religious entities. The effects of these entities, especially with vast energy reserves in their midst, was considered far worse than any damage the Husseins and the Assads could do to their 'people'. But the borders for these nations were purely arbitrary and did not in any way reflect the representation of the people in the region, only who had guns enough to stay in power.

That oligarchic control of WMD manufacturing cost Americans dearly over a 30 year period and it is this problem of primitive, monkey regimes using WMD that is the problem that will extend into the next two decades. Americans are delusional if they think religious totalitarianists of the Middle East will leave them alone on their own soil. The toties have already proved what happens when they develop aggressive WMD; they use it to attack their neighbors. So we will get drawn into another whirlpool not of our making at a much more destructive level.

It would be better if we engaged in nation-building that made it a crime to possess ANY form of WMD and have the force necessary to insure the disarmament of the region. And that might mean creating an independent state between Baghdad and Damascus which has zero tolerance of tribal or totie mass murder and injustice.

2018.04.20:08:08 |CD|<3 ⋈ |GW|>1-|JU|<2|TR|<2≈|OP|<2

Editorial Board, WaPost, 'How Congress can take back control of America's wars':

"This is far from the clarity of an old-fashioned declaration of war; yet the war against far-flung terrorist groups does not necessarily lend itself to one."

'Wars' are not the issue here, criminality is. The Committee supported version, S.J.Res59, has specific definitions of organizations like the Haggani Network and Al Nusrah as 'associated forces' of ISIS and the Taliban where force can be used because they have essentially declared war on American citizens. S.J.Res59 has appropriately limited AUMF countermeasures to specific organizations that have attacked Americans directly, although it also specifically allows U.S. force to protect Afghanistan citizens against terrorist force but not elsewhere 'associated forces' might operate. The repeal of previous AUMFs and the requirements for reporting are also appropriate even if the 'reporting' defined is technically an open, unclassified document that the enemies or their sponsors can read.

It is interesting that none of the 8 or 9 submitted AUMF resolutions have given authority to interdict with ANY force a biological or chemical attack with instruments of mass murder. That might involved use of force against sovereign supported 'militias' in half the world, but there is a noticeable lack of enthusiasm for allowing the president as CinC to destroy installations engaged in crimes against humanity even if that is authorized directly by Article I, Section 8, clause 10 in the Constitution. Are other AUMFs needed to defend North America against WMD criminal activity around the world?

2018.04.27:18:31 |CD|<3 ⋈ [GW]>1-[JU]<2|TR|<2≈|OP|<3

Witte and Gearan, WaPost, 'Trump- Merkel meeting is more business than pleasure for both leaders':

"Grenell shares Trump's deep skepticism about the Iran deal, calling it "a direct blow to the U.N.'s credibility" and the negotiations that led to it "a colossal and dangerous waste of time."

Macron emphasized the importance of keeping the deal during his meetings with Trump in Washington this week."

American and German relationships have traditionally been more business-like than social, nothing new. Most of the economic issues of two mutually beneficial integrated economies could probably be solved by a coin-toss between equal business partners.

The Iranian treaty, in which one side has many followers of the cult of Tagiyya among its Pasdaran leaders, is another international security issue altogether. One of the most obvious objections to the 'treaty' was the lack of IAEA inspector access to Pasdaran independent facilities that could have WMD construction components hidden inside. This happened in Libya, Sudan, Iraq, Pakistan, and Syria. The military installations can operate outside the sovereign authority of the Supreme Leader or the Guardian Council, as 'the Base' does on the Iraqi border. This is a serious international WMD danger to any society, Arabic, European, or North American.

The only way that this threat could be eliminated is by the IAEA inspectors having arrest authority for 'international obstruction of justice' by cultists attempting to hide evidence of WMD manufacture. The other objections can be set aside as the sovereign government of Iran adheres without Tagiyya deception to the treaty terms. It is only this one item that the international community should insist on; the ability of inspectors to appear at un-sovereign locations in a country with arrest authority for obstructionists at the specific location. Both Germany and America should be able to abide by the treaty except for that one item.

Objections to treaty:

3. The inspectors have limited monitoring powers.

Trump has complained that the International Atomic Energy Agency, the U.N. organization responsible for inspecting Iran's facilities, does not have sufficient monitoring powers over the nuclear facilities. He and other critics say the inspectors have no access to closed military sites where any suspect work might be done in secrecy.

Actually, the agreement does make some provision for inspecting military sites. But in requesting access, the IAEA must show Iran the basis for its concern. Iranian officials have repeatedly said the military sites are off-limits to the IAEA.

Further:

IAEA inspectors, with no arrest authority or personal security ability, are largely European experts. They were the ones who discovered the 2002 transfer of several tons of Polish insecticide neurotoxins to the Iraqi secret police at an airbase in Ramadi, Iraq. There is no possible good reason for insecticide concentrates to be in the hands of a 'cult', then or now. As for hiding the stuff, just spray it into five acres of desert sand. You could, by the way, find 50 times that amount of biotoxins in American landfills if you looked for them and that isn't even a crime, let alone a crime against humanity.

2018.06.17:07:57 |CD|<3 ◄|GW|<2↔|JU|>2 ≈ |OP|<2

Rep. Kinzinger (R-Ill) in TheHill, 'Singapore Summit a cause for optimism, however we must remain vigilant and show strength against Kim':

"Confronting the nuclear ambitions of North Korea is not for the faint of heart. The simple willingness to use military action makes diplomacy more effective, and as we move forward in talks with North Korea, I urge the president to work with Congress before making any future deals with Kim Jong Un."

Although a condition of War still exists in which ANY military force including WMD can be used, perhaps the Congress could add an AUMF protocol that allows the use of Overseas Contingency Operations for the 'de-militarization' of certain provinces in Korea on a long timeline that is independent of the CinC's automatic nuclear retaliation authority. The objective would be to set an American condition in which the Seoul government could change the DMZ according to the original, pre-imperialist, 1800s governance rather than the current 'border' along the DMZ. This might give the Seoul government the 'room' to negotiate territory exchanges for economic aid, while maintaining an American military safeguard on the peninsula.

The South is easily capable of trading a full 30 gigawatt power grid in the North for its nuclear and WMD facilities, even converting some weaponized uranium for use in its own nuclear power grid. They could, with U.N. consent, make Kim Jong-un a life-long governor of the 'Northern provinces' that currently make up the DPRK, insuring his 'dynasty' in the North.

The only problem with any 'peace treaty' is the imperialist mentality of Korea's Chinese and Russian neighbors who consider the DPRK a provincial extension of their borders. After all, the DMZ was created entirely by the socialist imperialism of Joseph Stalin and Mao Zedong, not some Korean referendum. The imperialism is still rampant in both countries and they will almost certainly attempt to destroy any North-South movement toward peaceful integration and democracy, especially if the local WMD is used to consume North American and east Asia defense resources.

TLO: The resource consumption by the U.S. is too desirable by the Chinese CCP for them to give it up in North Korea. Use of 'proxy' forces to weaken an enemy before their own strike is fundamental to Sun Tzu.

{8} Preventing terrorists from directing or supporting external operations against the United States homeland and our citizens, allies, and partners overseas;

2018.11.24:18:43 |CD|>3 ≈ |OP|>1....[WB]<2+|JU|<3 ⋈ [GW]>2

Applebaum, WaPost, 'Iran's regime could fall apart. What happens then?':

"In the case of Iran, anything even resembling a regime failure could have catastrophic consequences. Iran's economy is dominated by companies that are owned, openly or otherwise, by the radical Revolutionary Guard Corps. Most banks are owned directly by the state. The judicial system is dominated by clerics. And the educational system has also been twisted by decades of radical religious ideology."

If one were to check the current Iranian constitution, he might discover that many of its 177 Articles are parallel to the 7 in the American Constitution. Technically, the two We the Peoples should have enough in common that they would cooperate against crimes against humanity or crimes against the 'Peoples of the Books' such as Christians, Hebrews AND Shia Muslims. There is, however, no Iranian Constitutional basis for the overwhelming presence of the Pasdaran cult in the 'Expediency Discernment Council of the System' that can execute the Constitutional Supreme Leader's economic and veto powers without him even knowing it.

The Pasdaran are the senior officers of the Republican Guard who, much like the Chinese Central Military Commission, can own and control large segments of the industrial and financial sectors of their countries as independent entities within each nation. This unaccounted ownership of WMD is very dangerous to the future of a country and not only leads to its collapse through economic inequality, It allows these individuals to create a continuous war-need mentality in the country.

You don't have to cause regime collapse in Iran, only remove the Pasdaran cult mentality from leadership Councils like the Expediency and the Guardian by making them representative electoral rather than appointed. Power to the People?

{9} Ensuring common domains remain open and free;

2018.08.17:06:54 |CD|<3 ⋈ [GW]>1-|JU|>2|TR|<3 ≈ |OP|>1

Kiley, TheHill,'Cybersecurity: Cause for optimism, need for continued vigilance':

"Finally, the federal government must work more closely with private industry to ensure that if they share information critical to the mitigation and prevention of attacks, proprietary information is protected and the bureaucrats and politicians do not lay blame on those businesses."

Since this cyber aggression has already been shown to be an attack against We The People, it should come under the authority of Common Defense in which the individuals involved in some infrastructure can be held responsible for 'negligence' even if no actual cyber-attack was successful. In this day and age, cyber security should be universal in human, droid, and linkage categories. An organization that fails to maintain minimum established security protocols because 'they don't have time for it' should be held responsible.

But the same laws that define the 'negligence' should also have cybersecurity guarantees against third party access through 'laws' even in court proceedings. That is, the famous 'security disclosure' defense by the legal profession in which defendants seek to publicize 'classified evidence' at a legal proceeding would have to have sunset provisions where the negligence provision applies to the legal operators as well. Even an FOIA request for corporate cybersecurity data might be from of Common Defense 'negligence' by all judiciary participants in an attack-related event. Not easy, because a 'secret' court proceeding may be unconstitutional unless public review is available at some point. This smacks of a 'star-chamber' activity found in most totalitarian states, so some efforts to prevent security disclosures in a judicial context are very much needed in this century.

{10} Continuously delivering performance with affordability and speed as we change Departmental mindset, culture, and management systems;

{11} Establishing an unmatched 21st century National Security Innovation Base that effectively supports Department operations and sustains security and solvency.

2018.03.13:07:12 |CD|>3= |GW|>1 ⋈ |JU|>2 ∪ |OP|>3 |TR|<2

Shaban, WaPost, on Internet national security:

"Hunter said it could reflect "an evolution in the thinking" of the committee, perhaps an indication that it's going to approach transactions in which foreign people or entities seek to own 5G wireless technology with the same sensitivity and rigor that the feds currently "apply to military equipment traditionally."

This decision is almost certainly a reaction to the Beijing government passing laws in 2017 that forced the inclusion of 'firmware' in Chinese-made internet chips that allowed Communist Party government security agencies to access the device anywhere in the world AND record any data transmitted through that chip's internet equipment. Such a controlled chip in Chinese made equipment would have an enormous strategic advantage for Beijing economic and political interests. It is no accident that service and installation contracts with Chinese, Taiwanese, and Singapore internet system builders offer 'free' Chinese made equipment in their contracts.

If the American government were going to be serious about defending its people against cyber-warfare attacks, it might even consider nationalizing a cloned factory of the American chip maker (not the company) that was dedicated to making the 5G internet structure under strict DOD military specifications. This nationalized chip facility could then produce 5G routers, servers, fiber-optical amplifiers and other devices with built-in firewalls, encryption protocols and biometric access safeguards not accessible by foreign hackers or 'security' apparats.

Of course, the American government would have to admit by nationalizing a high-tech factory that government had the function of building 'secure' infrastructures, which many are ideologically opposed to.

[CD] 2018 Conclusions:

Human beings are a very dangerous species, especially if their 'tribal' economic value is decided by the amount of 'arms' the faction possesses. Many of the international police related conflicts with such tribalism involved prevention of WMD escalations to gain better net worth by one oligarchic tribe over another. Arms 'control' is seen as a product of this rather than a genuine desire to be at peace. In 2018, internet Interactive peoples in societies do not generally go along with this aggressive perception **if they know about it,** but the totalitarians have the ability to hide the WMD capability much more than democracies. This was one of Sun Tzu's fundamentals in making conquests through force and at least two thirds of humanity are unaware of the build-up of asymmetric lethality on the planet, now reaching something over a trillion dollars a year worldwide. The experimentation with chemical weapons in Syria and North Korea is being passed on to other Totalitarians such as the Iranians, Pakistanis east Europeans. American and NATO intelligence organizations collect this data because they would be foolish not to be able to reciprocate. The same is true of pandemic systems of germs, which may prove to be the ultimate weapon of genocide.

Table 1. FY2019 Defense Appropriations: House-passed H.R. 6157
amounts in billions of dollars of discretionary budget authority (numbers may not sum due to rounding)

Title	FY2018 Enacted Defense Appropriations				House-passed H.R. 6157
	Regular defense appropriation [Division C of P.L. 115-141]	Missile defense and ship repair [P.L. 115-96]	Total	FY2019 Request	
Base Budget					
Military Personnel	133.4	--	133.4	140.7	139.3
Operation and Maintenance	188.2	0.7	189.0	199.5	197.6
Procurement	133.9	2.4	136.3	130.6	133.0
Research and Development	88.3	1.3	89.7	91.1	91.2
Revolving and Mgmt. Funds	1.7	--	1.7	1.5	1.5
Def. Health Program and Other	36.6	--	36.6	35.8	36.2
Related Agencies	1.1	--	1.1	1.1	1.0
General Provisions	-0.9	--	-0.9	0.1	-0.5
Subtotal: Base Budget	**582.3**	**4.5**	**586.8**	**600.3**	**599.4**
Overseas Contingency Ops. (OCO)	65.2	--	65.2	68.1	68.1
Total	**647.4**	**4.5**	**651.9**	**668.4**	**667.5**

Source: Congressional Budget Office, "Estimate of H.R. 6157, the Department of Defense Appropriations Act, 2019," July 2, 2018.

2018.07.16:07:40 |CD|<3 ⋈ [GW|>3-[JU|<1|TR|>2 ≈ |OP|>1

Staniland in WaPost, 'The U.S. military is trying to manage foreign conflicts — not resolve them. Here's why.':

"As long as the U.S. government can limit the domestic costs of violence management overseas, few Americans will have incentives to pay attention to these low-level, far-flung wars."

Article I, Section 8, clause 11 gives the constitutional authority for declaring 'war' and virtually none of the current American military activities constitute a condition of 'war'. Violence management, as expressed in this article, would fall under clause 10, 'to define and punish Piracies and Felonies committed on the high Seas, and Offenses against the Laws of Nations.' That means pursuit and neutralization of cartel-level criminal attacks on humanity, which very few Americans object to, especially if they have been targeted by such criminal behavior.

Any police/military force engaged in violence management around the world that reduces the terroristic Offenses against the Laws of Nations (crimes against humanity) is a legitimate expression of American society, even if not directly authorized in each instance by the Congress. It is a well-known academic misperception of the human race to regard all military force as an automatic act of 'war', which normally involves, according to Sun Tzu's 'Art of War', total destruction of the enemy society.

CRS Insight, CRS-IN10855, February 2018, The 2018 National Defense Strategy

As such, it organizes DOD activities along three central "lines of effort"—rebuilding military readiness and improving the joint forces' lethality, strengthening alliances and attracting new partners, and reforming the department's business practices—and argues that all three are interconnected and critical to enabling DOD to effectively advance U.S. objectives. It also notes that programs designed to advance those objectives will be included in the FY2019- FY2023 budgets. Some further key points include

Building a more lethal joint force will require consistent multiyear investments to improve war fighting readiness, an optimally sized joint force, prioritization of preparedness for war as part of an overall deterrent and competitive posture, and the modernization of key capabilities. The latter includes nuclear forces; space and cyberspace capabilities; command, control communications, computers and intelligence, surveillance and reconnaissance (C4ISR) capabilities; missile defense; joint lethality in contested environments; forward maneuver and posture resilience; autonomous and unmanned systems; and resilient logistics (p. 6-7).

Strengthening allies and attracting new partners will require better burden-sharing amongst allies; expanding regional consultative mechanisms and collaborative planning; and deepening interoperability amongst allies and partners (p. 8-9).

Reforming DOD for greater performance and affordability will require prioritizing speed of capability delivery rather than the "exquisite" performance of systems and capabilities; better organizing the Department to enable innovation to improve lethality across the joint force; better budget discipline and affordability; rapid prototyping and fielding of equipment; and harnessing and

protecting the National Security Innovation Base (p 10-11). The
NDS sees harnessing that base as a source of competitive advantage

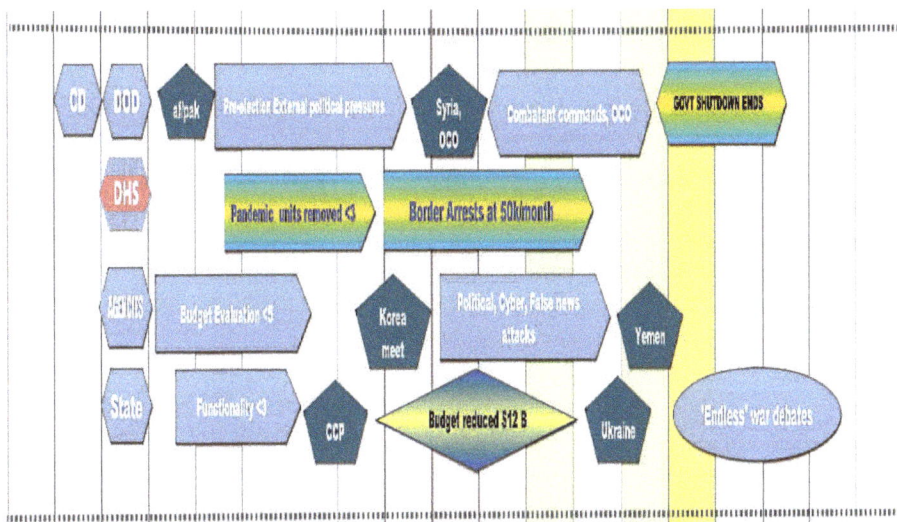

2018.05.06:08:12 |CD|>4 ≈|OP|>2 Ξ|WB|<1+|CD| ⋈|GW|>2

Anderson, Brookings Institution, in TheHill, 'Why war powers need an expiration
date':

"And while enemies may make more rhetorical use of a AUMF than this other
legislation, allowing their messaging to drive U.S. policy would be ill-advised."

One of the problems with the 'sunset provisions' and 'reporting clause' combinations
in the new AUMF is that an enemy proxy force through hostile state intelligence aid
would be able to scatter (as the Taliban and ISIS small forces have done) and re-
concentrate after the Authorization had terminated. That is a serious national security
issue, since some of them could be 'concentrated' in a constitutional democracy as
both Osama Bin Laden and Muammar Qaddafi managed. Remember, believers in the
Quranically false Caliphate world ruler doctrine will invariably attack humans engaged
in democracy, as will those who adhere to the Leninist world ruler concept. An absolute
sunset and detailed reporting AUMF serves them both, not human, let alone American,
security.

**It would be better if the AUMF sunset clause had the wording 'except when an
active, systemic crime against humanity is being perpetrated by members of the
named hostile 'entities'.** The new AUMF could also have a provision concerning the
48-hour reporting requirement that said the report of ongoing actions need only the
approval of the House and Senate Committees involved along with the Speaker and
Senate President. This would allow the ongoing actions concerning 'Offenses against
the Laws of Nations' (as put in Article I, Section 8, Clause 10) to remain hidden for
appropriate periods. These are criminal activities against humans, not necessarily 'war'
activities under the ancient War Powers Act, even if hostile WMD is involved.

Many in America worry about the President's authority as commander in chief and its ability to make unilateral attacks in a 'war' context, but the more serious problem is why the Congresses' Article I, Section 8, clause 11 'war' authority is used in **every** case of international conflict rather than use the authority of clause 10, offenses against the laws of nations, which would include asymmetric warfare and genocide.

2018.10.55:10:08 |CD|>2 ≈|OP|>2 Ξ |WB|<1+|JU|>2 ⋈ |GW|>2

Kheel, TheHill, 'Mattis: Russia's violation of arms control treaty 'untenable':

"At issue is the 1987 Intermediate-range Nuclear Forces (INF) Treaty, which bans nuclear and conventional ground-launched ballistic and cruise missiles with ranges between 500 and 5,500 kilometers. The treaty is credited with helping end the Cold War."

NATO might as well give up on this treaty the same as it had to do with the older ABM treaty. Dmitry Bulgakov has no intention of reducing the 4 battalions of Iskander-N missile battalions now being created at Kapustin Yar. The 9M729 missile has an effective, note effective, range of about 2000 miles, which makes it ideal for a 'cheap shot' at any maritime target area within 1200 miles of the Russian coasts (Black Sea, North Sea, Sea of Japan, Mediterranean Sea, etc). Deploying 4 battalions in mobile units gives individual, small target coverage of all of the coasts and border areas, including new Chinese and Korean mobile missile systems. Since other countries bordering Russia are not signers of the INF Treaty, Bulgakov would perceive a no-choice situation for Russian interests, along with protecting his expanded budget.

Unless all other nations agree to INF Treaty limitations in this century, there is no point in North America attempting to adhere to the technological limitations of such meaningless treaties. This would allow Americans to more rapidly deploy new mobil hypersonic 'Waverider' technologies, which can be in both an offensive Iskander-range mode or an ABM mode. A fully mobile version of the X-52A with its own launch controls might be used as part of any other U.S. arms platform, and even shoot down a 9M729 if we didn't abide by a treaty no one else is abiding by.

2018.11.18:10:04 |CD|>3 ⋈ |GW|<1-|JU|>2|TR|>3 ≈|OP|>2

Rebecca Kheel, TheHill, 'Trump and Congress on collision course with military spending':

"The National Defense Strategy Commission, a 12-member panel created by Congress to study and make recommendations on the U.S. defense strategy, recently released its final report.

The commission concluded that U.S. military superiority "has eroded to a dangerous degree" because of political, financial and international issues. Its report warned there will be "grave and lasting" consequences if Washington doesn't act quickly to reverse the damage and adequately fund the Pentagon."

Providing for the Common Defense, The Assessment and Recommendations of the Nation Defense Strategy Commission, November 2018:

Pentagon Reform: Necessary but Not Sufficient

> "Resourcing a strategy is not only an issue of providing reliable, adequate, and timely funding. It also entails ensuring that the available dollars are spent as efficiently and effectively as possible. This is more than a matter of treating taxpayer dollars with respect, as vitally important as that is. It is equally a matter of sharpening the U.S. military's ability to compete with its rivals by wringing maximum value out of the resources at hand.

This being the case, the NDS is correct to argue that the Pentagon's culture and way of doing business must change. Sustained reforms, implemented across every aspect of the Department's activities, are sorely need to bring one of the world's largest bureaucracies into line with 21st century business practices. This will be critical to fostering innovation, improving responsiveness and agility, enhancing the speed at which capabilities are developed and fielded, and improving the efficiency, effectiveness, and accountability with which the Department expends limited funds. Every recent Secretary of Defense has recognized these 60 imperatives, which has only become more pressing as America's competitive edge has eroded."

The Commission Report talks about the 'Pentagon's culture and way of doing business must change' but also notes that any massive attempt at fiscal responsibility by cutting the total budget won't work. **That is an accurate assessment from DOD in that the Congress cannot operate on its two-year electoral cycle (even though Defense appropriations are Constitutionally mandated at two years) because that in itself causes enormous waste in DOD.** What might be more useful is for the Congress to fund and law-up a new AI auditing system that operates parallel to each DOD department that makes purchases BUT reports through the IG offices instead of the local department's management. Modern AI accounting computers can flag many waste and fraud debits no matter how well the local 'slyde drool' manipulates the department expenses data.

The military may already have the 'system' for doing such real-time auditing regardless of where the DOD department is physically located. DARPA has several projects under way to upgrade military BARS type computers to 32 core capabilities. The transferable real time auditing software already available might fit nicely in such a mobile, plug-in system. 75 DOD abuse dollars saved for each dollar invested in BARS auditing computers?

Is national and world defense becoming too complex for the three branches in the Constitution to oversee and direct? The totalitarians of the world think so.

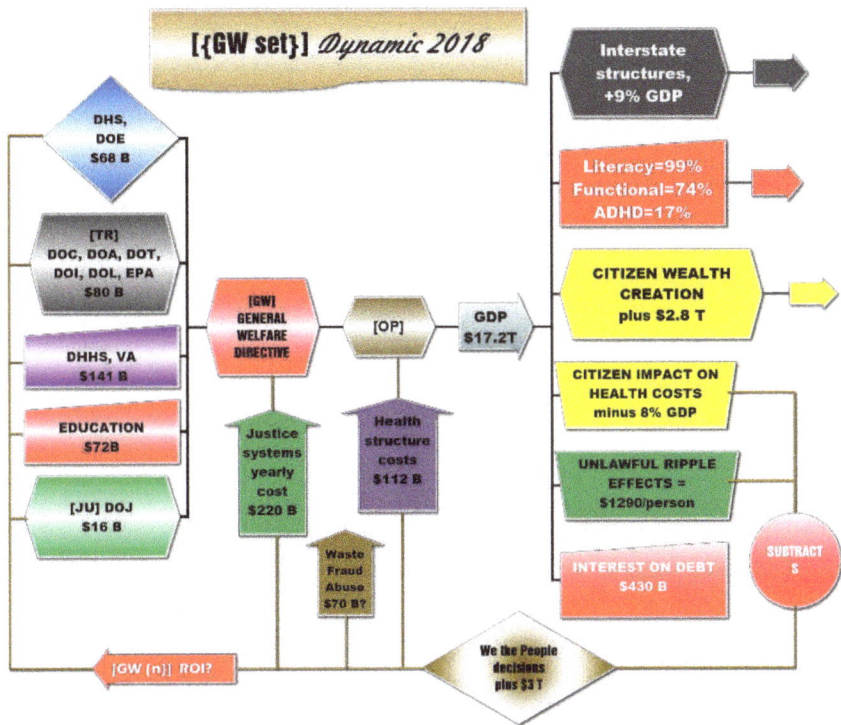

General Welfare [GW]

[{GW set}] *Dynamic 2018*

DHS, DOE $68 B

[TR] DOC, DOA, DOT, DOI, DOL, EPA $80 B

DHHS, VA $141 B

EDUCATION $72B

[JU] DOJ $16 B

[GW] GENERAL WELFARE DIRECTIVE

[OP]

GDP $17.2T

Justice systems yearly cost $220 B

Health structure costs $112 B

Waste Fraud Abuse $70 B?

[GW [n]] ROI?

We the People decisions plus $3 T

Interstate structures, +9% GDP

Literacy=99% Functional=74% ADHD=17%

CITIZEN WEALTH CREATION plus $2.8 T

CITIZEN IMPACT ON HEALTH COSTS minus 8% GDP

UNLAWFUL RIPPLE EFFECTS = $1290/person

INTEREST ON DEBT $430 B

SUBTRACTS

Figure 17. General Welfare [GW] dynamic

General Welfare is a Prime Directive of the Constitution because a society simply can't exist without it, or its co-directive Common Defense. It is a matter of balancing the two at any given time and the way the Congress and Executive does this is generally reflected in the {subsets} Article I has given to the Congress, especially the House which has sole appropriation authority.   These subsets actually have predefined 'functional codes' that determine which categories go with which subcommittees that have constitutional oversight. These were established with the very first appropriations in 1790 and have been added as the authority of federal system expanded. There are currently some 20 {functions} of government and those related to General Welfare are shown here. There are also direct Common Defense {050-150 functions} and also direct Justice {750-754 functions}and through {950}. General Welfare is considered here:

Codes	Departments	Cost	Constitutional Authority
250	General Science, Space and Technology	$29 b	Section 8.8
270	Energy	$15 b	Section 8.3, 8.1
300	Natural Resources and Environment	$42 b	Section 8.3
350	Agriculture	$18 b	Section 8.1, 8.3,
370	Commerce and Housing Credit	$41 b	Section 8.5, 8.3
400	Transportation	$93 b	Section 8.7
450	Community and Regional Development	$25 b	Section 8.3(?)
500	Edu, Training, Employment, and Social Service	$91 b	Section 8.3, 8.1, 8.2(?)
550	Health	$347 b	Section 8.1(?)
570	Medicare	$472 b	Section 8.3
600	Income Security	$541 b	Section 8.1, 8.2
650	Social Security	$773 b	Section 8.1, 8.18(?)
700	Veterans Benefits and Services	$125 b	Section 8.12

But note the classifications developed by popular consensus in various polls. They closely match the [CD] and [GW] domains except for constant worry about the 'economy' in general, even though there is no such constitutional category. The following {n} is a consensus of polls in 2018 concerning voter concerns prior to the midterm elections. There also is no {functional} category for climate change other than 270 and 300 because it is not considered a functional entity at this time in spite of its disastrous effects on weather, land use, immigration and energy.

{1}   The economy, tax cuts and jobs Act,

{2}   The availability and affordability of healthcare, pricing, ACA repeal and replace, Public Health Service Act have expired, artificial embryos, see [WB]

{3}   The possibility of future terrorist attacks in the U.S. see [CD]

{4}   The size and power of the federal government, cybersecurity, AI development

{5}   The Social Security system

Table 3.2 - OUTLAYS BY FUNCTION AND SUBFUNCTION: 1962 - 2025
(in millions of dollars)

[GW] General Welfare {SS}

Function and Subfunction	2011	2012	2013	2014	2015	2016	2017	2018	2019	2020 estimate
Total, Income Security	597,269	541,248	536,411	513,596	508,800	514,098	503,443	495,289	514,787	529,335
650 Social Security:										
651 Social security	730,811	773,290	813,551	850,533	887,753	916,067	944,878	987,791	1,044,409	1,097,184
(On-budget)	101,933	140,387	56,009	25,946	30,990	32,522	37,393	35,752	36,130	39,284
(Off-budget)	628,878	632,903	757,542	824,587	856,763	883,545	907,485	952,039	1,008,279	1,057,900

{6}   Illegal immigration. See [JU]

{7}   Hunger and homelessness

{8}   Climate change

{9}   The way income and wealth are distributed in the U.S.

{10}   Crime and violence

{11}   Race relations

{12}   Drug use, FDA Reauthorization Act, CARA, opioid deaths

{13} Unemployment

Table 3.2 - OUTLAYS BY FUNCTION AND SUBFUNCTION: 1962 - 2025
(in millions of dollars)
[GW] General Welfare {s-net}

Function and Subfunction	2011	2012	2013	2014	2015	2016	2017	2018	2019	2020 estimate
600 Income Security:										
601 General retirement and disability insurance (excluding social)	6,697	7,760	6,969	8,776	7,805	3,777	4,528	6,284	3,693	5,799
602 Federal employee retirement and disability	124,367	122,292	131,639	134,565	139,123	144,716	142,161	140,685	149,619	155,032
603 Unemployment compensation	120,556	93,771	70,729	45,717	34,978	35,159	33,320	30,948	29,900	29,913
604 Housing assistance	55,440	47,948	46,687	47,615	47,823	49,076	50,011	49,499	50,552	51,189
605 Food and nutrition assistance	103,199	106,871	109,706	102,936	104,797	102,300	99,702	98,065	93,587	95,074
609 Other income security	187,010	162,606	170,681	173,987	174,274	179,070	173,721	169,808	187,436	192,328

{14} The quality of the environment, Pandemic Act expires

{15} The availability and affordability of energy

Table 3.2 - OUTLAYS BY FUNCTION AND SUBFUNCTION: 1962 - 2025
(in millions of dollars)
[GW] General Welfare {scienc], [energy}

Function and Subfunction	2011	2012	2013	2014	2015	2016	2017	2018	2019	2020 estimate
250 General Science, Space, and Technology:										
251 General science and basic research	12,434	12,458	12,479	12,011	11,719	11,950	12,320	12,426	12,939	14,187
252 Space flight, research, and supporting activities	17,032	16,602	16,429	16,559	17,693	18,224	18,074	19,108	19,471	20,845
Total, General Science, Space, and Technology	29,466	29,060	28,908	28,570	29,412	30,174	30,394	31,534	32,410	35,032
270 Energy:										
271 Energy supply	8,084	9,017	9,038	4,056	4,710	2,021	2,827	1,444	4,110	2,563
272 Energy conservation	6,736	4,941	1,240	910	1,187	967	1,048	1,094	1,086	1,265
274 Emergency energy preparedness	-3,263	375	217	-140	449	234	-536	-878	-743	-32
276 Energy information, policy, and regulation	617	525	547	444	495	499	517	509	588	800

As far as the Chronicles are concerned, the [GW]{subsets} are necessary parts of a modern democracy even though they technically cover every minute of a person's life and require resources input from each citizen, even when the upper one percent do not pay much in taxes and the lower 15% do not earn enough to pay taxes. The perception of the domain requires a knowledge of the {subsets} in order to visualize the 'system' as a coherent whole. The 15 categories are shown with various related Opservationis in the Chronicles, although it was felt that prioritizing the [subsets} might distort the perception. Here are some [GW] samplings in 2018.

They are divided into the 15 {subsets} American polls deemed important without any operational research prioritization. Such things as the '{economy}', '{health}', and '{climate}' are undefined entities in the Constitution, even if covered by the General Welfare authority in Article I, section 8, clause 1. This is a sampling only; others can be found throughout the Chronicles.

2018.06.29:10:05 | ξ]<? [WB]>2⋈ [GW]>3⋈ [TR]<1 [LI]>3 ⋈ [JU]<1 ≈ |OP|>2-|CD|<3

Wagner, WaPost, 'No person in America should be too poor to live': Ocasio-Cortez explains democratic socialism to Colbert':

"So what that means is health care as a human right. "

Exactly how is **that done** within, note within, the existing Constitution? Easy to say and get votes saying it, but then what? Another bridge to nowhere?

{1}   The economy, tax cuts and jobs Act of 2017

2018.07.04:07:54 |GW|<3⋈ |CD|<1 |TR|<1 |LI|<1⋈|JU|>1 ≈ |WB|>3⋈ |OP|<2

Samuelson, WaPost, 'Trump's neo-isolationism won't work':

"To the contrary, power is being drained from nation-states to "market forces" or other global mechanisms that are difficult to control."

That is exactly the problem for We the People. America has been turned into an 'extraction' economy for a world economy rather than a North American 'internal cycle' economy. In the 1950s and 1960s, virtually all wealth generated by Americans was cycled through other North Americans in some way. Very little of that wealth was distributed worldwide, in spite of economic aid to Europe and Asia. Today, you have foreign extraction mechanisms controlled by such organizations as the Central Banks of China and Russia (net worth $8 trillion and $3 trillion) along with stateless sanctuaries like Qatar (net worth $400 billion) and Cayman Islands Monetary Authority (net worth $2 trillion), all of which are in a position to influence 'laws' in North America. But it might qualify as 'dumb' to isolate America from other North American economies; they are just too heavily integrated for mutual benefits.

But economic mutual benefit is not true if Ricardo models of free trade are manipulated around the world to protect wealth extraction from the United States (Middle East, China, Russia, India, etc) and especially is not true if such world interests are using the extracted wealth to control the political structure of We the People. There is no doubt the manipulations are under way when the 'security' services that detect the wealth extraction are under constant de-funding attacks. True, isolationism will not work. You must know thy enemy and you can't do that when isolated to the point you don't have economic 'eyes'.

2018.08.12:10:53 |OP|? ≈ ∑ |TR|>1 |LI|>2⋈|JU|>1....|GW|>2⋈ |CD|<3

Sheri Berman, Bernard College, in WaPost, 'Democratic socialists are conquering the left. But do they believe in democracy?':

"If democratic socialism is to revitalize the Democratic Party, it should have answers to questions that have bedeviled it in the past. What does the DSA's goal of socialism actually mean? If abolishing capitalism is its goal, as its adherents say, how are the growth, efficiency and innovation that are the prerequisites for redistribution to be achieved? And if reforms can't create a better world …..then how is socialism to be achieved? Is democracy, even when flawed, a means or an end? Will democratic socialists prioritize democracy if the votes for a "socialist future" do not materialize? Will they eschew the compromises and alliances necessary to protect democracy?"

'how are the growth, efficiency and innovation that are the prerequisites for redistribution to be achieved?

Lots of questions in which economics are linked directly to political power by both the socialists and the capitalists. Suppose 'redistribution' is not directly linked to politics but becomes a 22nd century, not 21st , infrastructure in which matter and energy transformation at a sub-quantum level and even health molecular change creates 'advanced' species that don't require ANY form of redistribution because it is built in at conception by new technologies now surfacing? Both the wealth-seeking totalitarian oligarchies of the past 500 years and the socialist totalitarian oligarchies of the past 100 years become meaningless under conditions of universal 'molecular' redistribution.

It is most likely the energy and genetic wars of this 21st century will be fought by capitalist and socialist oligarchies seeking to prevent a universal distribution of quantum-level perfection which doesn't need them for anything.

{4} The size and power of the federal government: cybersecurity, AI development, agency ROI,

2018.12.07:00:00 |CD|>3 ⋈ |GW|>1-|JU|>2 ≈ |OP|<3∑ |TR|<2 + |LI|<3|WB|<2

CRS in focus, Debt and Deficits: Spending, Revenue, and Economic Growth':

"The federal budget has not produced a surplus since FY2001. Reduced revenues and increased spending led to deficits in ensuing years, and the Great Recession and federal response produced deficits in FY2008-FY2010 (averaging 9.0% of gross domestic product [GDP]), which were the largest of the post-World War II era. Following a period of smaller deficits, real deficits have increased in each year since FY2015. The budget recorded a deficit of 4.0% of GDP in FY2018, which is larger than the average deficit from the preceding 50 years (2.9% of GDP from FY1968 to FY2017)."

TLO: Speaks for itself.

2018.08.20:07:31 |GW|>3⋈ |TR|<1 |LI|>3⋈|JU|<1 ≈ |OP|>2

Ron Charles, WaPost, Barack Obama's summer reading list is everything we need right now':

"Obama calls Rosling, a Swedish physician, "an outstanding international public health expert," and notes that "Factfulness" is "a hopeful book about the potential for human progress when we work off facts rather than our inherent biases." Given the huge cloud of distortion enveloping the country, this is just what the doctor ordered.

Hans Rosling, 'Factfullness':

"So if your worldview is wrong, then you will systematically make wrong guesses. But this overdramatic worldview is not caused simply by out-of-date knowledge, as I once thought. Even people with access to the latest information get the world wrong. And I am convinced it is not the fault of an evil-minded media, propaganda, fake news, or wrong facts.

My experience, over decades of lecturing, and testing, and listening to the ways people misinterpret the facts even when they are right in front of them, finally brought me to see that the overdramatic worldview is so difficult to shift because it comes from the very way our brains work."

Speculation:

Neurologically, people normally see the 'world' data significance as inversely proportional to the square of the distance from them. Attempting to see the world as one unified entity is admirable, but there actually are millions of homosapien 'subsystems' that an author (or a president) could get caught up in. That's one of the reasons for G20 style meetings that try to prioritize items so that the inverse square perception of a given head of state doesn't become a nationalistic obsession for him in relation to the other heads of state. But some leaders will wallow in the trivia of media 'events' or 'personalities' and then bet the farm that doesn't belong to them even when he is looking at four cards of a straight flush across the table.

2018.07.08:06:53 |GW|>3⋈ |CD|<1≈ ∑ |TR|<1 |LI|<3 ⋈ |JU|>2 |OP|>1

Kolesnik in TheHill, 'The Senate's grown-ups in the Trump-Russia probe follow facts, not politics':

"Understanding why it's a beacon requires a bit of intellectual alacrity. I and other followers of this probe have laid out hope that some U.S. government entity will provide a serious, sober revelation of what actually occurred. We're not there yet. Not even close."

A B-plus for the SSCI [Senate Select Committee on Intelligence] is certainly in order, even with the 'executive summery' mode it adopted as a constitutional oversight. The covert details in the ICA process, of course, need to be kept secure. But the SSCI really needs a mechanism in which it can determine whether a national security or even 'constitutional contempt' act whistle blower can be validated and made secure WITHIN the executive branch AND in all Congressional committees. That is, would the abuse of information about a threat to the Constitution itself, along with the threat, be a high crime and misdemeanor regardless of where it occurs? And who decides? Judiciary review of Congressional committees? Not likely under separation of powers theory.

But the SSCI could offer immunity conditions that guaranteed the 'safety' of whistle blowers (just appearing in closed hearing with attorneys might cost a patriotic 'snitch' $30,000) regardless of who they interact with in the Republic justice system. A DEA, FBI or CIA officer might have an agenda that contradicts his oath to defend the Constitution and could easily destroy the evidentiary path of a whistle blower, unless an alternate review was available. That would be true Congressional oversight, even if the item never became a public misdemeanor.

{5} The Social Security system

2018.01.09:00:00 |GW|>3⋈ WB|>3 |TR|<1 |LI|<3⋈|JU|>1≈ |OP|>2

https://en.wikipedia.org/wiki/Social_Security_(United_States) :

"In the 1937 U.S. Supreme Court case of *Helvering v. Davis*,[190] the Court examined the constitutionality of Social Security when George Davis of the Edison Electric Illuminating Company of Boston sued in connection with the Social Security tax. The U.S. District Court for the District of Massachusetts first upheld the tax. The District Court judgment was reversed by the Circuit Court of Appeals. Commissioner Guy Helvering of the Bureau of Internal Revenue (now the Internal Revenue Service) took the case to the Supreme Court, and the Court upheld the validity of the tax."

The Constitutionality of the old-age safety net has never been questioned in terms of its appropriateness under any Article, so it can be assumed that most such appropriations and {systems} are valid functions of representative government. No generation of Congress as challenged [GW] as a necessary function although there is endless debate concerning the [GD]{subsets}. Many of these could be separated out as {WB] subsystems, but perhaps not Social Security, which is a prepaid contract for extending life for some but not all.

2018.08.20:07:31 |GW|>3⋈ |TR|<1 |LI|>3⋈|JU|<1 ≈ |OP|>2

Ron Charles, WaPost, Barack Obama's summer reading list is everything we need right now':

"Obama calls Rosling, a Swedish physician, "an outstanding international public health expert," and notes that "Factfulness" is "a hopeful book about the potential for human progress when we work off facts rather than our inherent biases." Given the huge cloud of distortion enveloping the country, this is just what the doctor ordered.

Hans Rosling, 'Factfullness':

"So if your worldview is wrong, then you will systematically make wrong guesses. But this overdramatic worldview is not caused simply by out-of-date knowledge, as I once thought. Even people with access to the latest information get the world wrong. And I am convinced it is not the fault of an evil-minded media, propaganda, fake news, or wrong facts.

My experience, over decades of lecturing, and testing, and listening to the ways people misinterpret the facts even when they are right in front of them, finally brought me to see that the overdramatic worldview is so difficult to shift because it comes from the very way our brains work."

Speculation:

Neurologically, people normally see the 'world' data significance as inversely proportional to the square of the distance from them. Attempting to see the world as one unified entity is admirable, but there actually are millions of homosapien 'subsystems' that an author (or a president) could get caught up in. That's one of the reasons for G20 style meetings that try to prioritize items so that the inverse square perception of a given head of state doesn't become a nationalistic obsession for him in relation to the other heads of state. But some leaders will wallow in the trivia of media 'events' or 'personalities' and then bet the farm that doesn't belong to them even when he is looking at four cards of a straight flush across the table.

2018.01.09:15:24 |WB|>3⋈ |GW|>3⋈ |CD|<1 |TR|<1 |LI|<3⋈|JU|>1 |OP|>2

James V. Saturno, Megan Suzanne Lynch, Congressional Research Service, R41907, 'A Balanced Budget Constitutional Amendment: Background and Congressional Options':

"Summary

> One of the most persistent political issues facing Congress in recent decades is whether to require that the budget of the United States be in balance. Although a balanced federal budget has long been held as a political ideal, the accumulation of large deficits in recent years has heightened concern that some action to require a balance between revenues and expenditures may be necessary.

The debate over a balanced budget measure actually consists of several interrelated debates. Most prominently, the arguments of proponents have focused on the economy and the possible harm resulting from consistently large deficits and a growing federal debt. Another issue involves whether such a requirement should be statutory or made part of the Constitution. Some proponents of balanced budgets oppose a constitutional amendment, fearing that it would prove to be too inflexible for dealing with future circumstances.

Opponents of a constitutional amendment often focus on the difficulties of implementing or enforcing any amendment. Their concerns have been numerous and varied. How would such a requirement affect the balance of power between the President and Congress? Between the federal courts and Congress? Although most proponents would prefer to establish a balanced budget requirement as part of the Constitution, some advocates have suggested using the untried process provided under Article V of the Constitution for a constitutional convention as an alternative to a joint resolution passed by two-thirds vote in both houses of Congress. Although the inclusion of a balanced budget amendment as part of the congressional agenda has muted this debate in recent years, proposals for a convention are still possible, and raise concerns that one might open the way to an unpredictable series of reforms. The last American constitutional convention convened in May 1787 and produced the current Constitution.

TLO: Are they overlooking that the prime directive for Common Defense was transferred to the federals for the specific purpose of freeing up the budgets of the states? How do you 'balance' something when it varies by 205% per decade and might vary by two hundred percent during a war over several years?

2018.04.24:08:26 |GW|>3⋈ |CD|<1 = ∑ |TR|<1 |LI|<3⋈|JU|>1 |OP|>2|OP|>?

Lane, WaPost, 'Red America and blue America depend on each other. That's how it should be.':

"Cembalest calculates that if electoral college votes were allocated according to food and energy production as well as population, Texas would have 81 electoral votes instead of its current 38, North Dakota would go up from three to 14 — and New York would shrink from 29 to 19."

If the Electoral College Districts were allocated according to the 'wellbeing' of the citizens that calculated the food, energy use, health, and productivity of Americans, they might discover not just a well-known red-blue split but a 'purple' component that is much larger than either the red or blue. This would be a truer indication of the relation of people to GDP, especially since fully one quarter of the American GDP is parasitic services concentrated in California, New York, Texas and Florida. If you removed these international components because they do not produce food, energy or health, the true GDP is closer to $15 trillion with a 'purple' distribution and the big four (who do produce a lot of wellbeing internally) become interactive States rather than GDP subtracters from the rest of the States.

That only occurs if you introduce individual positive/negative health and productivity into the GDP calculation, which in turn would be necessary if the Electoral College district was itself 'representative' as Article IV, Section 4 of the Constitution requires. A purple Texas might have 29 Electors instead of 38, California becomes 40 instead of 55 because of its support of Malthusian Population Traps in its urban areas. Virginia, with 13 now, would become 19 under the wellbeing formula and Ohio would have 22 instead of 18 because its wellbeing increases with stable, productive populations.

Further:

The 'purple' formula at the College eliminates unrepresentative Population Traps from absorbing the wellbeing of the surrounding EC Districts (438 Electors) and States (100 Electors).   It is calculated on a much truer GDP basis than the author's red-blue regressive divide into urban traps absorbing the wealth of states around them.

CBO projections of the sources of deficit reduction in the FY2013-2016 budget,

Expiration of 2% FICA payroll tax cut: $95B (15.65%)
Other expiring tax provisions: $65B (10.71%)
Affordable Care Act taxes: $18B (3.97%)
Spending cuts ("sequestration") under the Budget Control Act of 2011: $65B (10.71%)
Expiration of federal emergency unemployment insurance: $26B (4.28%)
Reduction in Medic not counting economic feedback.
Expiration of tax cuts and the subsequent growth in the AMT: $221B (36.41%)
are payment rates for doctors: $11B (1.81%)
Other changes (mostly revenue, primarily reflecting economic growth): $105B (17.30%)

Economic Growth

Following the economic recession, now four years long, the urgent need for jobs and infrastructure, along with affordable housing and [LI] issues will be among the most important domestic policy issues for the next president.

Budget related issues

Note that the House of Representatives is solely responsible for appropriations under Article I Section 8 of the Constitution. If the laws passed in 2016 were examined under Preamble functionality as in the associated Congressional Resume, it can be noted that some 28 law groups, including appropriations involved health or wellbeing. Many other law bundles in [CD] and [GW] are also related to wellbeing from an appropriations cost reference. Items like VA expenses are health related, items like school nutrition are health related, so the actual number of appropriations involving health components in some way could go as high as 60 major entities for one year.

Résumé of Congressional Activity

SECOND SESSION OF THE ONE HUNDRED FIFTEENTH CONGRESS

The first table gives a comprehensive résumé of all legislative business transacted by the Senate and House.

DATA ON LEGISLATIVE ACTIVITY

January 3, 2018 through January 3, 2019

	Senate	House	Total
Days in session	191	174	..
Time in session	1,013 hrs., 29'	657 hrs., 46'	..
Congressional Record:			
Pages of proceedings	8,065	10,612	..
Extensions of Remarks	..	1,751	..
Public bills enacted into law	108	221	..
Private bills enacted into law	..	1	..
Bills in conference	1	1	..
Measures passed, total	641	816	1,457
Senate bills	145	105	..
House bills	224	557	..
Senate joint resolutions	7	2	..
House joint resolutions	1	1	..
Senate concurrent resolutions	14	10	..
House concurrent resolutions	15	18	..
Simple resolutions	235	123	..
Measures reported, total	*385	*610	995
Senate bills	252	11	..
House bills	114	529	..
Senate joint resolutions	1	..	..
House joint resolutions	..	..	..
Senate concurrent resolutions	..	..	..
House concurrent resolutions	..	2	..
Simple resolutions	18	68	..
Special reports	14	33	..
Conference reports	4	5	..
Measures pending on calendar	405	217	..
Measures introduced, total	1,967	3,257	5,224
Bills	1,540	2,670	..
Joint resolutions	18	22	..
Concurrent resolutions	28	52	..
Simple resolutions	381	513	..
Quorum calls	2	2	..
Yea-and-nay votes	274	326	..
Recorded votes	..	172	..
Bills vetoed	..	..	..
Vetoes overridden	..	..	..

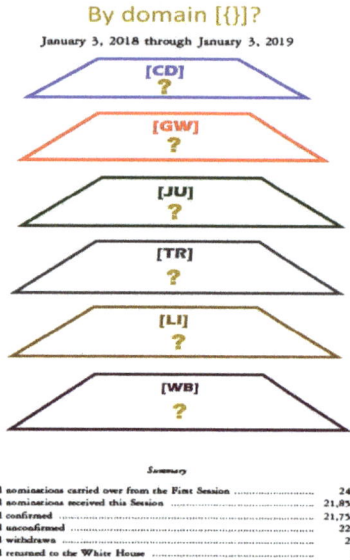

By domain [{}]?

January 3, 2018 through January 3, 2019

[CD] ?

[GW] ?

[JU] ?

[TR] ?

[LI] ?

[WB] ?

Summary

Total nominations carried over from the First Session	247
Total nominations received this Session	21,855
Total confirmed	21,751
Total unconfirmed	225
Total withdrawn	24
Total returned to the White House	0

TLO budget speculation:

While there is no national value added tax, it has been evaluated in many areas and compared to European VATs with considerable detail. Smaller Nations can use this effectively because many are at the same population density and size as American states. But the VAT is one of the most effective ways of insuring a fair distribution of healthcare cost throughout a society. Basically, every person, citizen or otherwise, has molecular degeneration over time and for others to correct this sometimes requires enormous resources of others. Any form of Keynesian or Complexity economic model indicates that you must 'put back' resources used in order to have equilibrium and this is exceptionally true of human health. At least such is the case for data through the end of the 20th century.

From Wikipedia, *Sales taxes in the United States,* 2018.05.00

> Sales taxes in the United States are taxes placed on the sale or lease of goods and services in the United States. While no national general sales tax exists, the federal government levies several national selective sales taxes on the sale or lease of particular goods and services. Furthermore, forty-five states, the District of Columbia, Puerto-Rico, and Guam impose general sales taxes that apply to the sale or lease of most goods and some services, and states also may levy selective sales taxes on the sale or lease of particular goods or services. States may also delegate to local governments the authority to impose additional general or selective sales taxes.

As of January 1, 2016, 5 states (Alaska, Delaware, Montana, New Hampshire and Oregon) do not levy a sales tax,[1] while California has the highest state sales tax rate at 7.5% (the territory of Puerto Rico has a higher 10.5% commonwealth tax that will be replaced by a value added tax in April 2016).[2][3] In some states, counties and cities impose additional sales taxes, and total sales taxes can be over 11%.

Sales tax is calculated by multiplying the purchase price by the applicable tax rate. Tax rates vary widely by jurisdiction and range from less than 1% to over 10%. Sales tax is collected by the seller at the time of sale.

Use tax is self-assessed by a buyer who has not paid sales tax on a taxable purchase. Unlike the value added tax, a sales tax is imposed only at the retail level. In cases where items are sold at retail more than once, such as used cars, the sales tax can be charged on the same item indefinitely.

The definition of retail sales and what goods and services are taxable vary among the states. Nearly all jurisdictions provide numerous categories of goods and services that are exempt from sales tax, or taxed at reduced rates. The purchase of goods for further manufacture or for resale is uniformly exempt from sales tax. Most jurisdictions exempt food sold in grocery stores, prescription medications, and many agricultural supplies.

Sales taxes, including those imposed by local governments, are generally administered at the state level. States imposing sales tax either impose the tax on retail sellers or impose it on retail buyers and require sellers to collect it. In either case, the seller files returns and remit the tax to the state. In states where the tax is on the seller, it is customary for the seller to demand reimbursement from the buyer. Procedural rules vary widely. Sellers generally must collect tax from in-state purchasers unless the purchaser provides an exemption certificate. Most states allow or require electronic remittance.

Suppose that all health-related entities, whether related to the Defense processes as Veteran activity, current injured or unit fatalities where combined in appropriations under a sales tax or a value added tax THAT HAD NO OTHER PURPOSE? The total healthcare cost in the U.S. was near $3.0 trillion. Some of the increase was due to the Affordable Care Act increase in coverage. Medicare spending in 2016 was $618.7 Billion with Medicaid (state support of healthcare with federal assistance was $480 billion and military health care including war casualties was about $44 billion. Private health insurance systems accounted for $991 billion and personal expenditures were at $329.8 billion. About 20 percent of each of these categories were for pre-natal and first year's health care. Or about $600 billion which is very close to what an 'end-product' sales tax would cover, judging from data on existing state sales taxes of 7%. Such data is nebulous because of the wide variety of tax structures in the states. For one thing the definition of 'end product' would exclude manufactured parts and possibly any item with an end value under $20 dollars which would eliminate most of life's daily necessities in food, clothing and transport.   This might pay for all medical care under the age of 18 months.

How do you make a tax fair unless the burden is proportionately distributed according to the gain by the individuals? [GW] taxes would be infrastructures equally used by all, so all should contribute. [CD] revenues are a reflection of the protection of wealth, so the higher the wealth protected, the higher the tax, but transnationals who benefit from American [CD]?

How does one determine the 'end value' of any item in a service or manufacturing process in order to add an impost that is not destructive of the produced item?

IT issues:

Improving student outcomes through an institutional approach that strategically leverages technology. Establishing a partnership between IT leadership and institutional leadership to develop a collective understanding of what information technology can deliver. Assisting faculty with the instructional integration of information technology. Developing an IT staffing and organizational model to accommodate the changing IT environment and facilitate openness and agility. Using analytics to help drive critical institutional outcomes. Changing IT funding models to sustain core service, support innovation, and facilitate growth. Addressing access demand and the wireless and device explosion. Sourcing technologies and services at scale to reduce costs (via cloud, greater centralization of institutional IT services and systems, cross-institutional collaborations, and so forth). Determining the role of online learning and developing a strategy for that role. Implementing risk management and information security practices to protect institutional IT resources/data and respond to regulatory compliance mandates. Developing an enterprise IT architecture that can respond to changing conditions and new opportunities.

Minimum wages:

{8} Climate change

2018.05.26:20:51 [WB] ⋈ [GW] +[CD] |TR| |LI|<2 |JU|<2 ≈ |OP|<1

Tzvi Kahn in TheHill, 'In Iran's water crisis, Tehran sows the seeds of its own decline':

"The regime remains unmoved. On April 22, Kayhan published an article titled, "His debauchery aside, Madani's primary crime was espionage.""

and

"If the water shortage persists, warned Isa Kalantari, the head of Iran's Department of the Environment, in a 2015 interview, 50 million Iranians will need to relocate to survive.""

If he had been engaged in espionage, he would have certainly followed the Pasdaran's own Taggayah philosophy of deceit and would have never done anything that even remotely appeared as politically incorrect or 'Western'.

As for the water shortages, saying they are 'periodic' might be correct, but under previous global warming cycles over the last 400,000 years, the drought 'period' can last a thousand years. Don't bother looking to the U.S. or E.U. for technical solutions on that little problem; they are going to be too busy building water infrastructures of their own over the next century.

2018.07.30:11:39 |CD|<3 ⋈ [GW]|2-[JU]|>2|TR|<2≈|OP|>3

Huminski in TheHill, 'Congress smartly moves forward on American national defense in space':

"The smart language on reusability also looks set to survive and become law. Under the conference version of the NDAA, the Evolved Expendable Launch Vehicle program becomes the National Security Space Launch Program. The NDAA also directs the defense secretary to pursue a strategy that includes reusable rockets in national security launches, mandates the continuation of certification processes to validate the use of these components, and requires justification for why a national security launch contract awards excludes reusable rockets."

Those reusable launch vehicles of the new Space Command might be fitted with 'environmental' pods that contain compressed hydroxil radicals to 'seed' in the stratosphere where the most dangerous, long lived methane compounds are located. These methane compounds when combined with various hydroxil radicals cease to be greenhouse warming conditionals. There is a possibility that removing 30% of the methane with 120 year life-cycles will reduce global warming temperatures by a full one degree, in turn slowing the process to a less disastrous level. But Space Command operating such re-use seed vehicles would have to be somewhat elitist; Totalitarian space forces, let alone ground forces, simply lack the necessary human empathy to carry out such a global security process with precision.

2018.11.27:08:36 |OP|<n ≈∑ [WB]|<3+|CD|<2 [TR]|<3 [LI]|<1[JU]|<1[GW]|<2

Editorial Board, WaPost, 'Our climate reality will catch up to us, no matter how hard Trump tries to bury the evidence':

"Cooking the next report will not change the facts. Mr. Trump and the Republican Party have been negligent stewards of the country's irreplaceable resources. Future Americans will not forgive or forget what these "leaders" did to them."

One study found that Chinese financial institutions supported construction of more than 50 coal-fired power plants abroad between 2001 and 2016. The authors estimate that these power plants release almost 600 million tons of CO_2 per year (more CO_2 than all but seven countries in the world) and that if these plants operate for 30 years on average, lifetime CO_2 emissions from the plants will be almost 18 Gt (roughly half of global emissions in 2017).

AND

Another study found that between 2000 and 2014, Chinese government entities spent roughly $100 billion on high-carbon projects abroad (coal, oil and gas) and roughly $60 billion on low-carbon projects abroad (mainly hydro).

It is interesting that the Chinese authoritarian government says it is 'completely committed' to the goals of the Paris Accord and yet can produce entire coal burning plants all over the world. Note: 'plants will be almost 18 Gt (roughly half of global emissions in 2017). That's 18 gigatons of CO_2 from new coal burners, some of which will be multi-fossil fuel burners.

Question: Why is it that a scan of American media publications shows a 90% partisan blame-game in their content rather than offering some mitigating solutions to global warming and cooling disasters? It is already accepted that American wealth redistribution mechanisms will not in any way change the growth in consumption of fossil fuels. How about a little media research on practical technical solutions such as mass tree planting, emission gas converters, standardized electric car mechanisms and home ethanol generators and their financing?

2018.11.01:00:00 |GW|<5⋈ |CD|<3 ∑ |TR|<2 |LI|<3⋈|JU|<3 ≈ |WB|<6⋈ |OP|<3?

https://en.wikipedia.org/wiki/Global_warming :

"Multiple independently produced instrumental datasets confirm that the 2009–2018 decade was 0.93 ± 0.07 °C (1.67 ± 0.13 °F) warmer than the pre-industrial baseline (1850–1900).[27] Currently, surface temperatures are rising by about 0.2 °C (0.36 °F) per decade.[28] Since 1950, the number of cold days and nights has decreased, and the number of warm days and nights has increased.[29] Historical patterns of warming and cooling, like the Medieval Climate Anomaly and the Little Ice Age, were not as synchronous as current warming, but may have reached temperatures as high as those of the late-20th century in a limited set of regions.[30] The observed rise in temperature and CO2 concentrations has been so rapid that even abrupt geophysical events that took place in Earth's history do not approach current rates.[31]"

and

In the scientific literature, there is an overwhelming consensus that global surface temperatures have increased in recent decades and that the trend is caused mainly by human-induced emissions of greenhouse gases.[287] No scientific body of national or international standing disagrees with this view.[288] Scientific discussion takes place in journal articles that are peer-reviewed, which scientists subject to assessment every couple of years in the Intergovernmental Panel on Climate Change reports.[289] In 2013, the IPCC Fifth Assessment Report stated that "is *extremely likely* that human influence has been the dominant cause of the observed warming since the mid-20th century".[290] Their 2018 report expressed the scientific consensus as: "human influence on climate has been the dominant cause of observed warming since the mid-20th century".

TLO: The notes at the Wikipedia site qualify as a valid consensus, so that the climate process becomes a major environment that affects all of the [domains] of the Constitution, primarily [CD] and [GW]. Over a 100-year period, this singular item has the ability to destroy ANY positive progression of We the People. There is virtually no chance of achieving Wellbeing as a human right if geophysical events begin to operate in a climate of a 5-degree F increase. The 5-degree combination of loss of energy infrastructures, agriculture land use, asymmetric warfare, imperialism or wealth concentration and human stress-procreation would result in world population reductions of 6 billion by 2140.

{9} The way income and wealth are distributed in the U.S.

2018.09.03:07:37 | ξ| <? |WB|<2 ⋈ |GW|<3 ⋈ |TR|<1 |LI|>3⋈|JU|<1 ≈ |OP|<2

Samuelson, WaPost, 'Where did our raises go? To health care.':

"Still, its [healthcare cost] chief flaw is that it is silently determining the nation's priorities without anyone assigning it that role. Medicare and Medicaid spending is squeezing most other government activities...... We recoil at disciplining health-care spending, because that seems inhumane."

Add in individual media costs (internet, cell, cable) of $1500 per year, consumer credit interest cost of $900 per year and maybe self-medication (pot, opioids, etc) costs of $4000 per year to the $5000 per year for health premiums. That $11,400 for four items is a very noticeable amount for the current $58,000 per year average income, which is actually quite good historically. It is also noticeable that all of these increase in direct proportion to any tax percentage reduction by the federal and state governments almost in the same year, so there is virtually no possibility of wage increases with tax reductions actually increasing the net worth of an individual. The process merely transfers wealth from government to an international market.

If all of these lifestyle conditions 'conspire' to prevent a person from being healthy because it is a 'fee-for-service' medical system, guess what? The fees will go up independently of any normal inflationary system (at a 9% rate instead of a 2.5% rate) because there are no economic or political checks and balances. About the only cure for that is a health system in which 'fees' are subject to a curative process rather than a treatment process. Basically, the costs increase as a function of profit per item rather than the limited profit of a cure per item group. You can multiply that 'universal' medical system where a fee's profit can be multiplied indefinitely for 300 million citizens and 40 million 'visitors' over the next 20 years.

Further:

Need something better than a system that guarantees yearly cost increases because no one is actually cured of anything like heart disease, mental illness, diabetes, genetic disorders or any of the other 3700 major medical conditions. Keep in mind molecular curative medicine was not really possible until this century.

2018.07.04:07:54 |GW|<3⋈ |CD|<1 |TR|<1 |LI|<1⋈|JU|>1 ≈ |WB|>3⋈ |OP|<2

Samuelson, WaPost, 'Trump's neo-isolationism won't work':

"To the contrary, power is being drained from nation-states to "market forces" or other global mechanisms that are difficult to control."

That is exactly the problem for We the People. America has been turned into an 'extraction' economy for a world economy rather than a North American 'internal cycle' economy. In the 1950s and 1960s, virtually all wealth generated by Americans was cycled through other North Americans in some way. Very little of that wealth was distributed worldwide, in spite of economic aid to Europe and Asia. Today, you have foreign extraction mechanisms controlled by such organizations as the Central Banks of China and Russia (net worth $8 trillion and $3 trillion) along with stateless sanctuaries like Qatar (net worth $400 billion) and Cayman Islands Monetary Authority (net worth $2 trillion), all of which are in a position to influence 'laws' in North America. But it might qualify as 'dumb' to isolate America from other North American economies; they are just too heavily integrated for mutual benefits.

But economic mutual benefit is not true if Ricardo models of free trade are manipulated around the world to protect wealth extraction from the United States (Middle East,

China, Russia, India, etc) and especially is not true if such world interests are using the extracted wealth to control the political structure of We the People. There is no doubt the manipulations are under way when the 'security' services that detect the wealth extraction are under constant de-funding attacks. True, isolationism will not work. You must know thy enemy and you can't do that when isolated to the point you don't have economic 'eyes'.

{10} Crime and violence

2018.02.27:07:30 |OP|>2 ≈∑ |TR|<3 |LI|>3⋈|JU|<1….|GW|>1

Gerson, WaPost, 'It's apocalypse now on guns':

"When I look at many of the people holding the guns, I don't really view them as legitimate protectors of my rights, or as qualified to make choices about the employment of violence in politics. I don't view America as halfway to tyranny. And I am grateful that Americans such as the Rev. Martin Luther King Jr. — who suffered actual oppression by government — made a principled commitment to nonviolent political change."

If one looks carefully at 'the people holding guns', he might find that the personality of someone with a Saturday night special in the middle of a subway robbery is very different from someone sneaking through the underbrush with a hog-stopper 357. Or the difference between an opiated sawed-off auto holder and the 'deputy' trying to protect against him with a pistol that is accurate to 25 feet. The point is that with 45 million 'holders' in the country, the defense against State tyranny is almost non-existent and the political use of weapons AND the abuse of guns is at a very low level. Charlottesville, Albemarle County, VA has maybe 60 violent crimes a year in a region with nearly 10,000 rifles. It's one major civil incident in 2017 had many displayed rifles on the street and yet the only violent act was with a rental car.

The idea of Americans 'holding guns' for political reasons or that they are irresponsible just doesn't exist, regardless of crowded urban street perceptions. In theory, an advancing civilization would have household 'weapons', including guns, in safe areas of the home and have the training necessary to maintain and use them. It is NOT the prohibition of dangerous devices in a Republic that should be the issue; it is whether the citizens are advanced enough, through literacy and consciousness, to use the 'weapon' effectively.

Further:

Having been given a human right in the 2nd Amendment as part of an advancing civilization compared to the rest of the world in 1789, it is necessary that the bearer of arms demonstrate he actually is 'advanced' on a day-to-day basis, something only modern psychiatric testing could do. Such as universal bio-medical diagnostics?

Of course, it could be noted that many Europeans and Asians consider it beneath their dignity to use or handle a tool or a weapon.

2018.04.03:07:30 |OP|<1 ≈ ∑ |TR|>3 |LI|>3⋈|JU|<1….|GW|<2

Noah Feldman in BloombergView, 'Second Amendment Repeal Would Hurt Constitution':

"To be sure, it's logically possible to think that the justices have the authority to decide the Heller case, which overturned restrictions on handguns in the District of Columbia, but that their judgement should be overturned by an amendment."

The Court in its Heller opinion was very specific in overturning a group of gun regulations in the District of Columbia BECAUSE those 'laws' effectively banned and criminalized the possession of ANY ballistic arms. The regulations, taken in total, and because of the admitted intent of banning weapons for ideological political reasons, was a clear violation of the 2nd Amendment's intent and reason for being in the Constitution. The opinions of the Court made that very clear, and specifically left open the question of the degree to which a community had the authority to control ballistic devices. Any reasonable regulation for public safety was acceptable, but not a fantasy ban of a constitutional 'right'.

From a practical standpoint, the District is one of the last places in the U.S. where weapons, especially rifles, should be allowed, and the Constitution gives the Congress the authority to control such devices on ANY federally related territory, including parks, military bases or even federal enclaves relinquished to the federal government by the 'several states' (see Article I, Section 8). Therefore, the repeal of the 2nd Amendment human right, and it is, by an amendment process is pointless.

We needn't go into the philosophical idea that the inability to possess AND control weapons, including some modern ones that qualify as Simple Weapons of Mass Destruction (SWMD: any combination of human molecular and device molecular systems that can cause permanent degenerative harm to many humans within a 30 meter radius), is a societal indication of an evolutionary failure because of the incompetence of its members.

2018.06.20:11:54 [ξ|<3 |WB|<2 ⋈ |GW|>3⋈ |TR|>2 |LI|<3⋈|JU|<1 ≈ |OP|>1

Berman, WaPost, 'Active shooters usually get their guns legally and then target specific victims, FBI says'

"Other research has similarly found tenuous links connecting shooting rampages and mental illness. In a 2015 study, Michael Stone, a clinical psychiatry professor at Columbia University, examined 235 people who carried out or attempted to carry out mass killings, and he concluded that about 22 percent could be considered mentally ill. An article published the same year in the academic journal Annals of Epidemiology found that "the large majority of people with mental disorders do not engage in violence against others, and that most violent behavior is due to factors other than mental illness."

That probably means the FBI profilers are using the DSM IV rather than the DSM-V (Diagnostic and Statistical Manual for Mental Disorders) which contains much more detail about PTSD. Stress disorders do not necessarily mean mental illness in the neurological sense, although one can trigger the other. The conclusion by the profilers that nearly all of the perpetrators had some form of developing stress disorder is probably correct; many of the mass shootings were proceeded by careful planning, which true mental disorder might not allow. But that also means warning signs were ignored and that might not be something modern societies can afford, rights and justice for all being involved.

Curative treatment as a mandated health 'right' for PTSD might be the solution.

2018.10.20:19:36 [WB]>2⋈ [GW]>3⋈ [CD]<3∑ |TR|<2 |LI|<3⋈|JU|<3 ≈ |OP|<2?

Bonnie Rothman in WaPost, 'Those 'superhumans' of the future Stephen Hawking feared? Look around.':

"For now, we don't seem too keen to engineer superhumanity. According to a Pew Research Center survey released in July, only 19 percent of Americans think it's acceptable to edit for intelligence. But it doesn't take a Stephen Hawking to see that we already live in a world of "significant political problems" and underprivileged humans who increasingly "won't be able to compete.""

Hawking was not really worried about super 'humans' coming into existence as much as mutations who are inherently predatory toward normal, 'self-improving' humans. True, only 19 percent of Americans think creating enhanced IQs was acceptable. But two Chinese universities, one thousandth of one per cent of the Chinese people, already have major laboratory editing facilities collecting DNA data on high IQ individuals. And you cannot study at these universities unless you are a member of the 'Party' or an offspring of a Party Member. There are 'elite' research structures similar to this in several western universities and military structures that are concerned with this as well.

But it is the 'mutations' that are the main concern, not the 'rational' child bearing brought about by literate pairs of humans. A genetically induced sociopath might be created as a DNA mutation because he, as a mutation, is less than a hundredth of one percent of the human population. A certifiable sociopath, with considerable IQ, from birth named Saddam Hussein managed to have violent humanity ripple effects of 700,000 deaths over 27 years and two trillion dollars of destruction around the world. A survey of DNA related ripple effects of violence in America might be as high as 3000 deaths a year and $100 billion in directly related economic effects.

A mutated predator bred in an artificial womb with 'selected' DNA sequences is a real possibility, just as Hawking visualized. Even a fairly rigorous Constitutional system of checks and balances on 'unnatural' genetic sequences might not protect future generations from the mutations that have already occurred.

2018.10.27:09:26 [CD]>3 ≈|OP|<4....|WB|<1+|JU|>2 ⋈ [GW]<2

Carless in WaPost, 'Brazil's version of Trump makes Trump look like Mr. Rogers':

"And, crucially, Bolsonaro has promised to wage war on Brazil's favelas, poor neighborhoods overwhelmingly populated by nonwhites, where most police violence already occurs. "I will give police carte blanche to kill," he has said. "Police that kill thugs will be decorated.""

Are the favelas really another version of the Malthusian Population Trap (MPT) that extreme politicians are reacting to? The density of the Rio de Janeiro favelas like Rocinha is something like 47,000 per square mile (Cudahy, Los Angelas: 22,000 per sq mi, and Caloocan, Philippines: 72,000 per sq mi) and actually consumes the energy, food and health resources of the Rio city region. The same MPTs might exist in Sao Palo and Sergipe.

Suppose the local cartel discovered that a density of 47,000 per sq mile was perfect (constant stress induces drug use) for a drug enslaved captive population? What would be the choices of ANY national government when confronted with a Malthusian Population Trap controlled by a drug cartel determined to 'improve' its holdings?

2018.12.13:20:35 |OP| $\approx\sum$ |WB|<n+|CD|<2 |TR|<n |LI|<1 ⋈ |JU|<n|GW|<4

Josh Horwitz in TheHill, 'Five gun violence prevention priorities for the incoming Congress':

"With the 116th Congress, we have an opportunity to create change and save lives. Universal background checks, extreme risk laws, an assault weapons ban, protections for those experiencing domestic violence and funding for gun violence prevention are of the utmost importance."

Taken together, these five items could be worded by a legislature in a state government to effectively ban ANY ballistic device or 'gun'. The 'law' language, including in popular referendums, has in many ways been so vague or undecipherable that a 'law' enforcement office or a prosecutor or even a psychiatrist would be allowed to determine whether a weapon is banned regardless of the 2nd Amendment. This has been true of well-meaning laws in several states and the ones in the District of Columbia and Chicago combined in such a manner that a gun could not be possessed at all. The Supreme Court tossed these laws simply because their vagueness effectively banned everyone from having a gun. That is a nowhere progression and always has been.

One possible solution is to differentiate between 'all guns' and 'simple weapons of mass destruction' (SWMD). The AR-15, AK-47, and several European pistols (banned in the country of manufacture, by the way) all have interchangeable trigger assemblies that have been modified by mass destruction junkies to make them near automatic as SWMD. It is almost as easy to make the trigger assembly with a 'safety' button built in that must be pressed each time the weapon is fired. That reduces the rapid fire capability by as much as two-thirds while increasing the aiming requirement for accuracy. That takes the gun out of the SWMD category altogether.

In order to be fair under the Second Amendment and not make unconstitutional ex post facto laws, a law requiring mandatory trigger safeties would have to be precisely written so that the modification only applied to the sale or resale of a gun after a specified date. A person could keep all the original weapons he wants in his hazardous material locker, along with medications, house cleaners, legal pot, 120 proof home brew and bug sprays. The mandatory hazards locker is also a gun safety need (negligent use of SWMD unless locked up) that might be considered by the state legislatures since it couldn't be constitutionally mandated by the Congress.

Would a simple safety switch requirement on firearm trigger pulls reduce the mass misuse and return weapons to a self-defense category as originally intended by the 2ns Amendment?

{13} Unemployment

2018.09.21:06:20 [TR]>3 = $\sum$ [LI]>1[WB]<2 ⋈ [GW]>1-[JU]<2....[OP]>2

Mellnik and Williams, WaPost, 'Is Canada 'ripping' us off'? Or is it the best U.S. trade partner?':

"For Trump to impose the 25 percent auto tariff, the U.S. Commerce Department must find that auto and parts imports threaten national security. .....“A car put together with American-made parts is not a national security threat," Toyota spokesman Ed Lewis said."

The trade between local industrial organizations only becomes a national security issue if any one of the manufacturing 'entities' in the North American Economic Union (Greenland, Canada, U.S.A., Mexico, Caribbean, Central America, Polynesia) becomes dependent on non-Union energy and materials in order to stay in business. If the auto parts subcomponents like the plastic coverings, touch screens or piston ring alloys are made outside the NAE Union and shipped in, they become dependent on the political and economic motivations of a hostile power. It would be more cost effective to have ALL of the components of a given product made within 1000 kilometers of the assembly plant itself and that would apply to all industrial processes within the Union (4 million total jobs?). The Lexus engine graphic in the article doesn't show a hidden transportation cost of perhaps $50 per engine because of the multiple assemblies. It might be better to have each of the locations shown as a 'final' assembly with the parts being made within a 1000 km of those assembly points.

The same rule might apply to medical and sport health equipment manufacturers, provided raw materials are available within the Union. Some things, like ethanol, might be regionally dependent and only be cost effective to produce in sunny regions of the Union like the Caribbean. They might qualify as an energy reserve area when the oil and shale deposits of Canada, Mexico and the U.S. are consumed in this century.

Further:

The idea for the big three of the Union is to build a common manufacturing distributed infrastructure that is independent of anything else over the next century and quibbling over 25% of a $10.00 item within the economic borders of such a Union might be counter-productive in the long run. But not if the sub-component materials can be shut off by a cartel somewhere on a moment's notice. Canada and Mexico can 'rip us off' at a 4 or 5 per cent level any time and it won't matter in the slightest unless they are doing it by bootlicking some totalitarian economic interest somewhere.

[GW] 2018 Conclusions:

General Welfare normally includes most of the items for what might be called 'wellbeing', such as healthcare, criminal justice violence and nutrition security. Many items, especially anything involving national infrastructures, are easily within the Article I authorities of governance. Some {sets} below can be calculated as just Tranquility for bringing peace and equilibrium ({4},{9})between the states, with climate change disasters {8} rapidly approaching a Common Defense problem on a national scale as well. It is noticeably becoming a popular consensus problem with its standing about halfway in the priorities people see. But We the People also see that the problems in General Welfare are becoming increasingly difficult to solve ({7},{10},{11},(13}) as population densities increase and become affiliated with non-citizenship.

These [GW] conditions are taken from various polls of people's concerns prior to the off-year elections of 2018. Off year elections are sometimes a better indicator of the concerns because they don't involve the personalities of contending leaderships. The {sets} for [GW] only:

{1} The economy, tax cuts and jobs Act,

{4} The size and power of the federal government: cybersecurity, AI development

{5} The Social Security system

{7} Hunger and homelessness

{8} Climate change

{9} The way income and wealth are distributed in the U.S.

{10} Crime and violence

{11} Race relations

{12} Drug use, FDA Reauthorization Act, CARA, opioid deaths: [CD]?

{13} Unemployment

{14} The quality of the environment, Pandemic Act expires

{15} The availability and affordability of energy

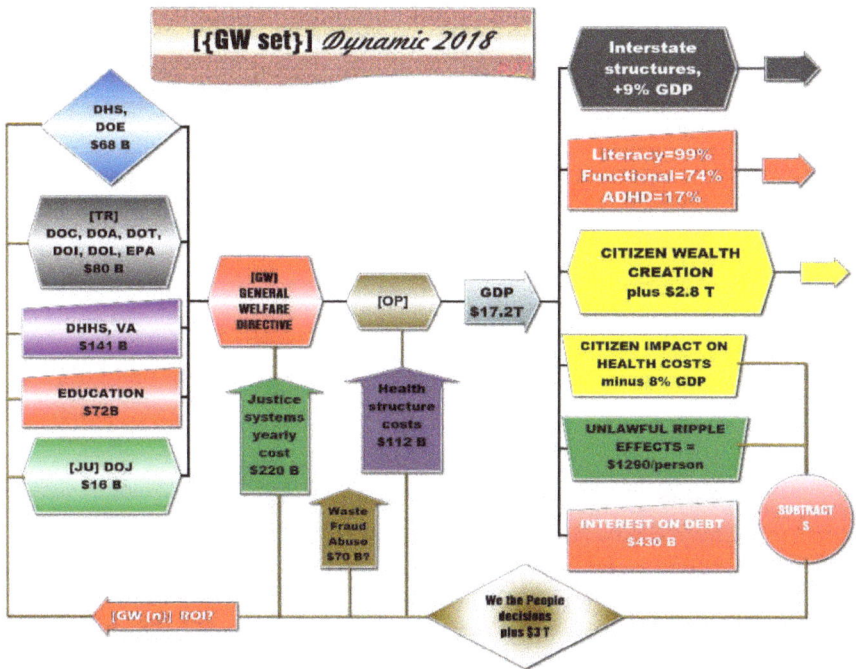

What has dismayed many Americans over the last few decades is that there seems to be no end to the problems in the society and yet the [CD] directive has actually kept those problems from becoming Posterity destroyers, with the [GW] set able to show enhancements of some magnitude over the same time period. The climate changes of the last century are beginning to show impact signs of increasing severity on America in that snow, windstorms, flooding and wildfire damages are becoming $100 billion a year costs to the Nation. It isn't an issue of blaming humanity for this; it is an issue of the [CD] and [GW] reaction to it. The combination of [GW] and [CD] balance has also improved the infrastructure, education and health care through the ACA and Chip subsystems. Considering minimum wages, same sex 'marriage' or contractual arrangements, BYOD usage (a police body camera is a BYOD) and internet identity theft major issues are sure signs that no survival or existential issues beset the Americans in 2018.

A graphic for the [GW set] might show many plus and minuses in various segments of society according to the original use of the 'dynamical system' definition: 'ability for adaptation, communication, cooperation, specialization, spatial and temporal organization, and reproduction. They can be found on all levels: cells specialize, adapt and reproduce themselves just like larger organisms do.' The [GW set] clearly does these things with varying degrees of success or failure, in this graphic of the set [TR], [JU] and [LI] set are shown in relation to General Welfare. Remember, General Welfare is noted as a prime directive in both the Preamble and the Article I authorities of Congress. It is also well noted in the Declaration of Independence, although not as a dynamical {se}t and the Declaration was not submitted to referendum like the Bill of Rights.

[TR] is a set in which Executive departments contribute toward a better [GW] and eventually to a better [OP] if they are organized well. Many issues between conservatives and liberals (or libertarians or anarchists) are ones the 'quanta' or 'exergy' value of each subset are measured or railed against. Exergy is an energy term that in the system of systems for [GW] is designated in dollar amounts and a very large segment of [GW] dollars is for [TR] related functions such as Agriculture, Transportation, Labor and various environmental processes. Justice [JU] is actually a combination of all three branches of government with its costs to society a direct taxpayer 'exergy' liability. It is more of an exergy value because many of the harmful ripple effects of predatory attacks on humans can't be measured in dollars , but in losses of [LI], [WB], and [TR] human capital. Human capital is an expression of the net worth an individual uses to create other wealth. The dollar cost of Justice for All, not just individual liberty [LI], can be quite high as a [WB] subset. But in 2016 the sum might not be as bad as places with severe Malthusian Population Traps such as Iraq and Syria or Venezuela. Katrina and Sandy were the nearest things came to the anarchical Traps

Just looking at the graphic indicates the slow drip, drip, drip of exergy costs entering society in the [TR] and [JU] sets. Health care costs, criminal justice costs, ADHD and mental dysfunction costs all drag on enhancing Posterity, even if some $2.8 trillion actually was produced as American and international wealth.

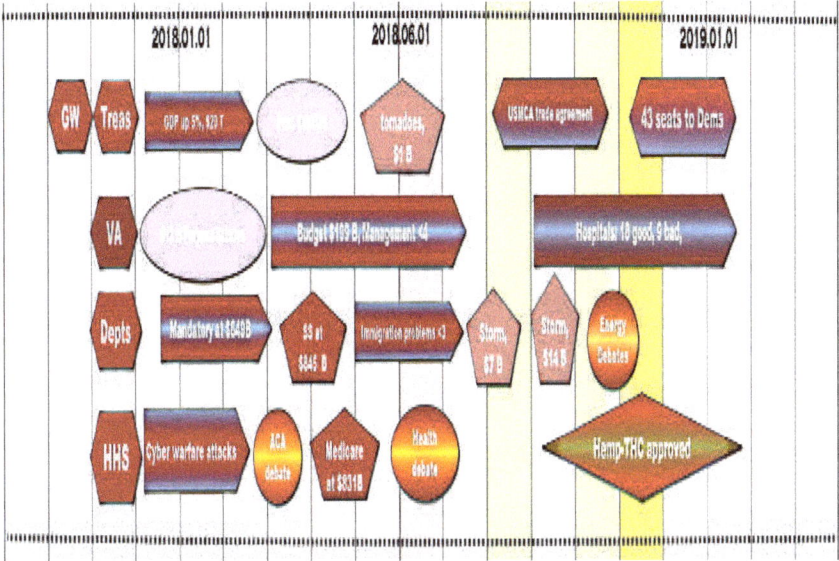

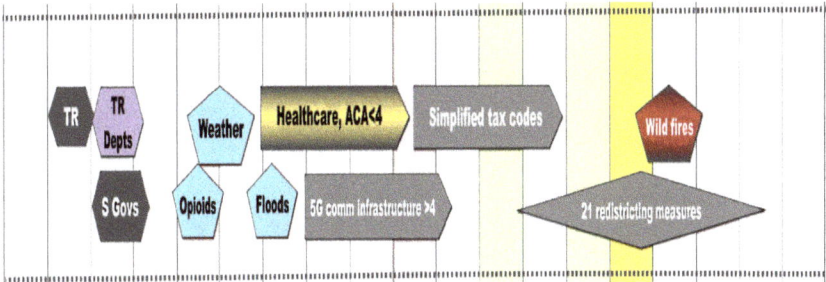

Liberty [LI]

The definition of [LI] had not changed in 2018, although the {elements} had moved into different positive and negative reconfigurations. Basically, Liberty [LI] is defined in America by the Bill of Rights in relations with government and is defined for interpersonal liberty by health and income or 'life, liberty and pursuit of happiness' with various interpretations and responsibilities attached. In America, the second Amendment on the right to bear arms (it is a human right because it was given by referendum to We the People in 1789) is a major contention since it can also violate many other rights during abuse. Liberty is the ability to be free of restraint, the ability to have 'consciousness', the ability to improve life, and perhaps the ability to have functional body parts. [Liberty] does not mean the ability to carry out primate parasitic aggression against other humans that violates THEIR [Liberty]; it must be maintained as equally valid for all. The main forms are:

Life liberty

Economic Liberty

Civil Liberty

Physical Liberty

These can be found in the Constitution as prohibitions on power, the Bill of Rights and a number of other Amendments, especially the 14th, which defined equal protection of liberty and equal due process of law concerning liberty. The combination can be seen in a Quality of Life Index.

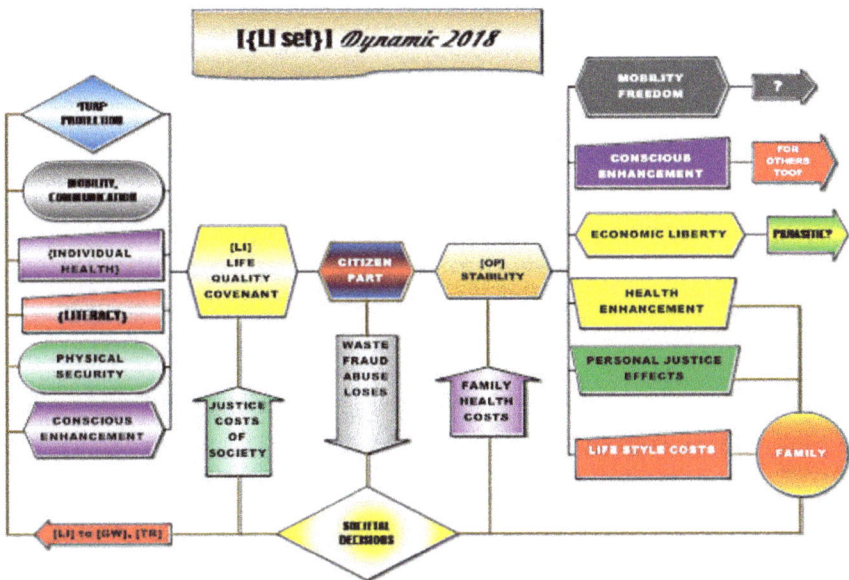

Figure 18. Liberty [LI] dynamic

{1} Life Liberty

2018.07.15:07:16 |LI|<3|TR|<2|WB|<2+|CD|<3 ⋈|GW|>1-|JU|<2≈|OP|<1

Julie Burkhart in TheHill, 'The terror of a future without Roe':

"Among other restrictions, Kansas has laws on the books requiring women to receive state mandated anti-choice materials that are purposely meant to discourage her from having an abortion, and then wait 24 hours before the procedure. Minors seeking an abortion must obtain dual parental consent, and women must be offered to view the ultrasound image of their fetus before obtaining an abortion."

This sounds a bit like someone reading a person their 'rights' during a pre-trial process. If the woman doesn't understand that she is creating life with her womb, how is she competent to make a choice that respects human life? Some women aren't even aware they 'accidently' created life until the second trimester. If the life being created has any of the 1400 birth 'anomalies' (Fragile X Syndrome, Downs Syndrome, Encephalopathy, diabetes, heart defects, etc) already detected by Genomic DNA mapping, it is almost certainly going to be an 'undue burden' to the citizens around the birth mother who is unaware of what she is creating.

Question: If a woman was designed by evolution to create life and she has a 'human right' to do exactly that, what are her 'citizenship' responsibilities in creating an entity that is certain to be a burden, spiritual, economic, or temporal, to others? Abortion is only a part of the procreation 'right', not an end value. If a woman has the 'right', what are the responsibilities within a human society that might carry the burden of the right? What is the real terror involved?

Note that the question couldn't be asked when Row v. Wade was considered, only after the DNA mapping was completed in this century.

2018.03.01:07:15 |WB|>3⋈ |TR|<1 |LI|<3⋈|JU|<4 ≈ |GW|>3⋈ |CD|<1 +|OP|>2?

Ignatius, WaPost, 'Are Saudi Arabia's reforms for real? A recent visit says yes.':

From the Serbian Numbeo database, contributed data with no warranty but reasonably accurate and is consistent with other general OECD indexes of this sort:

Top 60 Quality of Life Indexes computed from 11 lifestyle factors

Rank(1)

Country(2)

Quality of Life Index, higher better (3) https://www.numbeo.com/quality-of-life/rankings.jsp

Purchasing Power Index, higher better(4)

Safety Index, higher better (5)

Health Care Index, higher better (6)

Cost of Living Index, lower better (7)

Property Price to Income Ratio, lower better (8)

Traffic Commute Time Index, lower better (9)

Pollution Index, lower better (10)

Climate Index, higher better (11)

#..(1)	(2)	(3)	(4)	(5)	(6)	(7)	(8)	(9)	(10)	(11)
9th United States....	180.56	127.62	50.42	68.38	72.95	3.34	34.74	31.70	78.23	
31st Saudi Arabia...	149.58	131.46	63.31	60.19	47.86	2.79	34.01	71.72	41.02	
51st Russia...........	103.32	51.11	54.80	56.77	43.89	11.44	48.26	63.26	44.70	
58th Iran................	92.43	45.60	50.60	51.22	34.56	12.45	49.46	81.21	69.54	

Speculation: The new Saudi government set out to improve this Quality of Life Index on a yearly basis and if it is doing that, it doesn't have as far to go as some others. But are some of the others carrying out a war of attrition against the new Prince so that the QLI can't possibly increase?

TLO: intra-state relations do not always have domain values for the U.S. Generally, applying [JU], [LI], [TR] and [WB] effects locally will aid American [CD] and [GW] sets and in some combinations affect [OP] negatively, as in war and genocide. Note Item (3) comparative scales. But are all QLI items domain subsets in the U.S.A.?

Text- only descriptions on the internet won't let you 'see' the whole {set}.

The Quality of Life Index is a reasonably accurate assessment of [{LI}] in many sets and does reflect the four {forms}used here. Note that the comment made concerning a comparison of 'liberties' in Saudi Arabia and The U.S. is a comparison between totalitarian and democratic societies and that might be the best base line. Once the [{LI}] forms start to take hold as Liberty, the base line becomes the lowest levels of the QOL Index for a 'free' society, not totalitarian regressions. A form of the Standard Evolutionary Model?

{2} Economic Liberty:

Economy liberty is a difficult {subset} of [LI] because many people perceive themselves to be freer without a large personal income, but generally many things in life simply will not exist without a personal infrastructure of wealth associated Liberty. A person who cannot do 'work' to feed, cloth, or protect himself does not have liberty. A person who does work that consumes wealth of others also might not have liberty.

https://www.census.gov/library/visualizations/interactive/2018-median-household-income.html#

Real Personal Income for States: Percent Change, 2017–2018

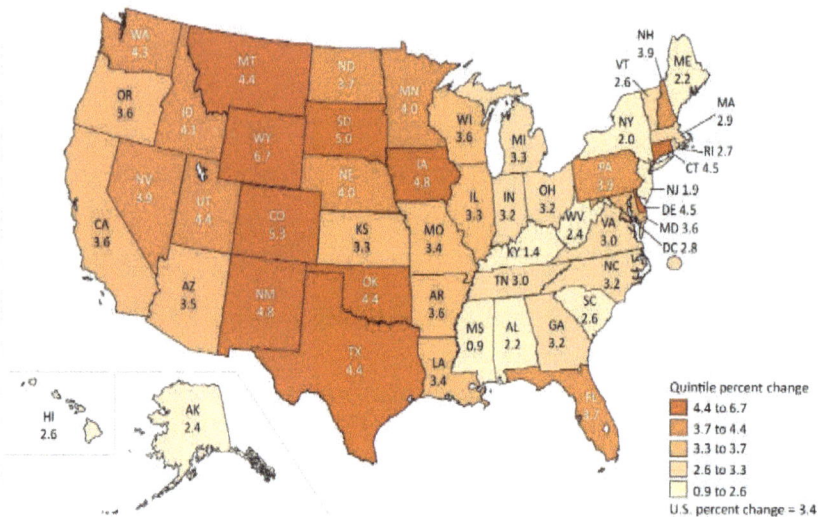

Quintile percent change
- 4.4 to 6.7
- 3.7 to 4.4
- 3.3 to 3.7
- 2.6 to 3.3
- 0.9 to 2.6

U.S. percent change = 3.4

U.S. Bureau of Economic Analysis

2018.09.03:07:37 [ξ] <? |WB|<2 ⋈ |GW|<3 ⋈ |TR|<1 |LI|>3⋈|JU|<1 ≈ |OP|<2

Samuelson, WaPost, 'Where did our raises go? To health care.':

"Still, its [healthcare cost] chief flaw is that it is silently determining the nation's priorities without anyone assigning it that role. Medicare and Medicaid spending is squeezing most other government activities…… We recoil at disciplining health-care spending, because that seems inhumane."

Add in individual media costs (internet, cell, cable) of $1500 per year, consumer credit interest cost of $900 per year and maybe self-medication (pot, opioids, etc) costs of $4000 per year to the $5000 per year for health premiums. That $11,400 for four items is a very noticeable amount for the current $58,000 per year average income, which is actually quite good historically. It is also noticeable that all of these increase in direct proportion to any tax percentage reduction by the federal and state governments almost in the same year, so there is virtually no possibility of wage increases with tax reductions actually increasing the net worth of an individual. The process merely transfers wealth from government to an international market.

If all of these lifestyle conditions 'conspire' to prevent a person from being healthy because it is a 'fee-for-service' medical system, guess what? The fees will go up independently of any normal inflationary system (at a 9% rate instead of a 2.5% rate) because there are no economic or political checks and balances. About the only cure for that is a health system in which 'fees' are subject to a curative process rather than a treatment process. Basically, the costs increase as a function of profit per item rather than the limited profit of a cure per item group. You can multiply that 'universal' medical system where a fee's profit can be multiplied indefinitely for 300 million citizens and 40 million 'visitors' over the next 20 years.

Further:

Need something better than a system that guarantees yearly cost increases because no one is actually cured of anything like heart disease, mental illness, diabetes, genetic disorders or any of the other 3700 major medical conditions. Keep in mind molecular curative medicine was not really possible until this century.

{3} Healthcare aspect of life Liberty:

2018.06.29:12:32 |CD|>2 ≈|OP|>2 Ξ|[LI]>2WB|<1+|JU|>2 ⋈ |GW|>2

Bever in WaPost, 'A plan to keep drug users from shooting up in public restrooms — and why it may be a bad idea':

"Jon D. Groussman, president of CAP Index Inc., a security consulting firm based in Exton, Pa., said that "in certain markets where you know you're having a problem, it's worth trying." But he added that closely monitoring public restrooms and sending employees to check on them periodically is typically "the best deterrent."

This problem might resolve itself in the near future. Some of the new bio-sensors for gas emissions are so sensitive that they can be incorporated into self-cleaning 'smoke detector' devices that can be place in bathrooms and detect ANY form of drug or hostile molecule arrangements. They may even be sensitive enough, with AI interpreters, to detect health problems by analyzing urine and feces gases in the bathroom.

Question: Since a person with chemical imbalances in his brain or organs almost always represents a misdemeanor imminent danger to others through various psychotic episodes, inability to drive devices, clumsiness, predatory de-inhibition, or sudden suicidal impulses, why would his expectation of privacy be true in ANY location?

{4} Civil Liberty related:

2018.06.28:12:23 Σ |LI|>3|TR|<2|WB|<2+| ξ |<n? ⋈ |GW|>1-|JU|<2 ≈ |OP|>

Ashley Baker in TheHill, 'Gorsuch's dissent in 'Carpenter' case has implications for the future of privacy':

"Rather than focus on the reasonable expectation of privacy analysis typically engaged in by the court in recent decades, Gorsuch's dissent argues that the court should follow a property rights-based theory of the Fourth Amendment. Under that theory, Carpenter had a property interest in his cell phone data. Gorsuch's decision to file a dissent may send a message to future defendants that without inclusion of a property-based argument his concurrence cannot be counted on."

Fourth Amendment, BOR:

"The right of the people to be secure in their persons, houses, papers, and effects, against unreasonable searches and seizures, shall not be violated, and no Warrants shall issue, but upon probable cause, supported by Oath or affirmation, and particularly describing the place to be searched, and the persons or things ..."

Note the 'and' between the two clauses. If one was an Originalist, the 'and' would mean that the 'to be secure in their effects' was a right in its own context and not dependent on the following clause involving government or judiciary warrants describing the 'effect'. As a stand-alone human right, ANY seizure of a person's effects (ie, property) by ANY party would be an abuse of the right. Since information about a person is created in real time by that person, it should be his property under copyright law at least, not ANY third party who may hold it and definitely not someone who reproduces it for his own use. That would be a clear violation of the individual's intellectual property rights and might even be extended to include his DNA structure since he is continually recreating it with new DNA cells in his body. Wither the DNA was originally created by the parents and might belong to them is another matter.

In this instance of Court analysis, the 'effects' right of electronic data might supersede any other persons right to the data, including governmental, so the Carpenter opinion might be perfectly correct.

Question: If the 'effect' information in a mobile device involved a probable cause that it would cause harm to others as an imminent threat, such as a cell phone triggering an IED or nerve gas canister, would the individual right still stand? In virtually any case of even suspected imminent danger to others, the individual rights are suspended and that too is perfectly correct from a Constitutional point. How would the Court interpret an imminent danger threat VS rights in a molecular (EMR, electronic, binary, DNA, etc) property context?

2018.10.09:10:14   [LI|>3? ⋈ |TR|<2|WB|<2+|CD|<1 ⋈ [GW|>1-|JU|<2 ≈ |OP|>1

John Soloman in TheHill. 'FBI's smoking gun: Redactions protected political embarrassment, not 'national security':

"So we can now say with some authority that the earlier redaction in Footnote 43 was done in the name of a national security concern that did not exist."

A condition of national security is an irrelevant argument during an official inquiry into possible criminal activity. As constitutionally legitimate officers of the investigating authority, they (Justice Department or FBI or NSA or any other) are bound by the 4th Amendment's 'shall be secure in their persons (that is, identity) .....and effects (that is, information they create) against unreasonable seizure. It is unreasonable at the point of meaningless disclosure. That would hold true in ANY investigative procedure UNTIL the personal information is revealed in a criminal court preceding, where it must be made open as part of a public trial according to the 6th Amendment.

There is nothing in the Constitution that bestows an 'investigative privilege' to any private citizen, including all media entities engaged in for-profit activities, so that the 4th Amendment can be set aside. Revealing ANY information about a person, except in a case of direct, imminent danger to others without their express consent violates the 4th Amendment protections and the security status of the data involved has no point.

2018.12.26:07:20 [LI|>3|TR|<2|WB|<2⋈|GW|>n|JU|<2

Lane, WaPost, 'I thought fraud in reporting was done for. I was wrong.':

"That [human distortion] includes journalism. Reporters and editors are as susceptible to motivated reasoning and confirmation bias as readers are, though we say, and believe, that professional norms and training equip us to resist distorting influences."

Lots of people want the world to appear exactly as their 'learned' view of it dictates. That would appear in the expressions of politics, economics, or ethnicity by both the left and right, with the frequency of the distortion increasing the more 'far-out' the individual becomes. That is why you have entire city populations with approximately the same sentiments on a subject even when the sentiments have no basis in reality. Some even call that the 'Galileo Effect' in which there is zero tolerance for sentiments other than the local prevailing one.

Claas Relotius may have become expert at enhancing the local Germanic beliefs about Americans or other cultures but he certainly isn't alone when it comes to the Galileo Effect.

2018.04.15:08:21 [LI]>3-[JU]<2 WB]<2+[CD]<3 ⋈[GW]<1≈ |OP]>3

Bowden, TheHill, 'Gingrich calls Mueller investigation 'breakdown' of constitutional law':

"This is why we have a bill of rights," Gingrich added. "I think what we're watching is a breakdown of the whole concept of constitutional rule of law. I think it's really very sobering, and a real threat to every American."

A Speaker, who had access to ALL national security Congressional Committee data, should know that the Common Defense authorities of Article I, Section 8 powers of the Constitution automatically supersede any individual rights as defined in the Bill of Rights or subsequent 'rights' in the Amendments. The rights, as amendments, are DEVOLVED from the Common Defense of the constitution, not co-equals if any political partisan group is engaged in an international activity that supports a non-constitutional economic or political interest of a foreigner, government affiliated or otherwise.

To advocate that a person occupying American soil, citizen or otherwise, has an unlimited personal right to earn a living through foreign revenue sources without being subject to the Common Defense authority of the Constitution is simply nonsense. Partisan political power exceptions to investigation has nothing to do with protecting the Constitution, no matter what 'party' is involved.

{5}   Physical Liberty related:

2018.03.04:10:02 ∑ [LI]>3[TR]<2|WB]<2+[CD]<3 ⋈[GW]-|JU]<2≈|OP]<?

Ana Marie Cox, WaPost, 'Trump actually thinks executing drug dealers would help. That's the problem.':

"There's no real need to explain why the execution of drug dealers is a bad idea, though it is a very, very bad idea. The country has already tried an aggressive enforcement approach to drug crimes — the four-decade-plus war on drugs — and among experts and law enforcement officers, it is almost universally acknowledged as a massive failure in economic and practical terms."

The 'war on drugs' never applied the necessary crime against humanity criteria the 1998 Rome Statute Section (k) against a WMD chemical distributor, whether it was permanently disabling drugs, radiation or poisons being created. Possibly wasn't systematized enough. Although many of the addicted distributors need treatment (regardless of skin tone) rather than imprisonment, the manufacturer and distributor of the WMD substances is not in that category. That form of genocidal predator, and his capital or media supporters, has engaged in a systematized attack on humanity no different from using VX neurotoxin bombs against Syrian towns. The neurological effects, whether slow or fast, are identical as far as a human brain is concerned and constitute a crime against humanity. It is not a matter of punishing or deterring a cartel-level WMD maker as it is permanently removing him and his co-conspirators from contact with the human race.

Speculation: since advocacy of leniency for a distributor of 'pleasure' is because the advocate needs that 'pleasure' (that is, he has adapted to the drug-food), could any person who wants easy availability of WMD devices be taken seriously as an advocate of Justice for all 'humans'?

2018.08.13:07:32 |OP|>3 ≈ ∑ |TR|>3 |LI|<3 ⋈ |JU|>1....|GW|>2 [ξ| >2 |WB|>2

Editorial Board, WaPost, 'An assault on minority voting continues in North Carolina': "Voting laws, including for felons, vary enormously across the country. In some states the right to vote is restored automatically when people leave prison; in others, including North Carolina, felons are required to complete their sentences, including serving probation or paying fines, before their rights are restored. Elsewhere, ex-felons face waits of several years before they can regain voting rights. In two states, felons may vote even while incarcerated."

The issue for a Federally related election is whether the person attempting to vote actually has the status of a citizen. Restoration of citizenship rights such as voting, driving, bearing arms, or mobility (ankle-bracelet, breathalyzer) should be conditional on proving that citizenship itself has been re-acquired, a federal Naturalization Clause activity, not a local regulatory process. That is, there is nothing that says the Naturalization Clause cannot require all persons convicted of high crimes and misdemeanors to take a verifiable citizenship test while attached to a biometric analyzer (aka polygraph, but more modern and accurate). This citizenship bio-test could even be a requirement for parole from an institution regardless of state and it is purely within federal jurisdiction.

The idea is that a person who violates the 'rights' of others by predatory aggression (robbery, fraud, misuse of lethal devices like drugs and guns, political defamation, etc) losses his own in proportion and these have to be re-earned by self-education with biotesting. That would also eliminate the easily abused skin tone test now common in the world by accurately taking the measure of a being's citizenship or empathy toward humans.

Further:

21 minutes ago:

Or how about you act like a civilized nation and take seriously the "inalienable" before "rights"? If you commit a crime, you will lose your freedom for a time. But voting rights should be irrevocable. What about the wrongfully convicted? Will they get to retroactively vote in all the elections they weren't allowed to participate in? One person, one vote - whether that person is a billionaire, a store clerk or a convict, whether they live in a rural town or a major city.

22 minutes ago: So, are you saying people lose their citizenship if they commit a crime and get put in jail? Or should? "biotest" for parole to answer what question? What will we require of those committing white collar crimes? The same citizenship test? Or, is this all about immigration for you?

14 minutes ago: They actually do lose their citizenship 'rights' if they go to prison in most states, even though 'citizenship' is strictly a federal process. The biotest would mean answering all of the questions in a naturalization citizenship test (currently 100 or so) while under biometric measure. 'fraud' was included in the comment for crimes, normally a white-collar activity. Immigration is only part of the citizenship problem, since demographic distribution of anti-social behavior is the same for citizens and the 22 million non-citizens who occupy U.S. space.

3 minutes ago: I don't see why they should have to take any citizenship test. Their rights should be reinstated when their time is up. Period.

1 minute ago:: I think everyone who registers Republican should take a citizenship test before being allowed to vote.

59 seconds ago:: I don't trust you... AT ALL.

11 minutes ago:: you forgot to talk about the brand on the forehead, that indicates current citizenship status.

5 minutes ago:: Actually, that is now done with a GPS implant under the skin, which any South American drug cartel boss can tell you how to insert them in their 'citizens'.

TLO [LI] for 2018:

The Liberty covenant is not really expressed in terms of the hypothetical wellbeing [WB] context even when about half of the American legislative process involves it. It was just not defined in the Preamble covenants like [LI] because there wasn't much anyone could do about it in 1787. Liberty is then measured in terms of the freedom and democracy an individual man or woman has, with individual wealth a component of those two {elements}.

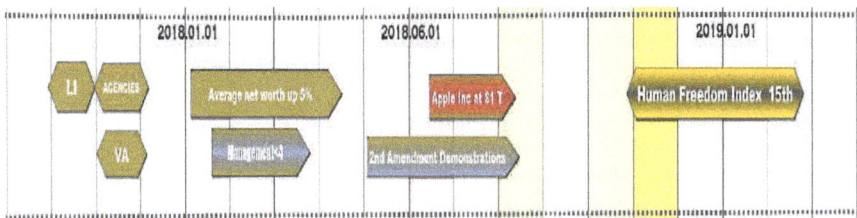

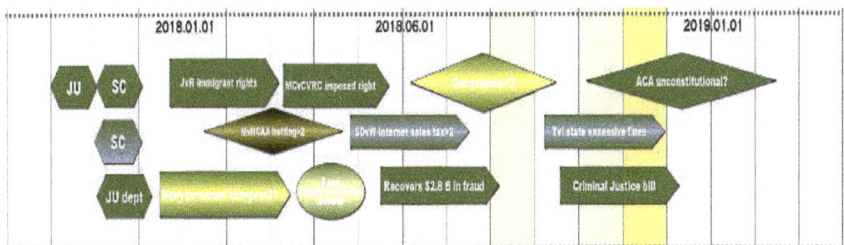

Even though [LI] can be measured against some combination of [GW] and [JU], it can also involve [WB] and [TR] in various combinations. Many modern indexes have been developed that quantify the 'Quality of Life' as shown in 15:07:16 and 01:07:15, with an index of the ability to move from one 'energy' state to another without obstruction from other people, a community, state, or a national government. Many such indexes on [LI] components are described at:

https://en.wikipedia.org/wiki/List_of_freedom_indices#

taken in combination with :

https://en.wikipedia.org/wiki/List_of_countries_by_wealth_per_adult

give a reasonable profile of liberty for the individual, but not any indication of how much the Liberty is used for anti-social behavior, which a small minority in each society rate as a 'right'.

Such life mobility, assuming it doesn't have the ripple effect of destroying life around the individual, shows up as a dollar net worth, a lack of indenture, availability of food and clothing, and personal safety. But it can also involve a very powerful altruistic 'freedom' to help others, which is natural for humans. It can also involve molecular freedom in which a person is free of the many thousands of 'system' degenerations that the mind/body can be born with or develop through its nutritional input.

The Constitutional environment of the six domains, according to most indices, place America quite high as far as personal liberty goes, as long as the calculation does not involve mental or physical health, which have not as yet been defined as part of the Liberty a person is enhanced by.

Further indicators of this:

2018.05.13:06:20   **[WB]n+|CD|<1…..[LI]|<2|TR|>3-[JU]>1+ [GW]>1=|OP|>1**

Wang, WaPost, 'For six decades, 'the man with the golden arm' donated blood — and saved 2.4 million babies':

"Harrison continued donating for more than 60 years, and his plasma has been used to make millions of Anti-D injections, according to the Red Cross. Because about 17 percent of pregnant women in Australia require the Anti-D injections, the blood service estimates Harrison has helped 2.4 million babies in the country."

Wonder what brought on the high percentage of hemolytic disease of the second newborn, HDN, in the first place? Something in the Aussie environment that caused the problem to approach a pandemic stage? It is only recently that HDN could be treated with a synthetic called RhoGAM (derived from Harrison's plasma) , so the 60 year altruistic blood donating really was remarkable. The post-natal ripple effects of HDN are pretty fierce on a newborn's body and mind, so prevention should be an automatic reflex for a good health system, if it can.

Speculation:

Should diagnosis of things like HDN be a designated human right in this century? 70 years ago, there might not have been too much you could do about the infant mortality and disfigurement of things like HDN or the other 1400 birth 'anomalies'. But that is no longer true. Molecular level diagnostics, some of which could be tough on the mom, could bring about treatment agendas not available before this century. But should such treatment be a 'right' with a corresponding mandatory 'responsibility' to be treated?

TLO:

Note the dynamic ripple effects of a single individual's molecular altruism. In America, suppose you multiplied that by the 10 million most capable of the process, as in gene therapies?

2018.10.17:09:53 |OP|>3 ≈∑ |TR|>3 [LI]>3⋈[JU]>1....[GW]>2 |CD|<3

Bernstein, BloombergOpinion, 'Madison Never Envisioned Minority Rule':

"But one thing I'd add is that we shouldn't forget how young representative democracy was at the time. It's hardly surprising that Madison et al. didn't work it all out properly. Even those who defend the constitutional system and Madisonian democracy in general – and I'm certainly one of them – should be clear that the original 1787 document had flaws that have only been partially repaired through amendment and interpretation. We should fight for the best, most democratic interpretation of Madisonian thought, not the government as it existed in the 1790s or the 1850s or the 1950s."

"The Framers worried about absolute rule by majorities. But they never would've imagined the opposite."

But they did. Most of the checks and balances in the Articles of the Constitution were clearly intended to prevent both a permanent majority from establishing itself AND to prevent the private ownership of power such as kings and nobles of Europe, Africa and Asia enjoyed. Remember, that the model for democracy that they Framers were using was that of the classical Greek city-states like Athens, Sparta, Corinth and Thebes. These city-states were so democratic that they could vote in a dictator during a crisis with 'king' powers and remove him when the crises passed. But the model proved true in every case since then; democracy cannot exist above a population size of a city-state. There are no examples of anything except a representative republic existing above the size of a major city anywhere in American history. The Framers were not thinking of a 'national' democracy because they knew it couldn't exist as anything more than the 'mob rule' they feared. American history has proved them correct.

The other half of the problem was the individual ownership of power, not exactly minority rule of kings, and that problem has not been completely resolved because a 'representative' can be elected by a propertied 'clan' of less than 10,000 in a given elective District of 600,000. Both mob rule and private ownership of power suppress the human rights (including health, education, and economic enhancement) a republic needs to exist, so neither was really intended to be dominate as the Framers worked out the Article compromises of the Constitution in1787. The only modern issue is whether private or foreign funding of political activity qualifies as 'ownership' that threatens a republic with its many small democracies.

[LI] 2018 Conclusions:

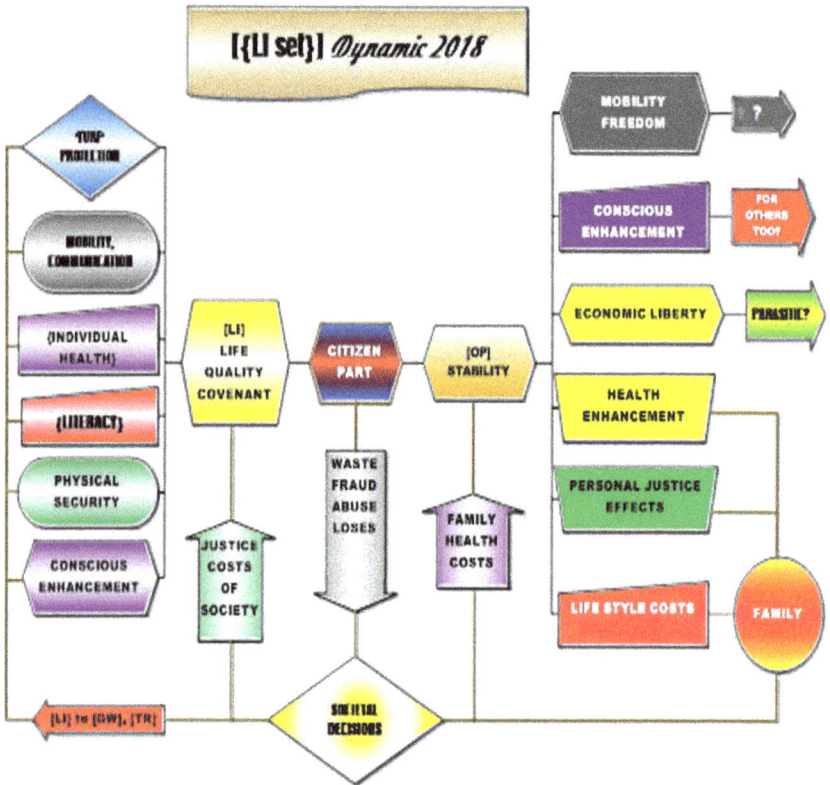

There are too many economic 'rights' conflicts in human societies in 2018 to further develop Wellbeing as a form of Liberty. This is true even though a Standard Evolutionary Model indicates that the stresses of environment can be greatly reduced by the mental and physical health of ALL members of each society. The inclusive health state of being has genetic ripple effects that frees the individual from desperate economic conditions as well as increases his awareness of his environment to the point he is able to administer his own health and wellbeing through the summed effect of the Liberty subsets used here; {Life liberty}, {Economic Liberty}, {Civil Liberty}, and {Physical Liberty}. But that is dependent on making sacrifices to all of the other domains, and you will **never** get a consensus on doing that. Neither could the Founders.

The continued pressures of foreign influences on the 2nd Amendment right of arms possession still maintained themselves even though it was not possible to remove a 'right' with renouncing the Bill of Rights itself. Very many believed that abolition of guns was an 'advance' for humanity even when most of those carrying them rated the activity in the same category as breathing. It was a device skill, like driving a vehicle or working a computer, nothing more. The Supreme Court appeared to agree that the 2nd Amendment was very close to a given right. .

The summing of these four processes can also be described by individual quality of life indexes that have become somewhat accurate in this century, although comparisons between different world societies might be a statistical stretch. You can have Physical and Life liberty living in as a sheep herder in some mountain vale by yourself and dozens of little societies in mountainous regions do this. There is also the conditions of Economic Liberty that are totally dependent on ones ability to acquire wealth from society while ignoring the other three conditions. In 2018, this had become very clear as some 100,000 people on Earth had economic freedom by ownership-control of 60% of the property or 'wealth' on the planet.

2018.02.08:07:10 [WB|n+|CD|<1…..|LI|TR|-[JU]<3+ |GW|>1=|OP|<2

Hall, WaPost, 'We are witnessing a democratic nightmare':

"Only when sectional and partisan battles gave way to new international responsibilities, and (relative) domestic harmony, in the 20th century could Republicans and Democrats define shared national interests and accept the need for permanent secret agencies to protect them."

The reason that Republicans and Democrats had 'shared national interests' was that their political constituencies were both being attacked by socialist one-party states (Germany, Russia, Japan, China, Cuba, Iran, Ottomans, etc.) BECAUSE the two parties had a shared Constitution that included such things as Liberty, Justice, and especially Common Defense and General Welfare. These are items that are intolerable to the one-party state because they prohibited a member of a ruling elite from attaining 'god' powers of life and death over every subject of 'his' national domain. The totalitarians still are haters of check and balance systems and still try to undermine anything that does that, such as investigative security agencies.

But if the bi-partisanship mentality has been heavily eroded by the closet toties in and out of government, those who have taken oaths to protect and defend the Constitution are obligated to consider all, repeat all, acts in terms of whether others are in the process of disavowing the Constitution and Bill of Rights and not consider their personal whims relevant. The investigative or security agency members certainly are not obligated to adhere to the partisan beliefs they may have been 'schooled' in to the extent that they hold Constitutional integrity itself in contempt. You can't have a democratic nightmare in a representative republic if its members are actually adhering to the Constitution and the 'rights' it creates. Only partisan extremism on the constitutional fringe can do that. .

The 2018.03.01:07:15 above described 'quality of life' conditions that people were using as a model and they generally summed parts of the four subsets here in various combinations. and then comparing them to other societies without showing any relationship between Liberty or any of the other domains or {subfunctions}

2018.12.16:11:43 has a good description of what happens to [LI] when the population density starts to overcome the resources of a region, an occurrence in many American cities during 2018 where the effects of the Recession could still be felt. As population density crept over about 7000 per square mile, Life and Economic Liberty decreased to the point Civil Liberty entered dangerous conditions with very large Justice ripple effects.. As the density increased to 9,000 per sq. mile, even physical Liberty or 'space' began to disappear, causing the overall Liberties to fragment.

This was not the condition of the majority of Americans as their economic and quality of life freedoms began to stabilize, along with some gains in civil Liberties, depending on where you were. There were few gains in the sum of the four freedoms here and many decisions made were failures because the Wellbeing conditions of health had not really improved, and the other forms of individual Liberty are dependent on staying in good health. Liberty [LI]., In spite of the four definition or components listed here, doesn't show really show where a Homosapien being is unless it shows him in a context of health such as the one produced by George Engel model. The context extends from community to basic molecules and a person is simultaneously in all of them.

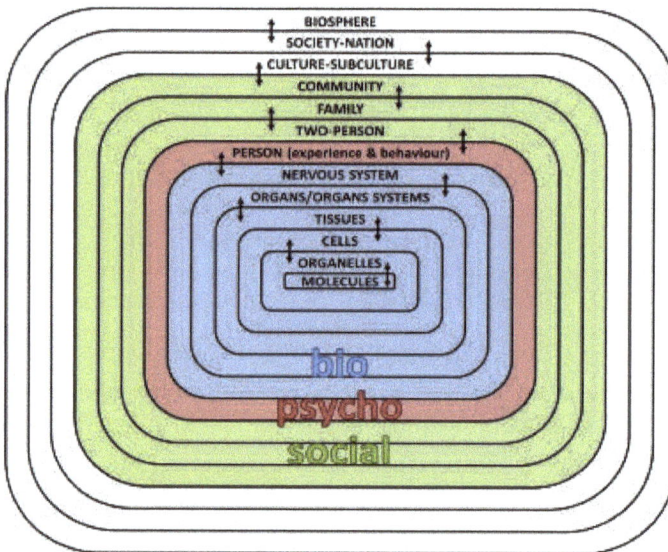

Figure 19.   Engel 'biopsychosocial' model, 1977

Our Posterity [OP]

This term, our Posterity, in the Preamble was originally set there by the Committee of Style as something of an after-thought and actually has no reference to it in the Federalist Papers that explained the dynamics of the three branches of governance to We the People. It was generally understood to mean giving something to following generations, but what if that was a dynamical process itself, such as found in a theory by a book *Generations* called 'Strauss–Howe generational theory' which described American history in terms of generation cycles that repeated themselves every 80 years or so. It described We the People in a dynamic sense but could not produce enough data to demonstrate the process the way statistical analysis can describe a population or a DNA Haplogroup. *Generations* was more a 'sense' of a Posterity process rather than a description of the domain [{OP}] that is used here and the same skepticism about that domain being definable also applies. The term as it is understood by Americans is used as the definition of the Domain,

'Posterity' for Americans means simply giving something better to a future generation. In some cases that could mean that you didn't pass on anything that made conditions worse for the next couple of generations. [OP] can become [OP]<n or [OP]>n. That was the common knowledge rule 'if it works, don't fix it'. That actually no longer applies in America because of the explosion of technical and molecular knowledge about humanity in this century. Posterity then becomes a 'least harm' optimization that sets the favorable conditions for 50 years in the future and that in turn almost certainly means healthcare and wellness of the thousands of molecular 'entities' in people. [WB]+/- as a sum of molecular subsets. One of the problems with 'don't fix it' in the health care world is that any of the individualized molecular systems in a person could stop working correctly and had to be fixed by someone else. This 'fix it' requirement based on the way molecular structures change and mutate has become a 21st century priority that clearly changing the way humans exist on earth. It was possibly even predictable that this *would* happen if one reads the Revelations carefully.

> Biblical Revelations 21:1:

> Then I saw a new heaven and a new earth; for the first heaven and the **first earth passed away**, and there is no longer any sea [separation of the two].

And also: Tao Te Ching: 16.1 and 16.2:

> Empty the self completely;
> Embrace perfect peace.
> **The world will rise and move;**
> **Watch it return to rest.**
> **All the flourishing things**
> **will return to their source.**

> This return is peaceful;
> **It is the flow of nature,**
> An eternal decay and renewal.
> Accepting this brings enlightenment,
> Ignoring this brings misery.

But a more general description of Our Posterity is located in https://en.wikipedia.org/wiki/History_of_the_United_States

With some 13 'eras' of events including the migrations of various haplogroups since the last Ice Age. This includes the Native American migrations form Siberia (native?), various European, and the forced migration of west-African haplogroups. The website describes in general how the six Preamble domains were interacting, including the various traumas of wars, xenophobic conflict and social Darwinist attempts at achieving Justice and Tranquility. But there is little discussion of [Our Posterity] simply because most of the problems were on a day-to-day time basis, not generational as Posterity requires. Unlike European and especially Asian societies, Americans did not have Posterity experiences to affect them and that might have been why the Constitution and its dynamics actually came into existence.

But into all of this event history, there were some dynamical processes that very definitely beginning to effect all of the domains simultaneously. One 'process' culminated on the Solvay conference of 1927 in which most of the scientific community with an accumulated wisdom of that period attempted to define the universe in 'quanta' terms rather than Newtonian or Galileon. Another process was the development of weapons of mass destruction (chemical, biological, mass kinetic guns, aircraft, nuclear, etc.) from about 1904 that in the following decades killed nearly 200 million people, with soldiers using the weapons only a small part of the lethality.

And a third that begin the end of Social Darwinist beliefs in 'might makes right' and 'survival of the fittest' appeared because the DNA mapping of the Human Genome that was completed at the beginning of the 21st century showed how absurd the concept of 'race' and individual superiority was. This DNA research culminated in a worldwide program involving the Ethical, Legal, and Social Implications (ELSI) of biotechnologies structure in 1996 as world DNA studies began to truly define what a human was made of.

https://en.wikipedia.org/wiki/History_of_genetics

Almost in sync with the increased availability of WMD, scientific knowledge of the universe, and technology awareness came the [our Posterity] dream come true, the internet of things where knowledge is almost immediately shared throughout the human race. Human evils also became immediately shared, with such things as direct political interference by totalitarian entities in the six domains of the Constitution. Note https://en.wikipedia.org/wiki/Cyberwarfare_by_Russia and the Iranian attack 'Operation Ababil' in 2012 and there after.

Posterity [{OP}] as a relation of [JU]

2018.04.21:19:03 |OP|<3 ≈∑ |TR|<2 |LI|>3⋈|JU|<3....|GW|>1

Will, WaPost, 'Gorsuch strikes a blow for constitutional equilibrium':

"Many conservatives have embraced populism where it least belongs, in judicial reasoning. They have advocated broad judicial deference to decisions because they emanate from majoritarian institutions and processes. Progressives favor such deference because it liberates executive power from congressional direction or judicial supervision."

Great little system. If you have both conservatives and liberals whose dogmas are so extreme that they do not reflect some aspect of Constitutional intent, then no matter how the 'law' is written by the Article I authorities, it will contain 'gibberish' reflecting the extreme of some partisans. The Article II presidential authorities can then interpret the 1000 page 'gibberish' from a purely unelected standpoint as devolved 'regulations' that the Article III judicial authorities must later determine if there is already regulatory precedence gibberish for the new gibberish. And at each step in the 'system', an unelected semantics attorney will advise the principals about the wording of the regulations at $600 per hour, possibly from a Moscow or New Delhi corner office thanks to the instant Internet.

Note that there is nothing in the Article III , Section 2 description of Judicial Power that prohibits the Court from interpreting Justice, a clear intent and purpose described in the Preamble, as the outcome of ANY 'controversy to which the United States shall be a party'. Gibberish does not supercede Justice, no matter who writes it.

Posterity [{OP}] as a relation of [TR]

2018.04.29:07:51 |OP|n $\approx \sum$ |TR|>3 |LI|>3⋈|JU|<3....|GW|<2⋈ |CD|<2

LaPlante and White, MITRE, in WaPost, 'Five myths about artificial intelligence':

"Myth No. 5: Artificial intelligence is a threat to mankind. "I fear that AI may replace humans altogether," Stephen Hawking told Wired in 2017. The truth is we simply don't know where AI will lead us, but that doesn't mean murderous terminators are going to start stalking the streets."

Don't bet the farm on that. Some of the new quantum-level nano technologies are creating AI implants that give a 'human' instant memory recall with a capacity four times that of the homosapien brain. Other AI nanobot implants can repair environmental damage from chemical, biological, or radiation devices that would make a soldier far more lethal than current ones. AI nanobots can also improve the strength, agility, and molecular purity of a being to the point that a current homosapien could not compete with it on an evolutionary scale. It is also possible that the nanobots could be passed on to a fetus and at some point, this new 'race' will forbid the birth of homosapien 'primitives' altogether. AI nano enhancement is a very probable timeline progression as something necessary to survive human induced catastrophes of the future, not a myth.

Posterity [{OP}] as a relation of [CD]

2018.08.17:06:54 |CD|<3 ⋈ |GW|>1-|JU|>2|TR|<3 $\approx$ |OP|>1

Kiley, TheHill, 'Cybersecurity: Cause for optimism, need for continued vigilance':

"Finally, the federal government must work more closely with private industry to ensure that if they share information critical to the mitigation and prevention of attacks, proprietary information is protected, and the bureaucrats and politicians do not lay blame on those businesses."

Since this cyber aggression has already been shown to be an attack against We The People, it should come under the authority of Common Defense in which the individuals involved in some infrastructure can be held responsible for 'negligence' even if no actual cyber-attack was successful. In this day and age, cyber security should be universal in human, droid, and linkage categories. An organization that fails to maintain minimum established security protocols because 'they don't have time for it' should be held responsible.

But the same laws that define the 'negligence' should also have cybersecurity guarantees against third party access through 'laws' even in court proceedings. That is, the famous 'security disclosure' defense by the legal profession in which defendants seek to publicize 'classified evidence' at a legal proceeding would have to have sunset provisions where the negligence provision applies to the legal operators as well. Even an FOIA request for corporate cybersecurity data might be from of Common Defense 'negligence' by all judiciary participants in an attack-related event. Not easy, because a 'secret' court proceeding may be unconstitutional unless public review is available at some point. This smack of a 'star-chamber' activity found in most totalitarian states, so some efforts to prevent security disclosures in a judicial context are very much needed in this century.

2018.06.15:06:58 |OP| ≈ ∑ |TR|>3 |LI|<3 ⋈ |JU|>1....|GW|<2

Will, WaPost, 'The Equal Rights Amendment is a farce that's ended in tragedy':

"Legislators sworn to "support and defend" the Constitution voted to clutter it with language the meaning of which they did not — could not — know. The meaning was irrelevant to the main purpose, which was to grandstand with an amendment the first, and for many advocates the sufficient, function of which was "consciousness-raising" — to "put women in the Constitution.""

The Equal Rights Amendment

Section 1. Equality of rights under the law shall not be denied or abridged by the United States or by any state on account of sex.

Section 2. The Congress shall have the power to enforce, by appropriate legislation, the provisions of this article.

Section 3. This amendment shall take effect two years after the date of ratification.

'Equality of rights under the law'? What does that mean? How would a Supreme Court asked to review an individual 'sex' act under the ERA be able to interpret it? A woman has something like 30 molecular structures that are completely different from a man's in order to satisfy biological evolution, including a couple of HARs (Human Advanced Regions of DNA sequences that differentiate humans from previous sapien or ape species) that are more pronounced than in males. Does a 'women' abandon all procreative functions of evolution in order to be 'equal' to a male? If not, then procreative activity involving sex becomes a 'privileged economic class', not an equal right.

Under modern molecular biology conditions, what is a human 'right'? Everybody keeps using the term 'rights', but what is an actual 'right'? The Founders in 1787 did not use the term in the Constitution, nor did the 27 grievances listed in the Declaration of Independence. The 'Bill of Rights' was Jefferson's and Madison's add-on to the signed Constitution in 1789 as protections for 'natural' rights people believed in at the time.

further:

But if you really want to throw mud into this quagmire, you can point out the added Bill of Rights was submitted to popular assemblies and referendum specifically called to ratify them, not legislatures, and only required a two thirds majority instead of the three quarters for 'Amendments'. Technically, if a 'right' is being added or removed, it has to be done by a two-thirds majority in popular referendum assemblies, not through the Congress or legislatures under Article V. That would invalidate the ERA and possibly the 14th Amendment or Civil Rights Act involving rights. Really need a renewable path for rights definition by a specially called Electoral College approved by states or popular vote in order to deal with modern procreative processes and health rights.

2018.05.03:05:34 |OP|>2 ≈∑ |TR|>3 |LI|>3⋈|JU|>1….|GW|>2+|CD|>1

Will, WaPost, 'Does Trump even understand the electoral college?':

"The electoral college gives the parties a distribution incentive for achieving geographical and ideological breadth while assembling a coalition of states ."

Since Article II, Section 1 Clause 2 hasn't changed, it is reasonably clear that the Founders intended that a body of people who were NOT the direct representatives of the current government, regardless of party, would be an electoral agency. A Elector, once created by a state legislature lawful order, was to act as an independent representative in a 'College' deliberative body. The constitutional intentionally removed the 'gerrymander' factor from a given federal election. The electors were duty bound ONLY to reflect the will of those they represented and largely have done so, although many are only so obligated on the first vote in all-or-nothing Districts. The 'College', in deliberative assembly, virtually eliminated both monetized oligarchic rule AND impositional mob rule by assuring a check and balance democracy. Tough to be anarchic from either the left or the right under those Elector conditions.

Speculation:

Suppose the Founders saw other purposes for a independent Electoral College than just representative screening of presidential elections, as in the 12th and 25th Amendments? Suppose an Electoral College was assembled for the purpose of Amending the Constitution with direct voting by populations to get representation on a specific national issue? For instance, the Vice President, already representing both the Congress and the Presidency, could be designated as an elected official to the United Nations through an Electoral College mechanism. Or a balanced budget Amendment could be created if an Electoral College were elected, genuinely elected, for that purpose with state consents through Article IV. Was Presidential succession the real purpose of the Electoral College or an afterthought by the Founders?

Further:

That is, two were intended to clearly represent the population of an entire state, regardless of political agendas and the others were intended to represent populations of a given Federal District regardless of the partisan makeup of the state Districts.

They could not vote for two people from the same state in order to maintain the national representation.

Elector clause: Each State shall appoint, in such Manner as the Legislature thereof may direct, a Number of Electors, equal to the whole Number of Senators and Representatives to which the State may be entitled in the Congress: but no Senator or Representative, or Person holding an Office of Trust or Profit under the United States, shall be appointed an Elector.

2018.08.13:07:32 |OP|>3   ≈ ∑ |TR|>3 |LI|<3 ⋈ |JU|>1....|GW|>2 | ξ| >2
|WB|>2

Editorial Board, WaPost, 'An assault on minority voting continues in North Carolina':
"Voting laws, including for felons, vary enormously across the country. In some states
the right to vote is restored automatically when people leave prison; in others,
including North Carolina, felons are required to complete their sentences, including
serving probation or paying fines, before their rights are restored. Elsewhere, ex-felons
face waits of several years before they can regain voting rights. In two states, felons
may vote even while incarcerated."

The issue for a Federally related election is whether the person attempting to vote
actually has the status of a citizen. Restoration of citizenship rights such as voting,
driving, bearing arms, or mobility (ankle-bracelet, breathalyzer) should be conditional
on proving that citizenship itself has been re-acquired, a federal Naturalization Clause
activity, not a local regulatory process. That is, there is nothing that says the
Naturalization Clause cannot require all persons convicted of high crimes and
misdemeanors to take a verifiable citizenship test while attached to a biometric
analyzer (aka polygraph, but more modern and accurate). This citizenship bio-test
could even be a requirement for parole from an institution regardless of state and it is
purely within federal jurisdiction.

The idea is that a person who violates the 'rights' of others by predatory aggression
(robbery, fraud, misuse of lethal devices like drugs and guns, political defamation, etc)
losses his own in proportion and these have to be re-earned by self-education with
biotesting. That would also eliminate the easily abused skin tone test now common in
the world by accurately taking the measure of a being's citizenship or empathy toward
humans.

Further:

21 minutes ago:

Or how about you act like a civilized nation and take seriously the "inalienable" before
"rights"? If you commit a crime, you will lose your freedom for a time. But voting
rights should be irrevocable. What about the wrongfully convicted? Will they get to
retroactively vote in all the elections they weren't allowed to participate in? One
person, one vote - whether that person is a billionaire, a store clerk or a convict;
whether they live in a rural town or a major city.

22 minutes ago:

So, are you saying people lose their citizenship if they commit a crime and get put in
jail? Or should? "biotest" for parole to answer what question? What will we require of
those committing white collar crimes? The same citizenship test? Or, is this all about
immigration for you?

14 minutes ago:

They actually do lose their citizenship 'rights' if they go to prison in most states, even
though 'citizenship' is strictly a federal process. The biotest would mean answering all
of the questions in a naturalization citizenship test (currently 100 or so) while under
biometric measure. 'fraud' was included in the comment for crimes, normally a white
collar activity. Immigration is only part of the citizenship problem, since demographic
distribution of anti-social behavior is the same for citizens and the 22 million non-
citizens who occupy U.S. space.

3 minutes ago:

I don't see why they should have to take any citizenship test. Their rights should be reinstated when their time is up. Period.

1 minute ago:

I think everyone who registers Republican should take a citizenship test before being allowed to vote.

59 seconds ago:

I don't trust you... AT ALL.

11 minutes ago:

 you forgot to talk about the brand on the forehead, that indicates current citizenship status.

5 minutes ago:

Actually, that is now done with a GPS implant under the skin, which any South American drug cartel boss can tell you how to insert them in their 'citizens'.

2018.09.29:07:19 |OP| ≈∑ |TR|>3 |LI|<2 ⋈ |JU|<2....|GW|>3

Kimberly Wehle in TheHill, 'Four legal takeaways from a sad day for the Supreme Court':

"Although the Senate Judiciary Committee isn't mentioned in the Constitution, it makes the rules on how the process unfolds. In this instance, those rules have favored the Republicans, who are in the majority. Because only a simple majority is required for confirmation these days, Republicans don't really need Democrats' "advice and consent." As a result, neither Democrats nor their constituents have meaningful power to influence the outcome."

We needn't go into a discussion of why the 67 million Independents are not represented in this procedure at all or whether the Senate Rules Committee could have protected the non-criminal and non-civil proceedings by an addition of a 'closed session' privacy hearing requirement for the affected parties in this advice and consent. The information disclosed by the parties involved could very easily been during a closed session of the Judiciary Committee since neither criminal or civil proceedings are required to determine SCOTUS eligibility. The consent procedure then becomes 'representative' when it is passed on to the full Senate even if there are only two 'Independent' members. Let any objections surface there after the Judiciary Committee, with earlier proper oversight by the Rules Committee, has approved the nomination.

But did the Committee actually determine if the nominee would follow the Article III, Section 2 'Law and Equity' authority throughout the realm of We the People, especially since he represents all of them in SCOTUS?

2018.10.03:06:36 |OP|? ≈∑ |CD|<3 ⋈ |TR|>3 |LI|<3⋈|JU|>1....|GW|<1

KC Johnson in WaPost, 'How partisanship and distrust leave Congress vulnerable to hacking':

"And Congress has consistently struggled to effectively defend itself against such intrusions, in part because the legislators and committees most exposed have fraught relations with the very intelligence agencies best equipped to protect them."

The problem with this is that as 'oversight' committees, the congress cannot actively seek the protections of the Executive agencies they look at. In order to protect individual members against foreign under-the-table influences, these Agencies, especially the FBI, would have to assign personnel to EACH Member and to EACH potential Member. That is nearly an impossibility, especially if the local candidate has a hidden agenda as a foreign 'sleeper' to interdict or subvert the security of the Americans. In the author's timeline, that has happened several times. Member security means that Capitol Hill would be crawling with ex-Agency personnel in critical positions for various Members, with many paid by the current Executive branch.

That's not necessarily bad; various Agency personnel have validated the oaths they have taken through background checks and polygraphs (beating a polygraph makes you a pathological liar, which might be worse than disloyalty) and there is no reason that security on Capitol Hill shouldn't include polygraphic screening for everyone including candidates. But citizenship testing for policy advocates as well? Try running the mandatory in-house citizenship with TS/SCI clearance test by any Congress in the last 40 years.

We don't need to turn the Capitol Hill into some kind of techno cyberfort with access scans on every corridor (you wear a need-to-know credential for each committee access, regardless of 'open' status), but certainly technical verification of belief in the Constitution and the oaths of office for everyone in the process might be a consideration, Agency security back-watchers included.

Posterity [{OP}] as a relation of [GW]

2018.05.23:10:43 |OP|>3 ≈ ∑ |TR|<3 |LI|>3 ⋈ |JU|>1....|GW|>2+|CD|>3

mba, WaPost, The recession is long gone. Where are the babies?':

"We're not there yet [Japanese depopulation]. But as it turns out — surprise! — having children is generally a good thing. If we're starting to turn away from it, we should start trying to figure out why."

'Why' might be the real question. Why create human life at all? Most societies around the world create babies as a reaction to a stressed environment because more were, note were, necessary to have some survive. But most of the old Biblical, Quranic, or Buddhist defined reasons for procreation under stress have disappeared. Just possibly, people in low birth regions of the world have decided that they need to create BETTER human life, not just more. Japan has been overcrowded since the 1800s and WWII may have been a reaction to the over-population compared to resources. That certainly wouldn't apply to Russia, where large families are nearly non-existent, but it is still an imperialistic state. China's economic boom in this decade almost certainly came about because of the 'one baby per family' policy where 400 million extra mouths to feed didn't happen.

The net effect is that many 'advanced' populations, as they become aware of their environment, start asking questions about whether the life they create is actually improved or improvable. A modern Internet-connected person needs only to flip through words like 'epigenetics', 'birth defects' or 'baby costs' to find out what is involved, and the idea of unplanned pregnancy might disappear. Unless the person can't read or write.

But each man or women in this century has to ask 'why' create life, not when.

2018.10.15:12:13 |OP|<3 ≈ ∑ |TR|<3 |CD|<4|LI|>3⋈|JU|>1....|GW|<2

Samuelson, WaPost, 'We're on mission impossible to solve global warming':

The emissions increases are almost certainly because of global industrialization, of which Americans are now, note now, only one of the contributors. Humans, by the way, emit CO_2 as they breath to the amount of 6 billion tons per year, or 6 gigatons (GT). Their industries are emitting something like 40 GT per year, more than enough to overwhelm the earth's global cycle of absorbing 27 GT of CO_2 per year. Note that the earth measures CO_2 in gigatons of matter, so the totals are colossal. The oceans have almost 40,000 gigatons stored and the earth surfaces, largely in trees, has another 3,200 gigatons, with about 750 GT floating in the atmosphere. The problem lies in the unabsorbed industrial GTs.

The key to lowering global warming is to reduce the industrial emission below 20 GT so that the natural absorption can actually work the other 20 GT. This is very tough to do because the amount of energy needed to do the sequestration of 20 GT of CO_2 would produce more CO_2 than it absorbs. It is not quite a lost cause if some technologies that convert CO_2 into its component carbon and oxygen atoms are developed using hydro or nuclear energy, which don't have a carbon footprint. But the scales involved are large. A single tree absorbs and stores 50 pounds of CO_2 a year, so absorbing one GT would require 40 billion new trees world wide. Not impossible, and beneficial for other reasons, but such a planting would require a commitment by ALL human societies. Good luck, considering human history.

Both reducing the waste of carbon based fuels (waste emissions by humanity at 3 GT?) by some form of carbon tax along with increasing the carbon capture by various means (4 GT?) could slow the future warming be perhaps 2 degrees F and avert the truly catastrophic effects warming causes of not having food growing lands for 9 billion people in 2070.

TLO: No posterity win at all unless a form of free energy sequestration is found and massively introduced world-wide.

2018.11.02:06:44 |OP|<4 ≈∑ |TR|<3 |LI|<3⋈|JU|>1....|GW|<2

Clement and Bahrampour in WaPost, 'Americans say they are less likely to fill out census than they were 10 years ago':

"Still, the discrepancy is striking and may increase concern that the share of households that respond to the 2020 count — without costly in-person follow-ups — will fall short of expectations. The mail response rate in 2010 was significantly lower than the share of survey respondents who said they would participate."

Pretty sad. The 10 questions on the D-61 form are used to determine the eligibility of a given area to have accurate representation in the Congress whether they are citizens or not. The lower the people participation in any given District, the more difficult it is to represent them whether they are a citizen or a U.S. National. But it might not be the question 9 concerning a persons 'race' that is the problem. And it may not be question 8, which singles out Latinos because they do not have a 'race' of origin. It could very well be that participation is not citizenship related but because question 4 asks for the telephone number of the residency and in the mobile device world, that is meaningless.

But giving the phone number in question 4 also gives the GPS location of the person on a 'public' record that any Russian or Chinese secret police agent might be able to access in census records. The census records themselves have proven to be unprotected by various hacker operations and no one in his right mind would answer a question giving someone else a GPS tracker option or an auto-dialer nuisance option.

The Question 4 telephone data should be replaced with the citizenship question that has the Congressional district as the location. That is, the participant isn't a very good citizen or even a U.S. National unless he knows what District he is in. But you live somewhere in the Nation with the privileges of citizenship, but you can't fill out a form determining representation required by the Constitution itself? Very sad.

2018.10.17:09:53 |OP|>3 ≈∑ |TR|>3 |LI|>3⋈|JU|>1....|GW|>2 |CD|<3

Bernstein, BloombergOpinion, 'Madison Never Envisioned Minority Rule':

"But one thing I'd add is that we shouldn't forget how young representative democracy was at the time. It's hardly surprising that Madison et al. didn't work it all out properly. Even those who defend the constitutional system and Madisonian democracy in general – and I'm certainly one of them – should be clear that the original 1787 document had flaws that have only been partially repaired through amendment and interpretation. We should fight for the best, most democratic interpretation of Madisonian thought, not the government as it existed in the 1790s or the 1850s or the 1950s."

"The Framers worried about absolute rule by majorities. But they never would've imagined the opposite."

But they did. Most of the checks and balances in the Articles of the Constitution were clearly intended to prevent both a permanent majority from establishing itself AND to prevent the private ownership of power such as kings and nobles of Europe, Africa and Asia enjoyed. Remember, that the model for democracy that they Framers were using was that of the classical Greek city-states like Athens, Sparta, Corinth and Thebes. These city-states were so democratic that they could vote in a dictator during a crisis with 'king' powers and remove him when the crises passed. But the model proved true in every case since then; democracy cannot exist above a population size of a city-state. There are no examples of anything except a representative republic existing above the size of a major city anywhere in American history. The Framers were not thinking of a 'national' democracy because they knew it couldn't exist as anything more than the 'mob rule' they feared. American history has proved them correct.

The other half of the problem was the individual ownership of power, not exactly minority rule of kings, and that problem has not been completely resolved because a 'representative' can be elected by a propertied 'clan' of less than 10,000 in a given elective District of 600,000. Both mob rule and private ownership of power suppress the human rights (including health, education, and economic enhancement) a republic needs to exist, so neither was really intended to be dominate as the Framers worked out the Article compromises of the Constitution in1787. The only modern issue is whether private or foreign funding of political activity qualifies as 'ownership' that threatens a republic with its many small democracies.

2018.12.18:06:49 |OP|>3 ≈∑ |WB|>3+|CD|<2 |TR|>3 |LI|<1 ⋈|JU|>1|GW|>2

Senator Warren in WaPost, 'Elizabeth Warren: It's time to let the government manufacture generic drugs':

"Public manufacturing will be used to fix markets, not replace them. The Affordable Drug Manufacturing Act would allow the government to manufacture generic drugs at lower costs or contract with manufacturers to produce the drugs at competitive prices. And if a potential manufacturer thinks it can do better, the bill provides that the license to manufacture the drug is continually offered for sale, with the only condition being that the buyer would agree to keep selling the product to consumers at competitive prices."

These drugs actually constitute a form of 'health infrastructure' that corrects the vast molecular distortions that occur in human bodies. With some 700,000 unique molecular subsystems that can go wrong at any time, human beings are at the evolutionary point where adding molecular and even quantum level enhancements is very close to a 'life right'. The manufacture of the enhancements shouldn't be a for-profit activity at all once the research and facility costs have been rewarded. That might even include such things as cannabis, nicotine, and alcohol. Molecular enhancement (and termination) should be a We the People decision making process, not an international for-profit cartel process at all.

How the Americans remove the drug infrastructure from private ownership to a public infrastructure like water and roads may have the greatest ripple effects of any process in this century. But molecular enhancement on an evolutionary scale requires some very well made Constitutional structures, not just Article I 'laws', so tread carefully with this.

2018.12.27:09:14 |OP| ≈∑ |WB|<3+|CD|>2 |TR|>3 |LI|<1 ⋈ |JU|<1|GW|<2

Binder, WaPost, 'five takeaways for 2018':

"Why doesn't unified party government endure? Call it the curse of overreach. Majorities exploit their newfound power to push hard on policy and procedure to advance their agendas. When they inevitably veer off-center to appeal to their base, the public acts as a "thermostat": When government activism increases, the public demands less, and vice versa."

Neither the 'curse of overreach' or the 'curse of gridlock' could exist if the American people started elected Independents who represented the majority in a given Electoral District. Many of the governance problems are created by people in both the Congress and Executive branches who are attempting to 'overreach' with their personal view of reality rather than serving a given District of Americans somewhere. That is the reason Americans keep trying to switch party control of the national direction; their choices of representation are limited to people who might represent 10 percent of a District or even a small economic oligarchy such as an international banking institution.

Speculation:

Would you have a perpetual condition of 'no-party' rule that formed and administered legislation in the interest of a non-polarized America if you had a substantial number of Independents in all three branches? If the extremes in both parties knew that they would have to deal with an Independent representative caucus that controlled just 20% of the votes in both Houses, would they be pulled toward a rational solution of a particular problem rather than always bowing to their minority sponsors? Would a 30% Independent caucus allow the Congress to actually plan taxation, regulation, and appropriation over a ten year cycle instead of the constant partisan destruction of the two year cycle?

Further:

Could ANY 'my way or the highway' agenda causing 20 years of gridlock exist if Americans were allowed to vote for someone with NO prior agenda, such as Independents profess and swear oaths to? Could ANY high ranking appointee in the Executive branch pass an 'advice and consent' review if Independents insisted on impeachment for administrative incompetence instead of for political affiliation?

Posterity [{OP}] as a function of [LI]

2018.02.27:07:30 |OP|>2 ≈∑ |TR|<3 |LI|>3⋈|JU|<1....|GW|>1

Gerson, WaPost, 'It's apocalypse now on guns':

"When I look at many of the people holding the guns, I don't really view them as legitimate protectors of my rights, or as qualified to make choices about the employment of violence in politics. I don't view America as halfway to tyranny. And I am grateful that Americans such as the Rev. Martin Luther King Jr. — who suffered actual oppression by government — made a principled commitment to nonviolent political change."

If one looks carefully at 'the people holding guns', he might find that the personality of someone with a Saturday night special in the middle of a subway robbery is very different from someone sneaking through the underbrush with a hog-stopper 357. Or the difference between an opiated sawed-off auto holder and the 'deputy' trying to protect against him with a pistol that is accurate to 25 feet. The point is that with 45 million 'holders' in the country, the defense against State tyranny is almost non-existent and the political use of weapons AND the abuse of guns is at a very low level. Charlottesville, Albermarle County, VA has maybe 60 violent crimes a year in a region with nearly 10,000 rifles. Its one major civil incident in 2017 had many displayed rifles on the street and yet the only violent act was with a rental car.

The idea of Americans 'holding guns' for political reasons or that they are irresponsible just doesn't exist, regardless of crowded urban street perceptions. In theory, an advancing civilization would have household 'weapons', including guns, in safe areas of the home and have the training necessary to maintain and use them. It is NOT the prohibition of dangerous devices in a Republic that should be the issue; it is whether the citizens are advanced enough, through literacy and consciousness, to use the 'weapon' effectively.

Further:

Having been given a human right in the 2nd Amendment as part of an advancing civilization compared to the rest of the world in 1789, it is necessary that the bearer of arms demonstrate he actually is 'advanced' on a day-to-day basis, something only modern psychiatric testing could do. Such as universal bio-medical diagnostics?

Of course, it could be noted that many Europeans and Asians consider it beneath their dignity to use or handle a tool or a weapon.

2018.04.16:08:28 **[WB]n+|CD|>2.....∑ [LI]|TR|[JU]>2+ [GW]>1=[OP]>2**

Barbash, WaPost, 'Arsenal of weapons, magazines, seized from pizza man who threatened school employee, police say':

"Another school employee alerted police to the message, which was left on an answering machine. The call prompted police to make a "welfare check" Saturday at the home of Robert Csak, 32, of Lindenhurst, N.Y. Newsday described Csak as a pizza delivery man. The apartment was sparsely furnished, with only a mattress, and a plastic chair and table. The officer, a military veteran, looked inside, saw the weapons and recognized them as illegal, Cameron said. Police then obtained a search warrant and seized them, Cameron said."

That appears to be the exact method for preventing misuse of weapons by people who do not have a 'right' to bear arms in that degree. But criminalization of ALL possession of weapons has clearly been overturned by the Supreme Court. In fact, should a non-criminal 'welfare check' on an individual be a police matter at all? Perhaps some psychiatric medical authority should have had responsibility to send a 'health inspector' instead of the police. In either case, removal of simple weapons of mass destruction would still be valid.

2018.07.01:09:24 **|OP| >4 ≈ ∑ |TR|>3 [LI]>3⋈[JU]>1....[GW]>1 ⋈ |CD|<3**

Woody Holton in WaPost, 'The father of our country didn't always know best. But he learned and changed.':

"Washington was beginning to realize that he was not going to win the war with a grand assault against the serried ranks of redcoats. In fact, that might be the best way to lose it."

One would have to overlook the 'grand assaults' Washington ordered at York Town which caused the final surrender of the 'serried ranks' in the Colonies. Of course, he had large ranks of French Regulars under Rochambeau along with his Volunteers and freed slaves. Washington's ego might have had less to do with anything than some think; he could assess the conditions he was dealing with through knowledge of the enemy (spies in the old North Church in Fortress Boston, perhaps?) and adjust accordingly, which is the best thing a commander in chief could do. Hint, hint.

But his 'father of his country' image doesn't come from his management of the Revolutionary War in the 1770s. It comes from his carefully acquired understanding of the absurdity of the Articles of Confederation in 1781. After the War, Washington was running his Mount Vernon Estate and begin collecting large sets of comments (now in the National Archives) from people like Franklin, Madison, Jefferson and other Founders. These documents and letters served as an intelligence database on what qualified as a 'republic' as opposed to a totalitarian/slave society, which was universal and worldwide in 1785. These summarized notes went with him to the First Constitution Convention in 1787 and because he and others removed their narcissistic self-interests from the scene, fathered a republic. Hint, hint.

Woody Horton:

I regret that this article was already too long for me to say more about what you call the other side of the story, but I do address it in my first two books, "Forced Founders: Indians, Debtors, Slaves, and the Making of the American Revolution in Virginia" and "Unruly Americans and the Origins of the Constitution." I try to do more than show that men like Washington and Jefferson oppressed African Americans and Native Americans, since everyone already knew that. Here's my focus: as blacks, Indians, and non-elite whites fought for justice, they powerfully influenced the movement for Independence and the adoption of the Constitution.

and

Check "Forced Founders" and "Unruly Americans" out of the library, buy them used - whatever! -Like Washington (and sadly, unlike Trump, it seems almost certain), you and I are still young enough to learn something new.

reply:

As an author, you might check out something that has recently (2006) been discovered called 'Human Accelerated Regions' of DNA sequences that identify a biped as a homosapien. One of the issues may be that much of the injustice and exploitation of 'humans' is caused by a lack of the HARs in some people. They have identified 49 for certain, but there are other sequences, possibly several hundred, that had been classified as 'junk' DNA but might be HARs that differentiate true humans from other animals.

Some of the atrocities that 'humans' have committed toward one another can be explained by a lack of combinations of HARs. Relying solely on the actions and/or reactions of people to their surroundings might not be a good indicator of that humanness. In such cases, historic interpretation, especially with re-writes, might be meaningless in a HAR genome mapping context.

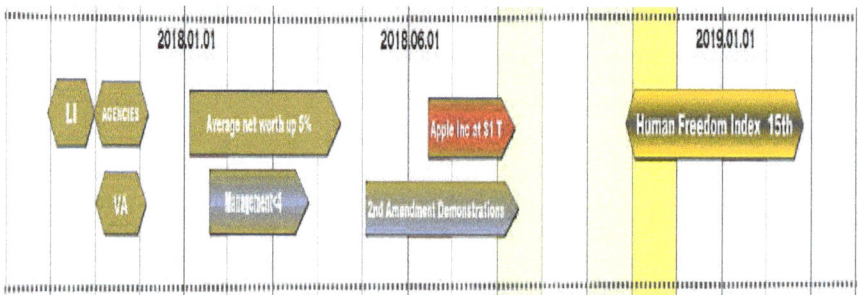

Well Being [WB] speculation

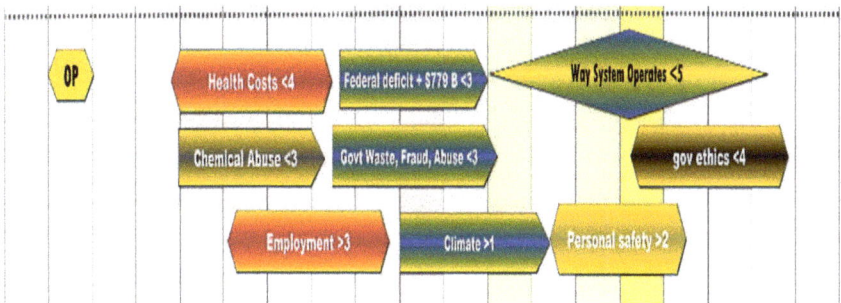

Health care 'system' process

One of the most promising developments in the 2000s has been the technical proliferation of ways of seeing a human being in all of its molecular glory. This has in turn led to many new treatments and 'cures' for many more Americans within the context of its 300 million known citizens and 20 million 'visitors'. This complexity progress of dealing with individual medicine at a cellular level (cancers, blood clots, fat tissue are the more obvious) means many medical people operate as specialists in one molecular group or another, but not necessarily as a 'whole person' evaluator. It takes no sense of a complex system to see that this gets more expensive by the year and not the decade. The brain development image shows the cell complexity growth in just two years of life. They happen to be critical years and considerable federal resources are allocated to them. Very appropriate for a General Welfare prime directive and certainly appropriate as a pre-emptive aid to Our Posterity. Sensing that does not take much skill by a Congressman who has seen that cellular process in his own family.

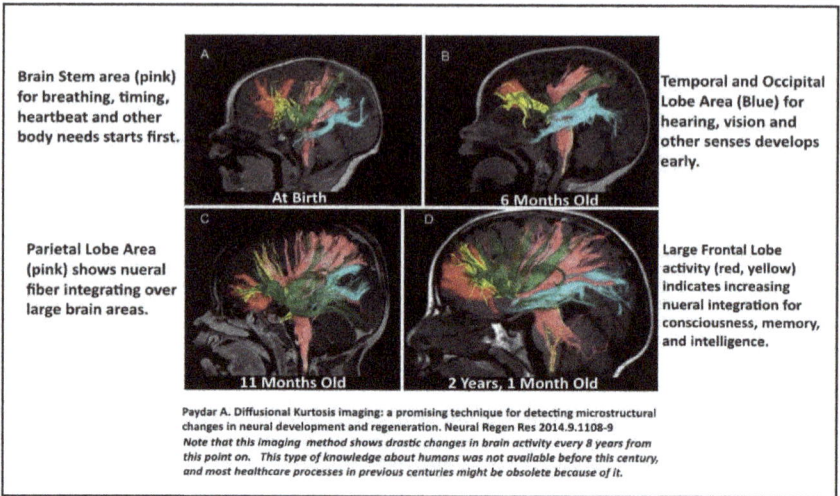

Brain Stem area (pink) for breathing, timing, heartbeat and other body needs starts first.

Temporal and Occipital Lobe Area (Blue) for hearing, vision and other senses develops early.

A — At Birth

B — 6 Months Old

Parietal Lobe Area (pink) shows nueral fiber integrating over large brain areas.

Large Frontal Lobe activity (red, yellow) indicates increasing nueral integration for consciousness, memory, and intelligence.

C — 11 Months Old

D — 2 Years, 1 Month Old

Paydar A. Diffusional Kurtosis imaging: a promising technique for detecting microstructural changes in neural development and regeneration. Neural Regen Res 2014.9.1108-9
Note that this imaging method shows drastic changes in brain activity every 8 years from this point on. This type of knowledge about humans was not available before this century, and most healthcare processes in previous centuries might be obsolete because of it.

With the U.S. health care system plagued by rising costs and inefficient delivery of care, the question of how to achieve quality care in a cost-effective way will be critical for any   president and congress.   .Note a general discussion of this at: https://www.cms.gov/Research-Statistics-Data-and-Systems/Statistics-Trends-and-Reports/NationalHealthExpendData/Downloads/ForecastSummary.pdf

Which is summed here as:

Total direct health care costs in USA in billions:

2010: $2,595.7

2011: $2,696.6

2012: $2,799.0

2013: $2,879.9

2016: $3,031.3

2017: $3,500.0

2018: $3,600.00

Increase per year is about $60 billion. Divided by 310 million people, this works out as a total added yearly cost per person of $193.   In ten years, the minimum increase might be $2000 per person without any significant increase in benefit to either his Liberty or Posterity. Worse, only half of Americans contribute to health care through one form of payment or another, such as insurance, Medicare withholding, or direct out-of-pocket fees. Virtually no emergency care is covered by the 'system' but is done anyway. This means that the 'taxpayer' pays increases of $193.00 per year not just for himself but as many as two other people. This is just one of the conditions of medical ripple effects; an individual's Liberty [LI] could be degraded by $600.00 per year.

Cellular medical care approaching a wellbeing 'system' is further complicated by the intense conflict over the Affordable Care Act of 2009 that resulted in the King V. Burwell Supreme Court decision on mandated 'taxation' to pay for medical care.

CHIEF JUSTICE ROBERTS concluded in Part III–B that the individual mandate must be construed as imposing a tax on those who do not have health insurance, if such a construction is reasonable.

The most straightforward reading of the individual mandate is that it commands individuals to purchase insurance. But, for the reasons explained, the Commerce Clause does not give Congress that power. It is therefore necessary to turn to the Government's alternative argument: that the mandate may be upheld as within Congress's power to "lay and collect Taxes." Art. I, §8, cl. 1. In pressing its taxing power argument, the Government asks the Court to view the mandate as imposing a tax on those who do not buy that product. Because "every reasonable construction must be resorted to, in order to save a statute from unconstitutionality," Hooper v. California, 155

2018.03.14:05:20 [WB]>3✉ [TR] [LI]

Achenbach and Rensberger, WaPost, 'Stephen Hawking, physicist who came to symbolize the power of the human mind, dies at 76':

"Physics was always the most boring subject at school because it was so easy and obvious. Chemistry was much more fun because unexpected things, such as explosions, kept happening," Dr. Hawking wrote in his memoir. "But physics and astronomy offered the hope of understanding where we came from and why we are here. I wanted to fathom the depths of the Universe."

Steven Hawking's neurodegeneration certainly didn't interfere with his perception of the depths of the universe. One wonders if his perceptive abilities were partially because of his awareness of the motor neuron disease and he was using it to focus his perception from outside the problem he was looking at, such as his 'arrow of time' concept. Neurodegeneration is a genetic process that covers such things as macrocephaly, ALS, and Alzheimer's that normally affect the entire brain and body. Didn't do that for him.

In this century, genetic mapping of a fetus might detect various forms of neurodegeneration that WILL develop later in life and it is just possible that the molecular combinations that trigger the degeneration might be removed at a very early stage. But not in the 1970s. Lots of mind 'energy' could be created among humans if those polyglutamine mutations weren't allowed to occur, but 'time' will tell.

Anyway, best wishes to Steven Hawking no matter what singularity he is now looking at.

2018.07.28:11:49 [ξ] <? [WB]<3✉ [GW]>3✉ [TR]<1 [LI]<2 ✉ [JU]<1 ≈ [OP]<2

Gopalan, TheHill, 'The case for treating cyber attackers like enemies of mankind':

"Surprisingly, aside from the U.S.-U.K. response, the international community's reaction has been passive acceptance of cyber-attacks. Partly, this is because cyber warfare is in a legal grey area and there is an asymmetry of capability. The absence of rules inhibits a strong response and that only benefits rogue actors. As a first step, cyber attackers must be characterized as hostis humani generis — that is, enemies of mankind. This term of art is employed against pirates, slavers and, recently, torturers."

While the term 'hostis humani generis' has been applied through history to human predators like pirates and slavers, it is possibly a reference to individuals who are genetically predisposed to consider humans 'prey'.

The DSM-5 defines Antisocial Personality Disorder (APD) as "[a] pervasive pattern of disregard for and violation of the rights of others, occurring since age 15 years, as indicated by three (or more) of the following:

Failure to conform to social norms with respect to lawful behaviors, as indicated by repeatedly performing acts that are grounds for arrest.

Deceitfulness, as indicated by repeated lying, use of aliases, or conning others for personal profit or pleasure.

Irritability and aggressiveness, as indicated by repeated physical fights or assaults.

Reckless disregard for safety of self or others.

Lack of remorse, as indicated by being indifferent to or rationalizing having hurt, mistreated, or stolen from another."

While APD or hostis humani can be learned, especially when taking wealth from others, it is most likely learned from one who has a Epigenetic or inherited predisposition to hunt or harm humans. Such inherent sociopaths have a remarkable ability to 'con' others into violent activity they personally take pleasure in causing. Saddam Hussein, Heinrich Himmler, Levrenti Beria, and Wu Zhifu are examples for hostis humani 'deception' murderers.

If a hostis humani is engaged only in cyber-attacks against humans, is he in the same category as someone who has deceived others into actual physical violent stalking of humans? And where is the point that a recognized hostis humani can be counter-attacked by legitimately defined Homosapiens under Common Defense, Liberty and Justice covenants of HUMANS in order to prevent further damage?

2018.05.21:19:38 [WB]>3 ⋈ [GW]<2 ⋈ [CD]<1 ∪ [TR]>2 [LI]>3 ⋈ [JU]>1 [OP]>1

Baron in WaPost, 'Antonin Scalia was wrong about the meaning of 'bear arms':

"In his opinion in Heller, Justice Antonin Scalia, who said that we must understand the Constitution's words exactly as the framers understood them, disconnected the right to keep and bear arms from the need for a well-regulated militia, in part because he concluded that the phrase "bear arms" did not refer to military contexts in the founding era."

People should keep in mind what the environment was like in the mid 1700s through the end of the century when the Constitution began to take effect in the new States, as did Justice Scalia. If you do a Wikipedia search on 'minutemen', you will find a description of what life was like at the time and the idea of bearing arms becomes clearer. Basically, the 'minuteman' was a farmer or storekeeper or teacher living in a spread-out community like Lexington, Massachusetts or Cowpens, South Carolina. This meant that he kept arms in the home so that he could carry it or 'bear' it to an assembly of militia that had been called up to defend a community. Militias of minutemen were common in nearly all communities, but a person did not become 'military' until he had actually joined the unit somewhere. Until then, he would just 'bear arms' from his home and maybe pick off something to eat along the way.

A western 'Posse' was also a deputized militia, even in 1950, with the members carrying sidearms and rifles that they brought from home, but in many cases they were assembled for law enforcement purposes, not as soldiers.

Bottom line is that the Founders believed it was necessary for all citizens to be ready to bear arms in defense of their communities or Nation if called to do that. **From an evolutionary standpoint, a modern minuteman would be able to handle any object he could use to defend his self, family, or community and that includes such things as autos, cell phones, first-aid kits, hazardous waste disposal kits, viruses cleaners and maybe in this century, simple WMD. A gun is just another object that needs bearing in an emergency that requires defense and an evolved person could do that.**

Wellbeing [{WB}] as a function of [{GW}]

2018.01.09:09:00 |WB|>3⋈ |GW|>2 |TR|<2 |LI|<2⋈|JU|<1 ? ≈ |OP|>2? |CD|<2

Ariana Cha in WaPost, 'Court to weigh if one parent has the right to use frozen embryos if the other objects':

"Cohen said the central issue focuses on how to balance one person's constitutional right to procreate with another's countervailing constitutional right to not procreate. The question parallels similar arguments used in other reproductive health cases, namely the Supreme Court's landmark 1973 abortion decision in Roe v. Wade. If women have the right to not be forced to be a gestational parent, do men — or women — have the right not to be forced to be a genetic parent?"

All of the Constitution's domains, plus [WB], are involved in this process. Note:
"The rapidly expanding world of assisted reproduction has triggered ever-more-complex legal fights, with disputes over parental rights and custody front and center."

If the rest of the human race is eventually going to 'absorb' the persons created by the frozen embryo combination, including forms that might not develop with homosapien DNA codes, does some form of judical 'arbitrator' from the State have a societal [GW] right to intervene? **A person has absolute rights up to the point that they affect everyone else, but is the time frame for 'effect' conception, post-natal, or even second generation?**

2018.05.03:21:42 |WB|>3⋈ |GW|>3⋈ |CD|<1 |TR|<1 |LI|<3⋈|JU|<1 |OP|>2

Tarlov in TheHill, 'Say it with me: Democrats are the party of health care':

"Yes, the road to get here has been treacherous. I remember the days when President Obama's health care law was deeply unpopular. I remember many stories of Americans who couldn't keep their doctors, suffered with rising costs and watched their insurers leave the exchanges. And we can never forget the gnawing drumbeat against ObamaCare from Republicans. In truth, not all of these problems have been solved and we must continue to work to improve the law (and try to surpass the negative messaging that is inevitable)."

Note: 'In truth, not all of these problems have been solved and we must continue to work to improve the law'. The problems of attempting to bring genuine healthcare to the entire country by 'improving the law' actually multiplied exponentially as the number of health-related research operations began examining the molecular structure of the Human Genome with its 700,000 molecular subsystems in a body. You have gene splicing, cloning, artificial wombs, AI medical nanobots, snake-oil merchants on every other website, opioid profiteering and constitutional subversion all going on at the same time you are making health 'laws'. It is no wonder that the parties and interests are zigzagging all over the socio-political-economic spectrum; they are not capable of establishing a rational 'system' under these rapidly changing circumstances.

The bottom line is that until a Constitutional referendum occurs that defines human life in a context of wellness, rather than endlessly treatable health with open borders, there is virtually no chance of a genuine improvement in a life the 21st century technologies are able to guarantee in the next few decades. It is delusional for all of the current party members to believe they can have an integrated wellness system without a carefully thought-out constitutional basis. The current parties are even less rational than the two parties that amended the Constitution with a prohibition on alcohol molecules without knowing what a human DNA molecule was.

2018.09.02:07:06   [WB]>3☒ [GW]>3☒ |TR|<1 |LI|<3☒|JU|<1 |OP|>2

Huckelbridge in TheHill, Roe v. Wade [abortion effects] comment:

And if Roe fell, the right to privacy would be undermined — the legal right that protects women's access to contraception.

There is no 'right to privacy' expressed or implied in any Constitutional Article, the Bill of Rights or subsequent Amendments. The 4th Amendment's 'secure' clause is close in preventing unreasonable search and seizure of 'effects', but a person has no Constitutional expectation of privacy if ANY public infrastructure is used for the individual lifestyle process. That is for the same reason that a person traveling down a six lane highway paid for with $3 million/per mile of taxpayer dollars doesn't have a private 'right' to do 90 miles an hour on it.

Access to Contraception, which is very possibly a woman's citizenship responsibility in creating life, is not even remotely in the same 'law' context of determining the termination of life that has achieved homosapien consciousness. That consciousness is developed in the third trimester and involves a social 'judgement' that automatically involves at least half a dozen other homosapiens, not just the life conceiver(s), especially if those conceivers are creating life for their own profit. **There really is no constitutional basis for determining the 'contracts' for conceiving life, so there is also no Constitutional basis for terminating it. In the Founders minds, sex with or without conception was a 'life, liberty, and pursuit of happiness' inalienable condition, not a right, and they wisely left it at that.**

But that is no longer true in this century. Since you can now, through DNA and molecular editing, change the birth conditions of the newly conceived, it is necessary to establish 'existence' rights that Roe v Wade related decisions were only dimly aware of. In this century, Roe v Wade is only a minor legal issue compared to endless editing and mutation of the human genome.

2018.09.20:08:05 |WB|>2 ≈ |GW|>2⋈ |CD|<3 |TR|>1 |LI|<3 ∪ |JU|<3 ⋈ |OP|<2

Chris Pope, Manhatten Institute, in TheHill, 'How the GOP fixed the worst of ObamaCare':

"Although ACA plans offer an important safety net for individuals with pre-existing conditions, they represent appallingly bad value for those who wish to purchase insurance before they get sick. Whereas working-age Americans incur annual median health care costs of $709, ACA plans have annual average premiums of $4,700 and deductibles typically over $3,900."

Comparing adult 30-somethings taking care of themselves to other age groups with chronic problems is meaningless. The average cost of healthcare in the U.S. is about $11,000 per person ($3.6 trillion per year) of which the 'big four' chronic conditions take considerable: Heart disease: $193 billion/year, Diabetes: $176 billion/year, Cancer(s): $171 billion/year and obesity: $147 billion/year. 'Undiagnosed' problems (read 'admin' costs for uninsured in emergency rooms) account for another $250 billion/year.

A healthy person with an annual cost of $709 (not likely in 2018) pays into the 'system' for 10 years at a rate that rewards him for being healthy (as it should) would not cover even one catastrophic illness, let alone a developing pre-condition, as in the 5th most costly health care hazard, environmental accidents ($108 billion/year).

Many chronic illnesses are self inflicted because of life styles (nicotine, caffine, alcohol, opioids, sugar, animal fat, etc) and start in the unprotected teens and go from there, so saying someone shouldn't be paying into a long-term federal 'system' IN SOME WAY is silly. But should those with chronic problems be penalized for their own negligence as well and who determines? Also, the ACA premium rates of $4,700 don't appear unreasonable if the total costs per problem are GOING TO BE $50,000 per year at some point, but a pre-emptive wellness 30-something doesn't need to pick up that whole tab.

2018.03.09:07:10 |WB|>3⋈ |GW|>3⋈ |CD|<1≈ |TR|<1 |LI|>3⋈|JU|>1 |OP|>2

Thiessen, WaPost, 'When will we stop killing humans with Down syndrome?':

"It is simply intolerable that so many joyous lives are being snuffed out. "All lives are a gift from God," Karen Gaffney says. "To me, that means that all lives matter, even if you will be born with an extra chromosome."

Genesis in the Bible:

26. Then God said, "Let Us make man in Our image, according to Our likeness; and let them rule over the fish of the sea and over the birds of the sky and over the cattle and over all the earth, and over every creeping thing that creeps on the earth."

27. God created man in His own image, in the image of God He created him; male and female He created them.

28. God blessed them; and God said to them, "Be fruitful and multiply, and fill the earth, and subdue it; and rule over the fish of the sea and over the birds of the sky and over every living thing that moves on the earth."

Note that an 'extra chromosome' might not be something that was intended by Genesis 26 and 27 because creating something in the image of God implies creating a near-perfect image life process. And the commandment 'be fruitful and multiply' was actually completed about the year 2000 AD. The ending of God's commandment and the requirement to make a perfect image implies that the new genetic editing technologies (CRISPR) can be used by mere mortals to do exactly that. Does that mean that everyone should be born with an extra chromosome or a genetically engineered reversed hypothalamus in order to be LGBT correct?

Does the end of Genesis 28 mean that mortals are not allowed to splice out a cancer gene sequence in the fetus so the 'perfect image' can be approximated? If mortals have dominion over the earth as of 2000 AD, does that mean they can edit the structure of the frontal lobe in the brain in order to double the level of consciousness a person is born with? And which mortals, given the editing toward a perfect image, decide who will have an IQ of 200 or be a fetus born free of all disease and malformation?

2018.09.29:12:16 | ξ| <2 |WB|<1 ⋈ |GW|>3 ⋈ |TR|<2 |LI|<3 ⋈|JU|<1 ≈ |OP|>2

Drs. Simon and Dimino in TheHill, 'To protect women and babies we need a new approach to labor and delivery':

"OB hospitalist programs overcome these delays by providing coverage and support to community OBs until they can arrive at the hospital or when the woman has no obstetrician, staffing hospitals on a 24/7 basis, including nights and weekends.

With a clinician onsite at all times, urgent health concerns and emergencies are quickly addressed by an OB/GYN with specialized training in those situations. In fact, an analysis by the nation's largest non-profit health system identified a 31 percent reduction in serious harm incidents before and after implementation of OB hospitalist programs."

Serious issue, although having community hospitals with birthing expertise all over the U.S. might involve some 3000 new physicians at $200,000 per year. Add in 1000 new OB support facilities at $700,000 each and the reality of doing that starts to sink in. If you added in pre-emptive, predictive DNA diagnostics and treatments to the pre-natal process in which society contributes 99% of the cost (see CHIPs programs), the safe birthing processes for all citizens, note citizens, might reach $10,000 each times about 1.4 million ladies.

That looks expensive and requires an additional 1000 OB specialists even if you had a cybernet of online experts available to each birth. But does careful, expert supported facility for birthing pre-empt a large number of deaths and birthing defects along with preventing a predictable disease later in life that might cost $120,000 per year (cancers, Downs, diabetes, obesity) for 15 years each? If the number of citizens involved is evenly distributed, does the problem remain a state responsibility or a federal one?

Wellbeing [{WB}] as a relation of [{CD}]

2018.07.29:07:47 |WB|>2⋈ |GW|>2⋈ |CD|<3 |TR|>1 |LI|<3⋈|JU|<3 ≈
|OP|>2| ξ] >?

Deane Walderman, Texas Public Policy Foundation, in TheHill, 'Medicare for all is a socialist's dream — and an American Nightmare':

"Instead of government-controlled, insurance-dominated healthcare, we need to return to our roots, to what made our country great: the free market. In 2017, the U.S. spent $3.4 trillion on healthcare for 323 million Americans, or $10,526 for every man, woman and child. Imagine if every family of four put $42,105 in an HSA every year! and simply shopped for and paid for their health care. No government stealing our money to pay its bureaucracy. No insurance company delaying or denying care. Just the old but right doctor-patient relationship with no one and nothing in between."

This is an absurd comment. The median income for a family in America is about $58,000 a year. There is no chance a family could save $42,105 a year and survive. Add in the fact that the U.S. healthcare is NOT a 'free market' because the medical related individuals, snake-oil types especially, contrive a 30-year pricing structure that is three times the normal inflation rate of the Nation and will bring about costs of $17 trillion by 2028. Such a 'system' excludes basic, life threat care to the point that Emergency Room treatments are all that is available to a 100 million people and increase at a rate of half a million a year even with Medicare and Medicaid. The current for profit 'system' brings about conditions of permanent debt indenture and servitude that are specifically prohibited by the 13th Amendment. The doctor-patient relationship is a meaningless fantasy in the century of curative instead of treatment healthcare.

True, the insurance bureaucracies siphon off 30% of the $3.4 trillion costs, but that is BECAUSE they are 'free market' oriented and have 'shareholders' on an international scale. There is also the issue of citizenship responsibility in that a person creates his own health problems by excess molecular distortions (drugs, alcohol, sugar, animal fats, etc) and then somehow expects others to pay to repair the damage so he can continue his lifestyle. Poll that idea to Americans sometime and see what they think.

If you want a government/private sector 'wellness system', not a 'treatment system', you would have to pay for it with an 8% sales tax that cannot constitutionally be used for anything else, unlike the income tax. You would have to have local medical courts of arbitration where a person could be fined for 'citizenship negligence' and medical shysters could be brought to trial. Such would have to be constitutionally defined, along with citizen responsibilities, as a human right that guarantees molecular health at conception and only citizens can give rights to each other, not a government. Very tough process, but ANY curative wellness process would be better than the 'free market' money hole that now exists.

2018.08.13:00:00 |CD|<4|LI|>3 ≈ |WB|>2+|JU|>2 ⋈ |GW|>1

Brown and Lindsay, CRS-R41981, 'CRS-Congressional Primer on Responding to Major Disasters and Emergencies':

Summary

The principles of disaster management assume a leadership role by the local, state, and tribal governments affected by the incident. The federal government provides coordinated supplemental resources and assistance, only if requested and approved. The immediate response to a disaster is guided by the National Response Framework (NRF), which details roles and responsibilities at various levels of government, along with cooperation from the private and nonprofit sectors, for differing incidents and support functions. A possible declaration of a major disaster or emergency under the authority of the Robert T. Stafford Disaster Relief and Emergency Assistance Act (the Stafford Act, P.L. 93-288, as amended) must, in almost all cases, be requested by the governor of a state or the chief executive of an affected Indian tribal government, who at that point has declared that the situation is beyond the capacity of the state or tribe to respond. The governor/chief also determines for which parts of the state/tribal territory assistance will be requested and suggests the types of assistance programs that may be needed. The President considers the request, in consultation with officials of the Federal Emergency Management Agency (FEMA), within the Department of Homeland Security (DHS), and makes the initial   decisions on the areas to be included as well as the programs that are implemented.

The majority of federal financial disaster assistance is made available from FEMA under the authority of the Stafford Act. In addition to that assistance, other disaster aid may be available through programs of the Small Business Administration, the U.S. Department of Agriculture (USDA), the U.S. Army Corps of Engineers, the Department of Transportation (DOT), and the Department of Housing and Urban Development (HUD), among other federal programs.

While the disaster response and recovery process is fundamentally a relationship between the federal government and the requesting state or tribal government, there are roles for congressional offices. **For instance, congressional offices may help provide information to survivors on available federal and nonfederal assistance, oversee the coordination of federal efforts in their respective states and districts, and consider legislation to provide supplemental disaster assistance or authorities.** Congressional offices also serve as a valuable source of accurate and timely information to their constituents on response and relief efforts.

Congressman direct help might be only feasible in Maryland and Virginia. Coordination with Washington's partisan systems would require a House and Senate secure network for EACH Member. No real control of funding distributions during disasters.   Link to FirstNet, CRS-R45179, somehow?

https://en.wikipedia.org/wiki/Essential_health_benefits :

Interpretation

The essential health benefits are a minimum federal standard and "states may require that qualified health plans sold in state health insurance exchanges also cover state-mandated benefits."[1]: 3 The act gives "considerable discretion" to the Secretary of Health and Human Services to determine, through regulation, what specific services within these classes are essential. However, the Act provides certain parameters for the secretary to consider. The secretary (1) must "ensure that such essential health benefits reflect an appropriate balance among the categories ... so that benefits are not unduly weighted toward any category"; (2) may "not make coverage decisions, determine reimbursement rates, establish incentive programs, or design benefits in ways that discriminate against individuals because of their age, disability, or expected length of life"; (3) must take into account "the health care needs of diverse segments of the population, including women, children, persons with disabilities, and other groups"; and (4) must ensure that essential benefits "not be subject to denial to individuals against their wishes on the basis of the individuals' age or expected length of life or the individuals' present or predicted disability, degree of medical dependency, or quality of life."[1]: 3–4

According to a Commonwealth Fund report in 2011:

As it stands, federal regulations for 2014 and 2015 do not establish a single, nationally uniform package of health services. Instead, the U.S. Department of Health and Human Services (HHS) gave states discretion to determine the specific benefits they deem essential. This approach was well-received by many state officials, who valued the opportunity to tailor benefit standards to reflect state priorities, and by insurers, who retained more control over benefit design. Groups representing consumers and providers were less supportive, however, expressing concern that the degree of flexibility found in the rules undermines the law's promise of consistent, meaningful coverage.[9]

Wellbeing [{WB}] as a Standard Evolution Model $\sum[\{OP\}] \leftrightarrow \xi$?

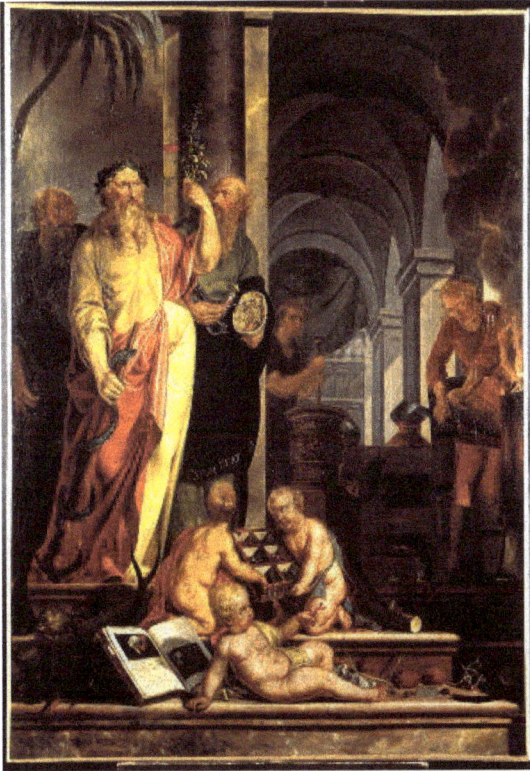

There is a common practice of attempting to group healthcare in categories so that it can be perceived in a total 'sense' of the individual's needs or even wellbeing of mind, body, and soul. That has been going on since the days of Hippocrates in 410 BCE where the body and spirit was described in terms of health as did Zhang Zhongjing in 220 CE but adding the concept of 'Ki' or life force. .This medical 'evolution' has been parallel to the hard sciences of the physicists and cosmologists and biologists as the devices of humanity improved. Many technologies appeared over a 2000-year period but only in this century has the process of standardization of human molecular 'parts' began to appear. Such things as the electron microscope, magnetic resonance imaging and a full understanding of microbiological processes have brought about a need to re-define George Engel's model of what some call biopsychosocial 'entities' and their interrelationships This is especially true since the process of Epigenetics created an increasingly ominous wide-spread experimentation with gene editing described as CRISPR

2018.12.30:10:20 |OP|>2 =WB|>3+|GW|>3✉ |CD|<3? |TR|<1 |LI|<3

Brad Plumer, Eliza Barclay, Julia Belluz, and Umair Irfan, vox, 'A simple guide to CRISPR, one of the biggest science stories of the decade....t could revolutionize everything from medicine to agriculture. Better read up now.:

"Further advances followed. Feng Zhang, a scientist at the Broad Institute in Boston, co-authored a paper in Science in February 2013 showing that CRISPR/Cas9 could be used to edit the genomes of cultured mouse cells or human cells. In the same issue of Science, Harvard's George Church and his team showed how a different CRISPR technique could be used to edit human cells.

Since then, researchers have found that CRISPR/Cas9 is amazingly versatile. Not only can scientists use CRISPR to "silence" genes by snipping them out, they can also harness repair enzymes to substitute desired genes into the "hole" left by the snippers (though this latter technique is trickier to pull off). So, for instance, scientists could tell the Cas9 enzyme to snip out a gene that causes Huntington's disease and insert a "good" gene to replace it."

TLO: Serious evolutionary matter, too much garage lab research….. Even with the Genome Map complete, there is no structure that is common to all researchers. No Evolutionary prohibition model at all.

2018.03.01:00:00 [WB]>3|Ki_ξ. ⋈ [GW]>3 ⋈ |CD|<1 |TR|<1 |LI|<3+[JU]>1 ≈ +|OP|>n?

Farre and Rapley, 'The New Old (and Old New) Medical Model: Four Decades Navigating the Biomedical and Psychosocial Understandings of Health and Illness':

https://www.ncbi.nlm.nih.gov/pmc/articles/PMC5746722/ :

By applying such reasoning to medicine, Engel defined the biopsychosocial model as encompassing information from the levels below and above the human being as experienced by each person—that is, the health professional seeks to integrate data from the human/psychological level with data from the biological level (below) and data from the social level (above) to construct the biopsychosocial description of each patient (Figure 19).

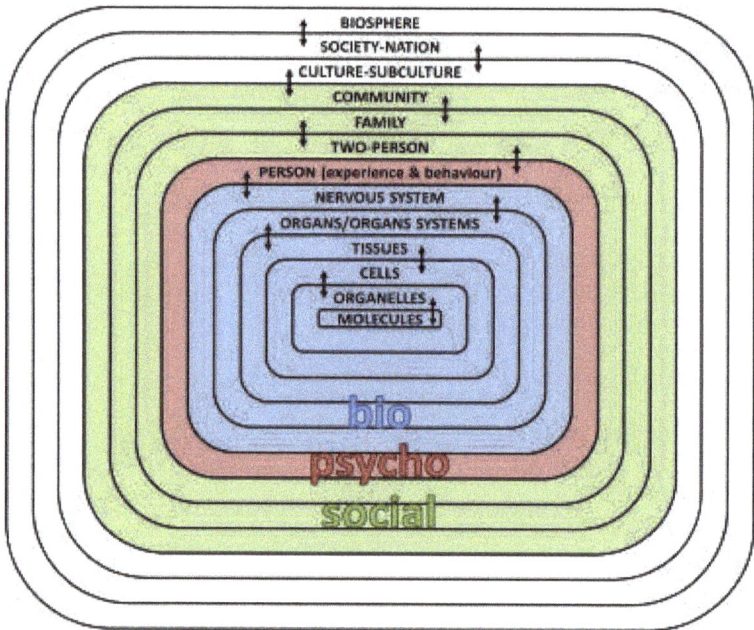

Figure 20.   Early health {wellbeing?} model

Schematic representation of the hierarchy and continuum of natural systems as applicable to Engel's definition of the biopsychosocial model---adapted from '*The clinical application of the biopsychosocial model*' {7}

TLO: Comprehensive model perception, but minute-to-minute instead of [{OP}]?

2018.01.01:00:00 |WB|>3↔|GW|>3⋈ |CD|<1 |TR|<1 |LI|<3+|JU|>1 ≈ +|OP|>n?

Note ACA model 42 U.S. Code § 18022. **Essential Health Benefits** requirements:

(a) Essential health benefits package. In this title,[1] the term "essential health benefits package" means, with respect to any health plan, coverage that—

(1) provides for the essential health benefits defined by the Secretary under subsection (b);

(2) limits cost-sharing for such coverage in accordance with subsection (c); and

(3) subject to subsection (e), provides either the bronze, silver, gold, or platinum level of coverage described in subsection (d).

(b) Essential health benefits

(1) In general, Subject to paragraph (2), the Secretary shall define the essential health benefits, except that such benefits shall include at least the following general categories and the items and services covered within the categories:

(A) Ambulatory patient services.

(B) Emergency services.

(C) Hospitalization.

(D) **Maternity and newborn care.**

(E) Mental health and substance use disorder services, including behavioral health treatment.

(F) Prescription drugs.

(G) Rehabilitative and habilitative services and devices.

(H) Laboratory services.

(I) **Preventive** and wellness services and chronic disease management.

(J) Pediatric services, including oral and vision care.

Also, single generation or less for infants, but perhaps five different phases of EHB for a generation. Reproductive healthcare as a 'right' is certainly multi-generational. But does the EHB or 'basic' mechanisms for 'ki' whole life represent something coherent or does a model have to go to a molecular or quantum level for that?

Overview of the Essential Health Benefits (EHB) Process

The 10 EHB Categories	State Selection of EHB-Benchmark Plans
Ambulatory patient services	• Each state selects its own reference plan, known as the EHB-benchmark plan
Emergency services	
Hospitalization	• EHB-benchmark plan must cover all 10 EHB categories
Maternity and newborn care	
Mental health and substance use disorder services, including behavioral health treatment	• All plans in the state must use the EHB-benchmark plan as a model
Prescription drugs	
Rehabilitative and habilitative services and devices	
Laboratory services	
Preventive and wellness services and chronic disease management	
Pediatric services, including oral and vision care	

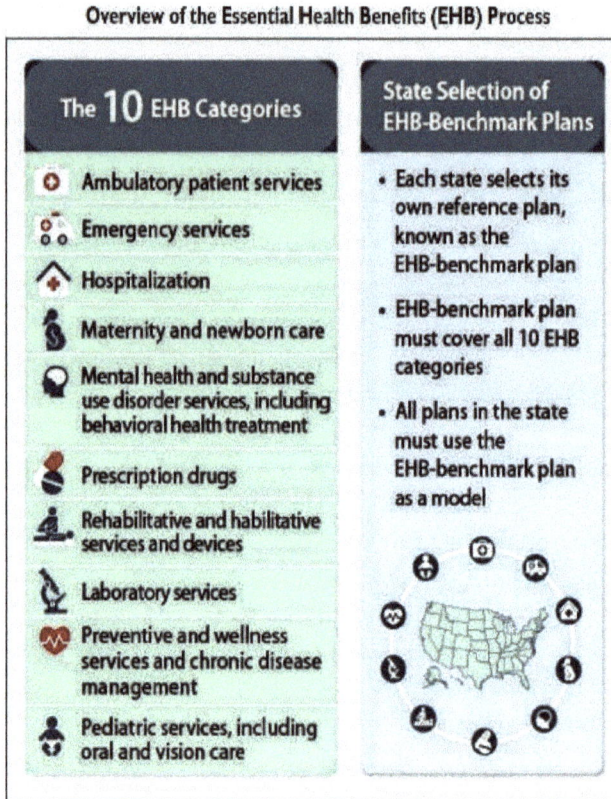

Source: Congressional Research Service (CRS) analysis

2018.01.09:15:24 |OP|>2 ≈ |WB|>3⋈ |GW|>3⋈ |CD|<1 |TR|<1
|LI|<3⋈|JU|>1

James V. Saturno, Megan Suzanne Lynch, Congressional Research Service, R41907, 'A Balanced Budget Constitutional Amendment: Background and Congressional Options':

"Summary

One of the most persistent political issues facing Congress in recent decades is whether to require that the budget of the United States be in balance. Although a balanced federal budget has long been held as a political ideal, the accumulation of large deficits in recent years has heightened concern that some action to require a balance between revenues and expenditures may be necessary.

The debate over a balanced budget measure actually consists of several interrelated debates. Most prominently, the arguments of proponents have focused on the economy and the possible harm resulting from consistently large deficits and a growing federal debt. Another issue involves whether such a requirement should be statutory or made part of the Constitution. Some proponents of balanced budgets oppose a constitutional amendment, fearing that it would prove to be too inflexible for dealing with future circumstances.

Opponents of a constitutional amendment often focus on the difficulties of implementing or enforcing any amendment. Their concerns have been numerous and varied. How would such a requirement affect the balance of power between the President and Congress? Between the federal courts and Congress? Although most proponents would prefer to establish a balanced budget requirement as part of the Constitution, some advocates have suggested using the untried process provided under Article V of the Constitution for a constitutional convention as an alternative to a joint resolution passed by two-thirds vote in both houses of Congress. Although the inclusion of a balanced budget amendment as part of the congressional agenda has muted this debate in recent years, proposals for a convention are still possible, and raise concerns that one might open the way to an unpredictable series of reforms. The last American constitutional convention convened in May 1787 and produced the current Constitution.

TLO: Are they overlooking that the prime directive for Common Defense was transferred to the federals for the specific purpose of freeing up the budgets of the states? How do you 'balance' something when it varies by 205% per decade and might vary by two hundred percent during a war over several years?

2018.03.01:07:15 [WB]>3⋈ [TR]<1 [LI]<3⋈|JU|<4 ≈ [GW]>3⋈ [CD]<1 +|OP|>2?

Ignatius, WaPost, 'Are Saudi Arabia's reforms for real? A recent visit says yes.':

From the Serbian Numbeo database, contributed data with no warranty but reasonably accurate and is consistent with other general OECD indexes of this sort:

Top 60 Quality of Life Indexes computed from 11 lifestyle factors

Rank(1)

Country(2)

Quality of Life Index, higher better (3)

Purchasing Power Index, higher better(4)

Safety Index, higher better (5)

Health Care Index, higher better (6)

Cost of Living Index, lower better (7)

Property Price to Income Ratio, lower better (8)

Traffic Commute Time Index, lower better (9)

Pollution Index, lower better (10)

Climate Index, higher better (11)

(1) (2) (3) (4) (5) (6) (7) (8) (9) (10) (11)

9 United States 180.56 127.62 50.42 68.38 72.95 3.34 34.74 31.70 78.23

31 Saudi Arabia 149.58 131.46 63.31 60.19 47.86 2.79 34.01 71.72 41.02

51 Russia 103.32 51.11 54.80 56.77 43.89 11.44 48.26 63.26 44.70

58 Iran 92.43 45.60 50.60 51.22 34.56 12.45 49.46 81.21 69.54

Speculation: The new Saudi government set out to improve this Quality of Life Index on a yearly basis and if it is doing that, it doesn't have as far to go as some others. But are some of the others carrying out a war of attrition against the new Prince so that the QLI can't possibly increase?

TLO: intra-state relations do not always have domain values for the U.S. Generally, applying [JU], [LI], [TR] and [WB] effects locally will aid American [CD] and [GW] sets and in some combinations affect [OP] negatively, as in war and genocide. Note Item (3) comparative scales. But are all QLI items domain subsets in the U.S.A.? This is an expression of the factors of life or 'Ki' model but needs work for an Our Posterity long-range model.

2018.06.05:10:58 |WB|>3⋈ |GW|>3⋈ |TR|<1 |LI|<3 ⋈ |JU|>1 |OP|>2

Editorial Board, WaPost, 'Health care is still a mess. Republicans are making it worse.':

"And costs are going up, fast. Federal health-care subsidy spending is set to rise by 6 percent per year for the next decade. This is not a result only of Obamacare subsidies; the federal government spends far more to subsidize the employer-based coverage most Americans get than it does Obamacare's individual market insurance plans."

CBO report 'Federal Subsidies for Health Insurance Coverage for People Under Age 65:

2018 to 2028:

"Net federal subsidies for insured people in 2018 will total $685 billion. That amount is projected to reach $1.2 trillion in 2028. Medicaid and the Children's Health Insurance Program account for about 40 percent of that total, as do subsidies in the form of tax benefits for work-related insurance. Medicare accounts for about 10 percent, as do subsidies for coverage obtained through the marketplaces established by the Affordable Care Act or through the Basic Health Program."

$1.2 trillion in 2028? That's only the government. The total cost of healthcare in the USA by 2028 will be something like $5 trillion and half of that might involve 'treatment' costs for medical anomalies that would be curable under a not-for-profit health system. **The 'system', in its entirety, is designed to extract wealth from individuals because they have no life-altering choices. That isn't the fault of Republicans and Democrats; it is the fault of a genetically programmed instinct humans have to exploit each other for wealth.** You will not bring about genuine 'wellbeing' or mind-body-spirit health so long as a 'system' is designed to indenture humans rather than cure them.

TLO for a Constitutional addition on Health Care or Wellness:

Wellbeing can be quantified as a summation of the relationships between the individual molecular, neural and Ki progressions of a human being. The above perceptions have been about these [CD] ⋈ [GW] balances and how they relate to a Wellbeing of a individual, which is a distinct entity in itself. It cannot really be the sum of its parts once it has achieved consciousness and engages in an empathic cooperation with other human entities. This is demonstrated by such things as 'quality of life' indices such as the Wikipedia one at:

https://en.wikipedia.org/wiki/Quality_of_life:

"Quality of life includes everything from physical health, family, education, employment, wealth, safety, security to freedom, religious beliefs, and the environment.[2] QOL has a wide range of contexts, including the fields of international development, healthcare, politics and employment. Health related QOL (HRQOL) is an evaluation of QOL and its relationship with health.[3] Quality of life should not be confused with the concept of standard of living, which is based primarily on income."

This concept is further defined in other indices such as a the Numbeo QOL index at:

https://www.numbeo.com/quality-of-life/country_result.jsp?country=United+States

which gives a 'consensus' based on a set of parameters that are sent to their database from individuals in the United States. This database has values like:

Quality of Life Index summation: 169.15 Very High

Purchasing Power Index   101.52   High

Safety Index   49.30   Moderate

Health Care Index   68.11   High

Climate Index   49.99   High

Cost of Living Index   72.76   Moderate

Property Price to Income Ratio   3.60   Very Low

Traffic Commute Time Index   32.31   Low

Pollution Index   35.12   Low

From TL2017, speculations

This Observationum refers to a constitutional change for adding a health right ONLY, not other rights and conditions, although the Authority for Use of Military Force, internal rules of the Congress, Economic warfare protection of citizens, 4th Amendment protections against surveillance abuse, 5th Amendment definitions of self-incrimination, and Tax Reform or balance are modern conditions not covered by the constitution of the 20th century or earlier. The justified fear of a 'runaway convention' has virtually gridlocked many Congresses from initiating a Convention or even sending an Amendment such as Tax Reform with an value added tax to the States for Article V ratification.

2017.12.02:09:34 is a lengthy observation on a balanced budget amendment to the constitution and shows some of the 21st century amendment procedure problems. It would be nearly impossible to balance the federal budget UNLESS either Common Defense OR General Welfare was reduced to about 10% of its current effects and costs. That, of course, leaves the American society wide open to dismantling by other states around the world.

2017.08.07:07:58 is concerned with a 'runaway' Article V convention that substitutes special interest issues for Posterity values, which is partially what happened in 1787. A special interest exclusion formula is discussed in it. The Heritage Foundation's *Heritage Guide to the Constitution* discusses this as well and notes that the Supreme Court had waived any requirement for an Amendment to have presidential signature and that two-thirds of both Houses in Article V meant 'of those present in session' was an Amendment quorum, not the full House and Senate membership. This was in the 1920s, and the concept of 'Representation' was not too well defined, or even desired, judging from the representation for the 18th Amendment on Prohibition. That Amendment also brought up the issue of a noble cause special interest in which there was no actual knowledge of genetic addiction that led to Prohibition. But everyone knew what the economic and spiritual effects of the addiction was.

That special interest 'gaming the system' would also be a major contention in any Amendment that involved a full Convention by the States; the 'representation' could be limited to special persons or candidates of each state. Such a mechanism, which almost certainly would have led to a 'runaway', would not have created a Wellbeing right, nor could the 'two-thirds present' quorum rule of the Congress, so a convention would have to have a much larger 'popular referendum' style of representation in each state. Whether Congress could Constitutionally create the 'conditions' within states for 'representation' was also an issue. Article V says Congress 'shall call a Convention for proposing Amendments' without saying it can make 'necessary and proper' laws governing such a Convention. Nothing whatever is said about adding a full Article, so perhaps the necessary and proper clause of Article I, Section 8 is all that would be required and there is nothing that says the Congress cannot 'empower' the Supreme Court to rule on the specifications of an Article representation issue, with appropriate presidential sign-off under his Article II Oath

The idea is, of course, to adhere to the original Founder's intelligence gathering on what qualified as 'checks and balances' and apply those rules throughout an Article VIII Convention process, especially where [OP] is involved.

Congressional Research Service, the Article V Convention to Propose Constitutional Amendments:

Contemporary Issues for Congress, 2017.04.11, Tomas H. Neale

Summary:

Article V of the U.S. Constitution provides two ways of amending the nation's fundamental charter. Congress, by a two-thirds vote of both houses, may propose amendments to the states for ratification, a procedure used for all 27 current amendments. Alternatively, if the legislatures of two-thirds of the states apply, 34 at present, Congress "shall call a Convention for proposing Amendments.... " This alternative, known as an Article V Convention, has yet to be implemented. This report examines the Article V Convention, focusing on contemporary issues for Congress.

CRS Report R42592, *The Article V Convention for Proposing Constitutional Amendments: Historical Perspectives for Congress* examines the procedure's constitutional origins and history and provides an analysis of related state procedures.

Significant developments in this issue have occurred recently: in March 2016, the Georgia Legislature applied for a convention to consider a balanced federal budget amendment, revoking its rescission of an earlier application; in April 2016, Tennessee took similar action. While both applications are valid, they may revive questions as to the constitutionality of rescissions of state applications for an Article V Convention and whether convention applications are valid indefinitely. Either issue could have an impact on the prospects for a convention. In other recent actions, the legislatures of Ohio, in November 2013, and Michigan, in March 2016, applied to Congress for an Article V Convention to consider a balanced federal budget amendment; these are the first new state applications since 1982 and are also the $33^{rd.}$ and 34^{the} applications for the balanced budget amendment convention. **If all 32 previous related state applications are valid, it is arguable that the constitutional requirement for requests from two-thirds of the states has been met, and that Congress should consider calling a convention.**

Internet- and social media-driven public policy campaigns have also embraced the Article V Convention as an alternative to perceived policy deadlock at the federal level. In 2011, the "Conference on a Constitutional Convention," drew participants ranging from conservative libertarians to progressives together to discuss and promote a convention. In December 2013, a meeting of state legislators advocated a convention, while the "Convention of States" called for a convention to offer amendments to "impose fiscal restraints and limit the power of the federal government." Also in 2013, the advocacy group Compact for America proposed the "Compact for a Balanced Budget," an interstate compact that would provide a "turn-key" application, by which, with a single vote, states could join the compact; call for a convention; agree to its format, membership, and duration; adopt and propose a specific balanced budget amendment; and prospectively commit themselves to ratify the amendment.

Congress would face a range of questions if an Article V Convention seemed likely, including the following. What constitutes a legitimate state application? Does Congress have discretion as to whether it must call a convention? What vehicle does it use to call a convention? Could a convention consider any issue, or must it be limited to a specific issue? Could a "runaway" convention propose amendments outside its mandate? Could Congress choose *not* to propose a convention-approved amendment to the states? What role would Congress have in defining a convention, including issues such as rules of procedure and voting, number and apportionment of delegates, funding and duration, service by Members of Congress, and other questions. Under these circumstances, Congress could consult a range of information resources in fashioning its response. These include the record of the founders' original intent, scholarly works cited in this report and elsewhere, historical examples and precedents, and relevant hearings, reports, and bills produced by Congress from the 1970s through the 1990s.

How does the Convention limit itself to a specific agenda such as Wellbeing when virtually every special interest inside and outside the United states would attempt to influence the delegates through 'covert' representation? It would be necessary, based on referendums and initiatives of the last decade to examine carefully the idea of representation verses pure democracy as Madison warned about even as he prosed the Bill of Rights. By 2000, what this referendum process actually did in a community was to isolate minorities from their Rights, especially voting rights. This might be an evolutionary 'norm' for humanity; everyone trusts and identifies with members of their own cave tribe more than anyone else. It is only dangerous to a larger society like a state or nation when the combined total of injustices to minorities, including genetic minorities represented a distortion of the national Justice covenant in the Preamble.

But suppose a modern molecular definition was applied to the injustice? There are thousands of minor molecular structures in a person, virtually all of them causing variations in what can be called normal. Other people don't have a problem with the variations unless they represent some form of open hostility such as conflicts concerning skin tone, which is actually a sensor for regulating body temperature. The stark black and white contrasts found in the USA as it evolved from migrations are an obvious example, but the same skin tone perceptions and conflicts have been applied by ALL human genetic codes including African and Asian to other genetic codes. The same perceptions can be applied to very many minor molecular aberrations caused by disease or environment such as Parkinson's (600,000), Downs Syndrome (1 million?), Schizophrenia (3 million Americans in varying degrees) in which the individual becomes a 'ward' of societies with limited citizenship. There are so many 'citizenship' variations that an initiative or referendum governance system like the Swiss have would be nearly impossible.

The net result is that a Constitutional referendum on a national scale would be very difficult because of the interjection of the minority representation problems of the American societies. Such health-related Amendments like the 18th, prohibition of alcohol use and distribution, were actually created by legislative groups in many states that managed the Article V three quarters approval without referendum. But they did not represent a majority of the American people, many of whom would have protected the source of their addiction by their votes. That is an overpowering interest of the addict, not the welfare of others and it doesn't matter what the addiction form takes; drugs, power, sex, or money. This again brings up the referendum issue as to whether people would vote for something that was in the interest of We the People rather than their personal minority. Madison and Hamilton didn't think so. Most of the initiatives of the last decade were so special interest biased that voters could not actually tell what they were voting for. California and Texas both had election 'roll-off' effects with huge referendum ballots that no one could read.

Most state level tax initiatives indicated that narrow majorities would approve the expenditure of funds *without* approving any means to pay for it. This was especially true when the means of paying for it empowered a legislature to tax without accountability, as was the case with several casino referendums. The money from the casinos, of course, did not go into public infrastructure processes afterwards as the initiatives said. Community level referendums for bonds or credit to purchase something generally worked well because the accountability for the revenue was clearly defined.

In order to add a full Article, not just an Amendment, to the Constitution such things as taxation power would have to be completely dedicated to the objective being added, but what about the removal of minority or special interests from a national referendum or Convention? If you had a state with a small population, it could come up with a special interest that would override a national need so that it would require that interest to be included in the Article. In a small 21st century population state, the political interests might not even be 'American' due to the internet.

How would a Constitutional Convention screen out special interests? One method might be through the Electoral College mechanism in which each delegate to the Convention was elected to authenticate specific sections of the new Article with human rights protections included. The 'Electors' would be the same as the Article II specifications of one per representative or 538 total.

Since a Human Right is involved in the Article, (the complete genetic protection of the newly created life), the Electors in the College would need a two thirds approval (355 Electors) of each section of the Article to be submitted to the states, which in turn would have to have a three quarters (38 states) approval or designate the states' Electors as approving. This would be true only if the states each voted to allow the Electors from their state to absolutely represent the people of that state and were given the Amendment voting power of the legislature in a Convention.

Aside: The Electoral College was created originally to elect a President and Vice president over great physical distances, but was it actually intended, as some Federalist Papers indicate, to maintain a Republic or representative form of government so that the original votes or will of the people couldn't be manipulated? Is it only now, in a high multiple technology period that its real use becomes apparent?

Congressional Research Service, *Electoral College Reform: 111 Congress Proposals and Other Current Developments,* Thomas H. Neale, 2009.11.04:

> John F. Kennedy, while serving in the Senate, was a leading defender of the Electoral College against proposals to establish a district plan variant in place of the current (then and now) general ticket or winner-take-all system of allocating electoral votes. In the course of Senate floor debate on this question in 1956, he paraphrased a comment by Viscount Falkland, a 17 century English statesman, declaring of the Electoral College, "It seems to me that Falkland's definition of conservatism is quite appropriate [in this instance]— 'When it is not necessary to change, it is necessary not to change.'" This aphorism may offer a key to the future prospects of the Electoral College. To date, policymakers have generally concluded that it has not been necessary to change the existing system, or perhaps more accurately, there has been no compelling call for change. **The first and only major constitutional overhaul of the Electoral College**

system to date, the 12ᵗʰ Amendment, was a direct response to turmoil accompanying the presidential election of 1800. This was a fundamental "crisis of regime" that, once surmounted, motivated Congress to propose a major reform, the 12 Amendment, in very short time. The fundamentals established by that amendment have remained intact for more than two centuries. As long as the Electoral College system functions well enough to avoid provoking a national crisis of similar scale, it may remain unchanged, if not unchallenged.

The twelfth Amendment as described in the CRS analysis indicates that the Electors in each state will 'assemble' in their state and verify the actual votes of citizens for president and vice-president. The Elector is then bound to vote as the popular vote for his district was made, establishing a 'representative' form of authority in each state. This is guaranteed by the Article IV of the Federal Constitution, so that this method of 'representative assembly' of electors would be correct. This doesn't sound very important in the 21ˢᵗ century with instant communications and BYOD everywhere; technically you could have validated citizen votes from cell-phones all over the United States including those 'offshore', but that might not come out as 'representative' where one is charged with a specific purpose such as an Elector at the College, especially if there already exists state representatives who determine the purposes of the Electors under their current constitutions.

For a discussion of current state legislative 'amendment' possesses from Ballotpedia.org, see

https://ballotpedia.org/2018_ballot_measures. $1.2 billion in contributions for state amendments?

Increasingly difficult to bring constitutional change by other than state legislature initiation as per Article V. A convention requires two thirds of the legislatures to approve a convention but the Congress, with Executive approval, can create the 'Mode of Ratification' for an addition which is not a mere Amendment. According to Article V, if the federal government, possibly all three branches approving, creates an Article Mode of Ratification, the 'equal suffrage in the Senate' becomes the state 'representation' authority and might be the criteria for ensuring representation by a full state population. The Mode of Ratification should then adhere to that of the current Electoral College.

Currently, there is a total of 538 electors, there being 435 representatives and 100 senators, plus the three electors allocated to Washington, D.C... The six states with the most electors are California (55), Texas (38), New York (29), Florida (29), Illinois (20) and Pennsylvania (20). The seven smallest states by population—Alaska, Delaware, Montana, North Dakota, South Dakota, Vermont, and Wyoming—have three electors each. This is because each of these states is entitled to one representative and two senators.

Constitutional Change methods

Constitutional Change Methods

Article V requires three fourths of the states to Ratify an Amendment. However, the addition of an Article containing a Human Right might require only the two thirds ratification as was originally employed.

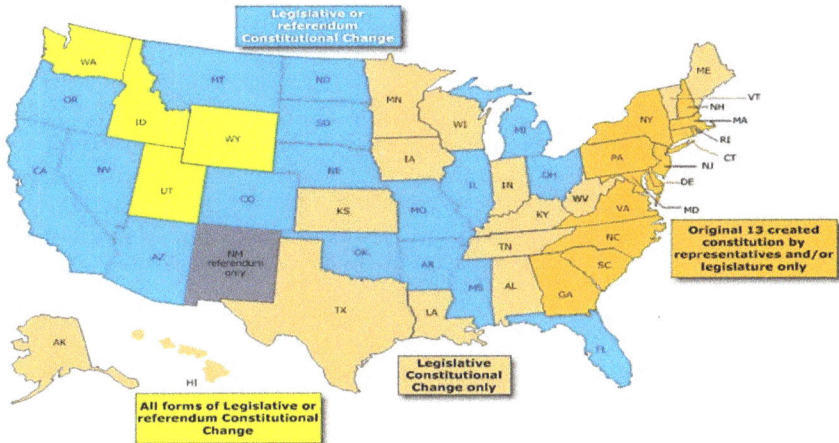

In a National Constitutional Convention, these 538 electors could easily qualify as representing the entire population of the US, subject only to approval by state legislatures who are also representative of the existing constitutions. A minimum of three Electors per state (territories too?) would be representative enough so that population intense states could not rule a Convention.

Other conditions might involve the process where constitutional Electors are 'free' to vote after three votes as designated representatives, (the inevitable need to compromise at constitutional conventions) or such things as a 'College' pre-qualification for local election as Elector. It would be silly for an Elector to vote if he were not 'savvy' about the American society AND had taken the constitutional oaths of citizenship in the Constitution already. It would also be silly to allow an Elector to be designated in a local district referendum election under false pretenses since he cannot be 'representative'. This would need a background investigation every bit as careful as a security clearance or presidential 'vetting' process along with a previous oath of office. It might even require biometric validation of intent, this being the 21st century of technology where foreign devices can be implanted for interdiction of legitimate constitutional activity, or instant 'payoff' by totalitarian elements.

It would require the Electoral College to operate in the manner of a closed session as is the case for many activities at the Kwedake Dikep's community, so that foreign influences could not interfere with its proceedings. Much of the original Constitution was formed by closed debate, not counting those debates at the City Tavern around the corner from Independence Hall in Philadelphia, but it was only being influenced by local governments who were not delegates. . The process would also require that a special Constitutional Convention Electoral College election be held in an off-year so that there would be no confusion with 'normal' democracy voting activity. This is important since the Electors to the College must be considered independently of the current representation in the government. That doesn't mean that one already elected to office can't be an Elector as well, especially if he or she is well versed in constitution history.

Since elections and referendums are held every two years now, an off year would have to be an odd number year and could involve preliminary referendums on the intent of sections in the new Article, in this case Article VIII, especially of the taxation empowerment and the concept of a 'right' in the Article .

Remember, at such a Convention you DO NOT want it to be associated with the election politics of the various legislatures because as much as ninety percent of their election activity does not involve [OP] or the passing of values to a next generation. It might even be necessary to isolate the Electoral College from any access by the public the same as many juries are isolated so that they cannot be intimidated during their deliberations on a {WB} Article VIII. One of the 'chaos' problems of the ACA was that it input from extreme corporate and state minorities that were not 'represented' and openly discussing their views in the media..

Note again the CRS Report showing the complexity of the issue, Electoral College Reform: 111 Congress Proposals and Other Current Developments: Pros and Cons:

> In addition to the electoral votes assigned on the basis of each state's House of Representatives delegations, the current system also allocates two additional electors to each state, regardless of population. Defenders maintain that this formula is an important "federal" component of the presidential election system, comparable to the two Senators assigned by the Constitution to each state, also regardless of population. Moreover, they note that these "senatorial" electors constitute only 18.6% of the Electoral College.

A 'mapping' of the Convention process, with much of the current legislation both state and federal already involved in Wellbeing processes, is shown in the 'convention map' timeline and is highly speculative.   Considerable ruthless caution is necessary on eliminating non-essentials to a Convention on rights that effect all persons and half the resources of We The people.   Note that both the 2012 and 2016 elections showed considerable referendum interest in Wellbeing related processes but also an extreme voter caution about where the [OP] should go. This caution was also shown as in the 2016 election of 'do nothing' representatives partly out of fear that things might turn out worse.

Even if it was decided by state laws that the Electoral College process was a lawful mechanism for a Constitution Convention, the states would then have to choose the 'intelligence agents' who would be qualified to be Electors. The reason for care in the picking of the 'representatives' of the Convention is very similar to the way the States were represented in the first Convention of 1787. They had gathered 'intelligence' about the way people were thinking in various parts of the country, much of which appeared in letters to Washington at Mount Vernon. Remember that you had a population of three million spread over an area twice the size of Western Europe and each Representative needed a literate, complex understanding of his 'territory' in order to be at a Continental sized meeting. Things are quite different now and an Elector might run the risk of trivial pursuit from endless media sources rather than see a forest instead of the trees.

How does a state define a Representative with the same perceptional modes of the First Convention but in a modern sense that takes into account 21st century technologies that can be both very damaging and very useful? The individual Elector would have to be literate in the Constitution processes (Rufus King, Massachusetts, and Charles Pinckney of South Carolina). There would have to be an awareness of his local people environment (John Langdon, New Hampshire, Dickenson of Maryland or John Blair of Virginia). Electors would need to be literate in scientific, medical and surveillance technologies involving citizens (Ben Franklin of Pennsylvania, Samuel Adams, Massachusetts) which was quite rare in 1787. But skilled in economics as a freedom basis of society? Many Convention delegates in 1787 knew about merchant economics, taxation being one of the reasons for the Revolution (Hamilton, New York, Madison, Virginia, Mifflin, Pennsylvania, or William Few of Georgia) and some Delegates were quite unsuccessful at being 'businessmen'.

Perhaps some common set of values would be required to be eligible as an Elector to a Convention in the 21st century that really wasn't required in 1787. A detailed knowledge of the six Covenants of the Preamble in some tested form might be required under modern circumstances. The Elector would have to have some minimum communication skills, political and environmental awareness AND a knowledge of bio-medical technologies and ethics AND have a long-developed empathy for an American community that was developing conditions of Posterity such as Ki ξ.

Would the minimum requirements as an Elector be defined as an **Elector Rule of Fours?**

> (1) 44% passage of the US Citizenship test at any time, including 4 questions in a second language of choice, with one fourth of Elector citizen costs paid by Federal, State, Community, and Self each.

> (2) A GRE General Test score of 144, a SAT score of 444, and a MCAT score of 444.

> (3) Residence in and paying taxes in the same Representative District communities for 4 years.

> (4) Spent 4 contiguous months in a public service occupation in a [TR], [WB], [CD] or [GW] system.

The other issue is how would the newly designated Electors 'represent' according to Article V, a segment of people on a given issue? The issue itself should be a reflection of the entire American people, not just some value that reflects an individual need. This sounds contradictory if one is looking at a solution for enhancing *individual* liberty through wellbeing. The enhancement comes from the *structure* of We The People, not the individual processes within that domain of sets. Indeed, even in a community spread over a large area, a 'representative' form might be needed to solve [sets] of mutual enhancements.

If one applied modern statistical methods to a 'population', and the rules apply to nearly all populations no matter what it is made up of, some rational approaches to an

Electoral representative might be found. One method involves taking a 'sample' from the group physically located somewhere in the manner of exit polling during an election.   The exit polls of the past view decades have become quite accurate in predicting the outcome of something much larger because of the ability to 'average' or sum the polling quickly. The sampling of a population after a vote simply says what exists at that moment for increasingly larger sections of We the People.

But suppose that an Elector was to 'represent' a district where the issue affected ALL of them equally, such as Wellbeing?   Then the polling wouldn't be as useful because it would show only the majority consensus for a given district, not necessarily all of those there. This has actually become a constitutional problem over the last two census because of the increasing diversity shown in populations.   The representative for a Convention would have to represent the district infrastructure on an issue and not necessarily the majority, so his vote, *but not the U. S. House Representatives,* might have to represent a larger area than just a given district on Wellbeing. So how would you do that?

2nd Convention Elector considerations

For a given state, and the Elector must simultaneously represent the State and the District that produced him, any issue of a convention would have to be screened by some formula in order that it truly 'represented' the entire population and not just individuals within it. The issue, regardless of which one, would have to be defined by the distribution of the Electors so that it was not submitted by adjoining districts. In order to be 'representative' of a state, the issue would have to be approved by Electors that were NOT from adjoining districts.   That is, something like the definition of life procreation as 'marriage' in a new Article would need the approval districts spread throughout the state but not adjoining each other in order to insure 'representation' at a convention.

The Issues Rule of Sixes:

> An issue which affects any of the six Preamble covenants, no matter how formed, must affect at least one-sixth of a Elector's population and then affect up to six Electors that are not physically connected within a state, then   affect the Electors of six states not connected within the USA. Ratification of a Rights Article section needs 66% of Electors approving.

The objective is to remove all individual motivation [think We The People as originally done] from an issue that a Constitutional Convention would consider in the manner that Washington brought a portfolio of the ideas for a new government to the 1787 Convention where the 'sampling' had been sent to him at Mount Vernon over a ten year period after the Revolution. There had not been too many individual motivations in the writings of Jay, Knox, Madison, Hancock, Adams and Franklin and there is no reason this creative problem solving shouldn't be kept intact at other conventions. It has only in recent years that Conventions have become individualized to the point that 'platforms' or structures do not follow a 'representative' rule. But a Constitutional Convention does not have the luxury of individual whims or needs; it MUST represent all of the people as defined in the manner of the original in order to be a legitimate process. Note that a Federal Congress can make such terms lawful and constitutional as majorities see fit.

Glorius but Mythical State of Being

To be Consitutional, Each Elector cannot be from any adjoining congressional districts. This allows an issue to be 'representative'. Same rule applies to States: six unjoined states for issue to go to Convention.

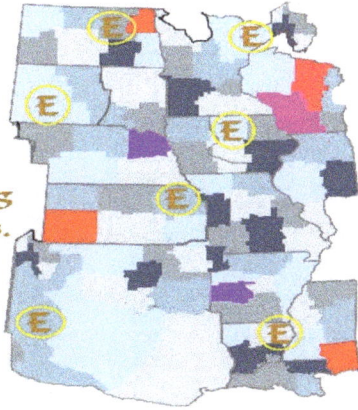

Article VIII
Constitution Convention Map

Starting Process	Information media for Article conditions	Election year conventions	Special Election for		Final vote of College
State legislature introduction. Set date, location for College, citizenship of Electors via Rule of Fours	Voting in legislatures of non- initiative states	Add to platforms, approve or disapprove sections, non-binding by law.	College Electors, held on second Tuesday of September	T H I N K I N G	Article VIII Ratification Sets Congress, Executive authority.

20nn odd year	20nn.06.nn	20nn.09.17	20nn even year	20nn.11.nn	20nn odd year	20nn.09.17

Initiate education on Article VIII	Voting in referendum legislature session to approve elections of Electors for Article VIII only.	Election year	National, State, Community elections	Electoral College convenes, debates sections
Local debates Congress sets aside internet, TV channel for debates. Congress Sets Rule of Sixes style conditions for Convention.	S.C. validates state Electoral representation.	Article VIII sections placed on primaries by states if required.	No Article VIII referendums, don't associate with political elections...	Closed sessions Set debate rules, committees of style, content.

{T1} Congress sets debate media systems, TV and internet channels full time use. Sets Rule of Sixes Electoral College representation.
{T2} States vote on Electoral College mechanism for Second Convention, insures 'Rule of Fours' citizenship for Electors, validates Rule of Sixes.
{T3} Supreme Court validates state Elector 'representation' through challenges.
{T4} Special Elector and alternates election, by legislature or referendum, in September of national election year, no other legislative agendas.
{T5} Convene Electoral College in summer of odd numbered year, debate Article VIII wording per state instructions.
{T6} Electoral College vote on Article VIII, two thirds is ratification of rights.

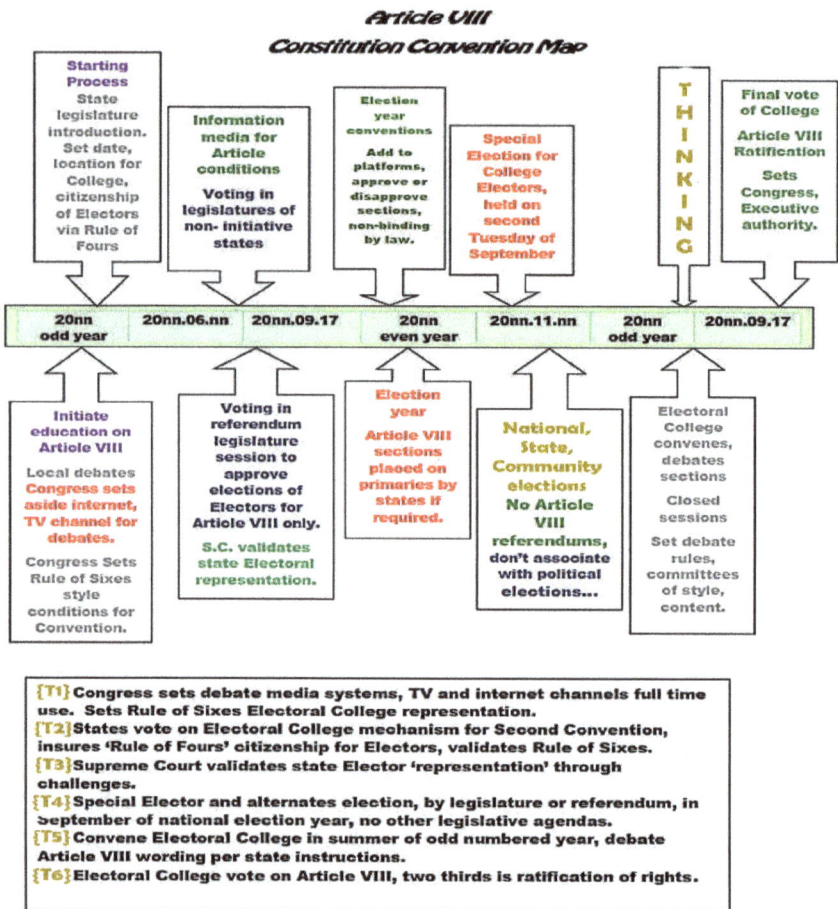

Figure 21.　Second Convention map

What, me worry? This entire process of a Constitutional Convention has not been shown to have any urgency as far as healthcare is concerned. The Patient Protection and Affordable Care Act of 2009 had a timeline of 10 years and has been proceeding according that timeline, with various sections being constitutionally validated by the Supreme Court and a reasonable coverage of many with chronic or genetic birth illnesses that wasn't there before. So why go to all this trouble to change the Constitution? It is the very nature of the beast, pardon, problem that needs to be addressed in terms of cost to the American society.

U.S. Center for Disease Control, 2018.00.00:

> January is National Birth Defects Prevention Month. Hospitalization
> for birth defects costs the U.S. over$2.6 billion annually. This cost
> is higher when including the financial and emotional impact of living
> with birth defects. In the United States, birth defects have led to more
> than 139,000 hospital stays during a single year (2004), resulting in
> $2.6 billion in hospital costs alone (1). Often, babies born with birth
> defects need special treatments or services to thrive, adding to the
> costs of their care. Families, communities, and the government share
> these costs. Examples of costs of certain birth defects are shown
> below:

> Heart defects: One study showed that overall hospital costs for
> people with a congenital heart defect were about $1.4 billion in a
> single year (1).

> Spina bifida: A 2012 study using data from Florida showed hospital
> costs for a typical baby born with spina bifida were about $21,900
> (ranging up to $1,350,700) (2).

> Down syndrome: The medical costs for a child with Down syndrome
> were 12 to 13 times higher than a child without Down syndrome. If
> a child with Down syndrome also has a congenital heart defect,
> families experience even higher medical costs

> Beyond the financial impacts, what are the emotional costs of birth
> defects?

There is a dot-connect between these disorders and the fact that the Genetic and Rare
(that is, Chromosomal) Diseases Information Center has a listing of nearly 7000
disorders that affect nearly 45 million 'citizens' in the U.S.A. Not only is this many
born with genetic anomalies, they have immediate effects on those around them in time
and effort to care for them or react to them. The one mentioned, Spina bifida, carries
an immediate cost of $21,900 dollars and a possible $1.3 million cost over the infant's
lifetime. Heart defects and Down's syndrome can be even worse in their ripple effects
on their surrounding families, possibly $2 million over several family lifetimes. Dot
connect these costs with the other 7000 disorders in 45 million people AND the fact
that many of these problems might be addressed by 'gene therapies' that are now
coming into existence IF they are detected early enough in the pre-natal stages. Is there
a [OP] savings of a trillion dollars of two generations if the genetic anomalies never
existed because of molecular corrections? What does that do to the Liberty, Justice,
and Tranquility covenants of America?

Prime Directives Interaction [CD] ⋈ [GW] → [OP]

Interactives through 2017

Interactions are conditions where the balance of Common Defense and General Welfare actually enhance or detract from Posterity. Many of the issues of either prime directive are dynamical enough to cross over into other sets and this has always been a perceptional problem from generation to generation or even from election cycle to the next. Taxation justice, Civil rights, criminal cartels, terrorism and world economics all have facets in Justice, Wellbeing, Liberty and interstate peace or Tranquility.

Political and Institutional Reform as a Process:

Many institutional reform processes exist in the American society and these have been going on nearly continuously. Examples are:
Justice Stevens on Reform through Amendments: 2014.04.14:07:24.
Tongue-in-Cheek reform of PACs: 201.05.22:10:42, 201.12.02:09:34.

2014.05.22:10:42,   [GW] [CD] [TR] [LI] [JU] [OP] :

> Re campaign money reform, try:
>
> Amendment XXVIII
>
> Section 1. In order to maintain Tranquility and Justice within the States, no transfer of funds for the purposes of election to public office will be lawful unless it is within 60 days of the date of the national elections, or when the transfer of funds for a political purpose is made in certified gold or silver bullion from a registered facility within the United States.
>
> Guess what happens when you must sign out 350 pounds of gold or silver for a political ad from a 'registered' and 'registering' facility in a local community.

Reform of 'Gridlock': 2014.11.17:07:02.

Possible Constitutional Convention: 2014.08.07:18:00, Confederate Constitution as a 'result' and 2014.12.02:09:34. as a 'reason' for a convention

Political polarization and partisan gridlock are rampant in government today. As economic challenges continue to dominate the conversation around the 2016 election, re-evaluating the current political structure may present an opportunity for the next president to stimulate economic progress.

Congressional Research Service, *Tax Rates and Economic Growth,* Jane G. Gravelle, Donald J. Marples, 2017.01.02:

> A review of statistical evidence suggests that both labor supply and savings and investment are relatively insensitive to tax rates. Small effects arise in part because of offsetting income and substitution effects (which make the direction of effects uncertain) and in part because each of these individual responses appears small. Institutional constraints may also have an effect. Offsetting income and substitution effects also affect savings. Capital gains taxes are

often singled out as determinants of growth, but their effects on the cost of capital are quite small. International capital flows also appear to have a small effect. Most expenditures that affect the productivity of labor and capital inputs (research and development, education, or infrastructure) are already tax favored or provided by the government. Small business taxes are also sometimes emphasized as important to growth, but the evidence suggests a modest and uncertain effect on entrepreneurship.

Paying for everything and still having some growth are the main exergy problems facing Americans on all levels. The 'income' taxation and fees system for revenue have clearly not been able to balance the rapidly growing needs of Americans with the world economic extraction of wealth from the United States. That is sometimes referred to as Asian Vulture Capitalism or AVC because it was not invented by John Locke in the 1600s, but by certain Asian Warlords 500 years earlier. It simply meant that you extracted whatever capital people could produce and then abandoned what was left to care for itself with less resources. Several Chinese, Thai, and Japanese imperial systems (but also Roman and Persian) fell apart as a result of the wealth disappearance from the general population.

The above study by the CRS on American tax rates is an indicator of this AVC process because the less tax/more wealth creation 'system' works ONLY if the more capital from less taxes re-appears in the local economy. That does not happen very well a 21st century world's economy, hence it is AVC motivated.

This has been an impact from China with its global production of manufactured goods at below costs in order to attract world economy capital: In an increasingly globalized world, the United States faces serious economic competition from growing powers like China, Russia and perhaps Brazil. The next American president will have to strategically manage this tricky relationship and decide whether it is a [CD] or [GW] issue.

Wonder how many senior members of the People's Liberation Army (PLA) are included in the 22, 000 offshore accounts uncovered so far? The implication is that members of the Chinese government are making international 'security zones' around the Chinese mainland (which extend not only into the air space of Japan and the Philippines, but also into Indonesia, Myanmar, Afghanistan and Russian Siberia) for THEIR member's protection. Could it be that a national military force was being used to extend the multi-generation protection of a wealthy elite to other nations rather than protect the citizens of that nation?

In this century, the wealthiest 2 percent of the world's population (including 31 billionaires in the Chinese National People's Congress) directly own or control 60 per cent of the wealth generated by human beings, something over 100 trillion dollars. Could it be that a military force is being formed to protect the 'assets' of the wealthy rather than the lives of citizens? Do Americans thank Marx or Keynes or Freidman for the economic concepts of Asian Vulture Capitalism run by totalitarianists?

Interesting that since World War I a century ago, the Americans are the only ones who have not fought for territorial gain in any of its conflicts. They have, in fact, opposed one party state imperialism in nearly every instance. Kaiser Wilhelm, Hideki Tojo, Hitler, Stalin, Castro, Mao, Milosevic, Saddam Hussein, Gadhafi, Mohammed Omar, etc., etc. China, through a nearly independent militarist society within its borders, has begun the usual, traditional imperialism cycle again, as has its allies Iran and Venezuela.

2014.02.29:00:00. The problem with Americans is they think the US military is the appropriate 'agent of change' for democracy rather than direct support of the genuine democracy institutions that are so despised by the totalitarianists.   But in order to believe that freedom made of a dynamical system of rights with power checks and balances magically grows like a flower, one would have to be a closet totalitarianist secretly in love with the power of the one-person state and secretly hoping that the democracy system will fail.

There is the problem of immigration, or cross-border economic activity is a major issue for Americans because apparently a good deal more wealth is leaving the Nation than being re-invested in it by transnationals who are 'feeding' their homeland. Not a [CD] issue when half a million people a year do it, but is it still a [GW] issue when perhaps 17 million are doing it?

One of those problems is the economic renunciation of 'citizenship' in that a person enjoys all the benefits of [CD], [JU] and [WB] without contributing to their maintenance. That might involve half those living in American in one way or another. 2014.05.01:07:05 is a discussion of 'citizens' coming across the borders with various germs that can harm other Americans and is an increasingly severe problem for [CD], not healthcare. 2014.07.13:00:00 discusses the children coming across the border and their 'protection' under the 14th Amendment. The issue is more serious in a Constitutional sense than in a local Tranquility sense but is a Posterity issue that might require a re-definition of the term 'citizenship' within the Constitution itself.

Perhaps affected by the lack of a single key issue, nationwide voter turnout was just 36.4%, down from 40.9% in the 2010 midterms and the lowest since the 1942 elections, when just 33.9% of voters turned out, though that election came during the middle of World War II and 12 million citizens were actually out of the country in non-voting, shot-at situations. The 2016 election lacked a "dominant national theme", with no single issue rising above all others. Some of the major issues of the election included income inequality, which could easily be the result of the ongoing AVC., and such items as the effects of the Patient Protection and Affordable Care Act (commonly referred to as "Obamacare" because it was working for him) and the above mention immigration or 'citizenship definition' problems.

Other [GW] problems included Medicare, the enormous government healthcare programme for over-65s and disabled Americans which has again risen in costs and was projected run out of money without tax reform.. Meidcare started in the 1960s and was a Democratic achievement under [GW] and [TR], But maybe not a [WB] success? It has two major [GW] burdens - the ever-growing cost of an inefficient healthcare system and the imminent retirement of the baby-boom generation, more and more of whom are becoming eligible for benefits. Not to mention becoming unemployed as far as the census is concerned That is multi generational and is a direct [OP], [GW] interaction mechanism affecting economic growth.

More do-it-yourself health care: apps and technology because of BYOD has quite possibly made people healthier, but it has also accelerated access to dangerous chemicals and that is still a wait and see, although 'rights' protections against molecular WMD by snake oil merchants on those BYOD have changed things. .. Technology has made do-it-yourself patient care much easier, a clear [WB] win. This goes beyond just a patient's ability to look up their symptoms online. There are apps to help with autism, apps that can simulate a check-up, apps that can monitor conditions. Wearables can motivate you to walk more or sleep more or check a diabetic's glucose level. But how does all this helping yourself make your health care better? How much is too much? And what does this mean for your privacy? Many healthcare data breaches and 4th Amendment violations by offshore people. [CD] or [JU} responsibility? Where is HIPACC when you need it?

Clear [WB] problem in doctor shortage. There aren't nearly enough of us to care for the U.S. population. By some estimates, the country is already short of tens of thousands of doctors, a problem that will only get worse as the demand for care increases with our aging population. Droids perhaps?

The fiscal cliff and after that, the budget deficit

Mr. Obama finds himself again contending with a bitterly divided congress that has been mired in parliamentary gridlock for the past four years and barely able to pass a sequestration bill to cut some spending. Analysts predict Congress would remain divided, with the Republicans in control of the House of Representatives and the Democrats keeping single-vote, and majority in the Senate. Not likely. Little chance of problem solving under those circumstances.

"There is no real prospect that this election is going to lance the boils, break the fever, bring us back to bipartisan policymaking," says Norman Ornstein, a prominent congressional scholar and co-author of *It's Even Worse Than It Looks: How the American Constitutional System Collided With the New Politics of Extremism.* "We're in for a long slog."

Iran remains the center of M.E. Common Defense and Justice problems, along with winding down US engagement in Afghanistan, ensuring stability in Iraq, (not a chance of success) promoting a resolution to the Israel/Palestine situation, fighting terrorism, ensuring open access to energy and preventing nuclear proliferation. The US is still trying to prevent Iran gaining a nuclear weapon. Iran maintains its nuclear program is solely peaceful, but no one believes that. See Chronicles 2014.01.08:21:08 and 2014.02.19:08:22.

With all of these [CD] and [GW] interactions it would be difficult to have a meaningful agenda, and it would especially be difficult to consider anything like a Constitution Convention on Wellbeing, even if one were looking down range into Posterity. A constitutional Dynamics for 2016 shows this to some degree in that a modest increase in GDP is being offset by thins like the overseas operations of the Defense and the loss of real value in the economy do to offshore wealth concentration, or AVC, and lack of revenue coming in. The waste, fraud and abuse in [GW] is not helping either, as it might be reaching $60 billion in 2018. The table on outlays indicates the functionality of 'big government' even though one can be very unhappy about cost abuses all around. But suppose one speculated on what the Federal dynamical system of systems would look like if a full Wellbeing directive was added to those systems by subtracting functions from the other two?

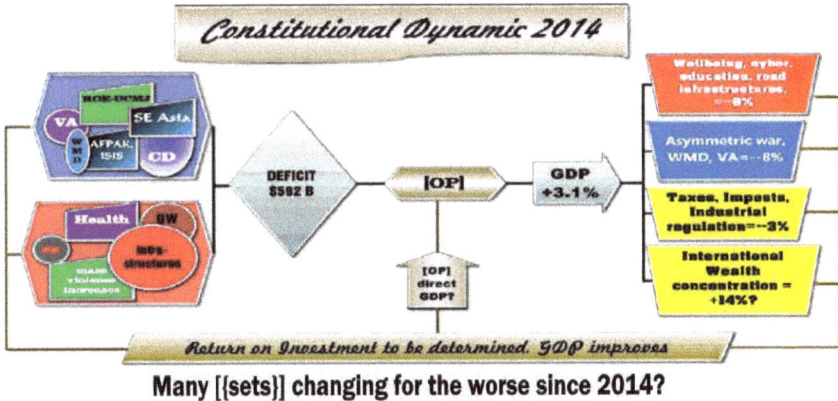

Many [{sets}] changing for the worse since 2014?

Note the breakdown of the 'Outlays by Agency' shown below and the subsequent mapping of the Agencies in terms of [CD] and [GW].   This is then projected into a speculative mapping of *three* prime directives including [WB] in 2025.

Table 4.1—OUTLAYS BY AGENCY: 1962–2021—Continued

(in millions of dollars)

Department or other unit	2014	2015	2016 estimate	2017 estimate	2018 estimate	2019 estimate	2020 estimate	2021 estimate
Legislative Branch	4,164	4,330	4,728	4,880	5,019	5,135	5,229	5,309
Judicial Branch	6,893	7,137	7,729	7,749	7,902	8,065	8,242	8,421
Department of Agriculture	141,808	139,115	153,773	151,485	153,011	149,038	146,833	150,987
Department of Commerce	7,895	8,958	10,527	10,545	11,074	13,120	16,948	13,134
Department of Defense--Military Programs	577,898	562,499	576,328	566,834	568,600	569,886	575,255	582,025
Department of Education	59,610	90,029	79,098	68,438	75,866	84,765	91,220	95,794
Department of Energy	23,638	25,424	27,416	30,373	30,194	31,194	33,163	33,516
Department of Health and Human Services	936,012	1,027,507	1,110,428	1,144,690	1,170,257	1,280,522	1,304,623	1,376,718
Department of Homeland Security	43,263	42,673	51,769	47,750	44,180	44,205	42,833	41,236
Department of Housing and Urban Development	38,527	35,527	28,691	40,738	40,184	38,802	38,025	36,060
Department of the Interior	11,279	12,340	14,022	15,040	15,265	16,581	17,031	17,060
Department of Justice	28,620	26,906	39,115	35,274	35,968	35,080	35,851	38,315
Department of Labor	56,774	45,217	43,546	50,962	53,960	52,433	55,571	56,062
Department of State	27,481	26,498	30,911	28,865	26,873	25,826	25,010	24,677
Department of Transportation	76,197	75,425	77,832	85,628	94,102	101,765	109,872	116,785
Department of the Treasury	446,892	485,623	540,376	618,290	726,582	827,296	906,536	973,682
Department of Veterans Affairs	149,074	159,216	177,812	180,220	178,842	191,684	199,894	206,184
Corps of Engineers--Civil Works	6,535	6,885	6,705	6,654	6,308	6,204	6,107	5,995
Other Defense Civil Programs	57,370	62,966	63,679	59,280	56,798	63,360	64,656	66,376
Environmental Protection Agency	9,399	7,007	8,340	8,693	7,870	8,081	8,382	8,673
Executive Office of the President	375	397	400	409	404	416	427	437
General Services Administration	-767	-890	-719	1,264	1,073	1,320	341	308
International Assistance Programs	18,742	20,950	18,042	26,430	29,371	28,161	27,370	25,931
National Aeronautics and Space Administration	17,095	18,268	19,153	19,256	19,069	19,290	19,750	20,245
National Science Foundation	7,083	6,837	6,895	7,026	7,732	7,926	8,065	8,358
Office of Personnel Management	87,517	91,734	93,883	96,115	99,502	103,519	107,708	110,974
Small Business Administration	194	-746	-378	960	858	1,101	1,119	1,133
Social Security Administration (On-Budget)	81,184	87,359	94,893	98,585	96,855	106,591	114,297	119,904
Social Security Administration (Off-Budget)	824,597	856,763	895,665	933,082	988,122	1,046,493	1,111,719	1,174,573
Other Independent Agencies (On-Budget)	9,069	15,942	22,072	22,335	22,501	25,158	25,729	33,207
Other Independent Agencies (Off-Budget)	-2,531	-1,710	552	1,180	-93	-1,448	-1,193	-1,454
Allowances			1,875	13,863	20,252	25,271	24,328	27,625
Undistributed Offsetting Receipts	-246,158	-257,594	-252,851	-255,632	-244,339	-246,511	-250,721	-258,020
(On-budget)	(-130,155)	(-145,618)	(-145,082)	(-150,158)	(-140,634)	(-141,410)	(-148,357)	(-157,085)
(Off-budget)	(-116,003)	(-111,976)	(-107,559)	(-105,674)	(-103,705)	(-105,101)	(-102,364)	(-100,955)
Total outlays	3,506,114	3,688,292	3,951,307	4,147,224	4,352,222	4,644,309	4,879,818	5,124,246

Interactives 2018

Suppose all of the Departments related to Wellbeing [WB] were actually placed in a set that was a prime directive and defined by Article VIII.   That would include all items of enhancement for the mind, body, and spirit of each citizen and ONLY citizens, such as Medicare, CHIP, ACA, education, and so forth. Would such a structure look like the map of 2025?

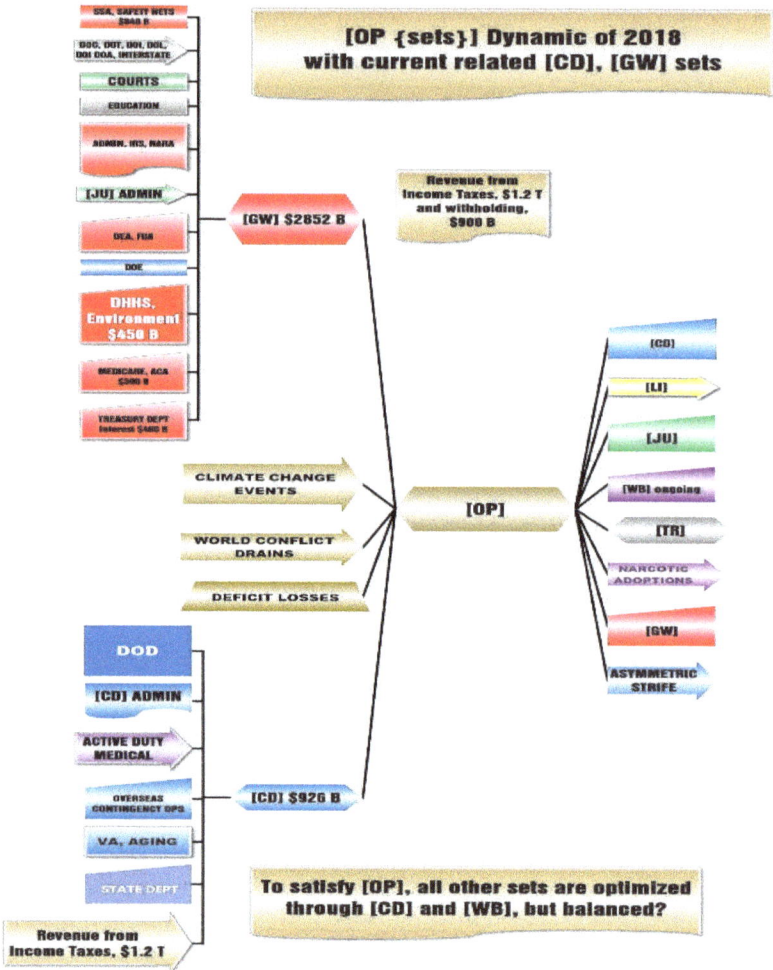

Figure 22.   Full [OP] conflict set 2018

Transitional element samples:

2018.02.15:07:15 |LI|>1|TR|<2|WB|<2+|CD|<3 ⋈[GW]>1-[JU]<2≈|OP|>3

Carney, TheHill, 'Immigration fight down to the wire':

2018.03.04:07:23 |LI|>3|TR|<2|WB|<2+|CD|<3 ⋈[GW]>1-[JU]<2≈|OP|<2

Minter, BloombergView, 'Killing Junkies Doesn't Work in Asia Either':

2018.03.13:07:12 |CD|>3= |GW|>1 ⋈ |JU|>2 ∪ |OP|>3 |TR|<2

Shaban, WaPost, on Internet national security:

2018.04.04:00:00 |WB|<2⋈ |GW|<2⋈ |CD|<3 |TR|>1=?

ScienceDaily, 'New coronavirus emerges from bats in China, devastates young swine
Identified in same region, from same bats, as SARS coronavirus

2018.05.07:22:20 |OP| ≈∑ |CD|>3|TR|>3 |LI|<2 ⋈ |JU|>1....|GW|>2

Ignatius, WaPost, 'Gina Haspel is tainted by her torture involvement. But she
understands Russia.':

2018.11.21:00:00 |CD|<3 ⋈ |OP|<4 ≈ |WB|<4?+|JU|<3 ⋈ |GW|<2

CRS report, CRS-R45392, 'U.S. Ground Forces Robotics and Autonomous Systems
(RAS) and Artificial Intelligence (AI): Considerations for Congress':

Summary

2018.12.09:09:04 |CD|>3 ⋈ |GW|>2|JU|>2|TR|>2 ≈ |OP|>3

Prime Minister Imran Khan in WaPost, 'Pakistani leader to the U.S.: We're not your
'hired gun' anymore':

2018.09.08:20:03 |CD|<3 ⋈ |GW|>1-|JU|>3|TR|<2≈|OP|>3

John McLaughlin in WaPost, 'Why so many former intelligence officers are speaking
out':

2018.07.13:06:09 |CD|>3 ⋈ |GW|>2-|JU|<2|TR|<2 ≈ |OP|>3

Lamothe, WaPost, 'Army to unveil details about new Futures Command in biggest
reorganization in 45 years':

2018.12.07:09:16 |TR|<2 + ∑ |CD|>3|LI|>1WB|<2 ⋈ |GW|>1-|JU|>2 ≈ |OP|<3

Charles Edel in WaPost, 'How democracies slide into authoritarianism':

2018.05.06:08:12 |CD|>4 ≈|OP|>2 Ξ|WB|<1+|CD| ⋈|GW|>2

Anderson, Brookings Institution, in TheHill, 'Why war powers need an expiration date':

Most of these samples involve Common Defense in a context of General Welfare with one or the other domain being more pronounced. The idea is to see them in some form of balance, even if the timeframe can extend out 10 years. This is difficult to do when appropriations for defense must be re-done every two years according to the constitution. That may be one of the reasons for the extensive use of Continuing Resolutions for Defense; it is easier than partisan 're-writes' of the budget. Perhaps the separation of the budget functions according a three-way mechanism involving Wellbeing or healthcare (Defence health is major) would cause the Congressional process to be partisan on one domain at a time rather than all or nothing. Note figure 22.

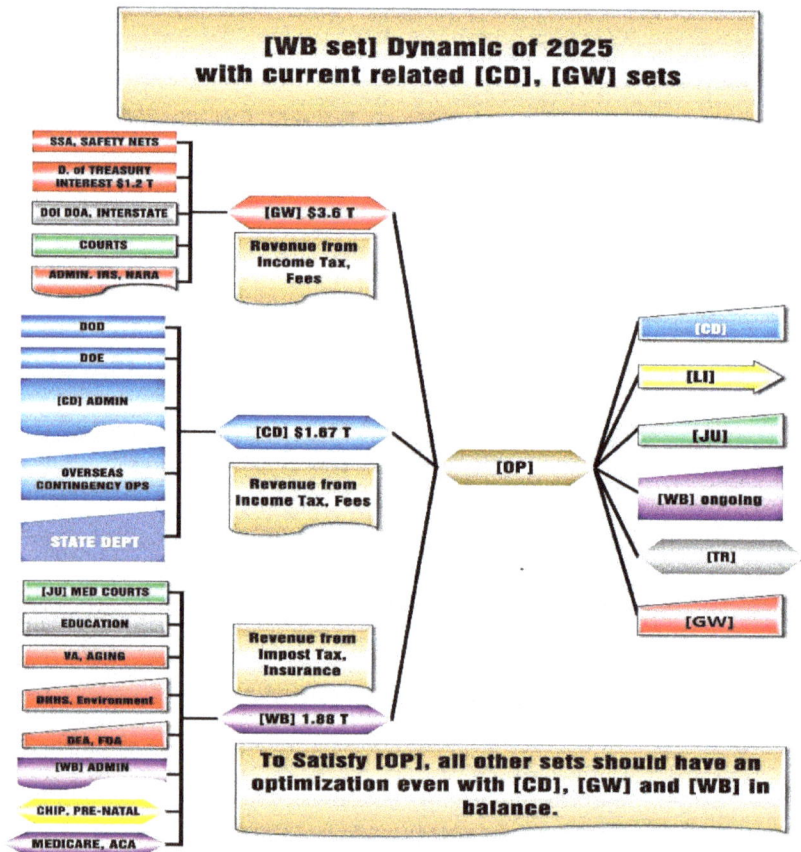

Figure 23.   [WB] sets separated from others in future

Comments from previous Chronicles still valid?

Suppose that Article VIII had a provision for the payment of all costs for life enhancement as a form of universal health. Would Article VIII have a Constitutional Section such as?

> Article VIII, Section. 9.   The congress shall have the power to appropriate revenue from all individuals, entities and devices for the maintenance and enhancement of the Wellbeing Right by attaching governance impost credits to any device or process within the jurisdiction of the Constitution. The Governance Impost Credits attached shall be solely for the molecular and/or genetic enhancement of human life through the General Welfare and Posterity covenants and may not be so excessive that the life and Liberty enhancement of any group of citizens is harmed within one generation of the Impost. All other taxation, imposts and duties, including from income and accumulated wealth, shall be for the Posterity enhancement of the Common Defense, Justice, and Tranquility provisions of Article I powers of the constitution and no Governance Impost Credits shall be added to or appropriated for the Common Defense, Justice or Tranquility purposes.

What the Section 9 of Article VIII wording would mean is that some form of transaction Impost would be used to cover all Wellbeing processes and the directives of Common Defense, Justice, and Tranquility (interstate activity) would be covered by income taxation and fee related revenue. This allows for the Wellbeing Imposts to be 'universal' since the processes of health and molecular enhancement are inherent in each individual as a 'human right'. It then allows for income or networth taxation to be applied proportionately to the benefit derived from non-Wellbeing processes like Common Defense and Tranquility or interstate commerce. This also makes Wellbeing a true 'Right' independent of economic exploitation.

This speculative Section 9 shows that the wording of Article VIII then becomes a critical matter for a Constitutional Convention and needs to have a Committee of Style made up of Electors that was just as open minded and creative as the original Style Committee in 1787. Such a committee would have to have Electors that had brought the consensus of many states and populations into the Convention through many referendums and state legislatures prior to the Convention and once convened, the three branches would combine to protect its deliberations from live for the moment or non-Posterity influences on all Sections.

These prior perceptions in the Chronicles have clearly carried over into 2018 even as an elective mid-term for presidencies . Some of the instances of the transitions between [GW] and [CD] have shown in the hypothetical Wellbeing dynamic system that [WB{n}] is becoming the main concern of We the People. Just a glance at the 2018 interaction samples shows this.

2018.06.01:06:28   [WB]<2⋈ [GW]>2⋈ [TR]>1 [LI]<3⋈ [JU]<3 ≈ |OP|<2

Wax-Thibdeaux, WaPost, 'Arkansas abortion pill restriction seen as both protecting women and a major rights setback':

2018.07.01:07:06 |LI|>5 ≈ |TR|<2|WB|<2-[JU]>2|OP|<1

Sarah Turberville and Anthony Marcum in WaPost, 'Those 5-to-4 decisions on the Supreme Court? 9 to 0 is far more common.':

2018.07.30:09:20 |WB|<2 ⋈ |GW|>2⋈ |CD|<3 |TR|>1 |LI|<3⋈|JU|<3 ≈ |OP|>2

Brnbaum, TheHill, 'Bernie Sanders's 'Medicare for all' would cost $32.6 trillion: study':

2018.09.09:06:50 |LI|>1|TR|<2|WB|<2+|CD|>3 ⋈ |GW|>1-[JU]<2 ≈ |OP|>2

Shafer in Wapost's Retropolis, 'The thin-skinned president [John Adams, 2nd president] who made it illegal to criticize his office': "Just one decade after adoption of the U.S. Constitution, the United States had survived its first constitutional crisis."

Sensing problems of 'balance' or transitions between {CD] and [GW] in relation to [OP] occurred even in the administration of the second presidency. And from then on. In times of severe crises such as the Civil War and World War II, the [CD] component became virtually the ONLY component and actually worked out provided the balance was re-instituted after the crises. In the decade of the 1970s, [GW] became the prime directive to the point that America barely had 'standing armies' anymore. This occurred again in the 2000s with [CD] minimized as the world asymmetric warfare mechanisms increased rapidly.

But with Wellbeing [WB] as a prime directive with significance equal to [CD] and [GW], this balance becomes something of a 'which comes first' issue. At least in 2018. With nearly half of the federal budget dedicated to some form of citizen health, along with increasingly usury costs of personal Wellbeing appearing in all of the Preamble Six domains as a variant of {Ki_ξ}, the balancing has become very complex. Do you aid [WB{n}] in all of its {ki_ξ} subsets to enhance [GW] then [CD] or must you take all resources for [CD{n}] in order to have some [GW{n}] and [WB[n}]?

Much of the partisan bickering of the three branches involves this three-way balancing perception and some of the partisanship involves the re-establishment of narcissistic Liberty [LI] as a prime directive for many IN the governing structure. Partisan control of wealth is becoming an increasingly major factor for this timeline and is affecting the Our Posterity covenant in unanticipated ways. Note the Congressional Research Service Reports:

2018.07.21:13:40 |GW|>n⋈ |CD|<n |TR|>4 |LI|<1 ⋈ |JU|>3 ≈ |WB|<2 ⋈ |OP|>2

CRS, R45129, 2018.03.15, 'Modes of Constitutional Interpretation'[by Supreme Court 'sensing']:

2018.12.07:00:00 |CD|>3 ⋈ [GW]>1-|JU|>2 ≈ |OP|<3∑ |TR|<2 + [LI]<3|WB|<2

CRS in focus, Debt and Deficits: Spending, Revenue, and Economic Growth':

2018.12.17:06:49 |OP|>1 ≈∑ |CD|<2 ⋈ [GW]>2 |TR|>3 |LI|<1 ⋈ |JU|>1

Devine, CRS, 'Congressional Oversight of Intelligence: Background and Selected Options for Further Reform': Potential Questions for Congress '

Complexity is increasing to the point individuals involved cannot perceive domains as true balanced timeline progressions?

End Interactives 2018

Math Stuff

Much of the Chronicle 'entity' studies through 2017 have simply recorded the sets of interactive processes that actually exist in the U.S. Capitol and how they relate to We the People in general. Only minor attempts were made to quantify the [XX] domains because of a suspicion that Newton was right in his perception concerning parallel structures in the universe. Some things might not have ripple effects or vectors that appeared in other items EVEN if they co-existed. In this Chronicle, some perceptional effort is made to express summed phenomena within a domain for wellbeing [WB] because of a surprising group of ripple effect on the six covenants, especially General Welfare [GW], after the 2009 Affordable Care Act 'system' was created. See: https://en.wikipedia.org/wiki/Patient_Protection_and_Affordable_Care_Act

Of special interest was the set of Essential Health Benefits (EHB) taken from a CRS summarization report. Each of the items that was to be covered by the ACA involved items that had massive societal effects if applied to 330 million people. 'Chronic disease management' alone required 2% of the healthy population along with the victims' own efforts. The very necessary EHB 'Emergency Services' also covered uninsured and foreign 'visitors' to an escalating cost as climate refugees begin appearing. But the question also arose as to what Essential Services could enhance the [WB] in both its individual and societal effects.

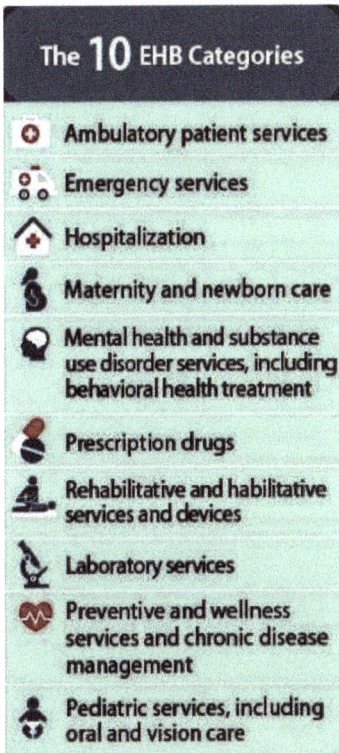

The 10 EHB Categories

- Ambulatory patient services
- Emergency services
- Hospitalization
- Maternity and newborn care
- Mental health and substance use disorder services, including behavioral health treatment
- Prescription drugs
- Rehabilitative and habilitative services and devices
- Laboratory services
- Preventive and wellness services and chronic disease management
- Pediatric services, including oral and vision care

That is, quantifying didn't necessarily show cause and effect. Much of the dynamics involved in the six covenants of the Constitution are something that a complex model might define as summed 'operators', perhaps as components of a Hamiltonian field such as in a domain transfer .. [{GW}]→ [{CD}]<n.. where some 'value' within {GW} is transferred to the domain of {CD} in order to achieve a balance within the domain [OP]. Both [CD] and [GW] are expressed as constitutional domains [n] of their own, but in this perception, they are {value sets} of the domains. For instance, a {GW} value might be hospitalization in the EHB, itself a subset of [GW], and some of the value might be transferred to the common defense {CD} set as a veteran's hospitalization value while maintaining the balance of the two domains. The Congress has appropriation models that do this type of transfer every Session, although the 'compromise' mechanism gives an appearance of chaos to the way each appropriation set is made. But from a visualization standpoint, the interaction of the various sets [{GW}] is so complex that individual Members of the Congress might only deal effectively with specific parts that their committee functions allow. There are serious complexity limits for any

perceptional mode, and it applies to human systems as much is complex perception applies to the 'ripple' effects of the Higgs Field in quantum mechanics or gravitational effects in cosmology.

https://en.wikipedia.org/wiki/Hamiltonian_field_theory#Explicit_time-independence

In a math sense, such a dynamic might require a field or matrix of some form that could show just the major subsets of the domain. The Hamiltonian field describes discrete 'entities' in terms of a coordinate field density in which some 'energy value' is move from one entity to another while continually showing the relation and change of state for the entities involved. Of interest is that a Hamiltonian field can show a domain subgroup affecting each other without it having a time-related coordinate. That is, a domain like Justice [JU] might have a coordinate position involving [GW] and tranquility [TR] in which each operates with a time coordinate that is different from the others. For instance, the [GW] ↔ [CD] domain relationship in the Prohibition Amendment to the Constitution where the narcotic alcohol was removed from society came in conflict with Justice, Liberty, and Tranquility **and** Our Posterity even though the narcotic use had become a serious [WB][CD][GW] effect. Over a 10-year period, the Prohibition process looked something like

..|WB|>3⋈|GW|<3⋈|CD|<2 →|TR|<1 |LI|<3⋈|JU|>1→ |OP|<3..

with [JU] and [CD] having time sequences independent of the others. But the alcohol use itself never actually endangered the integrity of the domains; it was an attempt to enhance [WB] without knowing what [WB] was. People at that particular point in history really didn't have enough information to know about DNA narcotic adaptions, only its ripple effects on their lives. That |WB|>3 effect then may not be true of the 2000s opioid epidemic that killed 30,000 a year, with a calculatable human capital effect on [GW] ↔[CD] in its entirety.

The Essential Health Benefits (as a [WB] dynamics subset) were defined by law in 2009 as those items necessary to maintain life in America in the first decade of the 5th millennium (1st millennium is earliest written knowledge base) but were they? There was no referendum or consensus about this, even with a well-defined political process about it for 20 years. And how do you 'quantify' them as essential elements of [wellbeing] as a 'domain' equal in importance to the current six or as a combination of the six? Complexity theory attempts to show relations between 'objects' that are interactive, but how do you do that without some form of comparison between a 'dollar' value and a 'time' value?

Even if one limited 'quantification of life' to some combination of the six current constitutional directives, he might still have to add a timeline AND a 'networth' value, maybe as human capital, to give meaning to the [wellbeing] domain. As a relational model, EHB would appear as:

- Ambulatory patient services (outpatient services) [LI], [JU]
- Emergency services [JU] [CD] [LI]
- Hospitalization [GW], [TR], [LI]
- Maternity and newborn care [OP], [LI], [JU]
- Mental health and substance use disorder services, including behavioral health treatment [LI], [JU], [CD], [GW]
- Prescription drugs [LI], [GW]

- Rehabilitative and habilitative services (those that help patients acquire, maintain, or improve skills necessary for daily functioning) and devices [LI],
- Laboratory services [CD], [GW], [TR]
- Preventive and wellness services and chronic disease management [CD], [GW], [OP]
- Pediatric services, including oral and vision care [GW], [OP]

From 2017.

Going back to speculation about the math involved in systems, which started in the 1970s for this analysis, is pretty traumatizing. It requires a person to look at his own perception at the same time he is trying to look at a summation of a 'system' called we the People, which is equated as the super-set 'Our Posterity'. The one thing that becomes obvious is that in order to maintain a purely 'open minded' problem solving perception, the person looking at Our Posterity cannot include any of his own needs in the perception as of importance. And this perception gets worse in a family environment or a group environment in which a responsibility for the survival of others becomes a prime part of the perception. A man or a woman 'system entity' just doesn't think beyond the environment of his locality in space-time or the 'entity' wouldn't be enhanced. So how does one devise a math, which would be the same perception for other 'entities' (like counting dollars is the same for all, except the greedy), to solve a problem for the Our Posterity super-set?

A system.

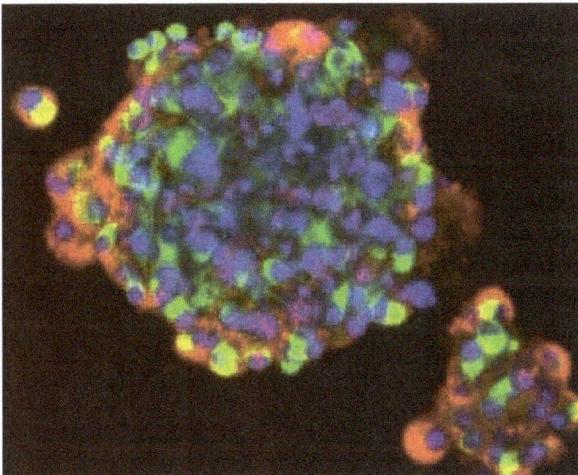

A group of molecular or quantum structures that operated as a single function that was dependent on its existence by co-existence with other systems with different functions. Each function is distinctive but requires co-existence. The stem cell image here is a good example of a dynamical human system in which groups of molecules form structures that interact for a purpose. In the case of stem cells, they actually *learn that function* [Ki_ξ (zhi) function learned as well?] and that makes them critical to all life because they can adopt to the needs of other cells in the human mind or body. But if the stem cell is a dynamical 'entity' that creates other larger more complex systems, what is the math expression for that?

System of systems.

Definition in use in the Chronicles: the reduction analysis of something into its various parts, each if which can be a system or entity itself. A human person is a system of systems that starts with a few conception molecules, begins multiplying through DNA programming into increasingly complex subsystems basically divided into body systems, mind systems, environment systems and spirit systems that integrate the other subsystems.

When the Human Genome mapping was completed in 2010, some 700,000 subsystems had been catalogued for humans. A human family develops as a system of systems and perhaps qualifies as the nucleus of positive energy or wealth development.

Dynamical System.

A set, usually defined mathematically, of unified systems that create an interactive environment for other combinations of systems. A solar system is a dynamical system, as is a galaxy of solar systems, or a human tribe or city state is. A group of city states becomes a set when they join in a common function. The Constitution then creates a Dynamical System through its Union of states.

The problem here is that a human system hasn't really been defined in terms of the sum of the 'Exergy' or life energy he produces, or whether that energy is translated into increasingly larger societal entities he is a part of. Taxation in dollars could be a way of defining that (the person's Networth Index the statistics people use) and has been for 7000 years since the formation of farming and literate communities as dynamical systems. How do you make numeric or mathematical 'constants' when all of the subsystems are in 'motion' or engaged in energy changes of some form? There is a need, then, to speculate on the type of energy that is being manipulated by the system of systems called HoSa or person. Especially true if one desires to remove the 'Exergy' from the Constitution's interstate commerce clause which can be calculated only in monetary units. [WB] energy just doesn't work in only that context. The process can easily slide into the obscurity of Bonini's Paradox.

Wikipedia, essay on the Exergy in the sense of thermodynamic laws of heat transfer or work, but it could also apply to the excess energy created in a brain or in what a group of people do, denoted by the small Greek letter ξ (zhi). Speculative....:

Exergy is a combination property of a system and its environment because it depends on the state of both the system and environment. The exergy of a system in equilibrium with the environment is zero. Exergy is neither a thermodynamic property of matter nor a thermodynamic potential of a system. Exergy and energy both have units of joules. The Internal Energy of a system is always measured from a fixed reference state and is therefore always a state function. Some authors define the exergy of the system to be changed when the environment changes, in which case it is not a state function. Other writers prefer [citation needed] a slightly alternate definition of the available energy or exergy of a system where the environment is firmly defined, as an unchangeable absolute reference state, and in this alternate definition exergy becomes a property of the state of the system alone.

A common hypothesis in systems ecology is that the design engineer's observation that a greater capital investment is needed to create a process with increased exergy efficiency is actually the economic result of a fundamental law of nature. By this view, exergy is the analogue of economic currency in the natural world. The analogy to capital investment is the accumulation of exergy into a system over long periods of time resulting in embodied energy. The analogy of capital investment resulting in a factory with high exergy efficiency is an increase in the natural organizational structures with high exergy efficiency. Researchers in these fields describe biological evolution in terms of increases in organism complexity due to the requirement for increased exergy efficiency because of competition for limited sources of exergy.

Embodied energy [human too?] is the sum of all the energy required to produce any goods or services, considered as if that energy was incorporated or 'embodied' in the product itself. The concept can be useful in determining the effectiveness of energy-producing or energy-saving devices, or the "real" replacement cost of a building, and, because energy-inputs usually entail greenhouse gas emissions, in deciding whether a product contributes to or mitigates global warming. One fundamental purpose for measuring this quantity is to compare the amount of energy produced or saved by the product in question to the amount of energy consumed in producing it.

In the International System of Units (SI), the unit of energy is the joule, named after James Prescott Joule. It is a derived unit. It is equal to the energy expended (or work done) in applying a force of one newton through a distance of one meter. However, energy is also expressed in many other units not part of the SI, such as ergs, calories, British Thermal Units, kilowatt-hours and kilocalories, which require a conversion factor when expressed in SI units.

The word "quantum" comes from the Latin "quantus", meaning "how much". "Quanta", short for "quanta of electricity" (electrons) was used in a 1902 article on the photoelectric effect by Philipp Lenard, who credited Hermann von Helmholtz for using the word in the area of electricity. However, the word quantum in general was well known before 1900.

The reason for evaluating 'systems' or entities in terms of quanta or other 'energy' sets is simple; energy levels in the physical universe are the basis for the molecular systems that constantly reform themselves base on the available energy at any given time. The same applies as the dynamical system becomes more complex and self-regenerating through DNA programing. Eventually it is the combined energy of each person that adds or subtracts molecular energy from its surroundings. The human entity becomes a dynamic system when he consciously organizes that energy use in terms of time and space. That is the universal concept of 'time is money'.

Into this discussion of defining space-time energy comes the idea of 'exergy', the excess of energy created by a work system or entity or human dynamical system. For lack of a better expression for humans who create value over and above what went into it, the prime directive idea of China, can be used. **It is a life force symbol Chi or Qi, ⅀ with three horizontal lines and a scrolled tail. Qi or Chi can also be represented in math by the Greek lower-case letter ξ (zhi) as a form of independent exergy that does transferable, note transferable, work by a person.** It, ξ, looks very much like the Chinese symbol for 'life force' or Qi_Chi, ⅀ , with three horizontal lines and a scrolled tail. It is a good perception of exergy or the excess of energy produced by the ability of a human to live. If a person 40,000 years ago is spending all of his waking moments hunting for food as the weather around him gets worse, he is not 'free'; he is strictly instinctive without the ability to acquire ξ (zhi). If a women is a tribal queen from 10,000 years ago where food is brought to her by others so she can produce life, she has become more 'free' and the level of ξ (zhi or chi) is increased to the point she can learn and teach about the environment around her. But does she impart Ki ξ (zhi) exergy to others? In a modern sense, if a person or his parents spend their lives paying for treatment of a genetic disorder, how do they create exergy or Qi over and above what they consume? Note that the expressions Ki, Qi and Zhi are being used interchangeably to make the point about work energy in a person.

The use of 'exergy' or ⤴ as a form of energy to define a person's Liberty or freedom is novel but well founded in spiritual or philosophical tomes like Sartre's *Being and Nothingness* or Noah Webster's essay, *A Citizen of America, An Examination into the Leading Principles of the Federal Constitution,* 1787.10.17 (a month after the Convention??):

> But I cannot quit this subject without attempting to correct some of the erroneous opinions respecting freedom and tyranny, and the principles by which they are supported. Many people seem to entertain an idea that liberty consists in *a power to act without any control.* .. $|LI| \to \infty$.. This is more liberty than even the savages enjoy. But in civil society, political liberty consists in *acting conformably to a sense of a majority of the society.* In a free government every man binds himself to obey the public *voice,* or the opinions of a majority; and the *whole society* engages to *each individual.* In such a government a man *is free* and safe. But reverse the case; suppose every man to act without control or fear of punishment—every man would be free, but no man would be sure of his freedom one moment. Each would have the power of taking his neighbor's life, liberty, or property; and no man would command more than his own strength to repel the invasion. .. $|\{LI\}| \leftrightarrow \{LI\}|<n$.. The case is the same with states. If the states should not unite into one compact society, every state may trespass upon its neighbor, and the injured state has no means of redress but its own military force.
>
> The present situation of our American states is very little better than a state of nature—Our boasted state sovereignties are so far from securing our liberty and property, that they, every moment, expose us to the loss of both. That state which commands the heaviest purse and longest sword, may at any moment, lay its weaker neighbor under tribute; and there is no superior power now existing, that can regularly oppose the invasion or redress the injury. From such liberty, O Lord, deliver us!
>
> But what is tyranny? Or how can a free people be deprived of their liberties? Tyranny is the exercise of some power over a man, which is not warranted by law, or necessary for the public safety. ..$|LI|< \to \infty$.. A people can never be deprived of their liberties, while they retain in their own hands, a power sufficient to any other power in the state. This position leads me directly to inquire, in what consists the power of a nation or of an order of men?
>
> .. $|TR|<2 = \sum |LI| >?$ →$|WB|>3$ $[\xi$ $]n?$ ⋈ $|GW|$ →>2-$|JU|<2?$ ..

The way Liberty is described by Webster as very close to the idea of individual exergy as: 'and the *whole society* engages to *each individual.* In such a government a man *is free* and safe.' Depends on who you talk to. It is the infrastructure of government without tyranny that cause a person to increase the ξ (zhi or qi, expressed as 3 horizontal lines and scrolled tail, .. [ξ] .. in his personal environment and that comes from being a cooperative yet independent citizen of that society. Liberty then becomes a spiritual entity as well as physical in some dynamic of its own, but within a social structure. The two, according to Webster, are not separable as systems. If you want to be a person enhancing Ki_ξ, then there must be a society that helps that. 'Ki' is as the combination of symbols for life energy, exergy, work AND the spiritual freedom acquired from those processes. **'Ki_ξ' or '[ξ_⩲]' or simply [ξ] is arbitrarily chosen in the Chronicles to represent all forms of energy that create a spiritual component of wellbeing [WB], possibly even with a monetary equivalence.** Strictly arbitrary for math purposes, but a GDNI domain of its own perhaps?

This is also, coincidently, an idea where personal freedom, [LI] in the Constitution, is also defined as an energy that is created by the work of the individual 'entity'. This energy excess can easily be found in the idea of wealth or power where the more one has of it, the 'freer' he is, nearly an absolute for the followers of John Locke in the 1700s who became Lords of Proprietorship. .. [ξ] ≈ |LI| → ∞ ... But Webster stated in 1787 that unlimited power causes everyone to loss ξ (Ki) because he must constantly defend against others without the 'system' infrastructure that balances power through representation. .. |JU|<2 ⋈ |TR|<2.. In this century, the ripple effects of molecular damage very easily distort one's ability to gain freedom or exergy energy, ξ, the zhi or qi life energy that is just as necessary as molecular feeding into physical systems within the mind and within the body.

Remember, this is an open-ended speculation with no pre-conditions in the mind, as were the original speculations with Washington in the 1780s. Liberty [LI] was then being described as a form of summed individual energy closely allied with the 'E Pluribus Unum' concept of "One out of many" or possibly a wellbeing of all. As: ..∑ [LI] ={WB+ ξ}..? The Preamble does not mention 'spirit energy' because that was a condition of religion which was thereafter prohibited from the Constitution because it was being 'politicized' all over the world. , the earlier uses of the Greek ξ (zhi) and the ancient use of the Chinese Qi or Chi, ⩲ all indicate the wisdom embedded in the six covenants of the Preamble and that qualifies it as the basis of any Our Posterity improvement. It would be very necessary to ensure that any [ξ_⩲] 'improvement' in the 'spirit' component was for all of We The People. Possibly?:

.. [TR]<2 = ∑ [LI] >3 →[WB]>3 [ξ_⩲]>2 ⋈[CD] [GW] →>2-[JU]<2→ [OP]>3 ..

End 2017.

Start 2018.

What would the so-called Standard Model say about all of this molecular level DNA and cell structure of human beings?

https://en.wikipedia.org/wiki/Mathematical_formulation_of_the_Standard_Model

Does it account for ALL of the energy combinations that can appear in Creation? Accounting for something in a model that can't be visualized by people going about their daily lives might be intellectually satisfying but not necessarily 'satisficing' in the operational research sense. Satisficing is a perceptional mode in which there is some form of optimization carried out by the 'system'. Its might appear as a method of universal health care in which the model, in this case one involving wellbeing that is evolutionary, can actually be translated into some daily value to an individual being.

An example is in figure 23 where a full medical database system from this century has 'fields' in which molecular conditions can be recorded for each individual, then translated into the existing medical procedures necessary as determined by either a legislative or executive or court system set up to do the 'satisficing' for the individual.

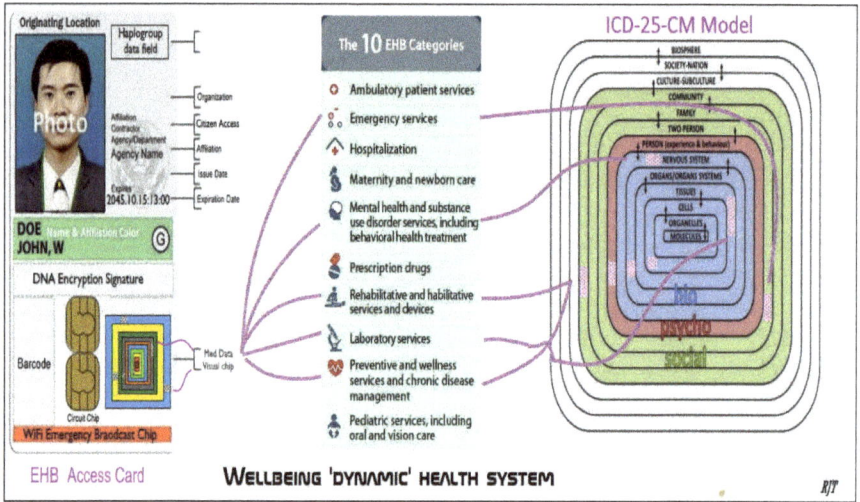

Figure 24.   Personal Wellbeing 'dynamic system'.

The math might work fine in the database, but it is a medical person who makes decisions about the [WB] component of [GW] and/or [CD], but then translating that into a working device in the real world? If the objective was to keep someone alive [{ξ}] anywhere in the world through some infrastructure of [CD], [GW], [TR], you couldn't even have fantasized about doing that before this century. The means just didn't exist before 2010 and in many places still don't, as anyone who has walked out of extreme climate, war, or poverty environments can attest.

Humans who wish to aid others could not even began to visualize a 'smart card that could aid them with such complexity as

.. $[TR]2 = \Sigma\ [LI] >3 \rightarrow [WB]<3 \rightarrow [\xi\ \xleftarrow]<4 \bowtie [CD]\ [GW] \rightarrow >2-[JU]>2 \rightarrow >[OP]?$ ..

where life-threatening wellbeing $[WB]<3 \rightarrow [\xi\ \Box\ ]<4$ starts to get reversed, especially when the life force for a person isn't definable in space-time.

Exactly how are people within the 'field' We the People perceiving these complex operators as part of their own Ki .. [ξ] .. or wellbeing or Liberty and Tranquility? Generally, there is a 'sense' perception of what is going on that is subject to continual updating with other information that allows for a 'biased' common sense perception of processes. This observational technique goes back as far as the Homosapien exists and doesn't always involve a purely quantitative interpretation, but a 'sense' of the total that is then broken down into parts. The idea of a wellbeing 'Ki' or 'Qi' cannot be quantified, yet it appears in continually in human thought and greatly affects the constitutional domains. Some examination of this perceptional mode is necessary for the domains to have value themselves.

Taking the example of TL2017 and arbitrarily adding a 'force' like Qi, .. [{ξ}] .. to a set of domains such as the six defined by the Constitution turns out to be quite difficult because even though one knows the entities exist, there is the classic problem of quantum mechanics in that one is only measuring the probability of a movement of something like Common Defense [CD], which is the sum of entire subsets of structures that are both positive and negative in the 'vector' they create as they move through time. This is especially true since major subsets of [{GW}] are almost entirely within a relation like ..[{WB}]>3 [ξ☐]>2 → [CD] ⋈ [{GW}].. where wellbeing of citizens is directly interactive with elements created by [{GW}]. The Essential Health Benefits 'emergency services' element is an obvious example of contributing to a domain operator; it directly saves lives caught by environments.

Assuming that one's perception of [{GW}] as a group of general welfare entities is in the form of the sum of {x}>n + {y}>n ↔ {t}<n, the idea that the sum is exactly equivalent to the subsets in some way won't work because each subset is dynamic and summing the 'dynamic movement' in some direction has a perception of its own that might not be relevant to a timeline. The timeline measurement is a common practice for nearly all economic activities in which the amplitude of 'something' is measured against time increments. That perception is very useful in many ways, note the negative going deficit spending compared to future time, with a high probability that wealth enhancement will simply cease at some point. 'Time is running out....' is a nearly continually applied expression.

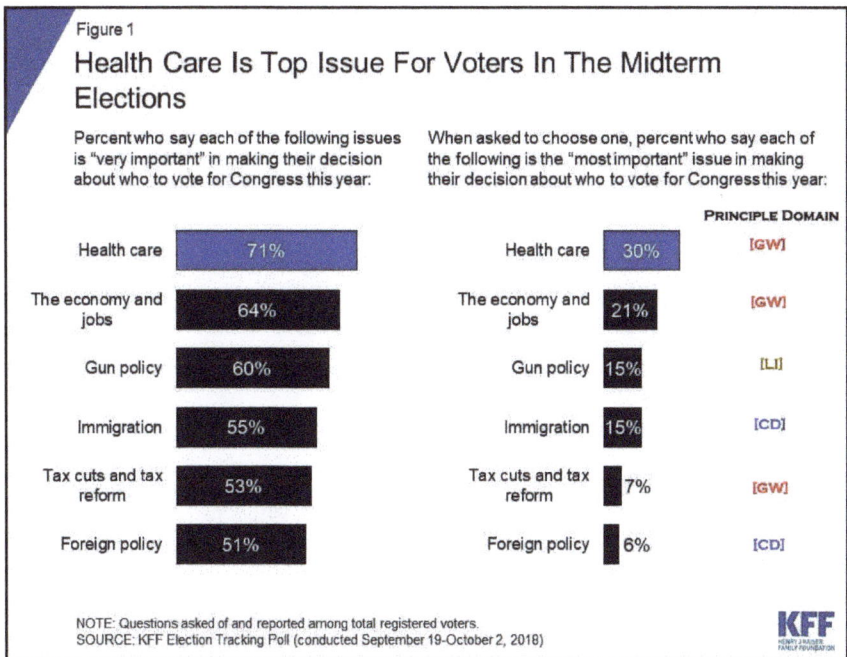

Figure 1

Health Care Is Top Issue For Voters In The Midterm Elections

Percent who say each of the following issues is "very important" in making their decision about who to vote for Congress this year:

When asked to choose one, percent who say each of the following is the "most important" issue in making their decision about who to vote for Congress this year:

Issue	Very important	Issue	Most important	PRINCIPLE DOMAIN
Health care	71%	Health care	30%	[GW]
The economy and jobs	64%	The economy and jobs	21%	[GW]
Gun policy	60%	Gun policy	15%	[LI]
Immigration	55%	Immigration	15%	[CD]
Tax cuts and tax reform	53%	Tax cuts and tax reform	7%	[GW]
Foreign policy	51%	Foreign policy	6%	[CD]

NOTE: Questions asked of and reported among total registered voters.
SOURCE: KFF Election Tracking Poll (conducted September 19-October 2, 2018)

KFF
HENRY J KAISER
FAMILY FOUNDATION

As this research involves the importance of referendums and popular consensus, it is necessary to visualize the Constitutional domains in terms of a population perception of priorities.   The Kaiser Family Foundation does a great deal of research in maintaining health or wellbeing related data and has produced a series of polls on that subject.   It is from the site: https://www.kff.org/health-reform/poll-finding/kff-election-tracking-poll-health-care-in-the-2018-midterms/ and shows that health care is very much on people's minds prior to the election of 2018.

The poll indicated that voters were concerned about both [GW] and [CD] but that what they were hearing about as issues from the federal candidates was immigration as the most important issue, and the president, economy, and the opioid epidemic in that order were next most heard. Discussions of repealing or enhancing the 2010 healthcare law were next in importance and that was reflected in the popular consensus of healthcare being the most important subset issue, although repeal was quite low in the scale. Healthcare costs were the major concerns because of their effects on personal economics as [LI] and [TR] and the well-publicized comparison of the costs being double what other countries' costs were.   This in some ways reflects the operator sequence ..|{WB}|>3 [ξ_🦅]>2 → [CD] ⋈ [{GW}|.. because the economy and jobs are necessary for the [{WB}] subsets to have meaning and immigration/foreign policy had become voter issues during 2018 that directly affected the ability of people to live safely as part of Common Defense.   Basically, healthcare is a major factor in *all* of the other domains and should qualify as a domain entity itself as [{WB}↔{ξ}≈∑ {CD}{WB}{TR}]; there is just too much quantifiable perception of it to be considered otherwise.

Attempting to express that in math symbiology is also an attempt to use its precision, but the problem I encountered was that a 'operation dynamic' perception of the whole and even complex renderings don't give a 'sense' of the progression, especially when |ξ_🦅] isn't measurable or quantifiable as an operator in a Hamiltonian field like scalars in the normal mechanisms. Ki is very much like an electromagnetic field in that you sense its presence the same as one would sense the presence of a field between two magnets or the way some animals navigate by sensing the earth's magnetic field. But many serious environmental traumas on human bodies have been mitigated over time by sheer [Ki] use. Human literature has had such examples of overcoming trauma by' will' or 'determination' that resulted in a healing of the trauma.   In fact, the examples are so numerous that one would think that spirituality was an 'entity' that could not be ignored by normal scientific reductionism even if it can't be measured in space-time coordinates. There is even a strong suggestion from those like Steven Hawking. who play with black holes that the time coordinate might be misleading even on planet earth's dynamics.

The term {WB}↔{ξ}≈∑ where wellbeing interacts with spirit to form a 'summed' operator happens too often to be ignored, the same as quanta are sensed rather than seen or heard. Virtually all of the ancient cultures had sensed systems of 'physical elements' plus an interactive 'void', so {Ki} is too well based perceptually to be ignored.   But there are also many examples of what happens when the Ki (or [LI] or [TR]) is *absent* from 'wellbeing'. In a Hamiltonian field or manifold, the operators like [CD] and [GW] co-exist with others but would { Ki_ξ} be an operator or an actual structure of the Field.?   Needs work.

Just as important is the reduction analysis of any of the covenants of the Constitution such as in the domain [CD]. Even if one quantified the largest elements of [{CD}], by going over the Defense budget of 2017-2019, he might be surprised as what qualified as pure Common Defense according to the authorities of Article I. Section 8 describes creation, maintenance and 'war' use of armies, navies, and militias which now includes costs of veterans (carefully avoided by congress during the Revolution), cyber warfare units, oversea contingencies and very recently a 'Space Force'. Visualizing this in its entirety might look like $[CD] \rightarrow \sum \{n1\}, \{n2\}, \{n3\} \approx [OP] >< n$

But this is also quantified by the amount of 'dollars' that the {nn sets} has through congressional appropriations. Worse, each of the {nn} elements have subordinate {element sets} that have parallel {WB}, [GW] and [TR] domain components that might be purely parasitic and distort any optimization that can be visualized. In the figure (table 1), the 'Defense Health Program' has a monetary value of $36B per year for active duty processes but also has ripple effects in [WB], [TR], and even [LI] since families are involved. How would you design 'optimization' math for the ripple effects of the original monetary value? This normally involves the math perception of metaheuristics or 'combinational optimization' where boundaries are defined for each element set and summed into some form of gain or profit or enhancement. See https://en.wikipedia.org/wiki/Mathematical_optimization for a general discussion. Any of the six Preamble covenants would qualify as domains that can be optimized, but [CD] ⋈ [GW] in terms of a future [OP] where they are 'balanced, ⋈' against each other as a necessary existential value of a successful society?

Table 1. FY2018 Defense Appropriations Act (H.R. 1625, Division C)
(amounts in billions of nominal dollars)

[OP]ₐ = l{CD}In?	FY2017 Enacted P.L. 115-31 Div. C	FY2018 Budget Request	House-passed H.R. 3219 Div. A	Senate Committee draftª	Final Bill H.R. 1625 Div. C
Base Budget					
Military Personnel [CB]	$128.7	$133.9	$133.0	$133.6	$133.4
Operation and Maintenance [TR]	$167.6	$188.6	$191.7	$192.6	$188.2
Procurement [GW]>? [TR]	$108.4	$113.9	$132.5	$126.7	$133.9
R&D [CB]≈[GW]>3	$72.3	$82.7	$82.7	$87.3	$88.3
Revolving and Management Funds [GW]?	$1.5	$2.1	$1.6	$1.7	$1.7
Defense Health Program [WB]>2 [TR] and Other DOD	$35.6	$35.9	$36.1	$36.3	$36.6
Related Agencies [GW]	$1.0	$1.0	$1.0	$1.1	$1.1
General Provisions [CB]ₐ	$-5.6	$0.1	-$2.0	-$0.7	$-0.9
Subtotal: Base Budget	$509.6	$558.2	$576.5	$578.8	$582.3
Overseas Contingency World l{CB}ᵇ Operations (OCO)	$76.6	$65.1ᵇ	$73.9	$65.0	$65.2
Grand Total	$586.2	$623.3	$650.4	$643.8	$647.4

Sources: H.Rept. 115-219, House Appropriations Committee, Report to accompany H.R. 3219, Department of Defense Appropriations Bill, 2018; Draft FY2018 Defense Appropriations bill and accompanying report published Nov. 21, 2017 by the chairman of the Senate Appropriations Committee, at https://www.appropriations.senate.gov/news/majority/fy2018-defense-appropriations-bill-released; and Joint Explanatory Statement to accompany H.R. 1625, The Consolidated Appropriations Act of 2018, at https://rules.house.gov/bill/115/hr-1625-sa.

Notes:
a. The Senate Committee draft bill includes $4.5 billion that the Administration added to its FY2018 budget request on November 6, 2017, after the House had passed its version of the FY2018 defense bill but before the Senate committee draft was published. The additional funds, to beef up missile defense programs related to North Korea and to repair two Navy destroyers damaged in collisions, were appropriated by P.L. 115-95, enacted on December 22, 2017.

b. The Administration's FY2018 OCO budget request includes $1.2 billion that was added to the original FY2018 OCO request on November 6, 2017. The additional funds are to support the Administration's decision to increase the number of U.S. military personnel who would be stationed in Afghanistan.

Such survival balance might require the subtraction of some elements like hardware from [CD], with their highly debatable costs, in order to satisfy an optimization of [WB]{Social Security}, {Medicare} or {urban infrastructure} which might look something like {aircraft carrier:$11Billion}⋈{Medicare:$7 Billion} + {Housing:$4 billion} rather than being able to afford all {sets}. Most political contentions of modern congresses are along these lines, with routine disregard for optimization of [OP].   Devil in the details as far as 'sensing' the balance between the two domains?   Is the optimization quantifiable in dollars only, without a human capital plus or minus? Perhaps only a Hamiltonian field with variable boundaries would be useful as a perception of the different {element] combinations within domains.

End 2018

Process Conclusions to 2018

TLO Epilogue to 2017

With a little backtracking since the Epigenetics research around the world was just developing, it was necessary to examine whether modifications of DNA really were going to change the concept of what qualified as Wellbeing or just healthcare. This appears to be the case, it can change Wellbeing in massive numbers of people, and registers high on the need to hold a Constitutional Convention in the near future. A general level book on genetic modification Epigenetics is shown here in an Epilogue simply because there is much more to come as far as Wellbeing is concerned.

Nessa Carey, *The Epigenetics Revolution*, How Modern Biology Is Rewriting Our Understanding of Genetics, Disease and Inheritance, p309, 2012.00.00:

> Transgenerational effects of epigenetic changes may be one of the areas with the greatest impact on human health over the coming decades, not because of drugs or pollutants but because of food and nutrition. We started this journey into the epigenetic landscape by looking at the Dutch Hunger Winter. This had consequences not just for those who lived through it but for their descendants. We are in the grip of a global obesity epidemic. **Even if our societies manage to get control of this (and very few western cultures show many signs of doing so) we may already have generated a less than optimal epigenetic legacy for our children and grandchildren.** [emphasis added]
>
> Nutrition in general is one area where we can predict epigenetics will come to the fore in the next ten years. Here are just a few examples of what we know at the moment.
>
> Folic acid is one of the supplements recommended for pregnant women. Increasing the supply of folic acid in the very early stages of pregnancy has been a public health triumph, as it has led to a major drop in the incidence of spina bifida in newborns[7]. Folic acid is required for the production of a chemical called SAM (S-adenosyl methionine). SAM is the molecule that donates the methyl group when DNA methyltransferases modify DNA. If baby rats are fed a diet that is low in folic acid, they develop abnormal regulation of imprinted regions of the genome*. We are only just beginning to unravel how many of the beneficial effects of folic acid may be mediated through epigenetic mechanisms.

Epigenetics involves molecular changes at a very basic human DNA level and that these changes have ripple effects for generations. The original Darmend Ripple Effect entity that has plagued humanity from day one, whenever that was. But note the emphasized Nessa Carey entry 'get control of this' and multiply by several hundred molecular 'entities. In 2008, the FDA published a document on this subject called *Animal Cloning: A Risk Assessment* that briefly covered this ongoing research and came to the conclusion there wasn't much [CD] danger then. SCNT is a process for cloning an existing 'entity' with a different DNA code in an embryonic stem cell, a process that could create 'perfection' in molecular structures, but the stem cells might not turn out as expected. What then? Is the changed stem cell through SCNT the same as the process that creates abnormalities? If the group of molecules after conception becomes abnormal and causes something like Downs Syndrome or various forms of Encephalopathy, are those exact causative molecules correctable? See an update on this process in 2018.04.20:00:00 and 2018.05.01:00:00

 In a family environment, the SCNT (Somatic Cell Nuclear Transfer) dynamic could vary the way things come out considerably, which can happen in normal procreation. But suppose there are abnormalities created by this, including by an unhealthy environment, that lead to family tragedies? Note the previous diagram on family interaction as a system with newly added SCNT conditions. SCNT is *artificially* inducing a change as cloning, but the same process happens during procreation as one of molecular abnormality.

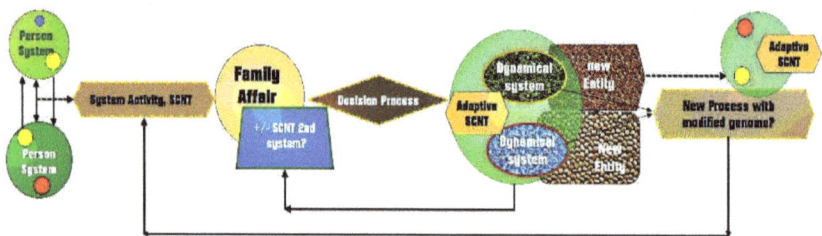

FAMILY SYSTEM VISUALIZATION, GENOME MODIFICATION
SCNT IS 'SOMATIC CELL NUCLEAR TRANSFER', BASIC HUMAN MODIFIER DYNAMIC SYSTEM

Once the SCNT process occurs in the child, the ripple effects increase from there on, in either a positive environment of mutual loving or into some relationship where the feedback is so negative that everyone is diminished in energy. But suppose there was a societal structure in this century in which the negative cycles caused by genetic abnormalities could be eliminated during the cell growth periods of the trimester or post-birth?

If We The People know that some SCNT process was going to create a prolonged harm to others, including insurance providers and tax payers, would it have a Justice right to intervene? It does with Typhoid, or Ebola,   but see **2018.12.03:00:00.** In the last two centuries, it did not because it would have been just 'bad seed' guess work based on misguided religious or economic fear. Justice, Liberty, and Tranquility could not be enhanced, and the ripple effects of something like Downs Syndrome or Schizophrenia could cause a Justice for All failure just because the SCNT process failed. There is no spiritual or Ki_ξ gain for anyone by the molecular adaptions of DNA that occur so randomly when they become dangerous.

Into this TLO comes the concerns for the two prime directives [CD] and [GW] which MUST be balanced from one generation to the next if the result is to be a 'human' society. Under the original General Welfare, 'bad seeds' were either tolerated, aided, or terminated by the community without much Justice until a Bill of Rights that everyone had 'agreed to' appeared. Even then, many attempts to manipulate SCNT occurred among the totalitarianists in the belief that something better would come from forced eugenic controls of 'race' superiority. Really? Racial superiority from a dice-rolled, randomized molecular process extending into Posterity?

At that point, one of crimes against humanity after about 1945, eugenic tyranny became not only a [GW] and [LI] issue, but a [CD] and [OP] survival issue in which you either eliminate the tyranny or it eliminates you.   That is even more prevalent in this century because the genetic technologies (12,000 research papers worldwide in this year) can create 'designer' babies, who in turn could very easily become slaves of their makers. There are many examples of this enslavement perversion by people in sending waves of immigrants into other countries as population 'dumping' or by creating Malthusian Population Traps that allow easy exploitation of those in the Trap.   'Anchor' or 'welfare' or 'designer' babies as slaves with little chance of Ki_ξ Liberty? Really?

This process of epigenetics then becomes an issue in which all six of the Preamble's covenants are directly involved, not the least of which is the suspicion that the desire to enslave might itself be an DNA malformation since the enhancement of ξ is lessened, and evolutionary control of epigenetics then becomes a Constitutional issue of considerable importance to [OP] as well. It involves a [CD] issue in that inherited diseases can now be manipulated as weapons. It involves a [GW] issue because the Ki freedoms of all We The People are affected by the dollar and emotional costs of molecular degenerations from poor or even no health.   It involves Tranquility [TR] in that there is no peace infrastructure for a state if its populations somehow create 'unbalanced budgets' and civil strife damage through both stagnation AND migrations. It becomes a Justice [JU] problem for the same population reasons affecting Tranquility,   with the note that much of the injustice is caused by the attacks of SCNT level DNA processes going wrong in less than seven percent of the population. How people are born into the world, epigenetics, determines the Ki_ξ Liberty he is capable of AND how his children might acquire that Ki exergy or energy AND their effects on Common Defense.

That combination makes the integration of sets for Our Posterity through Wellbeing a survival necessity well above the Article I 'interstate commerce' level of healthcare, let alone Wellness in which Ki_Zhi_ξ is created for all citizens.   Note the original description of the intent of the preamble:

> It described a people, not an individual king, or ownership oligarchy, as the basis for a system of systems. It described the systems of Welfare and Defence as necessary components of a people, which were obvious to all in that year, but added subsystems like Justice, Tranquility, and Liberty as conditions of a functioning human society.   No society had such a subsystem definition before, even as it might have included one or the other in its values. Societies of the Nile, Euphrates, Ganges, Yangtze, Han and Danube Rivers all had philosophies reflecting this or that form of Justice or Welfare or peace or dynasty progression. But none had ever linked all five to our, and note our, Posterity. A common path of evolution for a system of We The People?

This speculation is based on the accumulation of information about American Constitutional processes and the possibilities of a Constitutional Convention sometime in the future. Many of the Chronicles for the election year 2016 indicate just how difficult this process might be. The reason for such a Convention is now much more pronounced than before. Note Noah Webster's comment on tyranny in 'Math Stuff' above:

But what is tyranny? Or how can a free people be deprived of their liberties? Tyranny is the exercise of some power over a man, which is not warranted by law, or necessary for the public safety. ..|LI|< → ∞.. A people can never be deprived of their liberties, while they retain in their own hands, a power sufficient to any other power in the state. This position leads me directly to inquire, in what consists the power of a nation or of an order of men?

Genetic and medical technologies, along with the absolute control of wealth, energy and communications, could become a tyranny in which the possibilities of gaining Ki_ξ (zhi or qi life energy) by an individual person are minimalized except for a self-replicating elite like empowers or pharaohs or caliphs or czars. Americans can see this happening all over the world and see their own Ki_ξ (qi life energy) diminished by that process as energy and health 'costs' increasingly put them into a system of indenture without freedom. The 'order of men' is the Constitution and its human right protections are the defense against Webster's tyranny. An absolute tyranny of machine/man 'systems' couldn't be created as long as those protections exists and *are capable of being enhanced* through referendum Conventions.

If a Convention was convened in which the conditions of a Wellbeing human right were the only allowed consideration because of the Rule of Sixes and the Rule of Fours screening, would the Electors be able to produce an Article VIII that addressed the future needs of the Americans? Let's check back on the First Convention. Note this passage from Pauline Maier's *Ratification, The People Debate the Constitution, 1787-1788,* The Morning After, 2010:

> For an impatient man, Mason invested enormous attention in details. He knew they were important. They would determine whether the government would be a blessing or a scourge to future generations.
>
> Edmund Randolph also developed reservations about the Conventions proposal. Several of Randolph's objections coincided with Mason's: He too thought the Senate was too powerful, Congress's power too broad, and also that the federal judiciary would pose a threat to state courts. Randolph suggested letting state ratifying conventions propose amendments to the Constitution, which could be put into effect or rejected by a second general convention. Franklin seconded the motion, but Mason managed to have it set aside until the Convention could see the polished form of the Constitution being prepared by the Committee of Style.[35] The Committee of Style did not, however, solve the problems Randolph raised, nor those Mason listed on the back of its report.
>
> Nor did the Convention. Between September *12* and 17, the delegates went over the revised version of the Constitution one last time, considering a mass of changes, accepting some but turning down most. Twice they rejected efforts to increase representation in the first House of Representatives.[36] When North Carolina's Hugh Williamson noted that the Constitution included no provision for jury trials in civil cases, another delegate observed that jury trials were not proper in all civil cases. Maritime cases, for example, were

generally decided by judges specially trained in admiralty law. Mason saw the problem: A general principle would be enough, he said, and he thought that if a bill of rights that supported the right to a jury trial along with other civil rights were added to the Constitution, "it would give great quiet to the people." A draft could be prepared in a few hours using state bills of rights as models. Elbridge Gerry of Massachusetts moved to create a committee for that purpose; Mason seconded the motion. Connecticut's Roger Sherman said the existing state declarations of rights were sufficient protection; Mason answered that the laws of the United States would be paramount to the state bills of rights. He might have added—as the delegates well knew—that not all states had bills of rights. Still, not one state supported Gerry's motion.[37] Later the delegates rejected motions to protect freedom of the press, to include a phrase protecting the people's liberty against standing armies in time of peace, and, again, to guarantee jury trials in civil cases.

This passage about five September days in 1787 shows just how complex the process was and why so many things, such as 'Rights', that came later were left out. It was not just the desire to go home, although several delegates had already left for pressing home problems. Each of the items discussed as 'details' were accepted or rejected because of their relevance to the stated purposes of a Preamble or intent. Virtually no delegates introduced something of a trivial nature that was accepted in the Committee of Style final draft. The first section of each Article indicated the power being designated for each of three branches, novel as that was, and giving sometimes vague wordings to other sections.

The omission of 'Rights' and 'Protections' did not mean they weren't considered; everyone knew that an Amendment process *that could change specific details* was included and accepted. This author was having a little personal problem with this because his experiences in 20th and 21st century travel around the world on oceanographic ships and local history indicated that most people did not actually believe in 'rights' on planet Earth and he had a suspicion that those non-believers were genetically pre-disposed to some form of tyranny or abnormal power-greed. The Founder's omission might have been an indication of that genetics-based desire to oppress others, a flat contradiction to the building of Ki_ξ in the spirit component of people. But they didn't actually omit rights from the Nation; they left it up to popular referendum instead. Still, Alexander Hamilton and George Mason both had serious problems with the idea of tyranny by birth. Was popular referendum of rights a designed purpose or a random incidence from a systems dynamic standpoint?

 So if you are considering a 'Right' in this century and no other, it should have some form or structure that extended, not necessarily altered, the original idea of the Preamble Six and especially not tamper with the directives of [CD] or [GW] . That puts Wellbeing in a category of an addition in which each of the existing Articles has an addition to it, much like appending a Section nn to each Article. That is not an Amendment process, and even Amendments XIV (citizenship and due process for all) and XX (periods of Presidential and Congressional activity) might actually have qualified as Article level additions.

Preamble, Article VIII. Defines the purpose and intent of the addition and relation to the original.
Section. 1. Wellbeing as a Right. Defines the concept of a Human Right for all citizens.
Section. 2. Article I Authorities. Shows the extension of authorities of the Congress.
Section. 3. Article II Authorities. Shows the extension of authorities of the Executive.
Section. 4. Article IV state authorities. State and community rights and responsibilities.
Section. 5. Citizen Responsibilities. Defines the relation of a person to wellbeing of self and others.
Section. 6. Article III Authorities. Shows the extension of authorities of the Judicial.
Section. 7. Crimes Against Humanity (Criaghum) Prohibits genetic and molecular abuse.
Section. 8. Marriage and other contracts. Defines procreation as a right, and social contract rights.
Section. 9. Governance Imposts. Paying for the wellness costs to each citizen, it's not free.
Section. 10. Implementation. Extension of Article V and authority for future conventions 30 years ap
Section. 11. Termination of Existing Legislation. Prior century health, wellbeing laws obsolete.

This would mean that Electors in a Convention would have to create a Preamble, a Rights definition, the extension of authorities for the three Federal branches, a definition of States authority, citizen responsibilities, AND the mechanism for supporting the Right with revenue. There might also be a need for a Section prohibiting 'bills of attainder' so that previous 'law' and precedent are not extended. Note the brief structural perception used in previous Chronicles and research documents:

The Article VIII graphic taken from earlier Chronicles showed a summary of the needs in a Wellbeing addition where a Preamble states the relationship of the [sets] already enumerated and the new [WB] set as it is developing in this century. If the Sections of an Article follow in a [OP], [WB], [CD], [JU], [TR] and [GW] order with a principle intent of freedom [LI] or Ki_ʓ for all, would the wording of a Right have a Section 1. 'Wellbeing as a Right' that read like so:

> Article VIII, Section. 1. Each being, on his or her conception by a man and within a women but by no other means, shall be given the right to the fullest health that can be made available by the sciences and the American society for at least two years after conception. This right of genetic security for the newly created spirit is for the creational period of birth only and other General Welfare aid to molecular enhancement shall be a privilege of validated citizenship. The Wellbeing right shall not be usurped by any other act of a human or device. This right to genetic molecular health and genetic security shall have parity with other rights of validated citizens, provided other rights do not conflict with the Wellbeing provisions of human life or adhere to economic or instinctive gain after the birthing process.

Going back to the September authoring of the Constitution in 1787 as an example, it takes no effort at all to see what would happen if the wording of just one Section of an Article VIII was being considered by Electors in Convention. First, the Right only applies to 'validated citizens' and then only to life created by a human man and a human woman. Define those. Second, the time frame for the Wellbeing Care is from conception to two years, basically conception diagnostics, pre-natal care and post-natal care up to the age of the 'terrible twos'. But [WB] ceases to be a 'Right' at this time and becomes a societal privilege afterwards that can include treatments for any age or condition, but not guaranteed, especially if the lack of wellbeing is self-induced. Define that. Thirdly, [WB] shall have parity with other conditions of [JU], [LI] or [TR] but actually can supersede their conditions in order to improve Ki_ξ. What court decides that?

The same Convention debate almost certainly gets worse for an Article VIII Section 9 (shown above in Prime Directives Interactions because of the pressing need of 2016 tax reform toward functionality and fitness) in which revenue to the government is split into an 'Impost' system based on taxing transactions and an Income tax system based on a progressive structure. While taxation reform is a major consideration in a representative government, the issue sometimes gets side-tracked into an all or nothing debate on the size of government, which from a Complex Adaptive System standpoint is a serious issue. Note Chronicles 2018.08.07:18:00, 2018.12.02:09:34 and 2018.12.15:06:27. You cannot defend yourself or build a coherent physical structure as a 'system' if your 'size' doesn't reflect the conditions of your current, note current, environment. The environment relationship $[+OP]U[GW \bowtie CD]$ where CD and GW are reasonably balanced, and people are 'safe' enough that a Wellbeing condition can be considered are easily a 'government size' matter at any given time.

But what happens to the relationship if [+OP] has an added directive that is nearly equivalent to the balance of [CD] and [GW] and takes resources from both to achieve? From another look at Maier's *Ratification, the People Debate the Constitution, 1787-1788,* one could map the chapter 'Some Final Twists' and see how the various popular referendums approved the Bill of Rights in 1788. If you speculated about that process being introduced now, you might come to the conclusion that you were playing with quantum level fire. Nothing might be better than something.

But is nothing really an option? The world pressures of technologies like the internet and localized molecular manipulation is almost certainly going to be extended into the Human Genome through epigenetics along with weaponizations of new clone viruses and toxin chemicals. There are simply those who would put primitive 'race' superiority, which doesn't actually exist at a Homosapiens molecular level, into a policy of genocide with easily constructed genetic materials. There have been virtually no human aggression systems for 6000 years in which this primitive extermination mindset has not appeared, so a [CD] $\bowtie$ [WB] issue becomes the dominate criteria for creating genetic birth protections in this century and *protecting those advances for several generations* if some desired Posterity is to be achieved. The alternative [-OP] U [GW $\bowtie$ LI $\bowtie$ JU] sets inherent in doing nothing isn't really an option; the randomized creation of evermore dangerous Malthusian Population Traps (MPT) where mass destruction devices all over the world are produced cannot be a gain for humanity, let alone We The People.

It is important to remember that the MPTs around the world can become self-replicating in terms of the adaptions people make to them. Even small, urban MPTs have had genetic adaptions to stress and poor nutrition that are passed on through Mendel's gametes modification, creating asymmetric [CD] problems like 'lone wolf' violence. That gametes or SCNT processes in poor nutrition areas does not work well and continually produces mental and physical abnormalities over Posterity long periods. Anyone can see a news screen in 2016 and verify the ripple effects of human molecular distortion.

The better combination would be where there is a progressive increase in the wellbeing of people in regionalized non-Traps and aiding of those in Traps (North Korea, Indonesia, Indian Sub-content, Syria, Venezuela, etc.) until they can stabilize themselves out of the Malthusian Traps. For the advanced societies, the conditions might look like [+Op] U [WB] U [GW ⋈ CD ⋈ JU ⋈ TR] where introduction of the [WB] set moves much of the costs and resources from both [CD ⋈ GW] into a more protected human rights based Ki_ξ environment. Not an easy shift if there is no consensus of will.

Therein lies the Second Convention.

Glorious State of Being

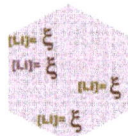

Family 'systems' slowly increase the [WB] function so that freedom or ξ ki increases in all communities in a state.

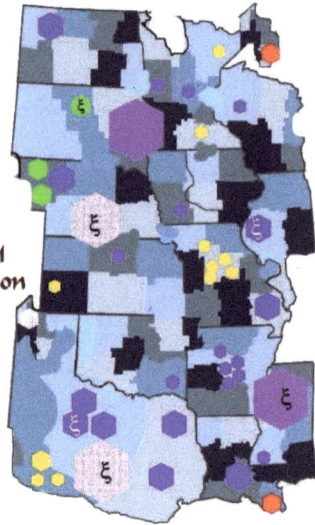

The speculative graphic of a timeline of [WB] effects through this century is very speculative but gives a general idea of what [OP] is desired when the Convention is initiated. It would mean a transfer of many resources into the protected 'rights' dynamical system while defending against obstructionist attacks from primitive societies. The 'primitives' would be those societies who wish for permanent totalitarian control and exploitation of life but don't have an evolutionary timeline of their own.

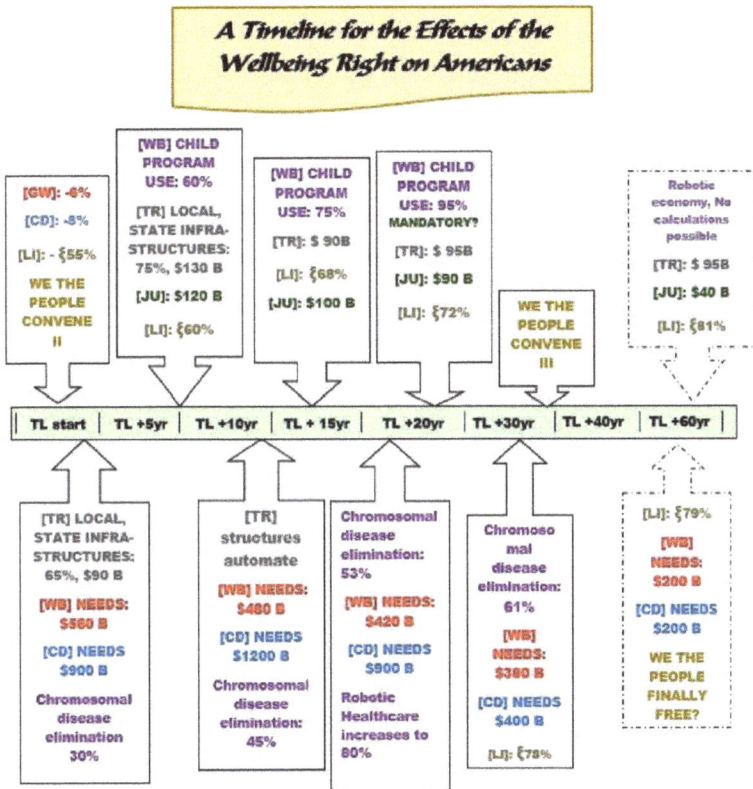

A Timeline for the Effects of the Wellbeing Right on Americans

	TL start	TL +5yr	TL +10yr	TL + 15yr	TL +20yr	TL +30yr	TL +40yr	TL +60yr

Above the timeline:

[GW]: -4%
[CD]: -8%
[LI]: - {55%
WE THE PEOPLE CONVENE II

[WB] CHILD PROGRAM USE: 60%
[TR] LOCAL, STATE INFRA-STRUCTURES: 75%, $130 B
[JU]: $120 B
[LI]: {60%

[WB] CHILD PROGRAM USE: 75%
[TR]: $ 90B
[LI]: {68%
[JU]: $100 B

[WB] CHILD PROGRAM USE: 95% MANDATORY?
[TR]: $ 95B
[JU]: $90 B
[LI]: {72%

WE THE PEOPLE CONVENE III

Robotic economy, No calculations possible
[TR]: $ 95B
[JU]: $40 B
[LI]: {81%

Below the timeline:

[TR] LOCAL, STATE INFRA-STRUCTURES: 65%, $90 B
[WB] NEEDS: $560 B
[CD] NEEDS $900 B
Chromosomal disease elimination 30%

[TR] structures automate
[WB] NEEDS: $480 B
[CD] NEEDS $1200 B
Chromosomal disease elimination: 45%

Chromosomal disease elimination: 53%
[WB] NEEDS: $420 B
[CD] NEEDS $900 B
Robotic Healthcare increases to 80%

Chromosomal disease elimination: 61%
[WB] NEEDS: $380 B
[CD] NEEDS $400 B
[LI]: {78%

[LI]: {79%
[WB] NEEDS: $200 B
[CD] NEEDS $200 B
WE THE PEOPLE FINALLY FREE?

The [WB] timeline could be seriously interrupted by various forms of WMD attacks, creation of non-human life forms, mutated evolution of super viruses, collapse of the energy economy through consumption without renewal, and various new technical innovations. But one innovation such as a matter transformer based on energy might guarantee the [WB] transition into a secure timeline for creation of Ki_ξ life forces well above the neurological levels available now.

The great Civil War of Humanities might be the clash between epigenetic enhancement for all life being created and primitives who wish to create another hierarchy of physical existence only, with their children at the top of the hierarchy of economic classes just the way it has always been.

For many societies, especially North American, the [TR] directive of the Constitution comes increasingly into play as communities attempt to incorporate [WB] with Justice for all and the [LI] rights of citizens. Protection of citizens, sometimes from primitive other citizens, in local communities allows families to create healthier, freer people rather than have oppressive economic and robotic mechanisms control them. Beyond that, their [OP] timeline would be what they make of it as a Nation.

Minimum Requirements for a Second Convention

[OP] and Ki extensions. Hope for ξ. Intent of and will for the Convention must be to bring about genetic and molecular protection for new life as a prime directive. The problem solving must be as open-minded as the first Convention but subject to modern philosophies compressed into a new Preamble of similar simplicity

[CD] Presidential CinC protection of Convention process against interference via Contempt of Constitution authority.

[GW]. Predetermination of location, information sites, funding by Congress. Set Rule of Sixes requirements for state Representative districts.

[JU] Judicial review of Rule of Sixes issue challenges. Contempt of Constitution warrant court created by Congress and Executive.

[TR]. State law authorization of Electors to have ratification authority in the Convention rather than return for state legislature referendums. . Set Rule of Fours for Electors requirements.

[LI]. Citizen Education, referendums in Rule of Six issue, and oaths of Electors prior to Convention. Citizenship definitions per state, requires setting aside individual needs in almost every instance of citizenship...

The need for the Second Convention is well established at this point early in the 20th Century. But there is also the need to defend against resource waste into reaction to primitive physical attacks and sophisticated economic attacks while building the [WB] ⋈ [GW] ⋈ [TR] infrastructures in North America. The Second Convention isn't necessary for defense and infrastructure, it is necessary to define a spiritual timeline beyond the Traps of resource consumption into stagnation of civilization.

Akhil Reed Amar, America's Constitution, A Biography, 2006, p44:

> Americans, Publius (James Madison) argued, must avoid continental Europe's fate by permanently unifying their New World landmass* as Britons had earlier permanently unified their island. When England, Wales, and Scotland were separate kingdoms, military competition between them invited invasion and foreign intrigue, triggering a heightened domestic militarization that threatened liberty. The indivisible union of England and Scotland at the outset of the eighteenth century gave island residents more room to breathe free.[100]
>
> Publius thus urged that 1787 America emulate 1707 Britain by forming its own more perfect, "strict and indissoluble" union.[101] What were the alternatives? The existing Articles of Confederation were unworkable yet virtually impossible to amend, given the high bar of state unanimity. With a little luck and a lot of help from the French navy; America had won her most recent war, but her prospects for the next big one, whenever and however it might arise, appeared uncertain at best. Experience had proved that the individual states could not be trusted to provide their fair share of American soldiers and the money to pay them and could not even be trusted to honor America's treaties with foreign powers. Without dramatic revision, the confederation could not fulfill its most basic purpose, which the Articles described as securing the several states' "common defense, ... Liberties,... and general welfare" against "all force

offered to, or attacks made upon them, or any of them" by hostile powers. To perpetuate the Articles' feeble regime would invite increased European military adventurism in North America and would leave Americans ill equipped to resist.[102]

Pretty good summery of conditions   that *still* exist in 2016, with the two prime directives and Liberty very much in danger from an entire array of random aggressions like the internet, foreign technological attack, modern chemical and bioweapon abuses and worst of all, the continued creation of multiplying genetic problems due to forced concentration of peoples without renewable resources. Very much like an aimless Confederation of peoples rather than an ordained Union with a positive evolutionary intent. With Tranquility, Liberty and Justice built into a new Convention looking at Wellbeing as a primary intent, the Union's Posterity is re-affirmed. But how well would the Rule of Four and Rule of Sixes checks and balances work?

TLO Epilogue for 2017

While many of the problems of We the People in 2017 were just carry overs from previous years, some became a consensus perceived by Americans. Healthcare, especially concerning the Affordable Care Act initiated in 2011, was still a major concern for most Americans because it affected their Liberty through indenture to health costs, the Common Defense through cross-border chemical destruction such as fentanyl and cocaine, and Tranquility because of the effects aggregate poor health had on state and community governments ability to function. Many of the problems are traceable through the Wikipedia yearly event survey

https://en.wikipedia.org/wiki/2017_in_the_United_States

along with a number of polling systems that showed the perception of the problems by Americans. That is not the same as the legislation going through States and the Congress or how complex the interrelations had become. The National Council of State legislatures (NCSL) had defined many state policy issues as having a federal component that '[{Tranquility}]' had to deal with. These were a consensus from 2016 to 2018, a legislative cycle that wouldn't necessarily appear in a Wikipedia event listing. They qualified as dynamical processes instead.

- {International trade}
- {Higher education}
- {Immigration}
- {Environmental regulations}
- {Federal infrastructure initiatives}
- {Data privacy}
- {5G technology}
- {Sports betting}
- {Disaster mitigation}
- {Medicaid}
- {TANF/welfare reform}
- {Opioids}
- {Prescription drugs}

Note that each of the conditions listed by the NCSL are {subsets} of the Preamble domains, ;legitimate in a model or not. . The order of the NCSL problem perception (and the resulting legislation) are of interest as General Welfare and Justice national processes, especially since a working model developed in one state is transferrable to others, if not nationally. Common Defense is, of course, a process attributed almost entirely as a federal process, although international trade, immigration and opioids were rapidly becoming defense issues at a state and community level. Many {items} like prescription medicine, Medicaid, welfare, and infrastructure involved the ACA 'system' in one way another and were clearly on people's minds as the attempts to repeal it proliferated after the 2016 election.

The interaction of activity on the ACA is described in the Epilogue in more detail because it had become the most significant issue of 2017 after some years of implementation.   Other issues, such as climate disasters, were also very much on people's minds even though the capital costs, human and fiscal, were not national in nature.

The following are from the attempts all through 2017 to alter or repeal the Affordable Care Act and involve [OP] observations on the effects of repeal and attempts to replace it with a consumer driven health system. It could qualify as an example of what can go wrong with society during the partisan 'reversal' mechanisms of political factions to erase the effects of the other faction.

2017.03.30:00:00   [WB]>2 ⋈ |GW|<4 ⋈ |TR|>3 ≈ |OP|>4

Krauthammer, WaPost, 'The road to single-payer health care':

"A broad national consensus is developing that health care is indeed a right. This is historically new. And it carries immense implications for the future. It suggests that we may be heading inexorably to a government-run, single-payer system. It's what Barack Obama once admitted he would have preferred but didn't think the country was ready for. It may be ready now. "

A human right like preemptive healthcare could only be established through a second Constitutional Convention, which is way overdue in the American timeline. But a wellness right of that magnitude affects all of the Articles of the Constitution and many of the Amendments in the Bill of Rights, so it would have to be submitted to specially convened representatives of We the People and ratified as an Article, not merely an Amendment.   That is the principle reason for the many false attempts to create a 'system' of healthcare;   the constitutional basis for doing that with the wonders of modern DNA based technologies doesn't really exist.   Anyone who thinks human life enhancement can be carried out through the Constitution's interstate Commerce Clause, the current authority for the ACA and the AHCA, is living in the 1700s.

But what would an Article VIII look like? Speculative Article VIII:

Preamble, Article VIII.   Defines the purpose and intent of the addition and relation to the original constitution.

Section 1. Wellbeing as a Right. Defines the concept of a Human Right for all citizens.

Section 2. Article I Authorities. Shows the extension of original authorities of the Congress.

Section 3. Article II Authorities. Shows the extension of CinC authorities of the Executive.

Section 4. Article IV state authorities. State and community rights and responsibilities.

Section 5. Citizen Responsibilities. Defines a person's relation to wellbeing of self and others.

Section 6. Article III Authorities. Shows the extension of authorities of the Judicial.

Section 7. Crimes Against Humanity (Criaghum) prohibits genetic and molecular abuse.

Section 8. Marriage and other contracts. Defines procreation as a right, and social contract rights.

Section 9. Governance Imposts. Paying for the wellness costs to each citizen, it is not free.

Section 10. Implementation. Extension of Article V and authority for future 30 year conventions.

Section 11. Termination of Existing Legislation. Prior century health, wellbeing laws obsolete.

2017.03.31:18:05   [WB]<4 ⋈ [GW]>2 [TR]>2 ≈ JU|<1 ⋈ |OP|>3

Peter Sullivan, TheHill, 'ObamaCare architect met with White House officials Thursday':

"After the collapse of the House Republican ObamaCare replacement bill last week, Trump said he thinks the health law will "explode" and Democrats will then come to the table for a deal.

Speaker Paul Ryan (R-Wis.), though, warned in an interview with CBS this week that he does not want Trump to reach across the aisle."

If you were looking for a problem-solving consensus, you could do worse. Emanuel's book *'Reinventing American health Care*' in 2014 had a chapter on the future of healthcare that optimistically described six megatrends (p319) for health in this century, which indicated an expectation of changes as part of the governing process. The megatrends are :

(1) End of Insurance Companies as we know them. (2015).

(2) VIP care for the chronically and mentally ill. (2020).

(3) The emergence of digital medicine and closure of hospitals. (2020).

(4) End of employer sponsored insurance (2025).

(5) End of healthcare inflation. (2020).

(6) Transformation of medical education. (2025).

You can add 20 years to each item in the timeline and still not be accurate, but items (1), (3), (4), (6) are well under way and are probably going into an irreversible change domain that can be enhancements to a national structure or bottom line disasters. Note that items (2) (3) and (6) are subject to massive interaction over the next 20 years and the very definition of molecular degeneration might have to be changed drastically in order to conform to the Bill of Rights and the 14th Amendment. Item (5) could only happen if the for-profit motivation of the Commerce Clause was removed from (1), (2), and (4). Item (3) with in-home and on-street droids instead of hospitals would also require a citizenship responsibility (item 6?) that neither the left or the right factions would tolerate because it would have to be 'mandated' by the national state, whatever the droids turn that into. And looming over all of these megatrends would be the need to pay for advanced 'universal' health care as a right that could consume two-thirds of the molecular capital (molecular energy summed into human capital indexes) of any and all persons, which in turn will cause most societies above a tribal level to disintegrate.

Anyone who thinks the Constitution's covenants of Justice, Tranquility, Common Defense, General Welfare, Liberty and our Posterity can be applied to wellbeing as a system (as opposed to trauma) in any given two-year legislative cycle is experiencing a poltergeist instead of a parakletos.

2017.06.09:21:51 |CD|<3 |TR| |LI| |OP|<2

Sullivan and Snell, WaPost, ACA repeal vs replace: "Senate GOP leaders have not yet identified which taxes they plan to keep to pay for things such as a longer Medicaid timeline and expanded tax credits.

But Lankford is one of many Republican senators who have already begun to openly embrace tax provisions the GOP once called some of the most onerous parts of the law.

Many GOP senators now view these taxes as a necessary evil in their quest to rewrite the health-care law while maintaining the deficit savings required by Senate budget rules."

While the House has the ultimate authority on taxation, it needs to be pointed out that somewhere in this process the strategic interests of the entire nation need to be considered on healthcare and it might be a representative group of states that can do this. No matter what 'cherry picking' is done, the states need to create a safety net that covers some $400 billion a year in healthcare costs from now to 2025. This is just the revenues of 'admin' and 'emergency' costs, not individual preconditions or lifestyle excesses. Interstate costs are more of a Senate process than a House process where representation districts are 600,000 people each. But states can be six Fed regions of governance too and might include border provinces in terms of health ($4 billion/year for 'aliens').

No matter what the district populations of 600k might ask of their 'representatives', the national concern would still have to have taxation coverage for 50 states and maybe 15 adjacent 'territories' that interact with that health system. Still need $400 billion a year taxation revenue to have ANY structure, even if it is 13th worldwide.

2017.07.16:06:05 |TR|<2 = |LI|>1WB|<2 ⋈ |GW|>1-|JU|<2 ≈ |OP|>3

Bolton, TheHill, 'Five key senators who will make or break healthcare reform':

"The Congressional Budget Office score of the bill, expected on Monday, could tip the balance one way or the other — as could pressure from President Trump, their home-state governors, doctors and hospitals."

Good luck to the five. The CBO is projecting that the Big Four (Medicare, Medicaid, ACA subsidies, and CHIP) will consume 7.8% of the entire GDP by 2035. All healthcare treatment systems, of course, subtract from the national wealth as well as individual net worth. There is no 'profit' to the dynamic system from an operations research standpoint UNLESS the 'system' is gradually restructured toward a cure process ONLY. The CBO will prove no matter what tinkering or replacement the conservatives attempt, the non-curative system will STILL consume an increasing amount of the GDP and will subtract at least another $600 per year from the net worth of individuals whether insured or uninsured.

These five senators, who clearly wish to see some 'system' operate from a national level in their states, are going to be disappointed by the CBO report because even with the Cruz amendment calculated in (it isn't on Monday), the Feds are still going to have to come up with a minimum of $600 billion a year in tax revenues, something at least 20 reasonably conservative Senators won't be able to handle. All five could realistically vote against the bill simply because the Big Four have not been made curative enough for their constituents to gain the Cruz Essential Services gain in net worth.

National healthcare is a very tough system analysis when you have 330 million people each with 700,000 molecular systems that could go bad anytime in life with a treatment cost that goes up at an inflation rate of 6% per year. The blame game does not work with something that complex.

2017.07.28:07:03 |WB|<2⋈ |GW|>2⋈ |CD|<3 |TR|>1 |LI|<3⋈|JU|<3   ≈ |OP|<2

Rubin, WaPost, 'Republicans' dream of repealing Obamacare ends':

"And what was the excuse for the rest of the Senate? They all had the power to stop a bill many openly trashed as a joke and conceded would do great damage. Nevertheless, all hoped someone else would do the dirty work of derailing it."

Virtually all of the conservatives had made long-term promises to repeal the ACA and were stuck with that promise. It would have been hypocritical for them to 'do the dirty work'. But the real issue is a Constitutional one when it comes to national level healthcare and this problem may be lurking in the back halls on the Capitol Hill. The Constitution's authority for doing healthcare by both parties is through the 'interstate commerce' clause 3. This in turn makes human wellness an ECONOMIC process without considering the Preamble's intent involving Justice (for all), Liberty (freedom from excessive taxation and indenture) and domestic Tranquility (state, local interaction). Clause 3 authority by itself has made people nervous as far back as the Clinton/Kennedy initiatives in the 1990s simply because human life is not just a commercial activity like making shirts or selling stocks.

 Some other specific Constitutional authority is needed for human wellness and it just might be that the difficulties in legislating such are because there really isn't an authority derived from a referendum by We the People such as when the Bill of Rights was voted into existence.

2017.07.28:07:03 |WB|<2⋈ |GW|>2⋈ |TR|>3 |LI|<3⋈|JU|<3 ≈ |OP|<2

Editorial Board, WaPost, 'The single biggest lesson from repeal-and-replace':

"Backstopping insurance markets, reducing uncertainty, relaxing some regulations, making the individual mandate less objectionable to conservatives, adopting automatic health-insurance enrollment — these are just a few of the ideas that could be in a compromise package."

Speculation:

It might be possible to make the individual mandate a preemptive care requirement that is scalable. Suppose there is a national safety net coverage for 'emergency' Essential Services found in all versions of the ACA and the 'repeal' HACA or BCRA that is tied to a mandated 'wellness' evaluation every 4 years? Emergency Essential Services (ES) in a facility might be automatically covered, giving insurance markets 'backstopping'. But the ES could also involve pre-emptive diagnostics that determine whether a person has not taken care of himself over many years.

Blood, DNA, Biopsy tests normally associated with emergency care can determine whether a person has been careful with his own health. Obviously, a heroin addict without income that lets his liver, kidney, and neurological systems fall apart is an emergency care process that society pays for and can't correct himself without the ES. But sugar, THC, and carbohydrate addictions leading to major body system failures might be considered negligence that only the individual is responsible for. That could involve a 'premium' of $10,000 instead of the ACA uninsured penalty but might not apply retroactively because of ex post facto conditions. As for 'regulatory' excesses, you can't have national 'fits all' laws with individuals in 50 separate state entities; some things should be left to states and communities, which in turn becomes a Constitutional Amendment issue involving 'citizenship'.

https://ballotpedia.org/Republican_effort_to_repeal_the_ACA,_July_2017

In the early morning hours of July 28, 2017, the Senate voted on an amendment from Senate Majority Leader Mitch McConnell (R-Ky.), also referred to as the "skinny bill." The amendment contained the following provisions:[22]

- A repeal of the requirement for individuals to enroll in health insurance
- A repeal of the requirement for employers to offer health insurance
- A delay of the tax on medical devices
- A suspension of federal funding for community health centers that include Planned Parenthood
- Greater funding for other community health centers
- An expansion of the ability of states to get waivers from ACA provisions

A repeal of public health program fund

The amendment was rejected by a 49-51 vote. Sens. Susan Collins (R-Maine), John McCain (R-Ariz.), Lisa Murkowski (R-Alaska) joined 48 Democrats in voting against the amendment.

This process was a nearly all consuming one that literally required nearly all of the Congressional man-hours through the first 100 days of the Trump presidency. Many of the repeal conditions did have national support because of the commitment to employer related health insurance. The entire process simply indicated the need for a national constitutional convention geared to healthcare ONLY and that there was too much fear of such a convention getting out of hand under the current political climate and international conditions. The net domain progression might be:

$\sum$ [WB]<2⋈ [GW]<2 [TR]>3 [LI]>3 [JU]><3 ≈ [OP]<2

Both [WB] and [OP] lose with so many uninsured or unhealthy individuals in the country. Attempts to maintain [LI] by libertarians and [TR] by states' rights advocates simply meant that Justice for all would be set aside.

The Russian undermining of the U.S. Election had also become a serious deterrent to holding a constitutional convention for ANY reason, even with the obvious needs for them.

2017.05.10:07:00 [CD]<2 [JU]<3 [GW]<1 [OP]?

Ignatius, WaPost, 'The Comey debacle only magnifies the Russia mystery': "In a book called "Spy the Lie," a group of former intelligence officers explain the behavioral and linguistic cues that indicate when someone is being deceptive. Interestingly, many of these are evident in Trump's responses to questions about Russia's covert involvement in U.S. politics. "

Wonder who, in the world intelligence system, is advising the White House about the uses of 'deception'? This timeline process from 2015 on doesn't make much sense. My CSI long range scanners say there is something else besides a 'Russian' investigation going on.......

2017.05.11:09:30 [JU]>3 [LI]<3|TR|>2⋈|WB|≈ |OP|>2

Hon. Adam B. Schiff (D-CA:28th) in WaPost, 'Only a special counsel can tell us.': "..... the American people would likewise benefit from a congressionally empowered independent commission, fully staffed and immune from political pressure, to carry on a separate, nonpartisan review of the facts."

Observation:

Noting that a judicial grand jury review is already empowered with full subpoena authority for a portion of this 'constitutional process', the entire matter might already have passed from a questionable review by extremely partisan Congress and Executive branches to the Judiciary Branch. That is how checks and balances are supposed to work.

The Article III authority of the Judiciary concerning 'Controversies to which the United States shall be a Party' is pretty clear about whether any constitutional controversy is subject to its authority and not necessarily the other two branches. There is no reason that the Congress cannot empower a Judicial independent court, not a commission, like the FISA system to investigate a crime against the constitution or its integrity such as foreign interference in American constitutional processes.

The Congress does not relinquish its oversight authorities with the empowerment of a closed court that can investigate free of a public two-year election cycle with the money involved in such a process. Further, there is nothing that says a judge of a five-man court could not also be a prosecutor providing Bill of Rights non-disclosure protections are in place. Public Roman circuses with $100 million media profits do not serve the Justice covenant of the Constitution when a process has endangered its own integrity, so neither the Executive or Legislative branches should have 'circus' authority for correcting it.

Can the Congress empower and fund a grand jury court to investigate free from any partisan minority?

[OP]>2, [JU]>1:There is also no particular reason that such a court could not give immunity for testimony on ANY subject concerning an attack on the Constitution or even assume guilt unless proven otherwise under immunity conditions.

[Shiff]: Given the taint accompanying the president's decision, only this step will give the public any modicum of confidence that the investigation will be conducted fairly, rigorously and independent of political influence and interference. And while Congress continues to press forward with its own vigorous probe,

[JU]>1: U.S. Constitution, Article III, Section 2: "The judicial Power shall extend to all Cases, in Law and Equity, arising under this Constitution, the Laws of the United States, and Treaties made, or which shall be made, under their Authority;--to all Cases affecting Ambassadors, other public Ministers and Consuls;--to all Cases of admiralty and maritime Jurisdiction;--to Controversies to which the United States shall be a Party;-- "

This is further amplified by a nearly all points attack by the Eastern Oligarchies as shown by:

2017.10.30:07:20 [OP] |WB|>2 ≈∑ |TR|>3 |LI|<3 |JU|>1 [GW]>2

Diehl, WaPost, 'China's Communist leadership has a model of totalitarianism for the 21st century':

"Perhaps most ominously, Xi envisions his updated police state as a model for the rest of the world. Twenty-five years ago, the liberal democratic system of the West was supposed to represent the "end of history," the definitive paradigm for human governance. Now, Xi imagines, it will be the regime he is in the process of creating. "It offers a new option for other countries and nations," he said during a three-hour, 25-minute speech that was its own statement of grandiosity. "It offers Chinese wisdom and a Chinese approach to solving the problems facing mankind."

The ideology expressed by Xi Jinping is actually a carefully researched process by Qu Qingshan and Yang Welmin along with compiled input from 80 government agencies and 230 university symposia. This research 'paper' started a year ago and was submitted to the 2300 congress delegates before it was added to the Communist Party constitution, not the People's Republic constitution as an 'Amendment'. Note that virtually all of the contributors to the research were believers in socialist one-party states to begin with and this almost certainly entered into their perception of 'evolution'.

Unfortunately, this constitutional convention outlined a 50-year plan based on systematic possession of power and wealth that has existed for 6000 years. Not exactly an improvement. At the least, it didn't involve the endless constitutional flip-flops of the West trying to satisfy one-percent minorities who don't believe in ANY constitutional future.

Further:

The 'liberal democratic system of the West' has proven over the last 20 years that it can become so diverse that it can only deal with the endless trivia of human societies, not an evolved system of governance. That is why you can have tribal societies that represent a tiny oligarchy in any region suddenly decide they deserve the status of 'national sovereign state' for that tribe's special interests. All you would wind up with under 'liberal democracy' is a massive number of medieval, circa 500 BC, city states each with the ability to manufacture genetic or biological or chemical weapons of mass destruction while the population 'indulges' in narcissism at each other's expense. This is evolution based on natural selection.

A 50-year Plan might have other domain progressions as well:

Police state: $|OP|n$ $|CD|>4 \approx \sum$ $|WB|<2$ $|TR|>3$ $|LI|<3$ $[JU]<1$ $|GW|<2$

Oligarchic: $|OP|n[LI|>3 \approx |CD|>2$ $|TR|<3$ $|WB|<4$ $|GW|>1$ $[JU]<1$

1.7 billion optimal:? Genocide? Democide?

Note that the [OP] is our Posterity but the other domains are the cumulative effects of the other countries' domains on it. The [CD] gains of the Oligarchies would require a negative going [CD] for America because of the cost differentials. It costs them a lot less to make bullets than the America [CD] structure for profit. The clear intention to remove all forms of liberal democracy from the planet was not apparent until about this decade, but it represents a permanent hostility to our Posterity. It might even make a wellbeing [WB] Posterity much more difficult.

Add in the technologies under development in this decade involving quantum computing, artificial intelligence, media interdiction of society, biological weapons through gene editing, space EMP weapons, and robotic drones contribute to a negative going Common Defense and General Welfare.

All of these combinations, along with opioid attacks against Americans

(2017.02.09:18:08 $|WB|<4$ $[GW]$ $|CD|<2$ $|TR|$ $|LI|$ $[JU]$ $|OP|<2$**), terrorism, and loss of infrastructure**

(2017.08.06:06:50 $|OP|>3 \approx$ $|TR|>3$ $|LI|>3$ ⋈ $[JU]<>1$ $|GW|>2$**) ,**

make [LI] and [TR] increasingly difficult, especially with many political factions attempting to attach quite trivial agendas to a national process.

Consensus on some [OP] problems on a world scale.

Business Insider, 2018:

Lack of economic opportunity and employment (12.1%)

Safety / security / wellbeing (14.1%)

Lack of education (15.9%)

Food and water security (18.2%)

Government accountability and transparency / corruption (22.7%)

Religious conflicts (23.9%)

Poverty (29.2%)

Inequality (income, discrimination) (30.8%)

Large scale conflict / wars (38.9%)

Climate change / destruction of nature (48.8%)

Consensus 2018, ABC News, Topics that worry Americans a great deal:

54% - The availability and affordability of healthcare

53% - The economy

51% - The possibility of future terrorist attacks in the U.S.

46% - The Social Security system

46% - The size and power of the federal government

46% - The way income and wealth are distributed in the U.S.

43% - Hunger and homelessness

43% - Crime and violence

39% - Illegal immigration

38% - Drug use

37% - Unemployment

34% - The quality of the environment

28% - The availability and affordability of energy

28% - Race relations

25% - Climate change

Random issue samplings, 2017

https://www.eurekalert.org/pub_releases/2017-01/natu-soa012717.php

The top issue for Republicans (47 percent), Democrats (40 percent), and independents (43 percent) is health care.

Unemployment is mentioned by 37 percent of Republicans, 25 percent of Democrats, and 26 percent of independents. The economy, in general, was mentioned by roughly a fifth, regardless of party.

While there is partisan agreement on some of the country's leading priorities, Republicans and Democrats disagree on the importance of other issues. For example, the second most common response from Republicans is immigration, named by 40 percent. In contrast, only 15 percent of Democrats listed immigration as one of their top five concerns.

Coming up with a solution to the public's priorities should be given a substantial amount of effort by the government, according to most Americans. However, the poll did not investigate what people specifically want to see accomplished for any of these problems. It is likely that, while health care is the top issue for both Democrats and Republicans, each group would prefer different resolutions.

Few expect much will be accomplished to solve these problems in the next year. The public views some problems as more difficult to deal with than others. Americans have little confidence in the government's ability to address poverty, racism, and the environment. There is more optimism for progress to be made on unemployment, immigration, and terrorism.

Fewer Americans regard the country as heading in the wrong direction than a year ago, although it remains a majority. In 2015, 69 percent said the country was on the wrong course and 30 percent said it was headed in the right direction. Now, 56 percent consider the country heading in the wrong direction and 42 percent say it is on the right track.

Republicans and Democrats have both had an about-face regarding the direction of the country. In the wake of Trump's election as president, 66 percent of Republicans say the country in headed in the right direction, up from 18 percent last year. Only 22 percent of Democrats now regard the country as being on the right course, down from 42 percent last year.

Record-setting hurricane season: The 2017 Atlantic hurricane season, which included 17 named storms and 10 hurricanes, may go down as the costliest hurricane season ever. In the United States alone, hurricanes caused more than $2 billion in 2017.

Opioid epidemic: Public health officials announced that drug overdoses have become the leading cause of death for Americans under age 50, with more than two-thirds of those deaths coming from opioid painkillers. President Trump declared the opioid crisis a "public health emergency" in October.

https://www.history.com/topics/21st-century/2017-events

U.S.-backed forces take Raqqa: After a four-month fight, the ISIS "capital" of Raqqa fell to a U.S.-backed coalition of Syrian forces, ending three years of ISIS control in the Syrian city. The defeat carried symbolic weight as the second major loss of territory for the Islamic State in three months. In July, ISIS troops were pushed out of the Iraqi city of Mosul.

Conclusion for 2017:

Outlook for a wellbeing convention is bleak, even as the complexity of the six Preamble covenants increases. Is it the accumulated pressures of population densities and movements that make the Common Defense and General Welfare interaction so difficult? Or is it the pressures of a form of universal Justice and Liberty that We the People are demanding? When a variety of external pressures, including totalitarian attempts to destroy liberal democracy as an evolutionary process, began to bleed away resources that both Justice and General Welfare need to maintain their domains within a society, some of the possible advances are set aside.

TLO Epilogue for 2018

Murray Gell-Mann, *What is Complexity?* Remarks on simplicity and complexity by the Nobel Prize-winning author of *The Quark and the Jaguar*, 1995:

> Since it is impossible to find all regularities of an entity, the question arises as to who or what determines the class of regularities to be identified. One answer is to point to a most important set of systems, each of which functions precisely by identifying certain regularities in the data stream reaching it and compressing those regularities into a concise package of information. The data stream includes information about the system itself, its environment, and the interaction between the environment and the behavior of the system. The package of information or "schema" is subject to variation, in such a way that there is competition among different schemata. **Each schema can be used, along with some of the data, to describe the system and its environment, to predict the future, and to prescribe behavior for the system.** But the description and prediction can be checked against further data, with the comparison feeding back to influence the competition among schemata. Likewise, behavior conforming to a prescription has real world consequences, which can also affect the competition. In this way the schemata evolve, with a general tendency to favor better description and prediction as well as behavior conforming more or less to the selection pressures in the real world.
>
> Examples on Earth of the operation of complex adaptive systems include biological evolution, learning and thinking in animals (including people), the functioning of the immune system in mammals and other vertebrates, the operation of the human scientific enterprise, and the behavior of computers that are built or programmed to evolve strategies-for example by means of neural nets or genetic algorithms. Clearly, complex adaptive systems have a tendency to give rise to other complex adaptive systems.

The basis of 'sensing' Gell-Mann's schemas in complexity mode has been established in the Chronicles as a useful mechanism, even if the full extent of the data per schema is overwhelming. One of the sensory mistakes is easily seen in the use of 'dogmas' to define long-term processes that change over a period. Note

https://en.wikipedia.org/wiki/2018_in_the_United_States

where a large number of items are 'significant' even when there is no dot-connect to a major system like the Six Covenants of the Preamble. There are many in the 2018 website that DO relate to the three branches, but not necessarily to the Constitution. Therein lies the complexity as shown in the following figure as a summarization of the 2018 progressions of the Six. The graphic summation takes the form

$[OP] \approx \sum [CD] > n[TR] > 3 [LI] > 3 \bowtie [JU] > 1[GW] > n \bowtie [WB] > ? + [\xi] > n?$ where Posterity is an approximation of the sum of the two prime directives and some combination of Justice, Liberty, and 'security' in [TR]. This is described by an observation in the Washington Post by the Krauthammers and shows this schema perception quite well.

[OP] is shown as a sum of the other domains, but it is a loop-back schema as well and the sum, except for [ξ] >n or Ki>n, leads to a Posterity.

$$\sum [CD]{>}n[TR]{>}3 \ [LI]{>}3 \bowtie [JU]{>}1[GW]{>}n \bowtie [WB] \ \approx \ {\rightarrow}[OP] \text{ can also exist.}$$

2018.11.29:21:36 |OP| ≈∑ |CD|>n|TR|>3 |LI|>3⋈|JU|>1|GW|>n ⋈ |WB|>?+ | ξ| >n?

Charles Krauthammer and son Daniel Krauthammer in WaPost, 'Charles Krauthammer: The enduring miracle of the American Constitution':

"The second miracle is the substance of it — the way that the founders, drawing from Locke and Montesquieu and the Greeks, created **an extraordinary political apparatus that to this day still works** and that has worked with incredible success for nearly a quarter of a millennium."

Note the Preamble as the intent of the Constitution:

We the People of the United States, in Order to form a more perfect Union,

establish (1) Justice,

insure domestic (2) Tranquility,

provide for the (3) common defence,

promote the (4) general Welfare, and

secure the Blessings of (5) Liberty to ourselves and

our (6) Posterity,

do ordain and establish this Constitution for the United States of America.

TLO: In 1787, combining those five items in nearly any order of priorities in a context of a long-term Posterity actually compresses about 70% of the world's knowledge into 52 words. None of the other Constitutions written since have managed such a statement of combinational wisdoms in so few words. The Founders were pretty sharp and had worked out some new ways of doing things, but were they really THAT perceptive?

But then again, 70% of the world's wisdom in 1787 has become maybe 50% now in the original five covenants and perhaps a Second Constitutional Convention with as much perception could add to it in this century.

The complex adaptive system of the Constitution as shown in the diagram and described by the little expression of Krauthammer shows just what a couple of centuries can do to an idea. Just the summing of $\sum[CD]{>}n[TR]{>}n \ [LI]{>}n\bowtie [JU]{>}n[GW]{>}n \bowtie [WB]$ as balanced schema is hard to visualize and attempts to reduce the domains into optimized {subsets} with components of other domains is a difficult modelling process. One can very quickly get 'lost in the weeds' with such a {} dynamic system and the history of the agencies of government show this to be a factor. There is also a tendency to use reductionism to visualize matter in an 'either/or' context, as a simplification that is usually inaccurate. The totalitarians don't even try to visualize this complexity anymore; they simply use brute force to simplify the {subsets} in their own sociobiological interests.

In this epilogue study, the idea of modelling interactive {subsets} was restricted to those involving the hypothetical Wellbeing domain and their interaction with other domains or external force agents such as totalitarian aggressors.

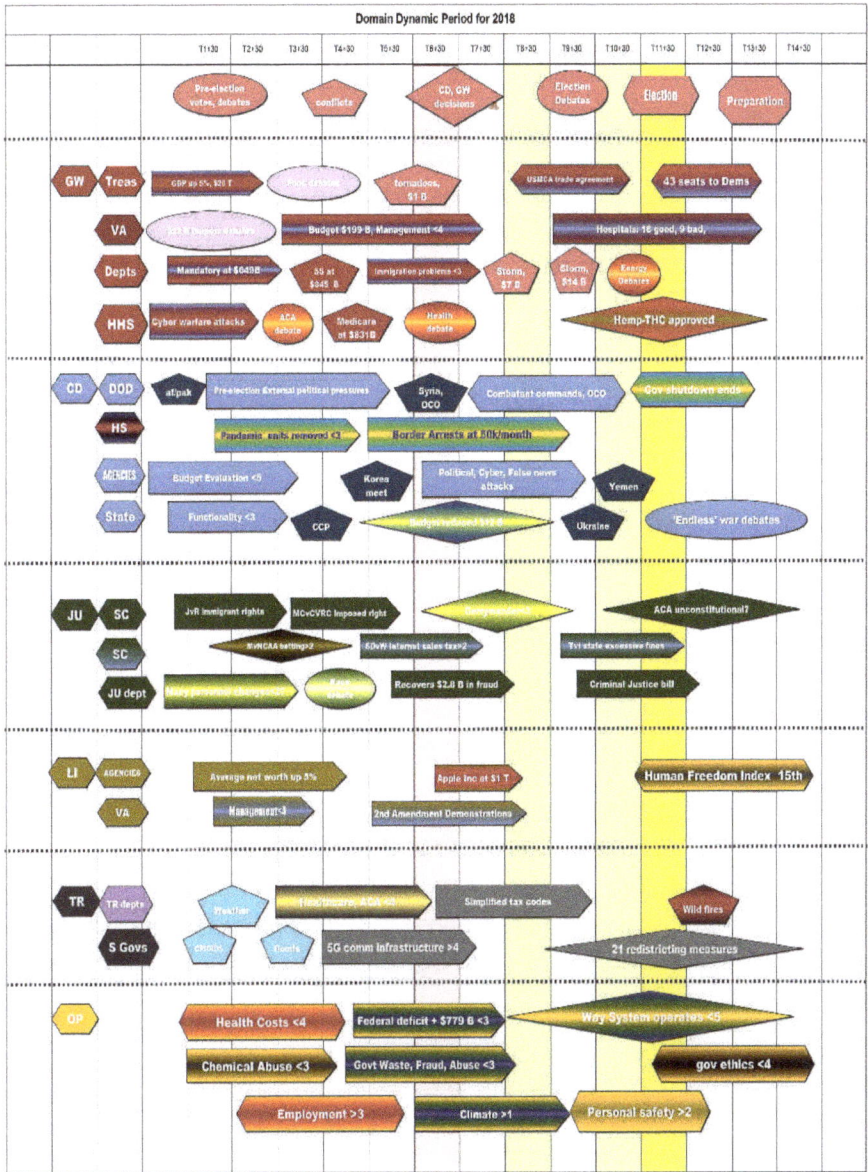

Figure 25.   Domain summary, too much CAS?

2018.02.08:07:10 [WB|n+|CD|<1.....|LI||TR|-|JU|<3+ |GW|>1=|OP|<2

Hall, WaPost, 'We are witnessing a democratic nightmare':

"Only when sectional and partisan battles gave way to new international responsibilities, and (relative) domestic harmony, in the 20th century could Republicans and Democrats define shared national interests and accept the need for permanent secret agencies to protect them."

The reason that Republicans and Democrats had 'shared national interests' was that their political constituencies were both being attacked by socialist one party states (Germany, Russia, Japan, China, Cuba, Iran, Ottomans, etc) BECAUSE the two parties had a shared Constitution that included such things as Liberty, Justice, and especially Common Defense and General Welfare. These are items that are intolerable to the one party state because they prohibited a member of a ruling elite from attaining 'god' powers of life and death over every subject of 'his' national domain. The totalitarians still are haters of check and balance systems and still try to undermine anything that does that, such as investigative security agencies.

But if the bi-partisanship mentality has been heavily eroded by the closet toties in and out of government, those who have taken oaths to protect and defend the Constitution are obligated to consider all, repeat all, acts in terms of whether others are in the process of disavowing the Constitution and Bill of Rights and not consider their personal whims relevant. The investigative or security agency members certainly are not obligated to adhere to the partisan beliefs they may have been 'schooled' to the extent that they hold Constitutional integrity itself in contempt. You can't have a democratic nightmare in a representative republic if its members are actually adhering to the Constitution and the 'rights' it creates. Only partisan extremism on the constitutional fringe can do that.

2018.02.22:21:13 |OP|<2 ≈ Σ |TR|<3 |LI|>3⋈|JU|>1....|GW|<2+|CD|>2

Evan Bayh in TheHill, 'New poll reveals why Founders would be worried':

"The bipartisan House Problem Solvers Caucus and several bipartisan groups of senators have each proposed plans that would marry these two ideas together, comprehensively saving the Dreamers and protecting the border. But Washington remains mired in disagreement, unable to move forward on any specific plan. That's not because a grand compromise on border security and immigration would mark bad policy. It's not because the compromise offends any particular constituency. It's just because, well, that's Washington."

The Founders would have been very worried because their checks and balances to reach a rational solution of 'federal' level problems had simply disappeared in this century. But they did debate the idea of putting 'citizenship' definitions in the Constitution but decided not to (thanks, Ben) because it was obvious the definitions would change over time. They nicely opted for an authority of the Congress 'to establish a uniform 'Rule of Naturalization' rather than birth citizenship. And this proved correct as wave after wave of immigrants stepped off a one-month boat trip. They would never have anticipated an immigration need for an Afghan translator serving our military or a need for asylum from Latin Conquistadors overrunning some county somewhere or a naturalization need for a skilled worker because our own society was too media-decadent to produce them. It really is time to create a 'uniform Rule of Naturalization'.

Speculation:

Suppose modern biomedical technologies on DNA Identification were used to create a 'green' card (555 nm, the exact middle of the color spectrum) that expressed a Condition of Naturalization? There are some 50 categories of alien residents created by the various waves and a single uniform ID card showing what the status is, including those with a presidential or gubernatorial pardon status, might be made a requirement for residency and work regardless of the time involved. That smart card would make the person or visitor an 'American National' which would cover all of the 43 million 'aliens' coming and going from the country. It happens that the military common access card (CAC) is already in wide use and is 'smart' with a 64 mbyte chip. There is no reason at all that a USNational card could not be created with DNA data concerning the Human Accelerated Regions (HARs) that truly identify a person as a homosapien, even if such data and health related to the HARs require 2000 mbytes.

Addressing two current 'wave' problems with three-year extensions is laudable, but a much more 'uniform' solution based on 21st century no-doubts DNA technology would go much further in solving the true Naturalization problem.

2018.03.14:09:02 [WB]n+|CD|<1…..|LI||TR|-[JU]+ |GW|<1=|OP|<2

The Editors, BloombergView, 'America's Next Big Drug Problem, Doctors and lawmakers need to take benzodiazepines seriously, before it's too late.':

"At the moment, Congress, the White House and the states are all considering stronger measures against opioids. That's overdue. On benzodiazepines, they should act now to avoid making the same mistake again -- by including them in their current deliberations and taking steps to rein in this other epidemic before it gets any worse."

1998 Rome Statute on the definition of a crime against humanity (criaghum):

For the purpose of this Statute, 'crime against humanity' means any of the following acts when committed as part of a widespread or systematic attack directed against any civilian population, with knowledge of the attack:

(1)(k) Other inhumane acts of a similar character intentionally causing great suffering, or serious injury to body or to mental or physical health.

(2)(a) 'Attack directed against any civilian population' means a course of conduct involving the multiple commission of acts referred to in paragraph 1 against any civilian population, pursuant to or in furtherance of a State or organizational policy to commit such attack.

A systematic distribution of a lethal toxin should be treated for what it is. That might put a doctor in the position of being considered a serial killer, but it is not possible to3/ suggest that there is a morally defensible 'mass treatment' distribution of a toxin. Doesn't matter who does it or why; it is still criaghum.

Khor, Third World Network, 2018.01.05, on digital technology processes

First, automation with artificial intelligence can make many jobs redundant. Uber displaced taxis and has now booked thousands of driver-less cars which will soon displace its army of drivers.

The global alarm over job losses was sounded a few years ago and is gathering speed. Scholarly studies warn that as many as half of jobs or work tasks in industries including electronics, automobiles and textiles, and professional services such as accountancy, law and healthcare, will be replaced by robots within one or two decades.

Second is a recent chorus of warnings, including by some of digital technology's creators, that addiction and frequent use of the smartphone are making humans less intelligent (as time and interest traditionally used to acquire broad and in-depth knowledge is now replaced by the narrow skills and short span attention required by social media) and socially deficient (as relations through social media replace direct human relationships).

Third is the loss of privacy, as personal data obtained from our internet use is collected by tech companies like Facebook and Google and sold to advertisers. The companies have the data on personal details and preferences of millions or even billions of individuals which can be used for commercial, and possibly non-commercial, purposes.

Fourth is the threat of cyber-fraud, other cyber-crimes and cyber-warfare as data from hacked devices can be used to damage computers and websites; empty bank accounts; steal information from governments and companies; send out false information; and engage in high-tech warfare.

Fifth is the worsening of inequality and the digital divide as those countries and people with little access to digital devices will be left behind or even lose their livelihoods. The internet can be used by big companies or tech-savvy small and medium sized firms to establish growing markets for their products, which is one of the major attractions of the digital economy.

2018.04.13:10:02 [GW]>1-[JU]>2|TR|<2-|CD|<2 ≈ |OP|<3

Brufke and Elis, TheHill, 'Proposal to amend the Constitution falls short in House':

"Further, said Kogan, the "ideal" level of debt may not zero, but rather a sustainable amount relative to the size of a nation's economy. Even many fiscal conservatives advocate for policy that carves out a path to reducing the overall debt burden instead of eliminating it altogether."

Unfortunately, any Wall Street economist will happily tell you that deficits don't matter. The reason such economists catering to hedge funds and retirement accounts say that is that since 1980, one half of all interest payments on the debt (current $300 billion a year) go to enhancing Wall Street funds that are dependent on a substantial yearly increase in the interest payments on the deficit. Those funds, coincidently, are held by nearly all employment relationships of the government down to a town level or contractor. That is, there is no incentive whatever to reduce the deficit because it would also reduce the interest payments a generation later when the retirement funds kick in for these individuals.

Rather than some 'balanced' budget amendment, which could be accomplished ONLY by reducing the Article I authorities of the Congress to appropriate General Welfare funds under Section 8 clause 1, it would be simpler to create a taxation system that incentivized deficit and cost reductions in government. That would require a tax schedule based on the GDP/deficit ratio to revenue/outlay ratio. That is, for every one percent increase in the deficit without a corresponding three percent increase in GDP , the taxation in each category would also increase one percent until there is a reduction in deficit for three consecutive years. The effect of this incremental increase in taxation, perfectly in keeping with both Keynesian and Friedmanist economic models, would give every segment of the economy reason to reduce governmental costs AND prevent them from accruing to future generations. You might not even need a Second Constitutional Convention to do that, although such would allow specific utilization of tax revenues rather than just to General Welfare OR Common Defense, the Achilles Heel of the current government.

2018.04.20:08:08 |CD|<3 ⋈ |GW|>1-|JU|<2|TR|<2≈|OP|<2

Editorial Board, WaPost, 'How Congress can take back control of America's wars':

"This is far from the clarity of an old-fashioned declaration of war; yet the war against far-flung terrorist groups does not necessarily lend itself to one."

'Wars' are not the issue here, criminality is. The Committee supported version, S.J.Res59, has specific definitions of organizations like the Haggani Network and Al Nusrah as 'associated forces' of ISIS and the Taliban where force can be used because they have essentially declared war on American citizens. S.J.Res59 has appropriately limited AUMF countermeasures to specific organizations that have attacked Americans directly, although it also specifically allows U.S. force to protect Afghanistan citizens against terrorist force but not elsewhere 'associated forces' might operate. The repeal of previous AUMFs and the requirements for reporting are also appropriate even if the 'reporting' defined is technically an open, unclassified document that the enemies or their sponsors can read.

It is interesting that none of the 8 or 9 submitted AUMF resolutions have given authority to interdict with ANY force a biological or chemical attack with instruments of mass murder. That might involve use of force against sovereign supported 'militias' in half the world, but there is a noticeable lack of enthusiasm for allowing the president as CinC to destroy installations engaged in crimes against humanity even if that is authorized directly by Article I, Section 8, clause 10 in the Constitution. Are other AUMFs needed to defend North America against WMD criminal activity around the world?

TLO: this could be a serious [OP] and [CD] omission of governance responsibility caused by the conflict of belief that all use of military type force involves 'war'. It is equivalent to saying a county sheriff could not cross over into another county to prevent an imminent threat by a criminal. A no-win for a society if [CD] is a prime directive.

2018.04.28:07:31 |WB|<2 ⋈ |GW|>2 ⋈ |CD|<3 |TR|>1 |LI|<3|JU|<3 ≈|OP|<2

Lena Sun, WaPost, 'Bill Gates calls on U.S. to lead fight against a pandemic that could kill 33 million':

"But even the best tools in the world won't be sufficient, Gates said, if the United States doesn't have a strategy to harness and coordinate resources at home and help to lead an effective global preparedness and response system."

Under conditions like the 1918 Pandemic where most of the world's medical personnel were drawn off to deal with World War I fighting, you could easily have a mutated

SARS infection introduced to several dozen 'supercarriers' (infected people who can wonder around without showing symptoms) climb aboard aircraft and hit a couple of hundred thousand people per day. The simulation in the article appears to show a SARS spread, but without the quite ruthless controls put in place in 2002, such a mutation might infect 200 million in a month.

If someone with a large computer system background got involved in a hardware development infrastructure like DARPA did for the Internet, they might be able to create a special world network of supercomputers that could only be switched on during a medical 'doomsday' scenario. They might even be able to create software similar to the Palantir system that can trace a viral bug with millions of dot connects so that health authorities will be able to shut the contagion in days rather than the weeks it took during the 2002 SARS outbreak. A system of massively parallel 50 petaflop servers in each of 2000 cities would go a long way toward predicting contagion paths and education on reacting to various pathogens. 2000 such units dedicated to a health system shouldn't be that tough in this century, especially if DARPA already has research funding for such things.

TLO: much more serious than people realize.

2018.04.24:08:26 |GW|>3⋈ |CD|<1 = ∑ |TR|<1 |LI|<3⋈|JU|>1 |OP|>2|OP|>?

Lane, WaPost, 'Red America and blue America depend on each other. That's how it should be.':

"Cembalest calculates that if electoral college votes were allocated according to food and energy production as well as population, Texas would have 81 electoral votes instead of its current 38, North Dakota would go up from three to 14 — and New York would shrink from 29 to 19."

If the Electoral College Districts were allocated according to the 'wellbeing' of the citizens that calculated the food, energy use, health, and productivity of Americans, they might discover not just a well-known red-blue split but a 'purple' component that is much larger than either the red or blue. This would be a truer indication of the relation of people to GDP, especially since fully one quarter of the American GDP is parasitic services concentrated in California, New York, Texas and Florida. If you removed these international components because they do not produce food, energy or health, the true GDP is closer to $15 trillion with a 'purple' distribution and the big four (who do produce a lot of wellbeing internally) become interactive States rather than GDP subtractors from the rest of the States.

That only occurs if you introduce individual positive/negative health and productivity into the GDP calculation, which in turn would be necessary if the Electoral College district was itself 'representative' as Article IV, Section 4 of the Constitution requires. A purple Texas might have 29 Electors instead of 38, California becomes 40 instead of 55 because of its support of Malthusian Population Traps in its urban areas. Virginia, with 13 now, would become 19 under the wellbeing formula and Ohio would have 22 instead of 18 because its wellbeing increases with stable, productive populations.

Further:

The 'purple' formula at the College eliminates unrepresentative Population Traps from absorbing the wellbeing of the surrounding EC Districts (438 Electors) and States (100 Electors).   It is calculated on a much truer GDP basis than the author's red-blue regressive divide into urban traps absorbing the wealth of states around them.

TLO:

Speculative imagery of the red/blue/purple Electoral College 'dynamic system' in which many Electors are obliged to vote for the majority pick of a given District in order to be representative.

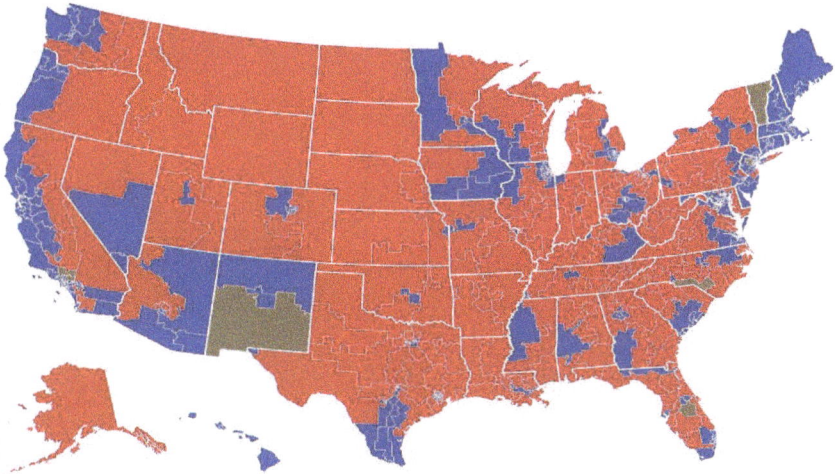

The current voting in 2016 indicated only a few 'Independent Districts' (shown in brown, not purple) because of winner-take-all. Without such a state law, the national vote might look something like this:

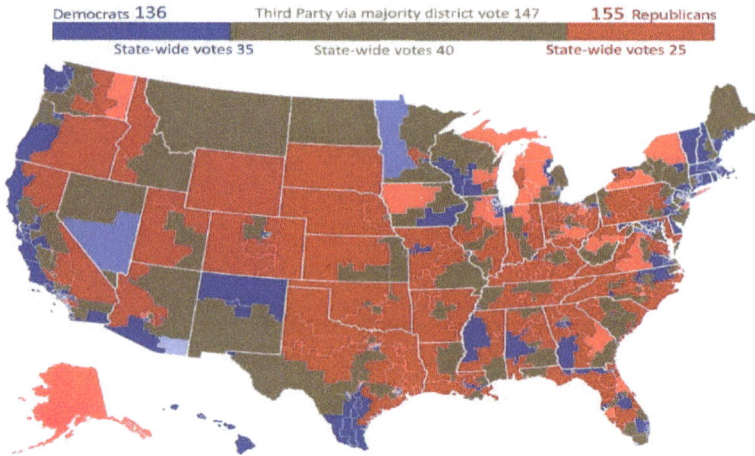

Democrats 136 • Third Party via majority district vote 147 • 155 Republicans
State-wide votes 35 • State-wide votes 40 • State-wide votes 25

The problem with this model is that a 'majority' of 270 Electors is nearly impossible, no matter what the candidates represent, so a president might be elected with both a popular majority of the turn-out AND an Electoral College vote of 146 out of 438, with perhaps 35 state level Electors added. Even with such a small turn-out vote, the Electoral College would STILL be representative of the country as a whole. A winner-take-all system might elect a president with half of the popular vote disqualified and with a popular vote of just 30%. Since the 'party' nomination process excludes all voters except party members, there can be no valid popular vote choice for the nation; it is pre-decided by 10 to 15 percent of the population in the primaries. Not representative enough.

This would also occur if the Electoral College was selected for a Constitutional Convention which, under checks and balances philosophy, might have been the Founder's original intention for the College; to be 'independent' but representative evaluators of a Constitutional change. The Founder's assumption that States would convene to amend the Constitution never materialized because of oligarchic control of power that inevitably develops. But no Constitutional changes in a half-century of traumatic technical, quantum, political and health changes?

2018.05.17:09:02 [WB]<2 ⋈ [GW]<2 ∑ [TR]>1 [LI]<2 ⋈ [JU]>3 ≈ [OP]<2

Honorable Markwayne Mullin in TheHill, 'Doctors need the whole picture on opioid addiction':

"This outdated law and its subsequent regulations, 42 CFR Part 2 (Part 2), keeps a patient's substance use disorder records separate and segregated from the patient's general medical record."

and

Not only does this segregation stigmatize the patients Part 2 was designed to protect, but in the modern-day digital world it creates a dysfunctional maze of bureaucratic rules that are impossible for physicians and administrative staff to navigate and even more impossible to enforce. Part 2 has created an inconsistent patchwork, where the level of care and privacy a patient receives depends upon the interpretation of Part 2 by the provider.

The 'outdated law' situation may be much worse than most on Capitol Hill think. It isn't so much a matter of stigmatizing a person as it is a matter of the individual having a 'citizen card' with his individual medical history on it. The absence of a 21st century medical data infrastructure is a much worse problem than just health histories leading to the 33,000 mis-diagnostic deaths each year. That's nobodies' specific fault; it just means that the EHR 'systems' that do exist grew all over the place as the technologies in the last 10 years developed. Spending $22 billion on new EHR systems over the last 10 years was fine, except that none of them can communicate with each other on an individual level. The Constitution's Article I, Section 8 easily authorizes the Congress to establish a medical information infrastructure, note infrastructure, including a modern 'health card' so that a person can be scanned by any first responder, provider, or emergency room anywhere.

As for the addiction records, the old data system is, as stated here, almost worthless. The Human Genome Project of the last 8 years has been systematically mapping the DNA structure of human beings and one of the findings is that people have 'inherited' AND 'adaptive' susceptibility to various substances. That includes sugar, nicotine, alcohol, opioids and so on. All of these involve the body 'learning' to adapt to various substances and this in turn involves a little gem called 'neuroplasticity'. **Neuroplasticity is the ability of the brain to remember or learn what substances are feeding it and this is the item that causes addiction if there is over-exposure to a substance**.

It is also the reason that treatment for addiction is so difficult, but the history could be a simple Neuroplasticity Index on a person's EHR card. The Neuroplasticity Index does not necessarily have to express the type of addiction publicly, only the genetic susceptibility to substances over time. Such an Index alerts anyone to a genetic problem as well as an environment problem; the higher the index the more caution in introducing other stronger substances.

As Albert Einstein said, don't make any laws that can't be perceived rationally, and fixing the records infrastructure rather than a symptom of the problem fits that idea.

2018.07.02:06:59   [ξ]<2 [WB]>1⋈ [GW]<2 ⋈ [TR]<1 [LI]>3][JU]<1 ≈ [OP]<2

Mincberg in TheHill, 'The Supreme Court's dangerous inconsistency on religion':

"Even before the Court's rulings in these two cases, serious concerns were raised about the inconsistency in conservative justices' views about government hostility towards religion in the two cases. Just about any explanation for the inconsistency has dangerous implications."

The 'inconsistency' could easily be based on whether a 'religion' advocated a theocracy in some way, which would be a clear violation of the intent and purpose of the Constitution. Islam is the only religion crossing American borders that has many advocates of a state religion or Caliphate, even though the Quran itself does not ordain such a Caliphate in any way. **The theocracy part of Islam is a man-made political philosophy having little to do with spirituality and therefore it is not inconsistent for the three branches of government, in a Bill of Rights framework, to be hostile to that political process.** The Supreme Court has also found certain practices of

English Puritanism and Italian Catholicism in advocating state religious laws to be unconstitutional. That is, the consistent hostility has been toward theocracy and that is exactly what the Constitution intended; religion was a personal, individual act and could not be forced on anyone through 'laws'.

In fact, the hostility toward theocracy has also extended to individuals who falsely used 'religion' to create cults of material worship that denies rights to others within the cult. The Supreme Court has not been inconsistent about banning state theocracy from the branches of government and unfortunately, there is only one religion that has false members who advocate it. The hostility toward theocracy should be consistent no matter what the source, including individual demagogues using it for material gain.

2018.07.05:07:04 |WB|n+|CD|<1…..|LI||TR|-|JU|<3+ |GW|>1 = |OP|<2

Rebekah Diamond in TheHill, 'Separating immigrant children from their parents is child abuse':

"As a pediatrician, I write this to urge all fellow physicians and health- care workers to officially report the abuse of immigrant children at the border and demand the immediate reunification of all families.

And as a mother, I implore all citizens to see beyond partisan lines and understand the simplicity of this issue: we cannot tolerate the abuse of innocent children."

The abuse didn't start at the U.S. border. If you cannot support the abuse of innocent children, **why doesn't your reporting procedure verify the systemic abuse of children in the community of origin**? Systemic abuse of children for economic or cultural reasons at its ORIGIN is a crime against humanity (ICC Rome Statute, Article 7 (d) Deportation or forcible transfer of population) and should be treated as such, not just the reaction to it a thousand miles away.

TrudyTruthTeller • 2 hours ago

Your comment is a complete detour from reality. Do you really believe the rubbish you posted? Firstly, this is an opinion piece, not a news piece, so this doctor is not attempting to "report" anything. Her piece is based on information we already know, not fantasies you are attempting to imply. You know nothing about these children, so stop trying to give this administration a pass on human rights violations that are proven by insinuating things you have no knowledge of.

 to TrudyTruthTeller an hour ago: All pediatricians in the United States are required by law to report indications of child abuse no matter where applied. The reporting mechanism has and is used to report abuse of asylum seekers anywhere in the world. That is the 'report' the author is discussing.

Attempting to suggest the problem originated in the United States is hypocritical in the extreme; it is a worldwide immigration human trafficking problem, not just American.

TrudyTruthTeller an hour ago

Clearly you don't know what you're talking about. I'm not going to waste my time with someone that implies "facts" that are figments of his/her imagination. These children are coming for asylum, because of the violence in El Salvador, they aren't being trafficked.

 to TrudyTruthTeller • 12 minutes ago : These children aren't being created by 'magic'

The Guardian (London) 'It's a crime to be young and pretty: girls flee predatory Central America gangs':

"Corrupt security forces, international drug cartels and warring street gangs have helped turn the Northern Triangle into the world's most dangerous region outside an official war zone. **And the threat of sexual violence against women and girls has become a growing factor behind the refugee crisis that is quietly unfolding on America's doorstep.**

Of the 32,142 female migrants detained by Mexican immigration agents in the first nine months of this year, almost one in three were under 18. Almost 15,000 12- to 17-year-old girls from Central America's northern triangle – Guatemala, El Salvador and Honduras – have been apprehended here [on their way across Mexico] since 2014.

TLO: TrudyTruthTeller is a 'Hollywood' moniker. Translation problems at the Cyber server in St. Petersburg or Tianjin?

2018.07.20:07:29 [WB]>2⋈ [GW]>4⋈ [CD]<3 ≈ ∑ |TR|<2 [LI]<3⋈[JU]<4 |OP|<22

Ignatius, WaPost, 'The intelligence community has never faced a problem quite like this':

"FBI Director Christopher A. Wray made a similar show of independence here Wednesday at the Aspen Security Forum, saying the Russia investigation wasn't a "witch hunt," as Trump claims, and affirming, "Russia attempted to intervene with the last election, and . . . it continues to engage in malign influence operations to this day."

Title 5, U.S. Code, Section 3331, oath of office for officials other than the president:

I [name] do solemnly swear (or affirm) that I will support and defend the Constitution of the United States against all enemies, foreign and domestic; that I will bear true faith and allegiance to the same; that I take this obligation freely, without any mental reservation or purpose of evasion; and that I will well and faithfully discharge the duties of the office on which I am about to enter. So help me God."

Constitution's Article II, Section One, Clause 8:

Before he enter on the Execution of his Office, he shall take the following Oath or Affirmation:—"I do solemnly swear (or affirm) that I will faithfully execute the Office of President of the United States, and will to the best of my Ability, preserve, protect and defend the Constitution of the United States."

Acts in renunciation of either oath would qualify as a contempt of the constitution but not necessarily 'high crimes and misdemeanors'. But the presidential oath does not say anything about 'all enemies, foreign and domestic'........

2018.08.06:06:58 [ξ]<3 [WB]<1⋈ [GW]>3⋈ |TR|<1 [LI]<3⋈[JU]<1 ≈ |OP|<2

Boot,WaPost, 'Republicans' hypocrisy on racism': "Nor is the response of leftist activists convincing when they argue that, as a minority herself, Jeong cannot be guilty of racism. Racism is "prejudice plus power," leftist activists explain. Actually, racism is defined as "prejudice, discrimination, or antagonism directed against someone of a different race based on the belief that one's own race is superior."

One out of every eight persons everywhere on earth is born with an accelerated form of Zenophilia, which is the neurological basis for 'racism', so ANY minority or group of Homosapiens with 100 people in it will have at least one born zeno. Zenophilia has little to do with race 'superiority' (a biomolecular or genetic impossibility) but is simply an inborn fear/hate of others who are 'different'. If you add in a neurological condition of sociopathia to the universal one out of eight Zenos, you will get a very dangerous homosapien who is quite capable of feeding a Zeno political, cultural, or economic hate agenda to everyone around him. If you have a white Zeno talking to a black Zeno or a yellow Zeno talking to a brown Zeno anywhere in the world, you will get approximately the same sociopathia or fear/hate reactions in the conversation. That Zeno conversation might not make sense to at least five out of the eight people around them, but they can be negatively influenced by it just like any other propaganda.

Perhaps humans should ask 'is he or isn't he the one out of eight who is Zeno?' when they interact with someone else. You should always ask that if there is a probability of sociopathia human hating in the interaction process for your own protection. Skin tone is an 'excuse' for a Zeno hate, not an end objective of superiority.

2018.08.21:06:20 |WB|<2✉ |GW|>2✉ |CD|<3 |TR|>1 |LI|<3✉|JU|<3 ≈ |OP|<2

Fransciso Toro in WaPost, ' Venezuela doesn't prove anything about socialism':

"Don't be fooled. All Venezuela demonstrates is that if you leave implementation to the very worst, most anti-intellectual, callous, authoritarian and criminal people in society, socialism can have genuinely horrendous consequences. **But couldn't the same be said of every ideology**?"

Sure. Oligarchic greed has happened regardless of whether a Marxist Socialism or Friedmanist Capitalism society originated it. The latter Roman Empire failed when a Senate oligarchy began selling the imperial crown to any gold, the Ming imperial cliques that degraded all government functions leading to foreign ownership of society, and the recent conversion of popular wealth into the hands of Iranian, Iraqi and Libyan cliques. All are examples. **The same transfer of individual wealth is being made by 200 Venezuelans in position to make laws of seizure.**

And one might even remember the 'Curse of the Ben', which was included in the acceptance speech of Ben Franklin in September 1787 during the final approval of the American Constitution. Even though he was strongly in approval of the final draft of the Constitution, he had his misgivings based on what he had seen while in Europe among the imperial houses there in the 1740s and 1760s. Ben wrote, while sitting in an office of the Christ Church next to its burial churchyard, the following as part of his urging the adoption of the newly drafted We the People intentions without the burden of oligarchical deficit spending that had been a genuine Curse in Europe and the Middle East:

Curse of the Ben, 1787.09.14: "There is no form of Government but what may be a blessing to the people if well administered, and believe farther that this is likely to be well administered for a course of years, and can only end in deficit Despotism, as other forms have done before it, when the people shall become so corrupted as to need despotic Government, being incapable of any other."

2018.09.19:07:01 | ξ| <4 |WB<21⋈ |GW|<1 ⋈ |TR|<3 |LI|>3⋈|JU|<1 ≈ |OP|<2

Itkowitz, WaPost, 'Senate passes sweeping opioids package, the set of 70 bills is one of the only bipartisan pieces of legislation to be approved this year.':

"While addictions to opioids are declining, heroin overdose deaths are rising. That's not because more people are using heroin, but because the drug is being laced with fentanyl - an incredibly potent, inexpensive and synthetic opioid. **The Centers for Disease Control estimates that of the 72,000 overdose-related deaths in 2017, 30,000 were caused by synthetic opioids**.

The Senate bill addresses the ease with which synthetic opioids are shipped from overseas, typically from China."

STOP Act in the 70 bill 'package':

Sec.1. Short title; table of contents.

Sec.2. Customs fees.

Sec.3. Mandatory advance electronic information for postal shipments.

Sec.4. International postal agreements.

Sec.5. Cost recoupment.

Sec.6. Development of technology to detect illicit narcotics.

Sec.7. Civil penalties for postal shipments.

Sec.8. Report on violations of arrival, reporting, entry, and clearance requirements and falsity or lack of manifest.

Sec.9. Effective date; regulations.

A quick check of other documents, such as the Congressional Research Service report, 'Drug Offenses: Maximum Fines and Terms of Imprisonment for Violation of the Federal Controlled Substances Act and Related Laws', indicates what this STAR Act also says. **Virtually all drug abuse 'seller' conditions are treated as offenses with severe penalties for ECONOMIC activity and not any form of mass murder as defined by war crimes or genocide. What such laws with penalties up to life imprisonment are saying is that serial or mass murder of citizens by chemical warfare means is a NORMAL human activity rather than a terminal crime against all humanity act.** You could spend $170 billion a year in treatment and legal costs and still not eliminate an attack on the American people at a rate of 70,000 casualties a year, or 400,000 victims a year if you count ripple effect deaths as well. Society respect for human life too good for someone who doesn't have any?

2018.10.20:19:36 |WB|>2⋈ |GW|>3⋈ |CD|<3∑ |TR|<2 |LI|<3⋈|JU|<3 ≈ |OP|<2?

Bonnie Rothman in WaPost, 'Those 'superhumans' of the future Stephen Hawking feared? Look around.':

"For now, we don't seem too keen to engineer superhumanity. According to a Pew Research Center survey released in July, **only 19 percent of Americans think it's acceptable to edit for intelligence.** But it doesn't take a Stephen Hawking to see that we already live in a world of "significant political problems" and underprivileged humans who increasingly "won't be able to compete.""

Hawking was not really worried about super 'humans' coming into existence as much as mutations who are inherently predatory toward normal, 'self-improving' humans. True, only 19 percent of Americans think creating enhanced IQs was acceptable. But two Chinese universities, one thousandth of one per cent of the Chinese people, already have major laboratory editing facilities collecting DNA data on high IQ individuals. And you cannot study at these universities unless you are a member of the 'Party' or an offspring of a Party Member. There are 'elite' research structures similar to this in several western universities and military structures that are concerned with this as well.

But it is the 'mutations' that are the main concern, not the 'rational' childbearing brought about by literate pairs of humans. A genetically induced sociopath might be created as a DNA mutation because he, as a mutation, is less than a hundredth of one percent of the human population. A certifiable sociopath, with considerable IQ, from birth named Saddam Hussein managed to have violent humanity ripple effects of 700,000 deaths over 27 years and two trillion dollars of destruction around the world. A survey of DNA related ripple effects of violence in America might be as high as 3000 deaths a year and $100 billion in directly related economic effects.

A mutated predator bred in an artificial womb with 'selected' DNA sequences is a real possibility, just as Hawking visualized. Even a fairly rigorous Constitutional system of checks and balances on 'unnatural' genetic sequences might not protect future generations from the mutations that have already occurred.

2018.10.26:22:30 [WB]<4 ⋈ [GW]>2⋈ [CD]<3 |TR|>3 |JU|<3 ≈ |OP|<2

Dr. Marion Mass in TheHill, 'Medicare for All' will never work, so let's stop pushing it':

"Consider: The number of health-care administrators — many drawing salaries well into the six figures — has risen by 3,200 percent between 1975 and 2010. (The number of physicians grew by 150 percent over the same timeframe.) This bureaucratic bloat diverts precious resources away from treating patients and inflates the cost of care. Reversing this administrative growth to all but the most critical positions could allow for a dollar-for-dollar offset in health-care costs.

Meanwhile, the clerical burden on doctors continues to grow. Doctors now report spending two-thirds of their time on paperwork."

This doesn't make sense. If there are 3200 percent more administrators, many of whom are in doctors' offices AND in the private insurance sector, how is it that a provider can wind up doing paperwork two-thirds of the time? Anyone who is familiar with the medical disease classification system known as ICD-10 knows that it lists a required classification of some 14,000 problems, along with an optional 70,000 insurance related codes that medical offices must deal with. This results to some degree in a national health cost of 'undiagnosed problems' of $270 billion a year, much higher than #2, heart disease treatments. Interpret as administrative costs for the 3200 percent increase in administrators, perhaps?

The 'market' solutions listed here will not work because modern communications will allow for pricing adjustments industry-wide on a given ICD-10 disease condition. This in turn guarantees that the costs per ICD-10 item will increase at a 6 or 7 percent level rather than the inflation level of 2%. There is no gain for Americans by just this process, but neither would a universal Medicare at an additional $4.0 trillion a year because there is still no attempt to remove the 'admin' costs from the system. **You would be better off manufacturing 800,000 AI med-bots that record everything they see in a health environment, including mistakes, and make up the ICD-10 (or ICD-15 in 2025) reports for both the private sector and the government HHS agencies.** Would intelligent med-bots with 500 terabyte memories drop $200 billion a year off the costs?

2018.11.30:11:37 |CD|>3|LI|<5 ≈ |OP|<2 Ξ|WB|<1+|JU|<2 ⋈ |GW|>2|TR|>3

Kyl and Morell, WaPost, 'Why America needs low-yield nuclear warheads now':

"In this way, Russia is intent on exploiting what it perceives as a U.S. nuclear capability gap on the lower levels of the escalatory ladder. That is because a high-yield, long-range U.S. response to Russia's first, limited use of a low-yield nuclear weapon against a military target is not credible. The Russians believe we are not likely to risk a global thermonuclear war in response to a "tactical" nuclear attack by them."

This is a well-known tactical strategy conceived by Vladimir Putin some time ago and in advanced stages of development now. The GRU assessments that America would not use large-yield, city busters (1 megaton and up) if others are using local, non-nuclear WMD as in Syria and Chechnya is correct. A variable yield nuclear 'tochka' can deliver a 50 kiloton (4 times Hiroshima) explosion 200 km, but Russian militaries still consider that 'tactical'. A European, American or Indian 'Pluton' style device is about 10 kiloton, but a version can be as small as 1 kiloton, which is **smaller than some chemical bombs** and has a destruction radius of half a kilometer. However, the small tactical can also be used as an anti-missile device and that might be its only value, especially if mounted in a hypersonic vehicle.

Russia, unfortunately, must also contend with 15 Chinese mechanized divisions near their borders which are also being equipped with DF-15 medium devices. The Chinese 'territorial occupation' philosophy which all 15 divisions are capable of involves concentration of force between enemy forces and Russia has no defense against this tactic except tactical nukes.

TLO: 'zeros' misplaced. 1 kiloton of kinetic energy is not the same as a 2000-pound bomb or one ton of kinetic energy equivalence. Destruction radius at ground level might not be much different, however. The availability of 'suitcase' nuclear devices is almost a certainty in this century; the human haters have no interest in whether Americans or Russians or Africans live or die. That interest won't get you into the history books.

2018.12.25:07:30 |CD|<3 ⋈ |GW|>1|JU|>2|TR|<2 ≈ |OP|<2 LI|<3

"It's difficult to find a good present for the leader of the free world," the news site wrote online. "We, at RT, have invoked our inner SNL [Saturday Night Live] writer to imagine what Donald Trump will find under the Christmas tree, where there is one box from us, this year."

They seem to know exactly what is going on in the U.S. media, based on the syntax used in the 'show'. That in turn might require close affiliation with people like Sterebriakov or Morenets over in the GRU offices near Opolchenie Street. But who can tell whether the RT employees and their GRU handlers were operating as 'rogues' since the disappearance and death of Colonel General Korobov in October? Can anyone show the GRU has a command and control or is it just following a general 'world deceit' program? Even the SBP (ninth directorate?) doesn't currently seem to know whether RT is acting on its own rather than in the interests of the State. But the sophistication is evident, far more so than American media.

TLO: It doesn't take much content analysis to realize the RT is an organ of the Russian government. Democracies that fail to counter such dis-information mechanisms are at a severe disadvantage on a world political media platform. Possibly a [OP]<2 simply by its unchallenged existence. But in America, it was also affecting [TR] at a <3 level and [JU] at a <2 level.

The preceding Opservationis are a sampling of the timeline for 2018 and are indicative of the complexity that humanity has created among their various haplogroups. One item that has been added is the Wellbeing {set} for Ki or {ξ 气 }, which designates the 'life force' or consciousness within the mind, body, spirit conditions of Wellbeing. This could be described as an energy component involving the product of human capital [WB], freedom [LI], peaceful co-existence [TR] and interactive Justice [JU] and it is undetermined whether such an energy is actually a {subset} or a resultant domain of human evolution. That is, 'Ki' is both individual and empathic among Homosapiens and there is evidence that this only developed a hundred thousand or so years ago as they 'evolved' into control of the physical environment. Control of the quantum environment may be the current evolution, so Ki might progress from a [WB]{subset} to a domain of its own.

At some point, the Wellbeing constitutional right with its {Ki} subset might become a 'consciousness' prime directive that directly loops back into all of the other domains and the earth environment itself. The [ξ_] life force relationship can appear in balance with the other domains as an essential part in each, but is it universal as part of an evolutionary model?

This combination appears in Math Stuff as:

.. [TR]<2 = ∑ [LI] >3 →[WB]>3 [ξ_]>2 ⋈[CD] [GW] →>2-[JU]<2→ [OP]>3 ..
where {ξ_ }, [TR], [LI] and [JU] are building blocks for the prime directives [CD] and [GW]. They, and [WB], all have a loop-back effect that is supposed to show in Our Posterity [OP]. The Ki is a component that is so influential that one can debate endlessly whether it is a {subset} of [WB] or something greater. Here, it is used as a {subset} because the other actual domains contribute to its existence in a constitutional representative Union, centralist or not. In this model, you could have progressions such as: [CD] ⋈ [GW] = [OP] or [WB] →[LI] [JU] [TR] or [GW] →[LI]+ [ξ_] but

not Ki or [ξ_气] by itself. It is the combination of the {subsets} within each domain as perceived or 'sensed' that allows an understanding of the We the People progression itself. Summing to the domains is perceptually accurate but reductionism into the subset details might not be.

Many of the [CD] issues have become an increasingly confrontational 'system' between intransigent imperial powers in Asia and Western democracies in general. Their view, based on Chinese success in controlling a major population through totalitarian methodology and central committee organization, has now put democracy itself in a 'suspect' status that should be diminished as a threat to oligarchic (central) rule. This has appeared in the increasing centralization of wealth in many countries where less than one percent of the world population controls 70% of the wealth. The historical progression of this type of totalitarianism has invariably resulted in warfare, asymmetric or total, as the elites contend with each other. Note the Iran/Iraq wars progression, which had all the symptoms of a medieval game of thrones. The Common Defense of democracies, plus Russia and Ukraina, contributed a loss of over $1.3 trillion to these Middle Eastern clashes with no resolutions in sight.

The Iranian success with asymmetric warfare by proxy armies led to a belief that it did not need to abide by an Agreement, not a treaty, on nuclear proliferation. This in turn led the United States to withdraw from the agreement as it constituted a [CD] failure. A similar failure occurred in older non-proliferation treaties with the exception of the New START treaty that went into effect in 2018. But nearly all such unilateral treaties are meaningless if other countries such as North Korea, Iran, India, and China can continue to develop WMD.

At the same time, American threat analysis determined a very real attack toward democratic institutions by cyber-warfare elements in Shanghai and St. Petersburg. This led to a reformation of American cyber defenses on the internet and the militarization of cyber-defenses in order to add a strike capability to the defense of internet activity, along with exclusion of foreign internet equipment in the United States. This [CD] progression might also involve [GW] and [JU] and even [TR] domains because of its economic and political ripple effects on the American society.

A Gallop Poll, taken in mid-October 2018, shows an unfortunate lack of interest by the Americans in their Common Defense domain as shown by one question asked in the poll:

Importance of Issues for Midterm Voting -- Registered Voters

How important will each of the following issues be to your vote for Congress this year?

Extremely/Very important percent

Healthcare 80%

The economy 78%

Immigration 78%

Way women are treated in U.S. society 74%

Gun policy 72%

Taxes 70%

Foreign affairs 68%

Way income and wealth are distributed in the U.S.   68%

The recent confirmation of Brett Kavanaugh to the Supreme Court   64%

U.S. trade and tariff policies   61%

Climate change   53%

Investigation into Russian involvement in the 2016 U.S. election   45%

'Russian involvement in Elections (cyber-warfare against democracies)' rated below 11 other issues, with foreign affairs, also a [CD] component, at 68%. Common Defense was not especially concerning, possibly because of the size and diversity of the Defense Department and its budget. The economy still rated as a very high concern even if the numbers indicated a quite good growth and stability index of about 3.0 percent. The economy was finally pulling out of the 2009 Recession, but people were still wary, as they were concerned about economic {sets} like {wealth distribution} and {taxes}. Few really believed the idea that tax reductions were an economic stimulus or that the taxes that had resulted were fair.

Foreign affairs (68%) involved the ongoing tensions with a parasitic totalitarian state like North Korea, which just might be heavily influenced both in nuclear testing and 'revolutionary' behavior by an equally totalitarian China. The [GW] domain involved intense trade restructuring with both the NAFTA system and the Pacific system of trade, along with European Union complexity and Ukraina/Russia {force subsets}. Other energy related conflicts, especially Libya and Venezuela, also involved American anti-imperialist defenses. These force concerns had many elements of what is known as a World War 'whirlpool' effect, but the force-incrementing into global violence did not happen in 2018. Such danger is noticeably not on the radar of the major political organizations during a congressional election year, even when the whirlpool was known to happen before both previous world wars.

The General Welfare Domain stayed the most major concern, with healthcare (80%), the economy (78%), trade policy (61%), and Taxes (70%) all components of voter interests.   These {subsets} all directly involve a person's life and may have appropriately had the primary interest of Americans in some combination. Climate change (53%) was beginning to effect Americans in 2018 in ways that were not obvious but the costs of various tornadoes, superstorms, draught and wildfires NOAA puts out yearly 'significant climate anomalies' graphic that shows the climate totals rather than individual events, but does not combine the costs to [GW] and especially not to [WB] or [Ki_ξ気].

U.S. Selected Significant Climate Anomalies and Events
for 2018

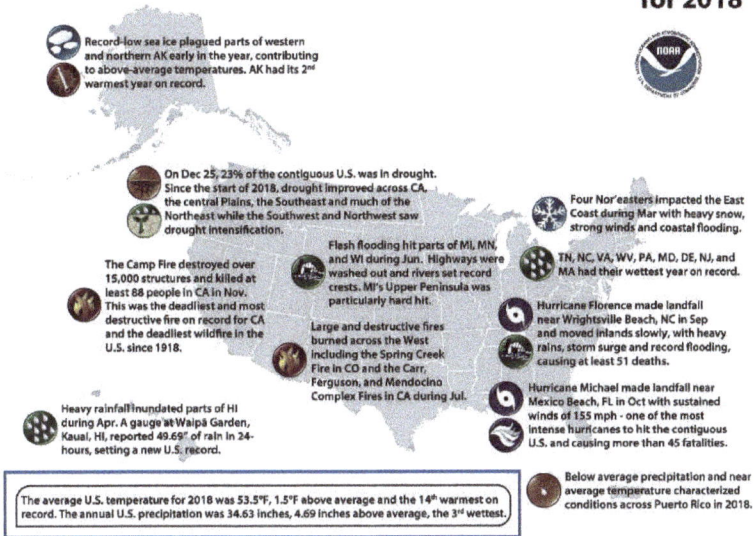

Record-low sea ice plagued parts of western and northern AK early in the year, contributing to above-average temperatures. AK had its 2nd warmest year on record.

On Dec 25, 23% of the contiguous U.S. was in drought. Since the start of 2018, drought improved across CA, the central Plains, the Southeast and much of the Northeast while the Southwest and Northwest saw drought intensification.

Four Nor'easters impacted the East Coast during Mar with heavy snow, strong winds and coastal flooding.

Flash flooding hit parts of MI, MN, and WI during Jun. Highways were washed out and rivers set record crests. MI's Upper Peninsula was particularly hard hit.

TN, NC, VA, WV, PA, MD, DE, NJ, and MA had their wettest year on record.

The Camp Fire destroyed over 15,000 structures and killed at least 88 people in CA in Nov. This was the deadliest and most destructive fire on record for CA and the deadliest wildfire in the U.S. since 1918.

Large and destructive fires burned across the West including the Spring Creek Fire in CO and the Carr, Ferguson, and Mendocino Complex Fires in CA during Jul.

Hurricane Florence made landfall near Wrightsville Beach, NC in Sep and moved inlands slowly, with heavy rains, storm surge and record flooding, causing at least 51 deaths.

Heavy rainfall inundated parts of HI during Apr. A gauge at Waipā Garden, Kauai, HI, reported 49.69" of rain in 24-hours, setting a new U.S. record.

Hurricane Michael made landfall near Mexico Beach, FL in Oct with sustained winds of 155 mph - one of the most intense hurricanes to hit the contiguous U.S. and causing more than 45 fatalities.

The average U.S. temperature for 2018 was 53.5°F, 1.5°F above average and the 14th warmest on record. The annual U.S. precipitation was 34.63 inches, 4.69 inches above average, the 3rd wettest.

Below average precipitation and near average temperature characterized conditions across Puerto Rico in 2018.

Please Note: Material provided in this map was compiled from NOAA's State of the Climate Reports. For more information please visit http://www.ncdc.noaa.gov/sotc

This climate [CD][GW][WB][TR] 'system' has only recently begin to register as a serious problem for Americans in 2018 but actually was not the combination's worst year according to https://www.climate.gov/news-features/blogs/beyond-data/2018s-billion-dollar-disasters-context because the billion dollar events were less than in the previous two years. The total physical climate damage for 2016 to 2018 was over $1 trillion dollars, with a human capital Tranquility effect much larger. Worse to come, as in a 'Warmaggeddon', not to be confused with an American music group? Americans didn't just ignore this environmental process and dealt with the series of events reasonably well, but at a loss to their combined infrastructure that was not a gain as far as Posterity was concerned. With some success in dealing with climate violence, they did not address the cause of climate warming, energy consumption, however.

As a national consensus, which would be necessary for any constitutional addition or modification, polled or voted referendum concerns like the 15 {sets} must be part of the analytical process. Some polls indicated the General Welfare [GW{sets}] as a group of concerns was determined early in 2018. These closely followed the Gallop poll before the election, but also involved {sets} related to [JU] and [LI], such as crime and the inevitable multi-ethnic 'race' interaction. The combined polls had an order of significance:

{1} The economy, tax cuts and jobs Act,

{2} The availability and affordability of healthcare, ACA repeal and replace, Public Health Service Act have expired, artificial embryos, see [WB]

{3} The possibility of future terrorist attacks in the U.S. see [CD]

{4} The size and power of the federal government, cybersecurity, AI development

{5} The Social Security system

{6} Illegal immigration. See [JU]

{7} Hunger and homelessness

{8} Climate change

{9} The way income and wealth are distributed in the U.S. [GW]+[JU]?

{10} Crime and violence

{11} Race relations [WB]

{12} Drug use, FDA Reauthorization Act, CARA, opioid deaths [CD]?

{13} Unemployment

{14} The quality of the environment, Pandemic Act expires

{15} The availability and affordability of energy

Items like hunger and homelessness, immigration, unemployment (at 4% in 2018?), and availability of healthcare all interacted with each other to increase a poverty level among Americans as the cost of living began to exceed the minimum pay levels available. In some complexity models, these negative-loop conditions could increase to a level that intensified Malthusian Traps all over the country. Some cities had population densities that were well beyond the level of surrounding regions to support them and this in turn required more and more national level (GW) and [WB] resources, even though the Traps were much worse outside the United States.

These Malthusian Trap urban areas also began to show as [TR] stresses in states that were 'maxed' out as far as their tax revenues were concerned. Several states had taxes on virtually every part of the economic activity (income, sales, license fees, utility fees, etc.) and this was becoming a serious impact on the economy even when drawing federal funds into the balance and not having to expend wealth in a Common Defense mode. The basic state and community services such as {education}, {transportation}, [healthcare] and [public safety] were all deteriorating in 2018 as the urban populations out-stripped available resources. The problem with Malthusian Traps is that virtually any environmental disaster can trigger it into a completely unstable 'chaos system' such as Syria, Yemen, Zimbabwe and Puerto Rico.

Many of these domestic problems were combining with international energy imperialism costs in a world economy that was essentially stripping wealth from Americans through manipulated trade imbalances, increasing defense costs. This combination, even with an increasingly robust economy, was causing more and more generated wealth to leave the American people and this in turn was causing basic wage/cost of living inequalities on an increasing number of people. At the same time, the healthcare system, even without the chaotic administration costs no other country had, was contributing to an increase in a 'poverty' class as the definition for it reached $35,000 per year. Items like [GW]<2 ⋈ [CD]<3, where '⋈' means the relational balance of the two domains and less than '<' means a *negative* progression of the domain for some {subset} group, were showing up in several commentaries calling for massive reform in [WB] throughout 2018 in the form of:

2018.10.26:22:30 |WB|<4 ⋈ |GW|>2⋈ |CD|<3 |TR|>3 |JU|<3 ≈ |OP|<2

Dr. Marion Mass in TheHill, 'Medicare for All' will never work, so let's stop pushing it':

There is a better alternative to cut health-care costs. Policymakers must take a scythe to the labyrinthine bureaucracy that is holding back health care, while at the same time pursuing transparency reforms that would allow the system to work more productively and efficiently.

Consider: The number of health-care administrators — many drawing salaries well into the six figures — has risen by 3,200 percent between 1975 and 2010. (The number of physicians grew by 150 percent over the same timeframe.) This bureaucratic bloat diverts precious resources away from treating patients and inflates the cost of care. Reversing this administrative growth to all but the most critical positions could allow for a dollar-for-dollar offset in health-care costs.

A timeline like [WB]<4 ⋈ [GW]>2⋈ [CD]<3 indicates that as the national security was going downward, the [GW] was still improving while Wellbeing, perhaps 18 {subsets} of the other two and Justice, was not. Much of this negative progression was from data about health that appeared in the category subsets of Precision Medicine where the individual person with some 7500 anatomical structures is diagnosed. Attempts to do this through a 'Medicare for all' dynamic system have proven nearly impossible for 320 million people, especially when some two million are added as 'immigrants' each year. With each decade since the 1950s, beneficial technology has increased the complexity of what governance perceives or analyses by an exponential value.

Fifteen major {subsets} that citizens are concerned about and half of them didn't even exist a century ago when the population was about 100 million? **Note again that the context of the Chronicles closely involves a popular consensus of conditions because of the need for that same referendum/consensus to produce an Electoral College 'image' that reflects the We the People referendum on Constitutional Amendment and Article addition.** The original mechanism, popular invalidation of the Articles of Confederation (1776) leading to a Constitutional Convention (1787 then Ratification of a Constitution (1789), had such a We the People image and there is little evidence that the process was a failure. For that reason, the Chronicles have attempted to 'sense' that image throughout the evaluation of a need for change in the form of an additional Wellbeing human right.

A popular referendum on an Amendment might work for many changes such as presidential succession, alcohol prohibition, or prohibiting a poll tax. Popular support for an Amendment as in these cases is not the same as a voted-on referendum of two-thirds involving a human right. Article V says three-quarters of the states or 38 approve an Amendment, but the rights in 1789 were approved by a two-thirds referendum and there is nothing in the Constitution that says that a new molecular Wellbeing right added as an Article couldn't be approved by 33 states if the Congress sets the conditions for a new convention.

Even the 14th Amendment giving birth citizenship and other due process 'rights' might have required a referendum of at least 33 states, not just a Congressional approval during a Civil War. An all-citizen healthcare program such as the Affordable Care Act *and* Medicare *and* Medicaid *and* Children's Health Insurance Program *and*

Supplemental Nutrition Assistance Program affect ALL of the Preamble intents, the Congressional authorities of Article I, The Executive authorities of Article II, the Judiciary Article III and the Bill of Rights. It is just too complex in a modern DNA health context to be written as a popular referendum. The complexity of the Preamble Six in 1788 almost led to Constitutional rejection even then.

Attempting to create a right such as wellbeing involving total health by referendum simply will not work any more than the attempts to create 300-Article constitutions through referendum around the world has worked anywhere. Still, very nearly all modern nations now have Constitutions that are an abiding agreement between the people and the governors, whatever form they take. But there are also totalitarian 'constitutions' such as the Iranian and Chinese which give absolute power without checks and balances by ANY entity, including the people

End epilogue 2018

Conclusions for 2018:

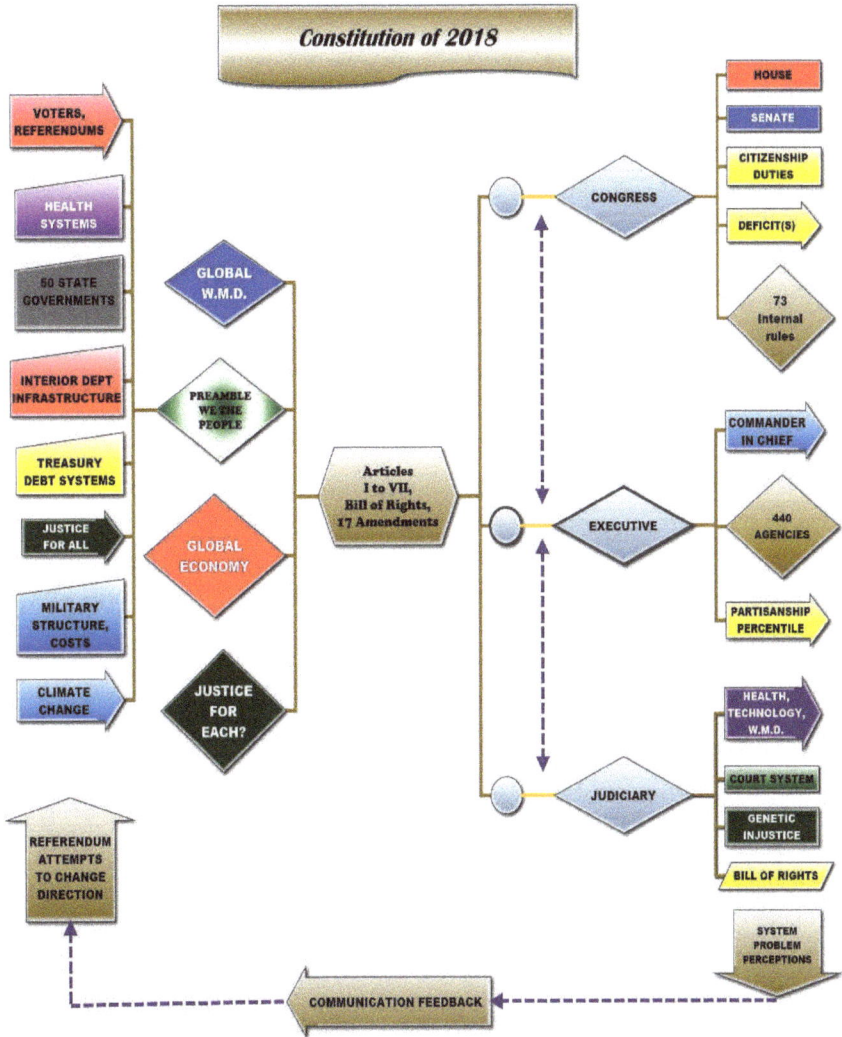

Figure 26. Constitution of 2018

None of the 21st century constitutional writings or implementations have anything that establishes healthy existence as a human right, physically impossible in most cases, although many do say that good health is an 'entitlement' due to each born citizen. But something that says a person has a human right to life-long wellness? No, and the American Constitution does not suggest that in any way simply because health was a 'divine' domain in 1787, especially with a yellow fever epidemic in the Caribbean trade ports approaching the Philadelphia site at the time. That is no longer true; the technologies for humanity to control its own Posterity through wellbeing become more real and available each day. It can even be visualized in a context that assumes there will be no wars of mutual extermination. The following graphic is, of course, purely speculative after a second Convention for a wellness right has completed its task.

Previously, the ACA set up by the Congress in 2008 had many of the complex issues of the Wellbeing 'system' imbedded in it, including mandatory payment systems to cover the costs in the hope that the total effect by 2018 would bring down the costs of the 'Basic Services' per person. This did not happen for a variety of reasons, including intense opposition by conservatives. Political and economic conditions came together in a manner that a dot-connect might perceive an almost unconscious desire by many elements in society to create a system of continuous bad health and health indenture. After all, there were four trillion dollars involved.

All of these problems in [GW]{health} were amplified by massive [CD] expenses that including illegal immigration, international deployments, veteran costs and increased WMD defenses. Most were necessary commitments to world peace (or world imperialism as the enemies saw it), but if you add in a healthcare drain of substance abuse ripple effects that were nearly \$800 billion a year, with abuse-related mental disorders involving 19 million people, the summed Posterity progression goes quite negative. About: Σ [OP]{n}$\rightarrow$<? The ripple effects of a dysfunctional healthcare system, which is 'profitable' for offshore entities, are becoming so common that they could actually be subject to genetic adaption, a serious Posterity negative progression. Genetic adaption, such as occurred with alcohol, rice and some carbohydrates (to diabetes?) over a 4000-year span would qualify as genetic adaptions, as would breathing less oxygen at high elevations. The 'effects of Wellbeing' graphic shows a possible reversal of this genetic trend after an appropriate wellbeing rights Second Convention. But perhaps some other conventions need to come first......

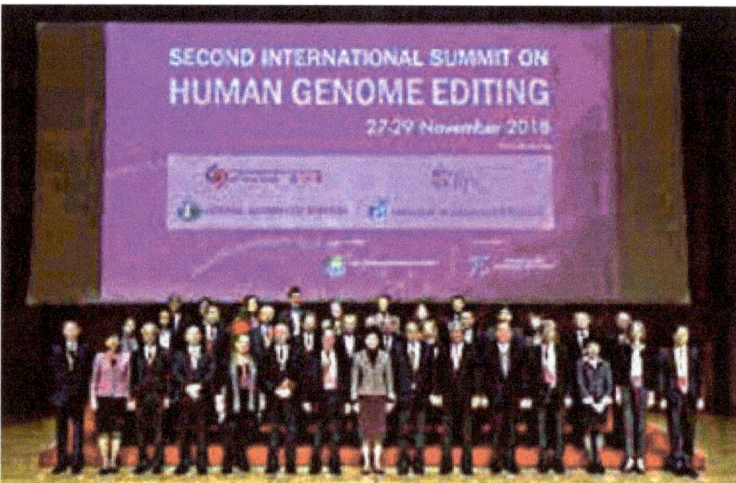

The Wellbeing model concept was coming under some suspicion because the expression for the Six or Seven domains, {>[ ](n)$\leftrightarrow$0$\leftrightarrow$<[ ](n)} , was valid without a pure time component {n}(t). For many processes that any given domain was involved in, there was NO initiating time. This was also something that had become a general consensus in the form of 'why the #&*!%? are they doing that NOW?'. Such could be applied to the 'logic' of just about any of the Preamble domains and to many of the Opservationis samples used in the Chronicles. Some were easily sensed as 'crazy' and it applied to all three branches of government when interacting .with each other and the public.

The need for the Second Convention in this decade had been established with the advent of vast medical, health, and genome technologies, along with the political and economic abuses of the cyber-space technologies that was directly affecting both Common Defense and General Welfare in ways not previously imagined. It devolved more into a matter of how to carry out such an epigenetic protection convention as Article VIII where (t) or a timeline (tl) became simply a dynamic point of an initiating referendum by We the People. At some point in 'time' or in the dynamic of the domains society would have to incorporate Wellbeing into its existence as an interactive entity . The dynamic model in its simplest would be something like Σ [OP]{n/t}$\rightarrow$> but not 0< where each of the summed domains began to acquire the 'Ki_ξ' factor of life forces into their priorities and this progressed to a series of positive Liberties for individual humans. **It is assumed that the nation improves as its citizens improve.** This might still come out as a timeline for all of the effects and it might look something like figure 26.

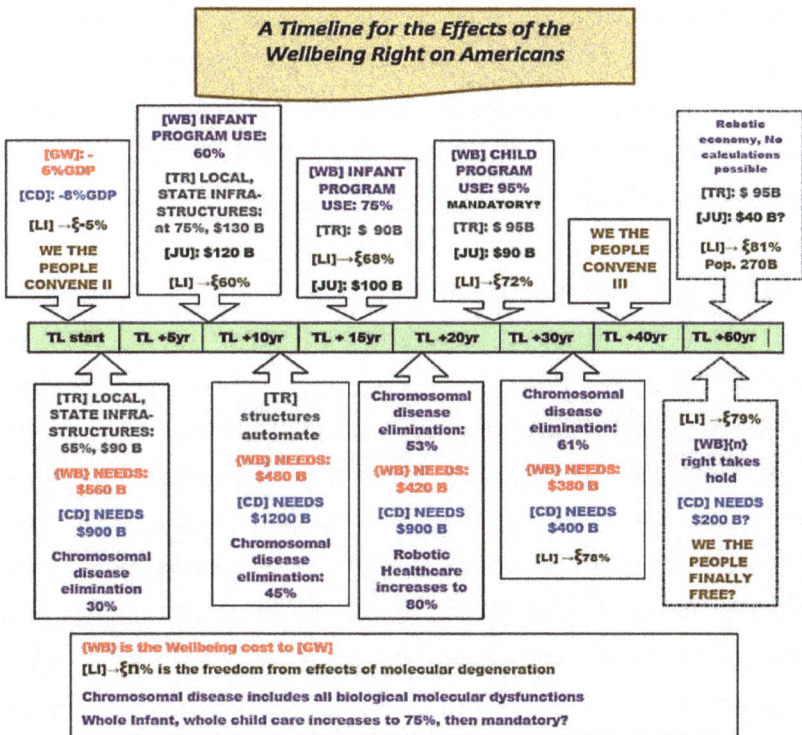

Figure 27.   Second Convention effects

The graphic shows a Second Convention that establishes the Wellbeing right and the possible aftermath in setting it up with Wellness from birth as a protected right rather than as a 20th century chaos buildup of impossible health conditions for those being born. This is reflected in the *additional* [CD] and [GW] costs after initiating. The term '[LI]$\rightarrow \xi$n%' signifies a possible increase or decrease in an individual's lifestyle 'freedom' because of the health environment's increase in effectiveness. Over a two-generation period, the costs of the ripple effects for [CD], [GW] and [JU] should become less as more and more people are born without genetic disorders which include adaptive disorders like obesity. If the '$\rightarrow \xi$n%' progression continues negative at perhaps $\rightarrow\{ \xi\}$-6% as it is now, then the chaos conditionals leading to existential decline, not just economic decline, would begin showing significance a generation from this 2018 decade. A four-degree F heat addition to the North American continent (along with the others) over two generations might make a [LI]$\rightarrow \xi$8% progression nearly impossible for the generations after 40 years simply because all societies would have to become totalitarian with robotic enforcement just to exist and totalitarians are inherently narcissistic. There is no 'future' when the homosapien dynamic recedes into a totalitarian, high-tech Dark Age.

Not a pleasant prospect, but a possible [WB]{n}<ξ81% in 60 'years' from initiation of the Wellbeing Right is quite possible as a transition. A < or less than 81% means that the total effect of the Wellbeing Right is *approaching* a high ROI and that has Epigenetic ripple effects that are truly Evolutionary PROVIDED that nearly all of the American 'races' participate as a true We the People. The Second Convention would require a commitment by a substantial majority of Americans even when the Constitution requires two thirds approval for a referendum on a 'right'. The People commitment would have to be closer to the three quarters approval required by an Amendment, something the Founders didn't have to do. Indeed, the true Constitution support after the First Convention was barely half We the People. Consensus is not easy and needs a representative form such as an 'enlightened' Electoral College to be successful. .

Just 'sensing' the complexity of a Wellbeing right would need considerable AI-droid aid in virtually all Standard Evolution Models that could be calculated by an average educated citizen with no 'cultural' barriers to his thinking. Such an infrastructure after the Second Convention might be expensive to initiate, as are all development processes, but 'Artificial Intelligence' entities already have a built-in ability to accelerate their own development the same as the homosapien species suddenly began doing a hundred thousand years ago. The [WB] progression also assumes that human hater WMD will not develop into a continuous genocide tool ([CD]<0?) the totalitarians now appear willing to create for asymmetric and parasitic warfare purposes.

The [CD], [GW] and [TR] structures for a Wellbeing right might appear daunting over the 20s decade, but just bringing the enormous costs of Chromosomal disorders under control and preventing any long-term care costs in the American society would be worth some 10 to 15 percent of the GDP that can be used to accelerate the [WB]{n/t} process for all. Would that lead to a permanent GDP cost reduction of 10 percent in each of 100 years? Does such a return on investment translate into more and more Americans enjoying the Blessings of Liberty to ourselves and our Posterity just as the First Convention intended?

Note Isaac Newton, Preface to *Opticks: or, A Treatise of the Reflexions, Refractions, Inflexions and Colours of Light,* 1704:04.01:

> To explain all nature is too difficult a task for any one man or even for any one age. 'Tis much better to do a little with certainty & leave the rest for others that come after you.

Note Charles Darwin, *Origin of Species,* 1859.11.24:

> In the long history of humankind (and animal kind, too) those who learned to collaborate and improvise most effectively have prevailed.

Erwin Schrödinger, *What Is Life? The Physical Aspect of the Living Cell,* 1944.05.00:

> In Darwin's theory, you just have to substitute 'mutations' for his 'slight accidental variations' (just as quantum theory substitutes 'quantum jump' for 'continuous transfer of energy'). In all other respects little change was necessary in Darwin's theory…

Figure 28.   Wellbeing Solutions

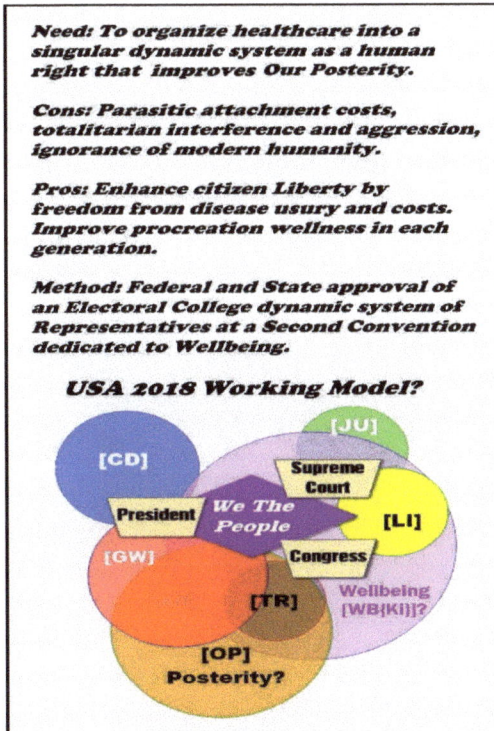

Glossary and Notes

While a glossary is not usually included in speculative literary efforts, the Chronicles involve many concepts that are not normally associated with the workings of Capitol Hill or the environment of the American People. Such things as North American words, operation research symbols and methods, or the rapidly advancing sciences of microbiology, the Human Genome with DNA evolutional mapping, new medical technologies, and totalitarian data technologies are rapidly impacting the Constitution and some things need to be defined in the context of the Chronicles research. This particular Glossary is also the chapter where the more common 'notes' chapter of many research documents are entered.

Note again that every effort is made to define a 'common meaning' in English for the terms used in the manner of online dictionaries and general information databases. The reason for this is to make each Chronicle more readable on a very complex dynamical system such as the Constitution. The individual Chronicle commentaries are themselves intended as speculative 'notes' on Capitol Hill sociological processes based on relevance to the constitution.

Kwedake.

N. or object. Pronounced kwe, dah, ke. An Iroquois Nation word of the north central North American region meaning 'the hill' or 'of the hill'. The Potawatomi local pronunciation of Kwedake means 'of or on the hill'. It represents the 200 foot high slope that arises from the joining of the Potomac and Anacostia Rivers and was known to have several fresh water springs and fair game in the 1500s and 1600s. The Kwedake was also an area of migration and meeting for tribes moving south from the Iroquois Nation and north from the Cherokee Nation. They were met here, sometimes in battle, by local tribes of the Powhatten, Potawatomi, and Dogues who fished, hunted and planted corn or tobacco in the Chesapeake region.

Dikep.

n. Pronounced dee' keap. A 1500s Iroquois Nation word meaning 'spring' or 'well' for acquiring water. The Potawatomi pronunciation of 'di'kep' also means fresh water spring as opposed to river water. The combination of the two words 'Kwedake Dikep' is used to say the 'Spring on (of) the Hill' of which there were several in the woodland slopes of what is now Capitol Hill, Washington, District of Columbia, the highest point in the land before the lowlands of the Chesapeake forests began.

Justice [1] [JU]

Fairness between individuals is so fundamental to human life that it is possible that humanity as societies couldn't have come into existence without it. It establishes the conditions under which people live in peace and respect with each other. It is also an innate, hereditary trait so common it may be found in genetic codes or alleles. Madison, Federalist 51: "Justice is the end [final intent or directive] of government. It is the end [final intent or directive] of civil society. It ever has been and ever will be pursued until it is obtained, or until liberty be lost in the pursuit." Aggression toward others is a natural human trait, but to harm others with that aggression without reason contradicts the deep-seated sense of Justice [JU] most people have. This is incorporated into the Preamble as a purpose and intent in order to insure the fairness of social behavior, both as an instinct and in conscious thought. Equal respect between individuals establishes the point where narcissistic aggression is met with an equal and opposite aggression defined as 'Justice for all'.

Older usages:

From the biblical passages of Deuteronomy, 0086.00.00:

> 18: Appoint judges and officials for each of your tribes in every town that Creation is giving you, and they shall judge the people fairly. 19: Do not pervert justice or show partiality. Do not accept a bribe, for a bribe blinds the eyes of the wise and twists the words of the innocent. 20: Follow justice and justice alone, so that you may live and possess that land Creation is giving you.

Modern Interpretation: One of the problems in the past has been that the concept of Justice has been used almost universally in all human societies with varying degrees of success and hypocrisy, but it has never actually been defined as a human value. It simply exists as part of them, like breathing. If one took the previous [JU] usages and attempted to quantify them, it might be seen as a dynamical system in which some 'energy' is transferred from one individual system to another or some 'energy sum' is transferred from one group to another for the purposes of creating equilibrium between systems. Injustice then becomes a condition where 'energy' is removed without establishing equilibrium and [JU] is not served unless the 'energy' is returned in some form that rebalances the equilibrium. [JU] energy transfer appears to be very similar to Helmholtz Energy in thermodynamics equilibrium, JU (in quants) approximates the system energy (in quants) minus the transfer conditionals and constants (in quants), but certainly needs work as an energy expression. On a general level, human aggression in ANY form needs to be balanced by [JU] return of value or a similar value to the people it is taken from. The rule of law is the mechanism by which the [JU] dynamic intent of the Constitution is produced.

Tranquility [2] [TR]

Or 'insure domestic tranquility'. In the Preamble that meant peace between the various states of the new Union. Historically, tranquility has also meant a state of mind very close to that found in the spiritual meditation states of virtually all religions.

One of the concerns of the Framers was that a government prior to that of the Constitution was unable, by force or persuasion, to quell rebellion or quarrels amongst the states, the same as it was everywhere on earth. The 'government' in 1786 watched in horror as Shay's Rebellion transpired just before the Convention, and some states had very nearly gone to war with each other over territory (such as between Pennsylvania and Connecticut over Wilkes-Barre). Note that the original 1600s 'Lords of Proprietorship' land grants created Virginia as all lands of the current States of Virginia, West Virginia, and Kentucky with the Carolina grants extending all the way to the Mississippi. Carolina as a thousand-mile-wide State? One of the main goals of the Convention, then, was to ensure the federal government had powers to squash local disorders or rebellions and to smooth Proprietorship tensions between states through [TR] related law.

But it might also be necessary to take into account that the term 'Tranquility' used by the Committee of Style at the 1787 Convention was a form of peaceful mind state that could be found with consistent meaning in nearly all spiritual scriptures. It is the quality or state of being tranquil; meaning calmness, serenity, and worry-free. The word tranquility appears in numerous texts ranging from the religious writings of Buddhism, where the term 'passaddhi' refers to tranquility of the body to similar definitions in other religions. In Islam, freedom from hypocrisy 'fitnah' or strife is tranquility, and in Christianity it becomes a state of secure, monastic meditation found in American churches. [TR] can also be closely associated with an empathy for earthly environments, and it may not be a coincidence that 'earthly environments' contain several thousand evolved plants with chemicals that affect the neurological tranquility of the mind or the wellbeing of the human body.

In a modern interpretation, [TR] can be defined as a form of individual freedom that contributes to personal security regardless of Proprietorship, materiality or instinctive aggressions. Tranquility is the 'peace of mind' guaranteed by the Bill of Rights and is co-existent with [JU] in all three branches of governance as intra-state, inter-state, and intra-individual entities of co-existence. The Article I, Section 8 terms 'uniform throughout the United States', 'interstate commerce', and 'necessary and proper' are extensions of insuring national Tranquility.

Common Defence [3] [CD]

Modern interpretation: [CD] means that all defensive protections are held in 'common' for all States within the Union. [CD] must be maintained in balance with other considerations, but must take primary value under conditions of attack, no matter what form the attack takes. Its qualities are therefore measured only against other prime directives such as General Welfare, with Posterity as a resultant prime. It is defined as a *focus* of societal energies to meet an opposing combination of energies, whether natural or unnatural.

Common Defense is an obvious process that human cave tribes practiced thousands of years ago and involved people defending each other against predators that appeared around or among them. In the modern sense, [CD] means allocating resources to maintain enough security so that the other covenants can take hold and flourish. Predatory attacks almost always come from societies or cults that do not have a form of Preamble Balance themselves.

Common Defence (spelled with a 'c' in the constitution) is used both in the Preamble to the Constitution and in the Article I, Section 8 powers of the congress without much fanfare. It was not until 1813, when Washington was burned to the ground because an enemy discovered there was no real common defense in this land that the idea became a reality. But it is a prime directive for the survival of any society because none have existed long without it. There is also the clear requirement that [CD] requires universal citizenship participation as each is able, including the sacrifice of [LI] and [JU].

Department of Defense

Secretary of Defense
Deputy Secretary of Defense

Department of the Army	Department of the Navy	Department of the Air Force	Office of the Secretary of Defense	Inspector General	Joint Chiefs of Staff
Secretary of the Army	Secretary of the Navy	Secretary of the Air Force			Chairman JCS
					The Joint Staff

Under Secretary and Assistant Secretaries of the Army — Chief of Staff Army

Under Secretary and Assistant Secretaries of the Navy — Chief of Naval Operations — Commandant of Marine Corps

Under Secretary and Assistant Secretaries of the Air Force — Chief of Staff Air Force

Under Secretaries Assistant Secretaries of Defense and Equivalents

Vice Chairman JCS
Chief of Staff, Army
Chief of Naval Operations
Chief of Staff, Air Force
Commandant, Marine Corps

Army Major Commands & Agencies

Navy Major Commands & Agencies

Marine Corps Major Commands & Agencies

Air Force Major Commands & Agencies

DoD Field Activities
American Forces Information Service
Defense POW/MP Office
Defense Technical Information Center
Defense Technology Security Administration
DoD Counterintelligence Field Activity
DoD Education Activity
DoD Human Resources Activity
DoD Test Resource Management Center
Office of Economic Adjustment
TRICARE Management Activity
Washington Headquarters Services

[WB]?

Defense Agencies
Defense Advanced Research Projects Agency
Defense Business Transformation Agency
Defense Commissary Agency
Defense Contract Audit Agency
Defense Contract Management Agency
Defense Finance and Accounting Service
Defense Information Systems Agency
Defense Intelligence Agency
Defense Legal Services Agency
Defense Logistics Agency
Defense Security Cooperation Agency
Defense Security Service
Defense Threat Reduction Agency
Missile Defense Agency
National Geospatial-Intelligence Agency
National Security Agency/Central Security Service
Pentagon Force Protection Agency

Combatant Commands
Central Command
European Command
Joint Forces Command
Northern Command
Pacific Command
Southern Command
Special Operations Command
Strategic Command
Transportation Command
Africa Command

[CD] to 2100 ?

Prepared by: Organizational & Management Planning, ODA&M, OSD
Date: January 2008.

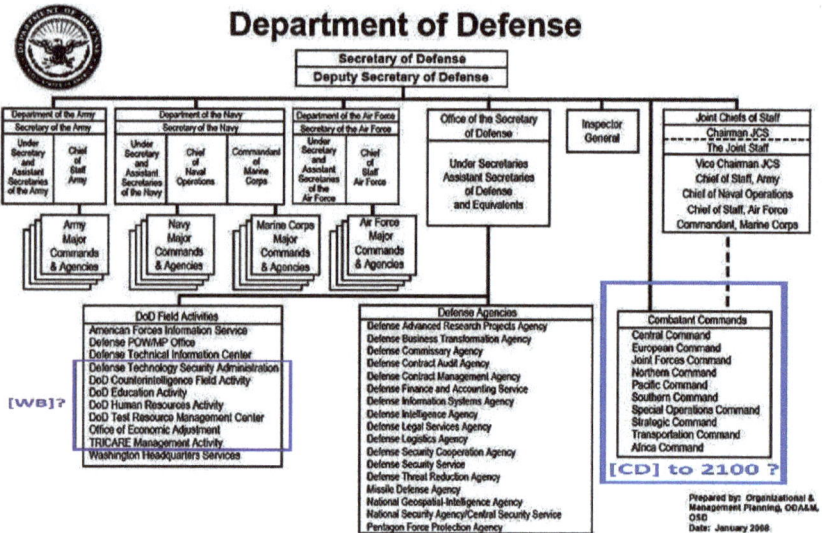

It doesn't take much TLO to determine that this enormous structure, even if it took a century to develop, can have negative cost sub-systems. From an operations research standpoint the issue might be whether each subsection is 'functionally optimized'. For one thing, the 'entities' in DoD Field Activities might also belong in a Wellbeing [WB] domain as wells as [CD]. But note the 'combatant commands' category that covers virtually the entire surface of the earth AND outer space. The commands might be able to 'functionally optimize' in order to get things done, but do the rest of the subsections do that too? This from a defense system with a couple of Navy cruisers and some Army regiments in 1904. Has this system prevented enough genocide on earth for 50 years to justify its expense to Posterity and would a future [CD] prime directive requires epigenetic defenses as well?

General Welfare   [4]   [GW]

Modern interpretation: General Welfare is a prime directive since its values of Welfare allow many societal processes such as food, clothing, shelter and even spiritual wellness to be maintained in order to enhance the structure of the society and its citizens through [LI, [JU], and possibly wellbeing. [WB]. Without this fundamental system, there is very little point to humans living together as a group in what in the 21st century could be called 'molecular' cohesion. Very many mind, body and spirit processes at a molecular level are Common to all living together and their 'welfare' is produced by a 'general' infrastructure. Schools, roads, medical facilities, government bureaucracy and communication mechanisms are all held as 'general' mechanisms of a functioning society. 'General' means for large segments of people, not individuals, and 'Welfare' has an ancient meaning in nearly all societies that one becomes 'better off' than he was (ye welled fare) within a community. This means that the minimum 'fare' of people in a community is increased over time, the reason for them to act together in common objective.

Welfare in today's context also means organized efforts on the part of public or private organizations to benefit the most vulnerable or exploitable segment of a population spectrum, generally referred to as 'public assistance'. This is not the meaning of the combined term as used in the Constitution, although it aids [LI] and [JU] for many. [GW] as a summed value is a much more fundamental evolutionary intent that was defined by the Founders in order to be a purpose of a much larger spectrum of people, therefore the infrastructure of a people is also included in the definition. This cannot be set aside in order to favor other intents of the Preamble; it must be balanced with the others. From 2012, the 'entities' or 'schemas' of the Complex Adaptive Systems perception can be found in the General Welfare or [GW] sets of the system of systems. Those separate entities when combined into the General Welfare prime directive shows just how much the directive has gone out of balance simply because of the size of each entities.

Codes	Departments	Cost	Constitutional Authority
250	General Science, Space and Technology	$29 b	Section 8.8
270	Energy	$15 b	Section 8.3, 8.1
300	Natural Resources and Environment	$42 b	Section 8.3
350	Agriculture	$18 b	Section 8.1, 8.3,
370	Commerce and Housing Credit	$41 b	Section 8.5, 8.3
400	Transportation	$93 b	Section 8.7
450	Community and Regional Development	$25 b	Section 8.3(?)
500	Edu, Training, Employment, and Social Service	$91 b	Section 8.3, 8.1, 8.2(?)
550	Health	$347 b	Section 8.1(?)
570	Medicare	$472 b	Section 8.3
600	Income Security	$541 b	Section 8.1, 8.2
650	Social Security	$773 b	Section 8.1, 8.18(?)
700	Veterans Benefits and Services	$125 b	Section 8.12

Social Security is included as [GW], although it has large components that are a pension system created to prevent starvation by the elderly. It might be improved as a mandatory entity with a 'savings' option that multiplied over the individual's lifetime according to the savings put in. That is the same as other pension systems except that the 'minimum' is a mandatory form of income tax. Other codes, such as 550, Health, might come under Authorities 8.1 or 8.3 or 8.18. But all would come under 8.1 which authorizes the taxation and appropriation for either General Welfare or Common Defense or both without specifying it exactly. Section 8.18 is also the famous 'necessary and proper' clause of the Constitution.

Codes 550, 600, 570, and 700 with an expenditure of $1.5 trillion all affect the wellness or health of individuals and might be treated as a Wellbeing 'schema' that is equivalent to a prime directive. Treating these codes as a directive might eliminate waste, fraud and abuse worth fifteen percent each in even one generation, so the definition of General Welfare needs considerable examination in this century.

Liberty [5] [LI]

Modern interpretation: Liberty can be measured as a form of energy in terms of the 'work' a citizen must put into his enhancement as an individual. It is separate from the 'work' energy required for [CD] or [GW] which the citizen contributes for 'common' and 'general' society and such 'work energy' is returned to him in the form of Posterity. [LI] is the work energy that allows the development of individual being within a context of his human environment and this energy is *not* expendable in the interests of the State or larger community, but in the enhancement of individual Tranquility.

Learning, religion, health and wealth are energy components of [LI] but not necessarily acquirable through the destruction of [LI] for others. Liberty is a total quanta energy form; subtracting any of it from others subtracts it from all.

Liberty is the combination of freedoms described in the Bill of Rights and the Amendments to the Constitution that allow an individual being to enhance himself and others within a human society. Liberty is altruistically given away in the form of personal wealth and energy to maintain the other social covenants of America. That is usually defined as sacrificing one's liberty [LI] for a larger value such as [GW] and [CD] and especially for posterity [OP], as in a military draft or very high taxation. It is a balancing component, neither total for the individual or totally removable from the individual being in the American society.

Other definitions held by societies: Freedom from government or private interference. The ability to exercise the rights enumerated by a Constitution or available or under natural, existential conditions. Note that in spite of popular belief, the Bill of Rights was intended to secure basic civil liberties in the absence of 'inalienable rights', which have never actually existed in spiritual or governance literature. Only the divine right to rule has ever been written there.

The state of being free within society from oppressive restrictions imposed by authority on one's way of life, behavior, or political views. Popular but not Preamble synonyms: independence, freedom, autonomy, sovereignty, self-government, self-rule, self-determination, civil liberties, and human rights. In instance of this; a right or privilege, especially a statutory one or the sum of rights and exemptions possessed in common by the people of a community.

Posterity [6]   [OP]

From the Latin posterus; 'coming after'. The modern definition [OP] has held very accurately with the ancient and old 'our Posterity', which means the successive development of citizens who are composed of improving molecular structures, all 700,000 of them, in the children of any given generation. There is the inherent meaning 'to ourselves and our Posterity'; leave something better for those coming after into the *entire* future, not just individual futures. But Posterity can also have an inverse square property in that the 'quant' of Posterity is equal to a sum of work energies inversely proportional to the length of time involved. In Posterity generation terms, the 'quant' created in the first generation might be progressively one third less in each succeeding generation, but never altogether disappears. The objective of 'our Posterity' is to optimize the 'quant' progression within the balance of [CD] and [GW].

At the time of the Constitution in the 1700s, biblical quotation was common and the term 'our Posterity' may have been derived from both the Bible and the influence of Isaac Newton's 1700s research on cosmic systems, *the Chronology of the Ancient Kingdoms,* which in turn was based on Newton's very private researches into the Bible as a mathematical or dynamic 'system'. Note the words of Paul in Biblical Acts 3:25:

> "You are the heirs of the Prophets, and of the Covenant which God made with your forefathers when He said to Abraham, 'And through your posterity [thy seed] all the families of the world shall be blessed.'

This was certainly known to Newton who was greatly concerned with various systemic timelines such as the *Chronology (1685-1710)* and *Observations Upon the Prophecies of Daniel (1690-1720)*. Much of these researches were based on Newton's suspicion that there were simultaneous systems at work in the universe he was measuring.

The Founders, in the deliberations at the Christ Church in Philadelphia and the City Tavern would have had great respect for the both the Bible and the 'scientists' of that period. Isaac Newton, by the time John Adams (1788), Franklin (1774) and Jefferson (1789) were visiting in London, was quite famous since his concepts on mathematics, optics and motion had been authenticated. Darwin and Mendel, with their evolutionary definition of 'our Posterity' that would eventually lead to the molecular definition of successive generations in modern society, had not yet defined genetic adaptions and progressions, which occurred in the mid-1800s. But there were many who talked of 'our Posterity' over the centuries; it is implicit on virtually all spiritual writings, medical writings, and the writings of 'rulers'. Only recently was [OP] also defined as an evolutionary molecular process, much to the horror of those who believed in an orderly universe.

Bryan Sykes, *DNA USA, A Genetic Portrait of America*, 2012, p317, concerning molecular hazards to our Posterity:

> To illustrate my point I have picked out 140 genes that help run eleven major body systems and shown their locations against the chromosome portrait of Mark Thompson, one of my African American volunteers. The composite portrait is the last in the gallery and I have put the detailed description of these genes in an appendix. These are only a tiny fraction of the total number of genes we need to keep going, but enough to convey the principle. In all of us they work equally from the two copies that we inherited, one from each of our parents. They have to cooperate properly, or we would simply not survive, as the example of severe inherited disease teaches us. So, whatever their own individual ancestry, whether African, European, or Native American, our genes must have found a way of working together. My pancreas functions on a combination of both African and European genes. Equally, "Rhett Butler," a white man from the South, depends on the DNA inherited from an unknown African ancestor for his heart muscles to work properly. "Ilsa Lund"'s digestive system, and much else besides, runs on DNA from her African ancestors. "Atticus Finch" needs his Mohawk genes to make sure his red blood cells do their job well.

Wellbeing [7] [WB]

The term 'wellbeing' has had many meanings in nearly all of the literature of the human race, but basically it involves the state of existence for an individual person that evolved some 70, 000 years ago with specific DNA material now associated with that Haplogroup. That Humane Genome is the construct of molecular systems that developed then and has progressed to the various 70 forms of humanity that have less than two percent difference in DNA sequences and are therefore called Cro-Magnons. The major subsystems of a human are Consciousness sets, Mobility sets, Cognitive senses such as sight, or hearing or emotion, reproductive sex, oxygenated blood systems and immune systems. Wellbeing is defined as the positive integration of these systems of Mind, Body, and Spirit into a singular whole entity. Wellbeing is an 'energy' value that is the sum of these components in space-time where the energy of the components is greater than that of the components themselves. Human Wellbeing is defined in terms of an energy or quanta sum greater than the parts, since other life conditions on earth did not evolve in that manner.

History has shown that the wellbeing integration of all of these components into individual entities that are conscious enough to enhance each other as 'nations' is what is defined as evolution or 'our Posterity'. The negative quanta of any of the major components can subtract from the total wellbeing of not just one person, who might not survive that diminished component, but several. This is where the term Darmend-Mendel Ripple Effect is seen to occur, where some lack of conscious wellbeing or physical wellbeing or brain wellbeing detracts from the survival of a person and might consume the wellbeing quanta or schema of others.

Wellbeing has been discussed continually in the last two centuries as a minor subsystem of the economics of Marx, Keynes, and Freidman along with being a subsystem of existential philosophies (Kumarila, Gautama, Lao Tzu, Sartre, Heidegger, neuroscience, etc.), medical technologies and/or political structures but never as a human right. That was simply because no combinations of Common Defense and General Welfare had a way of controlling evolutionary processes like wellbeing. It was only after the year 2000 that this changed drastically as a dozen different molecular technologies such as quantum electronics, genetic measurement, bio-medical analysis, energy use, and the forming of molecular systems became common through universal communication. All of these, when combined as the Chronicles have shown, have seriously stretched the original intents of the Constitution's Preamble to their limits.

Some Constitutional addition needed to be examined and this was done with a speculative Article VIII, which would have been the next Article in the Constitution. Since Wellbeing [WB] affected ALL of the other Articles and the Bill of Rights and several Amendments through XXVII, it could not be simply a 'rights' Amendment to the Constitution but a full Article which required a 'rights' referendum of convention.

But a wellbeing Article addition is not a simple process of giving a human right to the Homo sapiens who have successfully (sort of) occupied planet Earth. They have fulfilled a prophecy written somewhere around the birth of Christ:

Bible's Genesis 1:28 says:

> "Be fruitful and multiply and fill the earth and subdue it and have dominion over the fish of the sea and over the birds of the heavens and over every living thing that moves on the earth."

This fulfillment of a 'commandment' was done with enormous tragedy to the Homosapiens because of the continual belief among all human societies that 'might makes right' or that if you succeed by clever competition, you are automatically superior. It didn't matter how many molecular systems terminated in that 'superior' process as long as they weren't yours. That idea begin to disappear in the Molecular

Age of 2000AD when it became obvious that molecular deterioration or change could randomly defeat any 'superior' Homo Sapiens with as few as a thousand deformed molecules that are called carcinogens, disease, parasites, germs and so on. A right or dynamic system of wellbeing meant that a 'person' could be born free of such things in order to prevent the Darmend Ripple Effects from destroying other 'persons' nearby. Such a right also implied that a 'person' was responsible for himself and would not introduce carcinogens or diseases that others would have to expend their Wellbeing energy correcting. This was especially true whenever 'lasting peace' occurred between warring parties through [CD] and [GW].

Therefore, the modern definition of Wellbeing as a right used here is:

Any molecular process that contributes to the enhancement of a 'person's total being' of mind, body and consciousness. It is the positive molecular and quantum integration of the systems of mind, of body AND of the spirit that becomes better wellbeing for our Posterity [OP]. Wellbeing [WB] prevents a system that can be a negative integration as well, which in turn consumes the Wellbeing of others. It is actually a summed energy that is the *effect of successful molecular integration in a human*

Related Glossary and Notes

Apdicide.

From the DSM-IV description of Anti-social Personality Disorder in which an individual hatred of humans manifests itself in serial murder, serial rape or enslavement and inhumane cruelty. Apdicide is defined as some form of genetic mass or serial killing of or cruelty toward humans for pleasure from the individual's birth onward but usually appears in the late teens. While it doesn't meet the criteria of a crime against humanity or Criaghum because it is purely individual in nature, a group of APD afflicted individuals that have joined together in common tribal cause can easily commit Democide in the pay of a State structure or Criaghum as part of an ethnic imperative.

Asian Vulture Capitalism or AVC.

An 'economic' process known as Asian Vulture Capitalism (AVC) which has been practiced by certain national ruling political parties for a thousand years (including 'socialist') but is now greatly enhanced by the instant 'wealth deficits' the Internet allows in the United States, Asia, and the Middle East. It is a 'vulture' economic process because there is no capital feedback into the system that creates the wealth. AVC simply consumes the energy and wealth of a host society without benefit to the targeted society. This process caused the downfall of the Tang and Sung dynasties of China, hence its Asian origins, but the same process occurred in Colonial North America by England in the 1700s and by Soviet Russia in Eastern Europe during the 1900s.

Chromosomal abnormality.

Normally, humans have 46 chromosomes arranged in 23 pairs; the pairs vary in size and shape and are numbered by convention. Twenty-two of the pairs are autosomes, and one pair, number 23, is the sex chromosomes. Any variation from this pattern causes abnormalities. A chromosome from any of the pairs may be duplicated (trisomy) or absent (monosomy); an entire set of 23 chromosome pairs can be duplicated three (triploidy) or more (polyploidy) times; or one arm or part of one arm of a single chromosome may be missing (deletion). Part of one chromosome may be transferred to another (translocation), which has no effect on the person in which it occurs but generally causes a deletion or duplication syndrome in his or her children.

See:

https://en.wikipedia.org/wiki/Chromosome_abnormality

http://well.blogs.nytimes.com/2013/10/07/breakthroughs-in-prenatal-screening/?_r=0

Crime against Humanity or Criaghum.

Crimes against humanity, as defined by the Rome Statute of the International Criminal Court Explanatory Memorandum, "are particularly odious offenses in that they constitute a serious attack on human dignity or grave humiliation or a degradation of one or more human beings. They are not isolated or sporadic events, but are part either of a government policy (although the perpetrators need not identify themselves with this policy) or of a wide practice of atrocities tolerated or condoned by a government or a de facto authority. Murder; extermination; torture; rape; political, racial, or religious persecution and other inhumane acts reach the threshold of crimes against humanity only if they are part of a widespread or systematic practice. Isolated inhumane acts of this nature may constitute grave infringements of human rights, or depending on the circumstances, war crimes, but may fall short of falling into the category of crimes under discussion."

The Geneva Conventions generally involve conditions of 'war' and wouldn't necessarily apply to the interdiction of crimes against humanity (Criaghum), especially when the 'facility' for Criaghum is outside of a constituted or 'sovereign' authority as they are in Yemen, Bosnia, Somalia, Uganda, Darfur, Columbia, or Waziristan. The condition of 'war' does not apply to the Malthusian Population Traps found in many large cities even if systemic Criaghum is underway in their neighborhoods.

Question: Should the President of the USA have an explicit authority in the constitution to interdict Criaghum mechanisms anywhere in the world?

Cyberspace.

Cyberspace is the term developed at the start of the 21st century to define the nearly unlimited communication processes of the World Internet. It describes the *dimensional* aspects of the rapidly approaching Mobius field where one can go anywhere and yet remain at the point of origin. The infrastructure of cyberspace consists of the copper wire, fiber optic and wireless links to a finite set of computer nodes that have devices or people addressed by some electronic symbol. It is the principle entity by which the Constitution can degrade or enhance the relevance of all six of the Preamble's intents in the 21st century. As of 2010, cyberspace was a major agent in degrading of the Constitution's intentions, but also qualified as a major evolutionary advance for the Constitution if properly incorporated with Bill of Rights and [CD] type protections. As an evolutionary advance, it cannot be a purely economic process.

From https://en.wikipedia.org/wiki/Cyberspace

"Cyberspace is a global and dynamic domain (subject to constant change) characterized by the combined use of electrons and the electromagnetic spectrum, whose purpose is to create, store, modify, exchange, share, and extract, use, eliminate information and disrupt physical resources."

Darmend Ripple Effect or [DRE]

This term is used to describe the effects of genetic adaption by humans that Darwin and Mendel (Darmend) described so well in the 1850s. They triggered the idea of survival of the fittest known as 'natural selection', which worked well for very complex living things all the way from plants to dinosaurs to Homosapiens but the concept began to break down as molecular evaluation with increasingly sophisticated electron microscopes appeared. This allowed people to see what groups of molecules, including 'gametes' as Mendel called them, were really doing as they formed. It didn't take long at all to begin looking at DNA structures of people and the discovery that even simple alterations of DNA had catastrophic effects on the way an 'entity' or gametes in them would develop. Even 50,000 molecules altered in certain places of the brain caused a complete mutation inside, which then showed in the behaviour with other people. That is what qualified as the Ripple Effect of Darwin-Mendel's (and many others) research into human molecular structures.

This, the DRE listed here, is a hypothetical study of the negative effects of genetic or inherited mental or physical molecular degenerations that occur routinely among all species. This is not the same as environmental adaptions that Homosapiens or Hosa for short are so good at, or molecular injury from external conditions such as viruses, cancers, nicotine, words, guns or whatever. DRE is nearly a dynamic set of its own on the same order of magnitude as [CD] or [GW] in the Constitution but is more in the Wellbeing context because how you are born affects all of the other Preamble Six conditions. DRE is a dynamical system defined by the total 21st century molecular research that has occurred. Previous systems using genetics, such as Social Darwinism and Eugenics are now considered minor subsets of the research. But there is too much research into brain and body molecular systems to make other than general speculations about the 6000 or so molecular anomalies the research has found among the Hosa (short for HOmoSApiens). The DRE has many obvious effects on civilization; most mass killings, addictions and brain birth defects have very costly DRE that until now couldn't be understood.

But did Darwin show how 'consciousness' or Ki_ξ fit into all these ripple effects of humans?

Democide.

Democide, or acts of mass murder for political, economic, ethnic, or religious reasons by a governing or controlling entity, is a subset of the International Criminal Court's definition of crimes against humanity. It is the identification of the INDIVIDUALS engaged in Democide, regardless of affiliation in government that should be treated as criminal behavior.

State democide is mass murder by governing entities for political reasons [Punjabi of Pakistan, Belarusians, North Koreans], or economic reasons [Mexican cartels, Iraqi socialists, Iranian Quds Guard], or religious purposes [Al Qaeda, Taliban, Lord's Resistance Army], or ethnic tribal processes [Serbians, Sudanese]. A 'governing entity' is any large group that has acquired even minimal political power over others. Note that a government can carry out Democide against some society in order to defend itself *from* democide and this might be forgiven if both societies improve into a Posterity or generational effect. But rare, and almost always an effect of aggression.

Epigenetics.

The study of alteration of cell structures in Homosapiens through external of environmental conditions. This is a critical science developed in the 21st century after the DNA mapping of people was completed. This involves a subset system of the chromosome itself that can be altered by fetal development, environmental chemicals such as drugs or narcotics or diet. Even radiation can change the chromosome that leads to complex DNA and this in turn leads to an 'epigenetic factor' cause cell malformation like cancer, mental disorders, and diabetes. Epigenetics malformation may cause more than half of all healthcare costs that occur in human societies and is closely related to the DRE definitions used in this book

Economic models : Marx, Keynes, Freidman and Complexity.

When the world's trade systems really begin to appear during the feudal periods of Asia and Europe, around 1200, people also begin to define 'systems' of value exchange in the form of trade and metals exchange. This was a change from the barter system that Homosapiens had been using for the previous 40,000 years and really began to develop when farming communities appeared 7000 years. Somewhere around the 1700s, people began to define trade and the accumulation of wealth in terms of industrialization. Basically, the term 'economics' means that a being produces an 'entity' by using his energy and consciousness (wellbeing?) in excess of the food and empathic energy he takes in from his surroundings. This in turn is multiplied by his cooperation in a family or group and that combined 'entity' is generally referred to as micro-economics. When this group's efforts create a larger 'entity' that has excess 'entities' or profit, it is generally referred to as macro-economics because an entire society can become involved in the excess 'entity' wealth and its distribution. The American independent families qualify as one of the most successful 'entity' producing societies in history, using many forms of wealth creation and an unusual abundance of natural resources. By 2000 CE, the micro to macro to micro wealth production within the North American society began to break down as world multi-macro monopolies absorbed the wealth of the Americans without a return to them.

Marxian economics. Focuses on the role of labor in the development of an economy, and is critical of the classical approach to ownership wages and productivity developed by Adam Smith and John Locke. Marxian economics argues that the specialization of the labor force in creating excess wealth, coupled with a growing population as in Malthusian Population Traps, pushes wages down, and that the value placed on goods and services does not accurately account for the true cost of labor in producing an entity. The economics involved did not actually reflect the later government ownership of production ideology which would only work in crises conditions, only that an 'entity' produced should have its excess used for population equilibrium.

Keynesian economics. Refers to the concept that optimal economic performance could be achieved by influencing aggregate demand through activist stabilization (IE, no drastic slumps so that micro-economic system are more dynamic) and economic intervention policies by the government producing both infrastructure and many more wealth producing entities. Keynesian economics is considered to be a "demand-side" theory that focuses on changes in the economy over the short run. An economic theory of total spending in the economy and its effects on output entities and that inflation will eventually stall all entity creation.

Friedmanist economics. Several theories on monetary policy in which the total amount of money in a society affected the ability of the society and individuals to prosper, although this 'prosperity' was based on the perception by individuals on what to consume with the available money supply and not based on the availability of resources within a society. The theory was macro-economic extensions to micro-economic activity and involved the need for absolute individual freedom to determine the use of the acquired money. The idea was that if some, through a Social Darwinist evolutionary process, continually increased the monetary supply, the entire society benefits without any Constitutional interaction. That process had worked in the late 1800s according to his book, A *Monetary History of the United States, 1867-1960,* and was therefore valid for ALL historical periods. It did not take into account the sociobiological greed/power/property/greed cycle of a *world economy* with instant monetary *and* entity transfers that appeared after 2000 CE.

Complexity economics. Also known as 'Heterodox Economics' in which excess value, sometimes referred to as 'human capital or a total productivity of an individual, is multiplied by the 'teamwork' of a group of people. The analysis of dynamics considers other factors besides mainstream or orthodox schools of economic thought. Schools of heterodox or complexity economics include positive-growth elements of socialism, Marxism, post-Keynesian and Austrian, and often combine the macroeconomic outlook found in Keynesian economics with approaches critical of neoclassical economics. The output or product of a Complexity based economy was thought to be divided or distributed among the different social groups in accord with *the costs borne by those groups* in producing the output that is then re-cycled to *all* of the contributors, much the same as virtually all molecular structures re-combine energies to produce a total effect. Complexity entities, more or less, could be found in the "Classical Theory" developed by Adam Smith, David Ricardo, Thomas Robert Malthus, John Stuart Mill, and Karl Marx, but were latter historically re-defined as 20th century 'entities' by Keynes and Freidman. Complexity economics are an attempt to account for the 'dynamic' of various human capital values associated with the human productive activity while measuring the counter forces of societies. It basically involves studies where a group of people act to produce value where the sum is greater than or less than the sum of the parts, but such studies could not be applied to economics until this century technologies existed.

TLO Speculations on [OP] economics:

Rather than go into an extremely complex economics discussion, it would be easier to show what a common consensus of what the 'entity' of economics means. This is from the lengthy 31 page Wikipedia explanation of Economics. These elements of economics are consistent with most theories including Marxist, Keynesian, Friedmanist and also Complexity Economics. Each major 'system' of wealth mixes various elements of the 'consensus' compiled by Gregory Mankiw and re-stated in Wikipedia. Since all of the elements of the economic 'entity' have effects within the Constitutional dynamic, they are listed here with the Preamble set notation attached as TLO speculation.

Economics, Wikipedia, concerning definitions of

https://en.wikipedia.org/wiki/Economics

https://en.wikipedia.org/wiki/Complexity_economics

https://en.wikipedia.org/wiki/Keynesian_economics

Note that in spite of its pervasive integration with daily life, there is no direct constitutional authority involving a 'national' economy. The Article I authorities of the Congress give specific controls of tariffs, taxation, post roads, and monetary policy but not an authority to tell the Executive he has an inherent authority over it. That would have been physically impossible in 1789.

According to various polls cited in *Principles of Economics* by Harvard Chairman and Economics Professor Gregory Mankiw, economists have the following agreements by percentage. They, and the order of ripple effects on the Six covenants, are included here as examples of complexity, not defined [sets]

{1} CAS dynamic: A ceiling on rents reduces the quantity and quality of housing available. (93% agree) [GW] [WB] [TR] [LI] [JU]. TLO: Keynesian, Complexity

{2} CAS dynamic: Tariffs and import quotas usually reduce general economic welfare. (93% agree) [CD] [GW] [WB] [TR] [LI] [JU] [OP]   TLO: AVC vs Friedmanist vs Keynesian. Complexity not measured.

{3} CAS dynamic: Flexible and floating exchange rates offer an effective international monetary arrangement. (90% agree). TLO: [GW] [CD] [TR] [LI]   TLO: Freidmanist, AVC.

{4} CAS dynamic: Fiscal policy (e.g., tax cut and/or government expenditure increase) has a significant stimulative impact on a less than fully employed economy. (90% agree)   TLO: [GW] [WB] [TR] [LI] [JU] [OP] Friedmanist vs. Keynesian vs Complexity.

{5} CAS dynamic: United States should not restrict employers from outsourcing work to foreign countries. (90% agree). TLO: [CD] [GW] [JU] [OP] Freidmanist

{6} CAS dynamic: The United States should eliminate agricultural subsidies. (85% agree). TLO: [LI] [GW] [CD] [TR] [JU] Friedmanist vs Keynesian vs Marxian vs Complexity

{7} CAS dynamic: Local and state governments should eliminate subsidies to professional sports franchises. (85% agree) TLO: [TR] [LI] [JU]   Freidmanist

{8} CAS dynamic: if the federal budget is to be balanced, it should be done over the business cycle rather than yearly. (85% agree) TLO: [CD] [GW] [OP] Friedmanist vs Keynesian

{9} CAS dynamic: The gap between Social Security funds and expenditures will become unsustainably large within the next fifty years if current policies remain unchanged. (85% agree) TLO: [OP] [WB] [TR] [GW] [LI] [JU] Keynesian, Freidmanist, Marxian agree

{10} CAS dynamic: Cash payments increase the welfare of recipients to a greater degree than do transfers-in-kind of equal cash value. (84% agree). TLO: [WB] [GW [TR] [LI] Friedmanist vs Keynesian, no Complexity definition.

{11} CAS dynamic: A large federal budget deficit has an adverse effect on the economy. (83% agree). TLO: [CD] [LI] [JU] [GW] [WB] [TR] [OP] Keynesian vs Freidmanist

{12} CAS dynamic: A minimum wage increases unemployment among young and unskilled workers. (79% agree) TLO: [GW] [TR] [LI] [JU] Keynesian vs Complexity

{13} CAS dynamic: The government should restructure the welfare system along the lines of a "negative income tax." (79% agree) TLO: [WB] [TR] [GW] [LI] [OP] Complexity vs Friedmanist vs Marxian

{14} CAS dynamic: Effluent taxes and marketable pollution permits represent a better approach to pollution control than imposition of pollution ceilings. (78% agree) TLO: [CD] [WB] [TR] [GW] [LI] [JU] [OP] Keynesian vs Marxian

At one time during a closed economy, Keynesian economic cooperation between the government and the private sector was nearly a perfect balance of the Preamble's

Common Defense and General Welfare imperatives. This model remained valid with Complexity analysis but not with Freidmanist. The Marxist/Keynesian dogmas have created wild swings in 'prices' in the belief that they are creating wealth and that has not been the case in an electronic world economy. Friedmanist economies give the appearance on monetary wealth on a large scale, but such wealth is 'paper', not necessarily 'physical'. There is no serious evidence that entity-related taxation retards overall micro- or macro-economic growth, not in Keynesian, Friedmanist OR Complexity economics, assuming that the taxation is not of a parasitic nature.

Exergy

This definition is taken from a paper by Goran Wall and Dilip G. Banhatti, Exergy-*a useful concept for ecology and sustainability*, 2012, because it discussed the Exergy or use of solar energy by and for the Earth over millions of years and in terms of modern energy use and waste. It is also a generally held definition of the effect of energy use on societies and would therefore qualify as a way of viewing the [GW] and [CD] processes in terms of [OP] in the Chronology:

> Exergy is formed from Greek ex + ergon, meaning "from work". Some synonyms (from Wikipedia) are: availability, available energy, exergic energy, essergy, utilizable energy, available useful work, maximum (or minimum) work or work content, reversible work, and ideal work. Exergy is that part of energy which is convertible into all other forms of energy. It represents the potential of a system to deliver work in a given environment. The exergy E of a system of volume V having internal energy U and entropy S, and composed of many substances i (i = 1, 2, ...), each amounting to M_i moles (and having chemical potential $\mu 0i$ in the surroundings), is defined as: [equations not quoted here]

Note exergy 'represents the potential of a *system* to deliver work in a given environment'. Taking any one of the six covenants in the Preamble, it is possible to attach a 'work' value to the entire system, which just might be the input dollars minus the labor dollars minus the admin dollars equals a 'unit of ROI' which could be positive or negative energy. That is simplistic, but this **IS** an open minded speculation on Constitutional systems. This ROI unit, exergy, also closely defines the six Preamble directives as *systems* that operate to produce an effect. One might wonder if exergy is the 'work energy' Isaac Newton was looking for in the parallel effects of human systems, but exergy as used here really isn't gravity type of work...

See also: https://en.wikipedia.org/wiki/Second_law_of_thermodynamics

A speculation of the 'exergy' concept might be extended to 'human capital' in that humans routinely produce more energy than they consume, not counting poor health or wellbeing. costs. In their space-time, do humans transmit energy (Ki_ξ) to others, especially children, in the form of empathy or altruism?

$\{mind1\}+\{body1\}\rightarrow>1\{Ki\_\xi\}\leftrightarrow\{mind2\}$?

Ex post facto justice.

The constitution specifically prohibited the creation or use of laws under a condition of ex post facto which is Latin for 'after the facts' The reason for this is that legislatures and citizens alike would create conditions that were applied before a timeline event had actually occurred. This was called a 'Bill of Attainder' where a legislature could execute a person by making something he did 20 years earlier a crime. This little 'system' also involved appropriation of the 'guilty' person's property with a 'Corruption of Blood' so that the relatives of the 'guilty' one were also responsible. Communist and fascist seizures of power are the extreme examples of ex post facto appropriations of wealth, but there have been many instances of it worldwide base on religious beliefs.

The American Constitution specifically prohibits Ex post facto, bills of attainder and corruption of blood conditions by governments. But in the 21st century, such prohibitions will become extremely important because DNA mapping of individuals has the potential for enormous injustice and perhaps a total nullification of the [LI] and [JU] components of society. One of the Second Convention rights conditions would be protection against corruption of blood extremes where genetic lines are summarily attacked along ethnic, racial, or religious mechanism by citizens and foreigners intent on imposing *their* DNA sets.

Evolution, or systems of evolution, Quantum Standard Model?.

The following ten glossary items are extracted verbatim from the book '*Life Ascending, the Ten Great Inventions of Evolution*' by Nick Lane, 2009, as accurate but short descriptions of evolutionary cellular dynamical systems. There combinations resulted in other glossary items concerning Americans, including [JU] and [LI] but also are good descriptions of the system of systems called humans. Virtually all of the ten items are inherent in the mind, body, and spirit of a person and can be measured according to their system interaction. Humans cannot exist without this system of systems, so it is included to define an individual life. It is the positive combination of these items into one being that also requires a Constitutional intent of Wellbeing [WB] in this speculation.

a. The Origin of Life. The origin of life is one of biology's biggest conundrums. How prebiotic chemistry gave rise to biochemistry, how the first cells formed, what kind of energy first powered metabolism and replication -- all these questions are serious challenges. Remarkably, all are answered in broad brush stroke by the amazing properties of alkaline hydrothermal vents, which form naturally chemiosmotic, self-replicating mineral cells with catalytic walls. They concentrate organics, including nucleotides, in impressive quantities, making them the ideal hatcheries for life.

b. DNA. DNA is unique. RNA, chemically very similar, is far more unstable and reactive and couldn't encode organisms much more complex than a virus. For life to get going, DNA was needed. How a primordial RNA world gave rise to DNA and proteins is one of the great questions in biology. Yet a "code within the codons" gives suggestive clues to the origin of DNA and also points to life's origin in alkaline hydrothermal vents. A deep distinction in DNA replication mechanisms and other traits imply that bacteria and archaea emerged independently from a common ancestor in the vents.

c. Photosynthesis. Without photosynthesis life couldn't get very far. Photosynthesis provides both the fuel and oxygen for respiration -- and only aerobic respiration generates enough energy to support multicellular life. Oxygenic photosynthesis arose just once in the history of evolution, in cyanobacteria. The trick demands an elaborate biochemical scheme to extract electrons from water and thrust them onto carbon dioxide. Without that improbable pathway, we would not be here.

d. The Complex Cell. All complex life on Earth is composed of nucleated cells, known as eukaryotic cells. The eukaryote arose only once, and bacteria normally show no tendency towards morphological complexity. The last common ancestor of eukaryotic cells was a chimera, formed in a unique union between two prokaryotic cells called endosymbiosis -- a non-Darwinian mechanism whereby organisms converge rather than diverge. Without that chimera, evolution may never have progressed beyond bacteria, and again none of us would be here.

e. Sex. Sex is absurd. It costs a small fortune to find a partner, transmits foul venereal diseases and parasitic genes, and randomizes successful allele combinations. Worse, sex requires males, viewed by implacable feminists and evolutionists alike as a waste of space. Why we all have sex anyway was seen as the queen of evolutionary problems in the 20th century. Recent work shows that over time all complex species would degenerate like the Y chromosome without sex. The details help explain why sex first arose, enabling early eukaryotes to thrive.

f. Movement. Muscles set animals apart. They cause power grazing and predation and make food webs a reality. The proteins responsible for contractility -- actin and myosin -- are ubiquitous in eukaryotes and even in bacteria, propelling amoebae around, supporting plant cells, and helping bacteria divide. Actin forms dynamic cross links in much the same way that variant hemoglobin distorts red cells in sickle-cell anemia. Selection fashioned such spontaneous quirks into the might of muscle.

g. Sight. Sight may well have been the driving force behind the Cambrian explosion, when the first animals leapt into the fossil record about 550 million years ago. Thanks to a series of surprises in molecular biology, we now know how eyes evolved in great detail. Lens proteins and crystals were recruited from an astonishing range of sources, from calcite to mitochondria to stress proteins, but the ubiquitous light-sensitive protein rhodopsin probably evolved in algae, where it is used to calibrate light levels in photosynthesis.

h. Hot Blood. Endothermy drives a supercharged lifestyle, making our own 24/7 dynamism possible. Many small mammals eat as much in a day as a lizard does in a month. A big benefit is stamina, but there is no necessary connection between stamina and resting metabolic rate, and therapies like Velociraptor may have had the best of both worlds. One driver for endothermy may have been diets rich in carbon but low in nitrogen, such as leaves. Herbivores gain enough nitrogen from leaves if they eat a lot and jettison the excess carbon. Endotherms cleverly burn it off, gaining stamina while subsisting on a lower quality diet.

I. Consciousness. Consciousness is the most subversive evolutionary adaptation. It enabled us to transform the world -- but there are still deep uncertainties about what it actually is. We don't know yet how neurons firing in the brain can generate a feeling of anything: what, if anything, a feeling is in physical terms. This is what philosophers call the "hard problem," and some say answering it requires a radical overhaul of the laws of physics. The answer may lie in bees, which have complex neural reward systems -- they may not be truly conscious, but if they feel anything at all, they already possess the physiological rudiments of consciousness.

j. Death. Without death, natural selection would count for nothing, and life could never have evolved at all. Without cell death, or apoptosis, multicellular organisms are not possible. The key to both is mitochondria. They generate reactive free radicals that slowly undermine health, but in the short term optimise respiration, enhancing fitness when young. The penalty for vigour in youth is decrepit old age. There's hope. Birds leak fewer free-radicals, and live longer than mammals, without losing their vigour. The anti-aging pill may not a myth. End of direct quote.

Gene therapy.

Gene therapy is an experimental technique that uses genes to treat or prevent disease. This technique allows doctors to treat a disorder by inserting a gene into a patient's cells instead of using drugs or surgery. Researchers are testing several approaches to gene therapy, including:

(1) Replacing a mutated gene that causes disease with a healthy copy of the gene.
(2) Inactivating, or "knocking out," a mutated gene that is functioning improperly. and
(3) Introducing a new gene into the body to help fight a disease.

For more information, see:

https://www.nlm.nih.gov/medlineplus/genesandgenetherapy.html

HoSa.

HoSa is a short acronym for the descendants of Homo Erectus, which is inclusive of virtually all human species since achieving the ability to increase consciousness about 70,000 years ago. There were various sub-species of Homo Erectus all over the world from this or that migration, but the HoSa or Homo Sapien 'suddenly' appeared with new abilities and begin absorbing other species such as Floresiensis, Denisovans and Neanderthals. While the term 'Cro-Magnon' is used in the Chronicles, it is to refer to the more Eurasian species of HoSa and not necessarily the African and Asian descendants of Homo Sapien. The term 'HoSa' is used in order to perceive systems of systems from a DNA standpoint, not from a sub-species 'race' standpoint. The genetic history implies that all of the HoSa adaptions have approximately the same consciousness, sight, sex, instincts and self defense molecular structures. Until this century at least.

House and Senate Rules.

Article 1, Section 5, Clause 2: Each House may determine the Rules of its Proceedings, punish its Members for disorderly Behavior, and, with the Concurrence of two thirds, expel a Member.

This is carried out through the 'Rules Committee' and is known as the Jefferson Manual in the House of Representatives and as the Senate Manual in the U.S. Senate. This process is especially important in the Senate, where a filibuster rule can stop all legislation in the government. This is essentially a one–senator line item veto of legislation, something not even the President has. Cloture votes to close off filibusters peaked in 2008 with 112 votes to end filibusters, mostly on reactions to the recession and the introduction of the ACA. The Constitution gives exclusive authority to each chamber for its Rules and these cannot be challenged by other branches, hence their power in legislation.

Human Right, or Bill of Rights.

Human Rights are systems of respect between people that are mutually agreed to by formal referendum that creates them as such. A Human Right is a protection added into the Constitution during its referendum period of 1788 and generally added to other constitutions as ways of preventing the 'natural' predatory instincts of humans from becoming violent applications of totalitarian power. But a 'right' doesn't actually exist unless it is genuinely adhered to in the day to day respect for others as part of a social environment. A 'right' can be established in a family as a way of living together, in a community as mutual respect in transferring wealth or spiritual energy and in an economic entity as a human resource condition. But the principle that once agreed to, a right must be adhered to by all within its jurisdiction is fundamental to its success. Used in the Chronicles as in the Bill of Rights.

KI or Qi or Ki_ξ or Ki

The term Ki or Ki_气 is taken from the very large usage around the world of the Chinese concept of 'life force' and the European usage of the term Parakletos or 'holy spirit. that aids an individual. https://en.wikipedia.org/wiki/Paraclete with coordination of the mind and body. This is closely similar to the Asian idea of Qi (☐) or life force that aids the integration of mind and body. Since the concept of Holy Spirit appears in virtually all religious texts over a 5000-year period, it cannot be dismissed as non-existent any more than quantum theory because you cannot see the energy levels involved in 'particles'.

https://en.wikipedia.org/wiki/Zhang_Zai#The_meaning_and_characteristics_of_Qi_a ccording_to_Zhang_Zai

> Qì gōng (as in simplified Chinese) involves coordinated breathing, movement, and awareness. It is traditionally viewed as a practice to cultivate and balance qi. With roots in traditional Chinese medicine, philosophy and martial arts, qigong is now practiced worldwide for exercise, healing, meditation, and training for martial arts. Typically, a qigong practice involves rhythmic breathing, slow and stylized movement, a mindful state, and visualization of guiding qi.

For the purposes of this Chronicle, and not counting hints at it in other ones, the Japanese term 'Ki_☐ ' is used to express an energy component of the wellbeing domain that is not associated with the usage if wide usage if the 'Ki' term itself. The same applies to the term 'Ki_ξ' where the Greek letter 'xi' is used as an approximation of Parakletos. It is necessary for visualization to differentiate the symbol from many other linguistic usages. It takes the form [WB{ Ki_ξ}→ {mind}+{body}], where the independent subset { Ki_ξ} forms or amplifies the {mind} and {body} subsets that make up human health. That health is sensed at a molecular level in the Chronicles since such things as gene editing make the perception possible. Quantifying the [WB{ Ki_ξ] in terms of field theory will get you in trouble with every known physicist category because it complicates the sensing of the quantum world even more than it is, even though consciousness is the pre-curser of that perception. **For the purpose of Chronicle writing, the term Ki or the Greek small letter xi, 'ξ', is used to express any relation of spirit or neurological consciousness as a {subset] of mind and body health.**

MPT or Malthusian Population Trap.

This concern was originally developed by Robert Malthus in 1798 whose predictions that world populations would overwhelm resources were data based, not speculation. These observations saw the deterioration of societies all over Europe due to the intense crowding of the Industrial Revolution, something one Karl Marx picked up on in the 1800s. Most Americans didn't understand this because they could look around and see that their nearest neighbor was two miles away, but sailing to any world city would have shown the Trap.

By the 21st century, World technology resources have vastly improved the ability to feed and clothe people and make them healthier. Life expectancy went from about 59 to 75 on average. What has continually re-appeared is small enclaves within a larger population that had deteriorated into the 1700s population without resources 'community'. This has various names like 'ghetto', 'slum', 'jalap', 'pinminqu', but ALL human languages have the word for Malthusian Population Trap, MPT, within their borders. The question for Constitutional processes is just how much of a ripple effect MPT has on We The People and most research indicates it is considerable. From a [WB] standpoint, the question is whether the MPT becomes a genetic adaption over several generations with a result in some form of PTSD.

Optimization.

Many possible perceptions for 'optimization' including highest profits, lowest cost, best energy conversion level, human capital efficiency, etc., but for complex systems like the Constitution, the term means adding value to any one of the Preamble Six or Seven without substantial loss to any of the other covenants. For [CD] and [GW], the dynamic optimization is the balance of the two over time, optimizing one with serious cost to the other is not an optimization of the ultimate evolutionary goals of our Posterity. There are also many cases where optimization of a minor subset of something within [JU] or [LI] becomes the objective rather than the covenant. Individual optimization may be an economic processes idealized by various ideologies but such as {gluttony} can also be the knife that cuts the wrist.

Parasite, biological or organizational.

Synonym Discussion of PARASITE: An organism that lives on or within a host (another organism); it obtains nutrients from the host without benefiting or killing (although it may damage) the host. Humans are not genetically designed as parasitic, but are born with extreme adaptive capabilities that are normally symbiotic or complementary. Agriculture, forestry, water conservation and nutrient re-production are signs of symbiotic dynamical systems. A group of human beings interact with each other as mutually supportive 'entities' but can adapt to a parasitic existence. No human society has existed over generations or to genuine Posterity with parasitic attachments feeding on it.

TLO

Short designation for 'Time Line Opservationis', derived from Isaac Newton's research in the 1600s. Personal note or comment on the possible Preamble Six effects of an associated human process. Not the same as a Chronicle, which contains the original author's observation of a Constitutional process and sometimes in this century, the process that hasn't been defined by the Constitution, such as asymmetric warfare, electronic wealth transfer, healthcare and tribal genocide. A Chronicle and a TLO can be mixed, since they are CAS attempted insights into 'entities'.

Rule of Fours.

A somewhat arbitrary 'dynamical system' for defining the qualifications of an Elector to a Constitutional Convention. The 'fours' involve minimum values of a constitutionally aware citizen. Rule of Fours attempts to re-kindle the original problem solving mentality of the First Convention, but insure a general awareness of new technologies.

(1) 44% passage of the US Citizenship test at any time, including 4 questions in a second language of choice, with one fourth of Elector citizen costs paid by Federal, State, Community, and Self each.

(2) A GRE General Test score of 144, a SAT score of 444, and a MCAT score of 444.

(3) Residence in and paying taxes in the same Representative District communities for 4 years.

(4) Spent 4 contiguous months in a public service occupation in a [TR], [WB], [CD] or [GW] system.

Rule of Sixes.

A set of conditions for determining whether any condition of society warrants inclusion in an Article. Not the same as conditions for an Amendment, which might affect only one Article or Right. An Article affects all of the other Articles and Rights. The intent is to maintain the original Convention's problem solving ability for We The People, not individuals within We The People domains.

An issue which affects any of the six Preamble covenants, no matter how formed, must affect at least one-sixth of a Elector's population and then affect up to six Electors that are not physically connected within a state, then affect the Electors of six states not connected within the USA. Ratification of a Rights Article section needs 66% of Electors approving.

Spiritual 'system'.

These are documents relating to the spiritual essence of a Human Being. They describe a coherent energy within each individual that evolved from the various environments Man found himself in. The primary Spiritual Scriptures in evolved order are: Vedas, Tantras, Mahayana, Tao de Ch'ing, Testaments, Gospel, and Quran. There have been many attempts since the writing of the Quran in the 700s to define spirituality in terms of brain functions as these became more understood, especially in this century. But as a form of {energy}?

The original religious reasons concerning life itself were based on physical realties of 2000 years ago (only one out of three births reached the age of ten and eight births by a mother was a norm) and many of those realities as heavenly 'mandates' are being redefined into a new spiritual enhancement not previously understood or possible to measure. Odd that around 500 BCE, spiritual enhancement of a person was pictured simultaneously in five or six cultures as a Halo.

Set theory symbols used.

Set theory is used to express relationships between related 'elements' or 'entities', which in this Chronicles speculation are defined in terms of Complex Adaptive **Systems,** note 'systems'.   CAS implies a large number of entities that might not be closely related, where set theory would show a closer relationship and mathematics would attempt to show an *exact* relationship. The exact relationship is considered a perceptional error in the Chronicles because the idea is to see each part of the preamble as an open-minded domain.

 Because of this, and the close relationship with Venn chart perception in the Chronicles, slight variations of set notation are used. The normal system set notation is {} and is acknowledged but isn't complex enough for 'open-minded' perception. [] is used for open minded, but necessarily vague domains with a group of elements normally shown by a Hamiltonian symbol **H.** But here , A domain or manifold as large as General Welfare or Justice or Liberty is actually a group of sets which might have very complex elements or sets within the domain, so the brackets [] are used to express a Preamble covenant. This looks like:

[] brackets are a Preamble domain or covenant. May contain n elements summed together ex: [JU] or [LI] where [LI]= $\sum$ {wb x n} {ju x n} or whatever {subsets}.

{} is used for a set of elements.   ex: [{A} {B} {C}] From Georg Cantor's original definition.

⋈ or ⋈ are joined but balanced relations between domains or sets, NOT an equivalence in effects.
ex: [GW] ⋈ [WB] = {A ∪ B ⋈ C}

∪ or ↔ is a union of relationships, can be domains or sets or element combinations without attempting equivalence. The relationship exists without calculated progressions of effect. Ex: [GW]<2 ∪ [TR]>1[LI]<3

Ki_ξ is an 'energy' field **defined** as an entity or set that could be a domain. Taken from Newton's PM definition of 'simult relations' instead of functions.
ex: [WB] ⋈ [{GW x ξ} ∪ {A x ξ}].

⇒ or → implies that a set is related to another OR will be. Possible 'field' tensor.

∈ means an element of another condition. Not used here much because it implies subset only, rather than simultaneous balance {⋈} visualization.

$\sum$ or Σ is a summing of [domains] and their possible ripple effects on another domain, usually [OP]. Not necessarily positive adds(+) , but negative ripples as well (-).

→ used to indicate an 'influence' vector that implies a force on a given series of domains. Maybe a dimensional tensor.

↔ used to show a mutual 'influence' vector in that the following domains can be dynamic loops with instantaneous feedback of energy or work force or exergy which that can effect an optimization.

.. insertion indicator, not dynamic related, to replace widespread use of brackets [x] as author insertion. Items within **..XX ..** are inserted into text to show perception of a dynamic.

Example: .. |TR|<2 = ∑ [LI] > →|WB|>3 [ξ] ⋈ [GW] →>2-|JU|<2? ..

Set theory model visualization.

As of 2018.12.01, the set theory symbols are used arbitrarily, with a numeric 'value' from 1 to 6. While many 'elements' in set theory can be quantized with numeric values, there is the possibility that perception of the whole is distorted by the quantitative detail, hence the attempt at perceptional multivariate analysis.

One of the problems with '**sensing**' a complex entity is that there is no real 'symbolic' representation of the entity or domain with subsets. Merely color coding them is not perceptually valid for complex models, as those engaged in quantum research of bosons discovered. A fairly extensive color coding of 'spectrums' that include many more frequencies than visible light are now practiced with cosmic entity images that show many forms of energy radiation in the universe. But for human complexity that can be communicated, there are few methods. The Chinese and Japanese languages have quite complex ideograms to express ideas. The Chines word for philosophy is 'zhe xue' or:

哲学

But suppose you wished to add meaning to the kanji by adding a spectrum of colors that were understood to signify certain different things about 'philosophy'? Suppose green spectrums involved a degree of belief in a philosophy and reds involved a perception of 'value' in that philosophy process? Would the kanji then become something abstract like?:

哲学

or is that just too complex for visualization? The idea of sensing a complex entity with a standardized color spectrum might be useful in future operations analysis and certainly might help with differentiation of values in modern governance. What would a video 'language' of the future look like that relied on multiple senses including sight? Would the media language have a kanji 'noun' or subject with the spectrum pattern such as [WB {f(t) ▐ ▐ }] with various ▐ ▐ ▐ ▐ that described a degree or degrees of significance AND authenticity to the object? One 'visualization' that involves common knowledge authenticity might be a color spectrum 'tag' on a video display that shows the degree of confidence the display has, along with a time stamp. This is similar to the metadata fields now in use for literary activity, but with an immediate credibility display as well. . This would be especially valuable in the current Age of Deceit and Disinformation.

But there might be a more important complexity sensing for human health. If you took a human 'entity' with some 11 complex body 'systems', 11 functional mind 'systems' and a very many systems of life force ({Ki_ξ} used in the Chronicles) within the mind but dependent on energy from the body, the complexity perception requires a database with multiple 'whole-being' fields. In order for a doctor, EMT or an AI droid to measure the health status of any given individual , he or it would have to sense accurate data of many complex subfunctions at an organ, cellular and molecular level. This would involve a body-geographic locator of the molecules involved, then a code for the problem such as the International Classification of Diseases and some status condition spectrum that might tell the sensing entities what is happening in real time or over time. This perceptional formula of 11 body conditions, 11 mind systems and multiple life systems for [wellbeing $\{n1 \rightarrow n2 \rightarrow n3 \bowtie (t)\} \approx \{Ki\_\xi\} \rightarrow \infty$] might even take the form of a scaled **Mandelbox** set (3D, 4D and 5D, not the original fractal sequences) in which the geometry defines a near infinite series of health cell locations color-coded with status at each level.

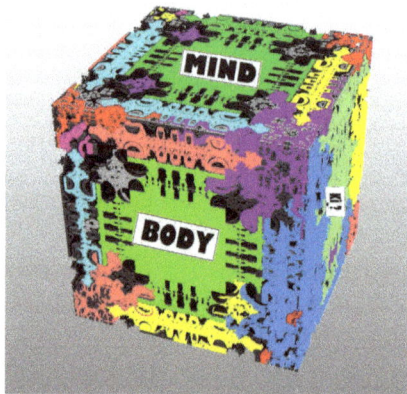

The mechanisms all currently exist for doing this in 2018. Set theory symbols can create models with appropriate algorithms on visualizations or 'sensing' that closely match real-time lifestyle models such as healthcare. But suppose you visualized the 'model' as a complex adaptive system with the objective look something like this? How would an auto accident victim appear in the blue molecular zones, the red neurological zone(s) and the green societal zones of the ICD Model? What zones would one born with Downs Syndrome or Schizophrenia or epilepsy appear in?

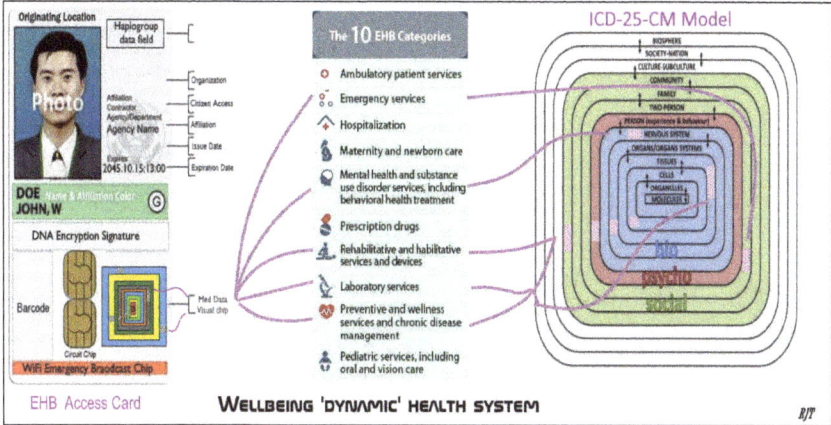

Originating Location | Haplogroup data field

The 10 EHB Categories

ICD-25-CM Model

Photo

DOE JOHN, W — Name & Affiliation Color ⓖ

DNA Encryption Signature

Barcode — Med Data Visual chip

Circuit Chip

WiFi Emergency Broadcast Chip

EHB Access Card

Organization
Citizen Access
Affiliation
Issue Date
Expiration Date

Affiliation
Contractor
Agency/Department
Agency Name

Expires 2045.10.15.13:00

○ Ambulatory patient services
Emergency services
Hospitalization
Maternity and newborn care
Mental health and substance use disorder services, including behavioral health treatment
Prescription drugs
Rehabilitative and habilitative services and devices
Laboratory services
Preventive and wellness services and chronic disease management
Pediatric services, including oral and vision care

BIOSPHERE
SOCIETY-NATION
CULTURE-SUBCULTURE
COMMUNITY
FAMILY
TWO-PERSON
PERSON (experience & behavior)
NERVOUS SYSTEM
ORGANS/ORGANS SYSTEMS
TISSUES
CELLS
ORGANELLES
MOLECULE

BIO
PSYCHO
SOCIAL

WELLBEING 'DYNAMIC' HEALTH SYSTEM

Would the costs to the individual appear in the white 'nation' zones as

$.. |WB|>3 |\xi] = \sum [LI] <n \rightarrow |TR|<2 \bowtie [GW\{xyz\}] \rightarrow <2-|JU|>2? ..$

Simple Weapon of Mass Destruction or SWMD.

A simple weapon of mass destruction is any molecular combination producing a device that is simultaneously lethal to humans within a 30- or 40-meter radius. This can be a fully automatic rifle or pistol, a grenade, a can of nerve gas, or an explosive device of any type. Larger explosive devices do not come under the definition of 'simple', only hand carried items are included in the term. But it can also apply to a group of humans engaged in a crime against humanity regardless of the devices used, such as 'terrorist weapons'. Distributed chemicals that permanently remove consciousness from the brain are SWMD. You will not solve the problem of Simple Weapons of Mass Destruction (SWMD) developed in the last century (and the worst SWMD are yet to come) in this country or any other until the term 'crime against humanity' is fully understood and ruthlessly defended against no matter what form it takes.

Republican form of Government.

Constitution Article IV. Section 4: The United States shall guarantee to every State in this Union a Republican Form of Government, and shall protect each of them against Invasion; and on Application of the Legislature, or of the Executive (when the Legislature cannot be convened), against domestic Violence.

This means that each state has a group of representatives to make laws and appropriate monies for their implementation, in the interests of General Welfare and Common Defense. By this guarantee, the Federal government has the authority to intervene when a local or state government no longer can be called 'representative', but that has never actually been done. Many other interventions concerning the guarantee of civil rights have occurred, but even during the Civil War, states in rebellion were still considered 'representative'. But in the instance of a one party political system in a locality within a state, could that 'party' actually be 'representative' under this guarantee? For that matter, if any Federal government branch became a single party entity, is it the duty of the other two branches to challenge the constitutionality of that branch?

Instrument of Government, 1653.

Omitted but used in earlier Chronicles. Some text closely aligned with Constitutional Article I, and II text. Ben Franklin copy was used?

Complex Adaptive System.

The following are general characteristics of a CAS:

1. Its experience can be thought of as a set of data, usually input —* output data, with the inputs often including system behavior and the outputs often including effects on the system.

2. The system identifies perceived regularities of certain kinds in the experience, even though sometimes regularities of those kinds are overlooked or random features misidentified *as* regularities. The remaining information is treated as random, and much of it often is.

3. Experience is not merely recorded in a lookup table; instead, the perceived regularities are compressed into a schema. Mutation processes of various sorts give rise to rival schemata. Each schema provides, in its own way, some combination of description, prediction, and (where behavior is concerned) prescriptions for action. Those may be provided even in cases that have not been encountered before, and then not only by interpolation and extrapolation, but often by much more sophisticated extensions of experience.

4.The results obtained by a schema or entity in the real world then feed back to affect its standing with respect to the other schemata with which it is in competition.

What distinguishes a CAS from a pure multi-agent system (MAS) is the focus on top-level properties and features like self-similarity, complexity, emergence and self-organization. A MAS is defined as a system composed of multiple interacting agents; where as in CAS, the agents as well as the system are adaptive and the system is self-similar. A CAS is a complex, self-similar collectivity of interacting adaptive agents. Complex Adaptive Systems are characterized by a high degree of adaptive capacity, giving them resilience in the face of perturbation.

Other important properties are adaptation, communication, cooperation, specialization, spatial and temporal organization, and reproduction. They can be found on all levels: cells specialize, adapt and reproduce themselves just like larger organisms do. Communication and cooperation take place on all levels, from the agent to the system level. The forces driving co-operation between agents in such a system, in some cases, can be analyzed with game theory. The number of elements is sufficiently large that conventional descriptions (e.g. a system of differential equations) are not only impractical, but cease to assist in understanding the system. Moreover, the elements interact dynamically, and the interactions can be physical or involve the exchange of information. Such interactions are rich, i.e. any entity or sub-system in the system is affected by and affects several other entities or sub-systems.

The interactions are non-linear: small changes in inputs, physical interactions or stimuli can cause large effects or very significant changes in outputs. Interactions are primarily but not exclusively with immediate neighbors and the nature of the influence is modulated. Any interaction can feed back onto itself directly or after a number of intervening stages. Such feedback can vary in quality. This is known as recurrency.

Such systems may be open and it may be difficult or impossible to define system boundaries, a serious issue in the Chronicles. Complex systems operate under far from equilibrium conditions. There has to be a constant flow of energy to maintain the organization of the system, but is it the energy that is the creator of the system or the entities that do it? **Complex systems have a timeline and sometimes parallel time**

lines. . They evolve and their past is co-responsible for their present behavior Elements in the system may be ignorant of the behavior of the system as a whole, responding only to the information or physical stimuli available to them locally, but in [CD] or [GW] is that equated with bureaucracy?

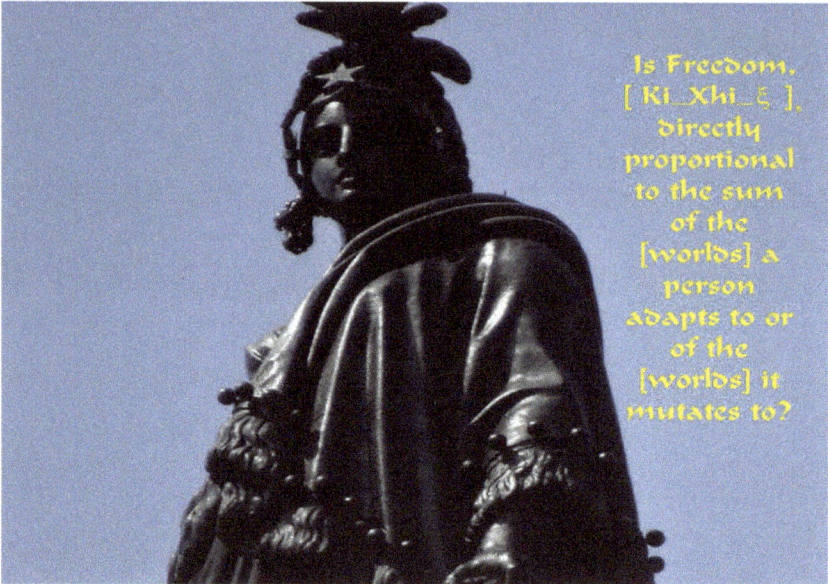

Is Freedom, [KI_Xhi_ε], directly proportional to the sum of the [worlds] a person adapts to or of the [worlds] it mutates to?

Traditional Index and bibliography not included for internet compatibility. That does not mean in any way that there were no contributors to this document. The Chronicles are intended more as a consensus of various disciplines communicated to We the People.